IMMUNOASSAY

IMMUNOASSAY

Edited by

Eleftherios P. Diamandis

Department of Pathology and Laboratory Medicine
Mount Sinai Hospital
Toronto, Ontario, Canada
and Department of Clinical Biochemistry
University of Toronto
Toronto, Ontario, Canada

Theodore K. Christopoulos

Department of Chemistry and Biochemistry
University of Windsor
Windsor, Ontario, Canada

Academic Press

San Diego   New York   Boston
London   Sydney   Tokyo   Toronto

Copyright © 1996 by ACADEMIC PRESS

Academic Press
A Division of Harcourt Brace & Company
525 B Street, Suite 1900, San Diego, California 92101-4495

United Kingdom Edition published by
Academic Press Limited
24-28 Oval Road, London NW1 7DX

Library of Congress Cataloging-in-Publication Data

Immunoassay / edited by Eleftherios P. Diamandis, Theodore K. Christopoulos.
    p.   cm.
  Includes bibliographical references and index.
  ISBN 0-12-214730-8 (alk. paper)
   1. Immunoassay. I. Diamandis, Eleftherios P. II. Christopoulos, Theodore K.
  QP519.9.I42I42   1996
  574.19'285--dc20
                              96-2001
                              CIP

PRINTED IN THE UNITED STATES OF AMERICA
       03   04 05 QW 10 9 8 7 6 5 4

This book is dedicated to Dr. Themistocles Hadjiioannou, Professor of Analytical Chemistry at the University of Athens, Greece. Professor Hadjiioannou is a distinguished analytical chemist and a most dedicated teacher who has introduced generations of students to the theory and practice of the measurement science (analytical chemistry). The editors are fortunate to be among his students and still benefit from the knowledge acquired through their work in Professor Hadjiioannou's laboratory.

CONTENTS

3   THEORY OF IMMUNOASSAYS

Theodore K. Christopoulos and Eleftherios P. Diamandis

4 **DATA INTERPRETATION AND QUALITY CONTROL**

H. Edward Grotjan and Brooks A. Keel

5   PRODUCTION AND PURIFICATION OF ANTIBODIES

Ailsa M. Campbell

7 INTERFERENCES IN IMMUNOASSAYS

James J. Miller and Stanley S. Levinson

8   **LABELING OF ANTIBODIES AND ANTIGENS**
Eiji Ishikawa

9 SOLID PHASES IN IMMUNOASSAY

J. E. Butler

12 RADIOIMMUNOASSAY

Tim Chard

13 ENZYME IMMUNOASSAY

James P. Gosling

14 FLUORESCENCE IMMUNOASSAYS

Theodore K. Christopoulos and Eleftherios P. Diamandis

17 NEPHELOMETRIC AND TURBIDIMETRIC IMMUNOASSAY

Daniel J. Marmer and Paul E. Hurtubise

18 SIMULTANEOUS MULTIANALYTE IMMUNOASSAYS

Larry J. Kricka

19 NONCOMPETITIVE IMMUNOASSAY FOR SMALL MOLECULES

Fortüne Kohen, Josef De Boever, and Geoff Barnard

20 FREE HORMONE MEASUREMENTS

Gyorgy Csako

21 AUTOMATION OF IMMUNOASSAYS

Daniel W. Chan

22 THIN-FILM IMMUNOASSAYS

Susan J. Danielson

23 IMMUNOBLOTTING TECHNIQUES

Jaime Renart, M. Margarita Behrens, Margarita Fernández-Renart, and José L. Martínez

24 DEVELOPMENT OF IN-HOUSE IMMUNOLOGICAL ASSAYS

Eleftherios P. Diamandis, Theodore K. Christopoulos, and Mohammad J. Khosravi

CONTRIBUTORS

Numbers in parentheses indicate the pages on which the authors' contributions begin.

Geoff Barnard (405), Regional Endocrine Unit, Department of Chemical Pathology, Southampton General Hospital, Southampton SO 16 GYD, United Kingdom

Edward A. Bayer (237), Department of Membrane Research and Biophysics, The Weizmann Institute of Science, Rehovot 76100, Israel

M. Margarita Behrens (537), Instituto de Investigaciones Biomédicas del CSIC and Departmento de Bioquímica de la UAM, 28029-Madrid, Spain

J. E. Butler (205), Department of Microbiology, University of Iowa Medical School, Iowa City, Iowa 52242

Ailsa M. Campbell (95), Institute of Biomedical and Life Sciences, University of Glasgow, Glasgow G12 8QQ, United Kingdom

John L. Carey (5), Immunopathology Division, Department of Pathology, Henry Ford Hospital and Health Care Corporation, Detroit, Michigan 48202

Daniel W. Chan (483), Departments of Pathology and Oncology, Johns Hopkins University School of Medicine, and Clinical Chemistry Division, Johns Hopkins Hospital, Baltimore, Maryland 21287

Tim Chard (269), Department of Reproductive Physiology, St. Bartholomew's Hospital, London EC1A 7BE, United Kingdom

Theodore K. Christopoulos (1, 25, 227, 309, 555), Department of Chemistry and Biochemistry, University of Windsor, Windsor, Ontario, Canada N9B 3P4

Gyorgy Csako (423), Clinical Chemistry Service, Clinical Pathology Department, W. G. Magnuson Clinical Center, National Institutes of Health, Bethesda, Maryland 20892

Susan J. Danielson (505), Johnson & Johnson Clinical Diagnostics, Rochester, New York 14650

Josef De Boever (405), Vrouwenkliniek-Poli 3, Universitair Ziekenhuis, B-9000 Gent, Belgium

Eleftherios P. Diamandis (1, 25, 227, 309, 555), Department of Pathology and Laboratory Medicine, Mount Sinai Hospital, Toronto, Ontario, Canada M5G 1X5, and Department of Clinical Biochemistry, University of Toronto, Toronto, Ontario, Canada M5G 1L5

Carolyn S. Feldkamp (5), Immunopathology Division, Department of Pathology, Henry Ford Hospital and Health Care Corporation, Detroit, Michigan 48202

Margarita Fernandez-Renart (537), Instituto de Investigaciones Biomédicas del CSIC and Departmento de Bioquímica de la UAM, 28029-Madrid, Spain

Dusica Gabrijelcic (355), RD Laboratorien GmbH, Am Klopferspitz 19, D 82152 Martinsried/Munich, Germany

Reinhard Erich Geiger (355), RD Laboratorien GmbH, Am Klopferspitz 19, D 82152 Martinsried/Munich, Germany

James P. Gosling (287), Department of Biochemistry and National Diagnostic Centre, University College, Galway, Ireland

H. Edward Grotjan (51), Animal Science Department, University of Nebraska, Lincoln, Nebraska 68583

Paul R. Hinton (117), Protein Design Laboratories, Mountain View, California 94043

Paul Hurtubise (363), Department of Pathology and Laboratory Medicine, Diagnostic Immunology Laboratory, University of Cincinnati Hospital, Cincinnati, Ohio 45267

Eiji Ishikawa (191), Department of Biochemistry, Miyazaki Medical College, Kiyotake, Miyazaki 889-16, Japan

Brooks A. Keel (51), Department of Obstetrics and Gynecology, University of Kansas School of Medicine, Women's Research Institute, Wichita, Kansas 67214

Mohammad J. Khosravi (555), Diagnostic Systems Laboratories, Toronto, Ontario, Canada M5G 1X5

Fortüne Kohen (405), Department of Biological Regulation, The Weizman Institute of Science, Rehovot 76100, Israel

Larry J. Kricka (337, 389), Department of Pathology and Laboratory Medicine, University of Pennsylvania, Philadelphia, Pennsylvania 19104

Stanley S. Levinson (165), Department of Veterans Affairs Medical Center, Louisville, Kentucky 40206

Daniel J. Marmer (363), Department of Pathology and Laboratory Medicine, Diagnostic Immunology Laboratory, University of Cincinnati Hospital, Cincinnati, Ohio 45267

José L. Martínez (537), Instituto de Investigaciones Biomédicas del CSIC and Departamento de Bioquímica de la UAM, 28029-Madrid, Spain

James J. Miller (165), Department of Pathology, University of Louisville School of Medicine, Louisville, Kentucky 40292

Werner Miska (355), Dermatology University Giessen, D 35392 Giessen, Germany

Jaime Renart (537), Instituto de Investigaciones Biomédicas del CSIC and Departamento de Biochímica de la UAM, 28029-Madrid, Spain

Bob Shopes (117), Tera Biotechnology Corporation, La Jolla, California 92037

Meir Wilchek (237), Department of Membrane Research and Biophysics, The Weizmann Institute of Science, Rehovot 76100, Israel

PREFACE

The value of good analytical methods in the advancement of science is well established. No fewer than five Nobel Prizes have been awarded to investigators who developed techniques capable of opening up new fields and facilitating the rapid expansion of knowledge. Examples of this phenomenon include the 1972 Prize awarded to Christian B. Anfinsen, Sanford Moore, and William H. Stein for their work on the structure and activity of ribonuclease; the 1980 Prize for work that led to the development of rapid DNA sequencing won by Paul Berg, Walter Gilbert, and Frederick Sanger in 1980; and the 1984 Prize to Niels K. Jerne, Georges J.F. Köhler, and Cesar Milstein for illuminating the cellular basis of immunology engendering the development of monoclonal antibodies. More recently, Michael Smith and Kary B. Mullis won in 1993 for their work in developing PCR techniques.

Another such technology is immunoassay. 1977's Prize to Rosalyn S. Yalow, Roger C.L. Guillemin, and Andrew V. Schally for radioimmunoassay thyrotropin-releasing hormone is an excellent example. Immunoassay is a classic example of a discovery that is based on a natural phenomenon (immunity) and used advantageously in a completely different context. To this end, the antibody, designed by nature to defend against viruses, bacteria, and parasites, is used as a unique analytical reagent armed with extraordinary specificity and binding affinity. Because of these two attributes, the antibody becomes a "dream" analytical reagent that is difficult to surpass.

Based on this phenomenon is a technology termed "immunodiagnostics," which employs thousands of people and is worth billions of dollars annually. In our view, this technology will continue to be used well into the 21st century. This technology will need people who understand it well and who will devote their careers to working with it, to discovering new aspects, and to expanding its scope. We hope that our new book will help in the training of this "new blood of immunodiagnostic specialists."

We are well aware that a few years may pass from the time the table of contents of a book is conceived until the book reaches the press. However, it is also true that for well-established technologies like immunodiagnostics, quantum leaps usually happen with time cycles of 10–15 years. We are thus confident that our book will serve as an educational aid for at least a decade.

We take this opportunity to thank all the authors for working with us over the past two years and to thank the staff at Academic Press, especially Monique Larson and Charlotte Brabants, who put forth a great deal of effort to produce a good book. We also thank Lisette Santos for invaluable secretarial help and our families who allowed us to use time usually devoted to them to work on this book.

Eleftherios P. Diamandis
Theodore K. Christopoulos

1 PAST, PRESENT, AND FUTURE OF IMMUNOASSAYS

THEODORE K. CHRISTOPOULOS
Department of Chemistry and Biochemistry
University of Windsor
Windsor, Ontario, Canada N9B 3P4

ELEFTHERIOS P. DIAMANDIS
Section of Clinical Biochemistry
Department of Pathology and Laboratory Medicine
Mount Sinai Hospital
Toronto, Ontario, Canada M5G 1X5

It seems that the progress in the field of clinical chemistry follows a periodic model. Each period starts with a breakthrough in analytical methodology, followed by the development of novel assays with improved sensitivity and specificity, for the detection and quantification of analytes that otherwise would be very difficult or impossible to measure with the existing techniques.

The analytical progress greatly facilitates the biochemical and clinical investigations and leads to generation of new knowledge related to disease mechanisms. This, in turn, necessitates the design of tests practical for diagnosis and monitoring of disease on a routine basis.

The utilization of enzymes as analytical reagents, the introduction of immunoassays, and, more recently, the advent of the polymerase chain reaction are examples of analytical milestones in the history of clinical chemistry and laboratory medicine in general.

Immunoassays employ antibodies as analytical reagents. The assays are based on the observation that in a system containing the analyte and a specific antibody, the distribution of the analyte between the bound and free forms is quantitatively related to the total analyte concentration. Immunoassays were first introduced in the 1960s by Berson and Yalow (1) for insulin and by Ekins for thyroxine (2).

In the first immunoassays (radioimmunoassays) the distribution of the analyte between the bound and free forms was monitored by adding a fixed known concentration of radioisotopically labeled analyte (tracer) followed by separation of the bound and free analyte and measurement of the radioactivity of, e.g., the bound fraction. The high sensitivity of radioimmunoassays is due to the high detectability of radioisotopes and the high binding affinity of antibodies. Any binding protein (e.g., receptors) may be used successfully for the determination of the analyte.

However, antibodies are most widely employed because of their exceptional specificity, stability, and versatility. Antibodies may be produced for a great variety of
low- and high-molecular-weight compounds.

Immunoassays were first applied, with exceptional success, to the determination
of hormones, the study of which was previously based on the use of biological
assays. This lead to a revolution in endocrinology and the introduction of new tests
for the diagnosis and monitoring of endocrine disorders. Futhermore, immunoassay
applications expanded to areas such as therapeutic drug monitoring, measurement
of enzymes, tumor markers, lipoproteins, vitamins, and many other metabolites,
and the detection and quantification of antibodies and antigens associated with
infectious agents.

In a period of over three decades of immunoassay utilization, several significant
improvements in assay design, reagents, and detection systems have emerged. Immunoassays with labeled antibodies were introduced (3, 4) (immunometric assays),
and shortly afterward the first "two-site" (sandwich type) immunoassays were
described (5). The development of hybridoma technology and monoclonal antibody
production (6), resulted in the design of new immunoassays with improved specificity
and sensitivity. In parallel, powerful computer programs for immunoassay data
reduction were created. Furthermore, considerable effort has been made to replace
radioisotopic labels with nonisotopic alternatives, thus avoiding the health hazards,
stability problems, and special requirements for licensing, handling, and disposal
of radioisotopes. Enzymes with chromogenic, fluorogenic, and chemiluminogenic
substrates have been employed. A plethora of assays using fluorescent and chemiluminescent labels have been reported as well. Today, the nonisotopic detection
systems offer equal or superior sensitivity and have mostly replaced the classical
radioisotopic labels in routine use. In parallel with the growth of nonisotopic immunoassays, new conjugation chemistries were designed and applied to the labeling
of immunoreactants (antibodies or antigens). The discovery and utilization of new
solid phases for heterogeneous immunoassays was another major advance.

The introduction of nonisotopic homogeneous immunoassays deserves special
mention; in these assays, the physicochemical properties of the tracer change upon
its binding to antibody, thus allowing direct monitoring of bound fraction without
prior separation of the bound from the free tracer. Homogeneous immunoassay is
the most widely used technique for therapeutic drug monitoring.

Immunoassays for measuring concentrations of free (biologically active) hormones have come to routine use (for instance, free thyroxine assay in the testing
of thyroid function).

Finally, the development of nonisotopic immunoassays, along with the increased
demand for higher assay throughout, resulted recently in the design of fully automated immunoassay systems with random access capability.

Current and future efforts in the field of immunoassay involve: (a) the development of multianalyte immunoassays, where a panel of clinically related analytes
can be determined simultaneously; (b) the design of immunosensors suitable for
real time monitoring; (c) The development of assays with even lower detection
limits (ultrasensitive immunoassays) so that more analytes will become accessible;
(d) The transfer of successful nonisotopcic technologies to DNA hybridization
assays; and (e) the utilization of recombinant DNA technology in the production and
engineering of antibody molecules with novel properties (e.g., catalytic antibodies).

Conceivably, during the next 5–7 years, we will likely witness the emergence of powerful new instrumentation capable of performing routine chemistry and immunological assays, and probably some hematological and microbiological assays as well.

Since the polymerase chain reaction can now be quantified using some variation of an immunological assay, we predict that PCR may also become part of hybrid instrumentation in the years to come. Immunoassays are powerful and well established and this fact allows us to speculate that they will continue to be used with increased frequency in the next century.

References

1. Yalow RS, Berson SA. Assay of plasma insulin in human subjects by immunological methods. Nature 1959; 184:1648–9.
2. Ekins RP. The estimation of thyroxine in human plasma by an electrophoretic technique. Clin Chim Acta 1960; 5:453–9.
3. Wide L, Bennich H, Johansson SGO. Diagnosis of allergy by an in vitro test for allergen antibodies. Lancet 1967; 2:1105–7.
4. Miles LEM, Hales CN. Labeled antibodies and immunological assay systems. Nature 1968; 219:186–9.
5. Wide L. Solid-phase antigen-antibody systems. In: Kirkham KF, Hunter WM, Eds. Radioimmunoassay Methods. Edinburgh: Churchill Livingstone, 1971:405–12.
6. Kohler G, Milstein C. Continuous culture of fused cells secreting specific antibody of predefined specificity. Nature 1975; 256:495–7.

2 | IMMUNE FUNCTION AND ANTIBODY STRUCTURE

CAROLYN S. FELDKAMP AND JOHN L. CAREY
Henry Ford Hospital & Health Care Corporation
Detroit, Michigan

1. CELLULAR AND MOLECULAR BASIS OF THE HUMORAL IMMUNE RESPONSE

The primary role of the humoral immune system is the elimination of foreign biomolecules and organisms, along with effete self-proteins and cells. This is accomplished by the binding of allo- and autoantigens with immunoglobulin. Subsequent responses, including activation of the complement and/or cellular immune systems, eventually lead to the phagocytosis and destruction of the target cell, virus, or protein.

To effectively accomplish this task, it is necessary that the immune system recognizes a very large range of non-self-antigens (foreign or alloantigens), usually at low concentrations. Failure to do so will result in immunodeficiency. Further, the immune system must manage to effectively respond to alloantigens without either overreactivity with self-antigens (loss of tolerance—autoimmune disease) or inappropriate response to immune stimulation (IgE production—allergy). Last, there must be an appropriate "damping" of a reaction when the desired effect (clearance) is accomplished.

These goals are accomplished by a combination of cell contact- and extracellular cytokine-dependent mechanisms. The elucidation of these pathways has closely followed upon the characterization of a wide variety of leukocytes (Table 2.1), cell surface membrane antigens (Table 2.2), and cytokines (Table 2.3). The following discussion focuses on the key cellular and biomolecular elements of the humoral immune response. For a broader discussion, the reader is directed to more extensive reviews of immune function and diagnostic immunology (1, 2).

1.1. Antigen-Presenting Cells (Refs. 3–7)

The plasma cells, derived from B cells, produce immunoglobulin. However, antigen-presenting cells (APC) and T lymphocytes are required for the effective stimulation and overall control of antibody production. The phagocytic leukocytes can be divided into two general functional classes: macrophages/monocytes and APCs. The former are responsible for the bulk clearance of effete self-molecules/cells or foreign antigens/cells. The macrophages do not reprocess antigens for presentation to the immune system to any large degree. These scavenger cells have high levels of receptors for immunoglobulin Fc region (FcR) and the third components of complement (thus aiding recognition of antibody- or complement-coated cells), but

TABLE 2.1   Selected Cellular Components of the Immune System

Cell type	Function(s)	Membrane antigen profile
T lymphocyte	B cell stimulation/inhibition Monocyte regulation Cellular cytotoxicity Hemato-lymphopoiesis Regulation	CD2+, 3+, TCR+, 5+, 7+, CD4+ 8-, or CD4−8+, HLA ABC+, Dr±, CD25±
B lymphocyte	Plasma cell precursor Antigen presentation	CD19+, 20+, 22+, surface immunoglobulin (sIg)+, CD32+, 35+, HLA Dr+, CD5±, 10±
Plasma cell	Immunoglobulin production	CD38+, 19−, 20−, 22−, sIg−, HLA Dr−, cytoplasmic Ig+
Monocyte/macrophage	Phagocytosis	CD4+, 11a+, 11b+, 11c+, 14+, 16+, 64+
Interdigitating dendritic cell (T-zone APC)	Antigen presentation to T cells	CD11a±, 11c+, 14−, 23±, 25+, 32±, 40+, 54+, 58+, 64−, MHC I, II+
Follicular dendritic cell (B- zone APC)	Antigen/immune complex presentation to B cells	CD11b+, 14−, 21+23±, 40+, 54± MHC II+

TABLE 2.2 Leukocyte Membrane Antigens and Their Functions

Antigen	Function	Leukocyte distribution
CD1	Unknown	Thymocytes, B subsets
CD2	CD58 ligand; activation of T cells	Most T and NK cells
CD3	Antigen-TCR binding signaling	Mature T and few thymocytes
CD4	MHC II receptor	T "helper" subset; monocytes
CD5	Unknown	Most T and B subset
CD7	Low-affinity IgM Fc receptor	Most T and NK cells
CD8	MHC I receptor	T cytotoxic/"suppressor"; some NK
CD10	Neutral endopeptidase	Pre B and act. B subsets; PMNs
CD11a	CD54 ligand; $\beta2$ integrin α chain	Leukocytes
CD11b	C3bi receptor; $\beta2$ integrin α chain	Monocytes; PMNs, T subset, NK
CD11c	C3bi receptor? $\beta2$ integrin α chain	Monocytes; PMNs, NK
CD14	Unknown	Monocytes
CD15	Unknown	PMNs, T subset
CD16	Low-affinity IgG Fc receptor III	PMN; macrophages, NK and few T
CD18	$\beta2$ integrin common β chain	Leukocytes
CD19	B cell activation	Pre B and B cells
CD20	Unknown	B and many pre B cells
CD21	C3d (CR2) and EBV binding, B activation	Mature "virgin" B cells
CD22	CD45RO ligand; B cell activation?	Most mature B cells
CD23	Low-affinity IgE Fc receptor II	B subset; follicular dendritic cells
CD25	Low-affinity IL2 receptor; T and B activation	Activated T and B and NK cells
CD28	B7 receptor; T activation	T cells
CD29	VLA/$\beta1$ integrin β chain; GPIIa	Leukocytes
CD31	PECAM adhesion molecule; GPIIa'	Platelets; B cells, PMN, monocytes
CD32	Type II IgG Fc receptor	B, PMN, macrophage, eosinophil
CD34	Unknown	Hematolymphoid stem cells
CD35	C3b receptor (CR1)	Monocyte, PMN, B and erythrocytes
CD40	Receptor for T cell CD40L, B activation	B cells
CD40L	Ligand for B cell CD40; B activation	T cells; follicular dendritic cells
CD44	Homing receptor for endothelium	Leukocytes, erythrocytes
CD45	Signal transduction control	Leukocytes
CD49a-f	VLA α chains; extracellular adhesion	Variable subsets of leukocytes.
CD54	ICAM; CD11a ligand; adhesion	T, B, dendritic cells and monocytes
CD56	NCAM; adhesion	NK cells, some T cells
CD58	CD2 ligand; adhesion	Leukocytes
CD62	P-selectin; adhesion	Platelets and precursors
CD64	High-affinity IgG Fc receptor	Monocytes
CD72	Ligand for CD5; T and B? activation	B cells
B7	Ligand for CD28; T activation	Activated B cells and dendritic cells
MHC II	Antigen presentation	B and activated T cells, monocytes
MHC I	Antigen presentation	T cells

Modified from Knapp *et al.* (27).

lower and more variable concentrations of histocompatibility antigens (HLA) and other cell adhesion molecules (e.g., CD54, CD58).

The APCs are much fewer in number and do not phagocytose cells and antigens to the extent of the professional macrophages. Rather, they "capture and process" antigen from molecular and cellular sources, presenting the antigen fragments on the cell surface in conjunction with class I and II major histocompatibility antigens

TABLE 2.3   Selected Cytokines and Their Functions

Cytokine	Source(s)	Function(s)
IL1	Macrophage	B and T activation; B differentiation and T proliferation
IL2	T cells (Th1)	T, B, NK, and macrophage activation
IL4	T cells (Th1)	T and B cell activation, proliferation, and differentiation (IgE isotype selection); macrophage, eosinophil, and NK activation
IL5	T cells	B cell activation and differentiation
IL6	Macrophage	B cell differentiation, NK activation, T cell activation and differentiation
IL10	Macrophage	Inhibit IL12 secretion and Th1 maturation
IL12	Monocyte, macrophage	Th1 cell differentiation
Gamma Interferon	Th1 cells	Stimulate B cell proliferation and IgG2a production; inhibit Th2 production
Tumor necrosis factor	Macrophage	Myelomonocytic and eosinophilic activation; B cell activation, proliferation, and differentiation; Th1 proliferation

Modified from Burke *et al.* (28).

(MHC). The APCs migrate to T and B cell zones in lymphoid tissue and "present" the antigens to effector and modulator cells of the T, B, and NK immune system. Further, the dendritic cells have unique pseudopodia or veils, which can extend out and enhance contact with T and B lymphocytes. These, in conjunction with other accessory membrane molecules and/or cytokines, are then responsible for eliciting the ensuing antigen specific immune response.

The lymph node APCs are divided into the dendritic cells, which present antigen to T cells, and the follicular dendritic cells, which present antigen to germinal center B lymphs. The B cells can also function as APCs (see below). The dendritic cells are leukocytes, and are derived from CD34+ marrow precursors (3). Cytokines are important in their maturation, as tumor necrosis factor alpha (TNFα) and granulocyte-macrophage colony stimulating factor enhance dendritic cell development, while blocking macrophage growth.

Dendritic cells and their variants (Langerhans cells, veiled cells) are found in the skin, afferent lymphatics, blood, and other nonlymphoid tissues. In the lymphoid tissues, the dendritic cells are usually found in the interfollicular regions. Long-lived variants in these locations are known as interfollicular dendritic cells. The dendritic cells usually do not have significant expression of receptors for C3 complement or the constant region of IgG (Fcγ), but they are rich in class I and II HLA molecules, as well as adhesion molecules such as CD2, CD11c, CD29, CD54, and CD58 (3, 7). Further, in line with their role of T cell stimulation (see discussion below), the CD40 and B7 antigens are strongly expressed on the dendritic cell membrane (5–7).

Follicular dendritic cells are APCs located in the primary (unstimulated) and secondary follicles (stimulated, with germinal centers). While these areas are thought of as "B cell" zones, a significant minority of the cells are T cells, macrophages, and APCs. The latter are rich in Fcγ receptors, which bind and present antigen to resting and activated B cells. The follicular dendritic cells can hold these antigens for many months, probably playing a crucial role in sustaining the humoral immune response by stimulating new and memory B cells (8).

The role of APCs in T cell activation can be seen in two phases: the stimulation of resting, "naive" T cells (primary response) and the activation of memory T cells (secondary response). Both dendritic cells and, to a lesser extent, B cells can present antigen to T lymphocytes. Effective presentation by either requires not only antigen–MHC complex, but other stimulatory cell-to-cell contact and the proper cytokine environment.

Last, B cells may also serve as APCs *in vitro*. They constitutively express class II MHC (HLA Dr), and have an antigen-specific receptor (immunoglobulin). Such B7+ B cells are able to stimulate T lymphocytes in an antigen specific manner. However, small resting B cells do not have the costimulatory binding proteins (B7; see below) necessary for productive activation of T helper cells. In such a scenario, the T cells become unresponsive, and it has been argued that such B cell APCs play an important role in the induction of peripheral tolerance or anergy to self-antigens (9).

Dendritic cells present the HLA–antigen complex to the T cell antigen receptor (TCR). While the latter can recognize both the antigen and the HLA molecule, binding and the subsequent intracellular responses are greatly augmented by binding of either CD4 to MHC II or CD8 to MHC I molecules. However, if only this TCR/CD4(8) and antigen/MHC II(I) binding occurs, it is most likely that the T cell will become nonresponsive or anergic. Indeed, this may be an effective way of inducing peripheral tolerance to self-antigens, particularly for Th1 helper T cells (9). Effective APC activation of T cells requires costimulation by the B7 antigen on the dendritic or B cell binding the T cell's CD28 or CTLA-4 antigen. T cells stimulated in such a way will coexpress a ligand (CD40L or T-BAM) for a B cell antigen, CD40 (see discussion below). Only when these costimulatory cell contacts are made does activation of the T cell to antigen occur.

1.2. T Cells

1.2.1. T Cell Receptor and Accessory Adhesion Molecules

The TCR antigen is a member of the immunoglobulin superfamily. Unlike immunoglobulins, the TCR is usually composed of one alpha and one beta subunit (α and β). A small fraction of T cells express another set of TCR gene products, delta and gamma (δ and γ). Like the immunoglobulins, accessory molecules are necessary to transfer the binding of antigen to TCR signal into the cell. The most critical accessory molecules for T cell activation are the B7–CD28 or B7–CTLA-4 complexes. The antigen–TCR–CD3 complex, along with MHC–CD4 and B7–CD28 binding, usually suffice to activate the T cell. However, investigators have shown that CD2–CD58, CD11a–CD54, and CD4–MHC II or CD8–MHC I adhesion significantly augment the stimulus provided by the TCR-Ag and B7–CD28 (or B7–CTLA-4) binding. Some of this may simply be due to stabilization of the cell-to-cell contacts, although intracellular signaling after crosslinking of HLA–CD4 or HLA–CD8 has been demonstrated.

1.2.2. Cytokines and T Functional Subsets

The major T helper functional subsets, Th1 and Th2, are believed to come from the same progenitor cell (Th0). The Th1 cells secrete interleukin-2 (IL2), γ-

interferon (γIFN), tumor necrosis factor (TNF), and IL12. The Th2 cell secretes a reciprocal set of cytokines: IL4, IL5, IL6, and IL10 (9). The Th1 cell will drive B cells to preferentially secrete IgG2a, inhibiting Th2 function. IL12 is a particularly important cytokine in this process, as, without it, the generation of Th1 cells is blocked (10). This probably reflects the role of IL12, along with IL1 and TNF, in inducing production of γIFN, which is required for Th1 maturation. IL12 is usually produced by monocytes, macrophages, and accessory cells due to parasitic and bacterial infections. As a positive feedback mechanism, γIFN stimulates further production of IL12. The Th2 cells inhibit IgG2a, but stimulate IgE and IgG1 synthesis. IL4 plays a key role in this process. In addition, IL4 and IL10 inhibit monocyte and macrophage production of IL12, thus blocking Th1 maturation and related immune responses.

1.3. B Cell Stimulation and Immunoglobulin Production

1.3.1. Activation

The primary stimulus for B cell activation is the binding of the membrane-bound immunoglobulin to the antigen via the hypervariable region. In the case of humoral responses to multivalent antigens such as polysaccharide, these lead to effective cross-linking of cell surface immunoglobulin, and T cell-independent activation. However, antibody production to most antigens is "T cell-dependent." In this phase, the antigen must be presented in conjunction with a MHC molecule on an APC, and the B cell costimulated by cell contact as well as cytokines. Such regulatory features are useful, as they preclude spurious alloimmune responses or destructive autoimmune reactions. Several variations are possible, the most common being antigen–MHC II presentation by an APC to a B cell in the presence of T–B cell contact by B7–CD28.

In general, cross-linking of B cell membrane immunoglobulin leads to increased levels of cell contact molecules (CD25, HLA Dr, CD40, B7), along with an increased responsiveness to cytokines important to complete activation (9). Perhaps the most important T–B cell contact activation step is the binding of the B cell CD40 antigen to the T cell CD40L (T-BAM) (9). The T–B cell adhesion (CD4/HLA Dr, CD11c/CD54, and CD2/CD58) is quite important in augmenting the antigen–immunoglobulin binding for B cell activation (9). Interaction with APCs is also required; usually this occurs via the Ag–MHC–sIg and/or B–sIg–(Ag-Ig)–Fc receptors on follicular dendritic cells. Such contact enhancement is the same whether it is delivered from Th1 or Th2 cells.

1.3.2. Proliferation and Maturation

T-cell-dependent B cell activation and differentiation occurs primarily in the germinal centers of lymph nodes, spleen, and tonsils. The B cell activation sequence in the follicles is postulated to occur as follows (8). After MHC II–Ag–sIg and CD40–CD40L binding, and, in the presence of the proper cytokines (IL2, IL4), the B cells begin to proliferate rapidly. In this process, they enlarge, and are morphologically called blasts. The latter give rise to terminally proliferating cells (centroblasts), which may also undergo somatic hypermutation of the immunoglobulin genes. These centroblasts then give rise to nondividing cells (centrocytes), which, as the name implies, are smaller.

Continued survival and maturation of a centrocyte depends upon whether its sIg can effectively bind any antigen–MHC II complexes on the follicular dendritic cells. If it can, then CD40–CD40L, soluble CD23 binding, and/or IL4 binding by the centrocyte will prevent cell death (apoptosis). This is due to induction of synthesis of the bcl-2 protein by such a stimulated centrocyte. The presence of soluble CD23/IL4/IL6 will also drive such a B cell toward terminal maturation, creating a plasma cell (9).

1.3.3. Th1 and Th2 Cells, B Cell Proliferation, and Isotype Switching

The differential application of cytokines will drive B cell activation and differentiation toward IgG production (Th1, IL1, -6, -12) or IgE production (Th2: IL4, γ-interferon). Th1 cells and their cytokines stimulate B cells to mature and secrete IgG2a antibody. In particular, γIFN inhibits IgG1 gene transcription, while IL4 is responsible for enhancing IgG1 and IgE gene transcription (9). Further, plasma cell maturation and secretion of immunoglobulin requires a combination of IL4 and IL5.

The postulated mechanisms of immunoglobulin isotype switching (isotypes are defined in detail in Section 2.2) are complex and controversial (11). Briefly, the heavy-chain class switch is due to a deletion of a large segment of DNA intervening between the constant region exons and the new heavy-chain exon DNA. This appears to be accomplished by a "looping out" of the intervening DNA, followed by deletion and reannealing. An uncharacterized "switch recombinase" enzyme system catalyzes this process.

2. ANTIBODY STRUCTURE

2.1. Function and Structure

Immunoglobulins share a common structural unit and at the same time exhibit the diversity needed for their central function in the immune response. Immunoglobulins are the major secretory product of B cells and the major component of the system of humoral immunity. Their synthesis is initiated by exposure of the organism to a foreign antigen which, after cellular processing, stimulates individual B cells which have receptors that recognize an epitope on the antigen. This binding stimulates clonal proliferation and subsequent antibody synthesis.

The remarkable structure of the immunoglobulin molecule is central to its function as a modulator of the immune system. Furthermore, recent advances in molecular biology demonstrate the mechanism by which this unique structure provides the vast diversity required.

Immunoglobulin molecules are bifunctional proteins having unique recognition sites which specifically bind antigen, as well as functional sites remote from the antigen binding site. The latter participate in various effector functions such as complement activation, stimulation of mast cells to release histamine, and removal of antigens in circulating immune complexes. In this way antibodies participate in many different reactions which make up the immune response. The development of our understanding of immunoglobulin structure and function has been reviewed extensively(12–14).

As a group, antibodies are heterogeneous proteins which can be classified into a small number of classes and subclasses based on the presence of certain common antigenic determinants shared by the members of the group. Each subclass comprises individual populations of similar proteins with unique amino acid sequence, each one of which is the product of single B-cell clone. Heterogeneity within a class was first noted as variable electrophoretic mobility of the major classes of immunoglobulins.

2.2. Basic Structure

The basic structural unit of all classes of immunoglobulins is a symmetric four-chain heterodimer made of two identical heavy chains (H, MW 50,000 Da each) and two identical light chains (L, MW 25,000 Da) which form the characteristic Y-shape (Fig. 2.1). Each L chain binds a H chain with one or more disulfide (–s–s–) bonds. The two H chains likewise are bound by one or more disulfide bonds in the "hinge" region, all of which contribute to the chemical stability of immunoglobulin molecules. Immunoglobulin heavy chains μ (IgM) and ε (IgE) do not have a hinge region, but contain additional amino acids in an additional constant domain in the general location of the hinge. In addition, intrachain disulfide bonds in both light and heavy chains contribute to the secondary structure. Initial descriptions of antibodies were according to their electrophoretic mobility, primarily in the gamma region, where they show broad heterogeneity of electric charge.

2.3. Heavy Chains

Immunoglobulin classes (IgG, IgA, IgM, IgD, IgE) are major subgroups of immunoglobulins originally defined serologically by antigenic differences in the H-chain constant region. The different heavy chain forms are designated γ, α, μ, δ, and ε. It is now known that different heavy chain constant regions are coded by different genes, although there is some homology among them. Subclasses within the five heavy chain classes further divide immunoglobulins into subgroups (IgG1, IgG2, etc.). Four IgG subclasses also show differences in the number of disulfide bonds in the hinge region and in the number of amino acids in the hinge region. Heavy chains of IgM and IgE contain additional amino acids which form an additional constant domain between $C_H 1$ and $C_H 2$. IgA and IgM classes occur naturally as polymers of the basic four-chain unit and contain additional polypeptides which facilitate the special effector functions of the immunoglobulin class (e.g., secretory fragment of IgA). The term *isotype* is used to describe antigenic determinants which are shared by all members of the same class of antibody and are present in all individuals of the species (IgG, IgA, IgM, etc.). The term *allotype* refers to allelic forms within a class or subclass. Genetic loci for allotypes are located in the constant region of H and L chains.

2.4. Light Chains

Myeloma tumors (malignant proliferation of a single B-cell clone) produce a predominance of a single antibody. Some myeloma tumors also produce excess light chains of a single type (Bence–Jones proteins). These pathologically occurring monoclonal proteins were the source of information of immunoglobulin structure in the prehybridoma days.

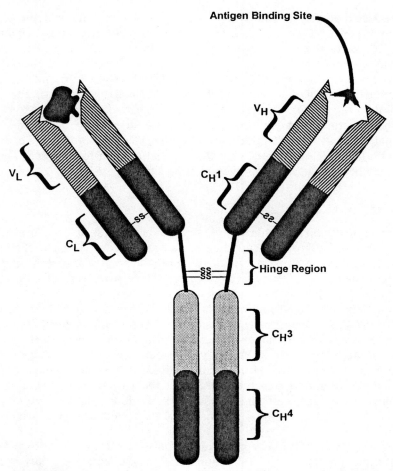

FIGURE 2.1   Monomeric subunit of immunoglobulin molecules. The figure shows the basic four-chain subunit common to immunoglobulins. Heavy chain and light chain domains are indicated. Heavy chains are held together by a variable number of disulfide bonds (–SS–) in the hinge region. Light chains are bound to the amino-terminus of heavy chains by disulfide bonds. Antigen binding sites are formed by the variable domains of light and heavy chains. The disulfide bond cross-linking sites and number of C-terminal regions will vary within and between the immunoglobulin classes.

In humans there are only two light chain types, κ and λ. Any single immunoglobulin molecule can have either κ or λ light chain type, but not both (the unique product of a single B-cell clone). Since developing B-cell precursors attempt to arrange the κ light chain genes first, humans usually have a mild predominance of cell-bound and intracellular kappa light chains (1.5 to 2.0 : 1). Other species have κ and λ chains in different characteristic ratios. Within the λ L chains, two allotypes have been observed. No allotypic forms of κ light chains have been found.

2.5. Variable and Constant Regions

Both L and H chains contain regions of amino acid sequences which show very little variation among immunoglobulins (constant region), while other sequences

vary a great deal among individual antibodies (variable region). Isotypic and allotypic loci are genetic variations in constant regions of both H and L chains. The
constant regions of the two H chains, the carboxy-terminal end of each peptide
chain, form the "tail" of the Y-shaped intact antibody (C_H, C_L) (see Fig. 2.1). The
variable regions are the amino terminal ends of both chains (V_H and V_L). In the
intact Ig molecule the variable regions of L and H chains together form the antigen
binding sites at the ends of the arms of the Y. The term *idiotype* is used to describe
the epitope(s) formed by the unique three-dimensional antigen binding end of each
monoclonal antibody. The definition is based on serological evidence, i.e., binding
of anti-antibody which competes with the original antigen for binding. Thus, the
idiotype may be at or near the antigen binding site.

2.6. Three-Dimensional Structure

The immunoglobulin molecule in three dimensions is made up of several globular
domains, each containing corresponding sequences of both H and L chains (e.g.,
V_H, V_L, C_H1, C_H2). The domain is a folded β sheet structure formed by alternating
antiparallel sequences connected by loop regions. This structure is called the "immunoglobulin fold" (15).

The most important contribution to antibody flexibility is the hinge region between C_H1 and C_H2 domains. Movement of the "arms of the molecule" have been
demonstrated by x-ray crystallography using bivalent antigens (16). In fact, Fab
fragments rotate relatively independently. Between contiguous domains are short
helical sequences which give the molecule additional flexibility (elbow bending).
In the modular (domain) structure described, the variable domains of both H
and L chains are folded, with the hypervariable regions relatively exposed. The
hypervariable regions of H and L chains make up a cleft or trough which is the
antigen binding site.

The importance of antibody structural flexibility in effector functions is recognized, but remains subject to investigation. Clearly, segmental flexibility at elbows
(between domains) and hinge regions is a factor in the accomplishment of certain
effector functions such as linking of multiple antigens on a cell surface, agglutination,
or surface immunoglobulin binding of the "bunch of tulips"-shaped C1q. In addition,
internal movements between H- and L-chain domains facilitate a good fit in antigen
binding and increase the effective affinity. It is now not considered likely that
antigen binding per se triggers conformational changes that signal secondary func-
tions(17, 18). Since the main contributor to segmental flexibility is the hinge region,
it is easy to appreciate that different IgG subclasses show different flexibility.

2.7. Fragments

Early studies on antibody structure were facilitated by the discovery that digestion
with certain proteolytic enzymes resulted in predictable fragments. Papain digestion
cleaves disulfide bonds near the hinge region, yielding a crystallizable fragment
consisting of the constant portions of two H chains (Fc) and two fragments which
bind antigen (Fab). Each of the latter contain the variable region from both H and
L chains. This Fab fragment is univalent (can bind only one antigen) (Fig. 2.2).

Pepsin digestion splits IgG at a different site in the hinge yielding a bivalent
fragment which contains both binding sites $F(ab')_2$. This fragment can be cleaved

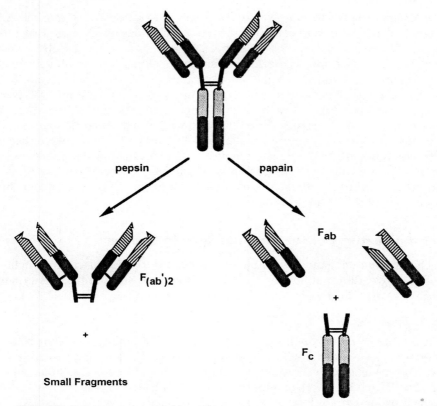

FIGURE 2.2   Pattern of protein fragments after enzymatic cleavage. Proteolytic cleavage of immunoglobulin in the hinge region by pepsin results in a fragment containing both antigen binding sites, $F_{(ab')}2$. The constant regions of the heavy chains are digested into small fragments. Digestion with papain results in two types of fragments, one containing a single antigen binding site (F(ab)), the other containing the constant regions of the heavy chains which crystallized (Fc). Characterization of these fragments led to the discovery of the Y-shaped structure of immunoglobulins.

into two identical univalent fragments almost identical with Fab. Pepsin digests the Fc fragment into small fragments which generally are not recovered. In general, enzyme cleavage occurs in connecting regions between the globular domains.

Though they were most important in the development of understanding of antibody structure, Fab fragments continue to be useful in the development of immunoassay components. Their smaller size, univalency, and ability to bind antigen can be exploited in assay design. In addition, the lack of the antigenic sites in the constant regions can improve specificity in two-site immunoassays by reducing interferences by heterologous antibodies (anti-species antibodies which may be found in some patients' sera; see also Chapter 7). This is also true with cellular immunoassays, where the lack of Fc components precludes nonspecific binding to cellular Fc-receptors.

2.8. Carbohydrates

Immunoglobulins are glycoproteins which contain 3–12% by mass carbohydrate as oligosaccharide side chains depending on the Ig class. Oligosaccharides are bound to asparagine in primarily *N*-glycosidic linkages or to serine in *O*-glycosidic linkages in one to five locations. In each site, the oligosaccharides may vary in structure and length. The variable amounts of carbohydrate may account for electrophoretic microheterogeneity observed even within a monoclonal protein of a single class.

Carbohydrate is found in higher concentration in the secretory piece of IgA, the hinge region and the constant region of H chains (C_H2), but not in L chains or the variable regions of the H chain. The biological role of the carbohydrate is not known, although there is speculation that it functions in the secretion process. Other roles for the carbohydrate are participation in binding to Fc of macrophages and elimination of antigen–antibody complexes. The so-called glycoforms may vary in the sera of individuals with diseases in which IgG has been implicated, such as rheumatoid arthritis, systemic lupus erythematosus, and Crohn's disease, but the importance of this is not known(19).

2.9. Structural Features of the Immunoglobulin Classes

Though immunoglobulins all share the characteristic four-chain structure described above, different immunoglobulin classes show structural diversity, some of which is related to specific functions associated with the class (Table 2.4).

2.9.1. IgG

IgG is the predominant immunoglobulin class (75% in humans). The prototypical monomeric four-chain structure made up of two γ H chains and two either κ or λ L chains has a molecular weight of approximately 150,000 Da. Four subclasses (IgG1, IgG2, IgG3, IgG4), or allotypes, are distinguished by genetic polymorphisms (alleles) within certain loci in the C_H and C_L domains.

The distribution of light chain type and carbohydrate composition varies among allotypes. IgG subclasses also differ in the number of disulfide bonds and number

TABLE 2.4   Immunoglobulin Classes

Characteristic/Function	IgG	IgA	IgM	IgD	IgE
Molecular weight (Da)	150,000	400,000	900,000	180,000	190,000
Heavy chain	γ	α	μ	δ	ϵ
Number of subunits	1	2	5	1	1
Allotypes	G1, 2, 3, 4	A1,2			
Additional components		Secretory peptide, J chain	J chain		
B cell integral membrane protein			+	+	
Fix complement	+		+ +		
Bind macrophage Fc receptors	+		+ +		
Opsonization	+				
Mucosal immunoglobulin secretion		+			
Histamine release from mast cells					+
Early (primary) humoral immune response			+		
Late (secondary) humoral immune response	+				

of amino acids in the hinge region. For example, IgG3 has a longer hinge region containing 11 disulfide bonds which results in an increase in molecular weight and increased rigidity compared to IgG1.

IgG subtypes also vary somewhat in their functions. IgG participates through various C_H domains in various mechanisms of the immune response by fixing complement and binding Fc receptors on macrophages. IgG also crosses the placenta and confers immunity on the newborn.

2.9.2. IgA

IgA occurs as a monomer of two α H chains and two κ or λ L chains, or as a dimer of the basic unit (Fig. 2.3). There are two subclasses, IgA1 and IgA2. Secretory IgA contains an additional peptide, the secretory piece (SP), which is not homologous with any other sequences in the immunoglobulins. The SP is synthesized in the mucosal epithelial cells and may appear independently of IgA, especially in patients who cannot synthesize IgA. In addition, IgA and IgM contain a polypeptide segment of 15,000 Da, called the joining chain, or J chain. This protein appears to be bound by disulfide bonds to α or μ H chains in the IgA or IgM multimeric forms and is thought to function by joining the subunits. The J chain is not essential to polymerization, however, as it is not synthesized in some lower vertebrates which also have polymeric immunoglobulins.

IgA is the predominant immunoglobulin in mucous and other secretions of the intestinal, respiratory, or gastrointestinal tracts where it appears to be the first line of humoral defense against microbes which are ingested or inhaled.

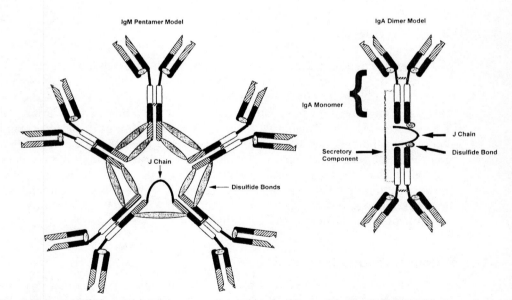

FIGURE 2.3 Polymeric structures of IgM and secretory IgA. Five four-chain IgM monomers are joined by disulfide bonds in the C_H3 domains and by disulfide bonds to the J chain to form a pentamer with 10 antigen binding sites. For secretory IgA, the IgA dimer is joined by disulfide bonds and the J chain. An additional secretory component is joined by noncovalent and disulfide bonds.

2.9.3. IgM

IgM is a pentamer of four-chain subunits linked by disulfide bonds between C_H3 domains of the μ chains and by disulfide bonds to a J chain (Fig. 2.3). The IgM subunits lack a hinge region, but contain an extra 130-amino acid domain in the position analogous to the hinge region of IgG. The molecular weight of the pentamer is 900,000 Da.

IgM is the first immunoglobulin to be synthesized after exposure of an individual to antigen, later to be replaced by IgG of the same specificity by a gene-switching mechanism to be described in detail later. IgM is the major immunoglobulin exposed on the surface of B cells and also functions by efficiently binding complement in the initiation of the complement cascade.

2.9.4. IgD

Along with IgM, IgD predominates on the surface of B-cells at an early stage of development. IgD is a four-chain monomer of 180,000 Da. This immunoglobulin is of relatively low concentration and is relatively labile to thermal and enzymatic degradation.

2.9.5. IgE

IgE has the lowest concentration of the immunoglobulin classes and participates in allergic reactions, during which it binds with very high affinity to mast cells which release histamine when the IgE is cross-linked by specific antigen binding. The four-chain monomer has increased molecular weight due to a relatively high carbohydrate content.

3. ANTIGEN BINDING

Antigen recognition and binding are probably the most unique features of antibody structure, and provide the flexible mechanism which functionally couples the entrance of a foreign antigen with the complex immune responses which protects the organism from infection. Binding occurs at the ends of the "arms" of the Y structure, distal to the loci which participate in many effector functions (e.g., complement binding and binding to Fc receptors). The spectrum of effector functions elicited reflects the immunoglobulin subclass distribution in the individual as well as the location of the antibody synthesizing cells. The mechanism by which the tremendous diversity of antigen binding specificity is achieved within the population of immunoglobulins which have, for the most part, a similar structure has been a matter of intense interest and investigation.

3.1. Antigen–Antibody Interaction

Most antigen–antibody complexes have the characteristics of other well-studied protein–protein interactions. The free energy of binding is a function of the amount of surface of each protein (antigen and antibody) which is hidden within the complex from exposure to solvent(13, 20). It has been estimated that at least 600 Å^2 of buried surface is associated with a stable complex. The antigen–antibody bond occurs through multiple noncovalent bonds—electrostatic, hydrogen, hydrophobic, and Van der Waals. Long-range forces such as electrostatic and hydrogen bonds are important in the rate of formation of antigen–antibody complexes at the points of contact. The short-range forces contribute significantly to bond strength by reducing the rate of complex dissociation. Cross-reacting antigens show a wide range of affinity depending on the balance of attractive and repulsive forces within the binding site (21). Typical dissociation constants for antigen–antibody reactions are $>10^{-9} M$.

3.2. Antigen Binding Site

The antigen binding site is formed from the amino-terminal ends (variable domains) of L and H chains. The two chains are folded to form globular variable domains, V_H and V_L, similar to the folded domains of the constant regions. Looped segments called complementarity defining regions (CDRs) at the ends of the molecule are formed by hypervariable regions which are brought close together in the three-dimensional structure.

In individual antibodies, V_H and V_L form a cleft or trough of somewhat variable size (approx. $2 \times 2 \times 1$ nm deep) as observed by x-ray crystallography, into which the epitope fits and binds with high affinity. The actual points of contact in the few antigen–antibody systems which have been studied are 4–6 to 16–17 amino acid residues, usually charged(13). Deep within the site, hydrophobic residues predominate. As the cleft may be larger than the original epitope, it is clear that any antibody can conceivably bind other epitopes, especially those with similar structure, as long as the charged residues in either the antigen or the antibody in the binding site are compatible (no electrostatic repulsion). Heteroclitic antibodies have been described which have binding sites that can accommodate amino acid changes in antigen causing an increase of several orders of magnitude in binding affinity. There have been detailed studies on only a few antigen–antibody pairs, but the results can be extrapolated to understand cross reactivity and specificity in immunoassays.

3.3. Hypervariable Regions

Analysis of amino acid sequences of variable domains of both H and L chains showed that even within so-called variable regions many sequences are homologous among different antibodies. However, approximately 15 amino acid positions separated into three general locations ("peaks") showed extreme variability (22). This finding suggested that these hypervariable "hot spots" represent the amino acids involved in the formation of the unique antigen binding site of each clone. Subsequently, it was demonstrated that the hypervariable region indeed forms exposed loops at the ends of the molecule (CDRs). The CDRs are flanked by relatively conserved framework regions (FR).

3.4. Idiotype

Each immunoglobulin has unique epitope(s) formed by hypervariable region, probably near or part of the antigen binding site, called idiotope. These antigenic determinants, together called idiotype, were discovered with the use of antibodies to immunoglobulins. Binding of anti-idiotype antibodies to the immunoglobulin can often be blocked by the hapten against which the antibody is directed, suggesting that the idiotype is near the binding site. Private idiotypes are thought to be unique epitopes. Public idiotypes are epitopes which are shared by individual members of a genetically closely related group, such as inbred mice, and probably include a family of very similar, but still unique, antibodies. The study of idiotype/anti-idiotype interaction has been stimulated by the hypothesis that such interaction is a mechanism for immune self-regulation. Also, since anti-idiotypes presumably fit closely into the idiotype binding site, they may mimic the external antigen structure. If this were true, anti-idiotypes might be useful in the design of therapeutic agents and vaccines. However, recent studies of crystallized anti-lysozyme/anti-idiotype complex suggest that idiotype mimicry does not always occur (23).

3.5. Antigen

An epitope or antigenic determinant is a group of amino acids or other chemical groups exposed on the surface of a molecule, frequently a protein, which can generate an antigenic response and bind antibody. The amino acids forming the epitope are not linear in amino acid sequence, but they reside close together on the surface of the tertiary structure. Although some researchers hypothesize that there are a limited number of structures which are highly antigenic (24), others propose that there are overlapping epitopes over the whole surface of a protein, any one of which can be antigenic. Surface access is the most important feature (20).

4. ANTIBODY STRUCTURE AND IMMUNOLOGIC DIVERSITY

4.1. Theories of Antibody Diversity

An abiding question in immunology was "how does the immune system provide the necessary diversity through known genetic mechanisms?" Theories range from speculation that all necessary genes for every antibody preexist and that expression of the gene is somehow directed by exposure to the antigen (germ-line theory), to the idea that there are a more limited number of genes for antibodies and that needed diversity is achieved by gene mutation in either somatic or germ-line cells (somatic mutation theory). Current information about antibody structure and molecular genetics currently supports a third mechanism, gene rearrangement.

Consistent with earlier knowledge describing variable and constant domains in both light and heavy chains, it has now been shown that there are three separate, unlinked genetic loci for the C regions of H chain and κ and λ light chains. Each C locus is linked with a set of V genes. Thus, in any given B cell, one C gene rearranges to be near one V gene and fuses to form the gene for H or L chain. Additional gene segments containing information required for messenger RNA transcription are also fused in the process, resulting eventually in complete genes for immunoglobulin chains. In this way a limited amount of DNA in segments widely separated by noncoding DNA can be manipulated during B-cell differentiation to produce the tremendous number of different H- and L-chain genes which will combine to form one unique antibody per B-cell clone(25). In addition, somatic mutations occur throughout the genome. With this variety of possible B-cells circulating, the immune system awaits exposure to antigen to initiate clonal expansion and antibody secretion(12).

4.2. Light-Chain Gene

Kappa light chain rearrangements have the simplest sequence of events (Fig. 2.4). As there is only one class of κ L chains, there is only one exon coding for the constant domain. The variable region is coded in two gene segments, variable (V_κ) and joining (J_κ), each of which is found in multiple copies. The first step in gene arrangement is V/J joining in which one V and one J segment are fused to form the V gene and at the same time intervening DNA is deleted. In the primary transcript of V and C genes, the messenger RNA still contains additional introns which are subsequently excised. Lambda light chains follow a similar sequence, but as there are multiple copies of C (corresponding to subclasses), each with an associated J segment, there are more possible combinations for the final rearranged gene.

4.3. Heavy-Chain Gene

In contrast to the small number of segments spliced to form the L-chain gene, the H-chain gene is made of four different segments, V, J, D, and C. Nine gene segments correspond to one gene for each H-chain class and subclass and within these segments there are separate exons for the subclass domains, e.g., C_H1, C_H2, and C_H3. There are 6 J_H segments and at least 20 segments of a fourth type of segment, the diversity (D_H) segment, which lies between the V and J genes.

DNA rearrangement begins with V/D/J joining, then linking to one of the C segments. As described above for the light chain, gene moving and fusion results in the deletion of intervening DNA. Additional diversity is also achieved at this step since the joining is somewhat imprecise, causing the junction to vary by a few nucleotides. Short sequences of random nucleotides (N) may also be inserted at the points of joining.

4.4. Isotype Switching

The arrangement of gene segments for the C region isotypes occurs in the order of immunoglobulin synthesis during B-cell ontogeny, μ, δ, $\gamma3$, $\gamma1$ (11). $C\mu$ and $C\delta$ are close to each other and may be expressed in the same cell early in development. Later during development additional rearrangement occurs to move the C gene for another isotype, e.g., $\gamma1$, close to the V/D/J gene and in the process delete $C\mu$ and $C\delta$, a process called isotype switching (11, 26). This mechanism explains the early presence of both IgM and IgD on the surface of pre-B cells. When cells differentiate to synthesize IgG, IgM and IgD synthesis is suppressed and further H-chain gene rearrangements are inhibited. Thus, the identical antigenic specificity, a function of V regions, can be present in antibodies of different isotypes

5. CONCLUSION

5.1. Relationship between Antibody Structure and *in Vivo* Function

In the immune response, structure *is* function. The unique structural characteristics of the immunoglobulin achieve the needed coupling between a multitude of specific antigens and a more limited number of specific effector reactions which

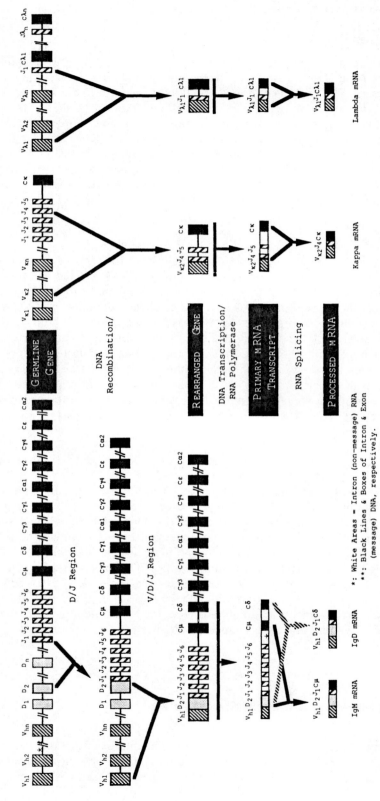

FIGURE 2.4 Gene rearrangements of heavy- and light-chain genes illustrating proposed mechanisms for immunoglobulin diversity. Individual gene segments for V, D, J, and C regions are sequentially selected and joined to form a rearranged gene for a single light chain and single heavy chain. Unused sequences are excised. After messenger RNA transcription, additional introns are removed, and the exons forming the final mRNA are spliced together. (figure adapted, with permission, from Ref. 29.)

protect the organism. The latter is accomplished by structural diversity among the immunoglobulins which is genetically conserved. Delicate and appropriate responses reflect the distribution of immunoglobulin forms and their associated functional capabilities as well as the location of the cells which synthesize them. Important structural and biochemical features are binding specificity and the effector functions which take advantage of the physical flexibility of the immunoglobulin molecule.

5.2. Relation of Antibody Structure to *in Vitro* Actions

The most important features of antibody structure in *in vitro* assays are binding specificity and affinity. Current knowledge of binding site structure and the potential for the binding of alternative epitopes offers understanding of the observations of nonspecific binding and cross-reactivity. Antibodies in competitive binding assays are typically used at high dilution, a condition in which the reaction can be assumed to be essentially univalent and second order. The Fc portion of the molecule frequently has little role in the design and function of these assays except in those which use some effector function such as complement fixation as a detection device or staph protein A as a separation.

In solid-phase and two-site immunometric assays, structural flexibility begins to play a role allowing relatively free antigen binding even in constrained circumstances. Sandwich assays introduced new interferences due to the presence of antigenic sites in the heavy chain which can be linked by antibodies or other biological binders.

The era of monoclonal antibodies and genetic manipulation of antibodies for experimental and analytical purposes takes advantage of our knowledge of the advantages and disadvantages of natural immunoglobulin structure and chemistry to optimize new bioactive molecules for specific applications.

References

1. Colvin RB, Bhan AK, McCluskey RT, Eds. Diagnostic Immunopathology, 2nd ed. New York: Raven Press, 1994.
2. Shoenfeld Y, Isenberg DA. Natural Autoantibodies: Their Physiological Role and Regulatory Significance. Boca Raton: CRC Press, 1993.
3. Knight SC, Stagg AJ. Antigen-presenting cell types. Curr Op Immunol 1993; 5:374–82.
4. Scott P. Selective differentiation of CD4+ T helper cell subsets. Curr Op Immunol 1993; 5:391–7.
5. Lederman S, Yellin MJ, Covey LR, Cleary AM, Callard R, Chess L. Non-antigen signals for B-cell growth and differentiation to antibody secretion. Curr Op Immunol 1993; 5:439–44.
6. Linsley PS, Ledbetter JA. The role of the CD28 receptor during T cell responses to antigen. Annu Rev Immunol 1993; 11:191–212.
7. Steinman RM. The dendritic cell system and its role in immunogenicity. Annu Rev Immunol 1991; 9:271–96.
8. Liu Y-J, Johnson GD, Gordon J, MacLennan ICM. Germinal centers in T-cell-dependent antibody responses. Immunol Today 1992; 13:17–21.
9. Parker DC. T cell-dependent B cell activation. Annu Rev Immunol 1993; 11:331–60.
10. Trinchieri G. Interleukin-12 and its role in the generation of T_H1 cells. Immunol Today 1993; 14:335–8.
11. Harriman W, Völk H, Defranoux N, Wabl M. Immunoglobulin class switch recombination. Annu Rev Immunol 1993; 11:361–84.
12. Roitt I. Immunology.St. Louis: C. V. Mosby, 1985.
13. Goodman J. Immunoglobulin structure and function. In: Stites D, Terr A, Eds. Basic and Clinical Immunology, 7th ed. Norwalk: Appleton and Lange, 1991: 109–21.

14. Eisen H. Immunoglobulin molecules and genes. In: Immunology, 2nd ed. Philadelphia: Harper and Row, 1980: 338–80.
15. Amzel L, Poljak R. Three-dimensional structure of immunoglobulins. Annu Rev Biochem 1979; 48:961–97.
16. Schumaker V, Phillips M, Hanson D. Dynaminc aspects of antibody structure. Mol Immunol 1991; 28:1347–60.
17. Poljak R. Structure of antibodies and their complexes with antigens. Mol Immunol 1991; 28:1341–45.
18. Nezlin R. Internal movements in immunoglobulin molecules. Adv Immunol 1990; 48:1–40.
19. Rudd P, Leatherbarrow R, Rademacher T, Dwek R. Diversification of the IgG molecule by oligosaccharides. Mol Immunol 1991; 28:1369–78.
20. Colman P. Structure of antibody-antigen complexes: Implications of immune recognition. Adv Immunol 1988; 43:99–132.
21. Tedford M, Stimson W. Molecular recognition in antibodies and its application. Experientia 1991; 47:1129–38.
22. Wu T, Kabat E. An analysis of the sequences of the variable regions of Bence–Jones proteins and myeloma light chains and their implications for antibody complementarity. J Exp Med 1970; 132:211–50.
23. Bentley G, Boulot G, Riottot M, Poljak R. Three-dimensional structure of an idiotope-anti-idiotope complex. Nature 1990; 348:254–7.
24. Atassi M. Precise determination of the entire antigenic structure of lysozyme. Immunochemistry 1978; 15:909–36.
25. Tonegawa S. Somatic generation of antibody diversity. Nature 1983; 302:575–81.
26. Coffman R, Lebman D, Rothman P. Mechanism and regulation of immunoglobulin isotype switching. Adv Immunol 1993; 54:229–70.
27. Knapp W, Dörken B, Gilks W, Eds. Leucocyte Typing IV. Oxford: Oxford University Press, 1989.
28. Burke F, Naylor MS, Davies B, Balkwill F. The Cytokine wall chart. Immunol Today 1993; 14:165–70.
29. Parslow, TG. Immunogobulin genes, B cells, and the humoral immune response. In: Sites D, Terr A, and Parsolow T, Eds. Basic and Clinical Immunology, 8th ed. Norwalk: Apppleton and Lange, 1994:81–3.

3 THEORY OF IMMUNOASSAYS

THEODORE K. CHRISTOPOULOS
Department of Chemistry and Biochemistry
University of Windsor
Windsor, Ontario, Canada N9B 3P4

ELEFTHERIOS P. DIAMANDIS
Department of Pathology and
Laboratory Medicine
Mount Sinai Hospital
Toronto, Ontario, Canada M5G 1X8

1. BINDING THEORY

The Scatchard model (1) is the most widely used mathematical approach to the quantitative description of the multiple equilibria taking place when a binder (e.g., an antibody) binds reversibly to a ligand molecule, L (antigen, analyte). The Scatchard model focuses on the individual binding sites of the binder and applies the law of mass action for each site, s, defining the association constant (affinity constant) K and assuming that the affinity of each particular site for the ligand is not influenced by the extent of occupancy of the other sites (independent and noninteracting binding sites). Thus,

$$s + L \leftrightarrow sL \tag{1}$$

and

$$K = \frac{B}{F(N - B)}, \tag{2}$$

where B and F represent the concentrations (molarities) of the bound and free (unbound) ligand respectively, and N is the total concentration of the binding sites. N is given by the product of the total binder concentration times the number of binding sites per binder molecule. $N - B$ represents the concentration of unoccupied (free) binding sites on the binder molecule.

The mass conservation of the ligand requires that

$$T = B + F \tag{3}$$

where T is the total ligand concentration. Solving Eq. (2) with respect to B/F gives:

$$B/F = K(N - B). \tag{4}$$

The plot of B/F vs B for various ligand concentrations and a constant binder concentration (Scatchard plot) is a straight line with a slope of $-K$ (Fig. 3.1). The x-axis intercept corresponds to an infinitely high ligand concentration (saturation of the binder) and gives the total concentration N of binding sites. A solution of a monoclonal antibody usually yields a linear Scatchard plot. Figure 3.1 shows simulated Scatchard plots representing the binding of a ligand to various concentrations of a binder. The lines shift to the right with increasing binder concentration, whereas the slope remains constant. Figure 3.2 demonstrates how the presence of nonspecific binding can distort an otherwise linear Scatchard plot. Nonspecific binding is defined as a low-affinity, unsaturable binding of the ligand to reaction vessels or other solid phases involved in the binding experiment. The following binding model (2) incorporates the nonspecific binding:

$$B = \frac{NKF}{1 + KF} + nF. \tag{5}$$

The first term of the above equation can be derived by rearranging Eq. (4) and describes the specific binding. The second term accounts for the nonspecific binding which is proportional to the free ligand concentration (n is a constant). Equation (5) can be written as:

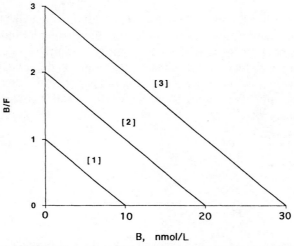

FIGURE 3.1 Simulated Scatchard plots for the binding of a ligand to various concentrations of identical and independent binding sites: [1] $N = 10^{-8}$, [2] $N = 2 \times 10^{-8}$, and [3] $N = 3 \times 10^{-8}$ M. $K = 10^8$ M^{-1}.

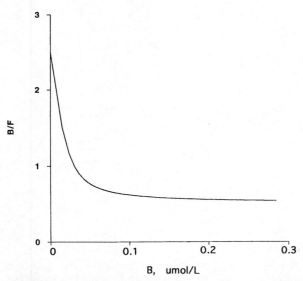

FIGURE 3.2 Scatchard plot for the binding of a ligand to a single class of binding sites ($N = 2 \times 10^{-8}\,M$, and $K = 10^8\,M^{-1}$) in the presence of nonspecific binding. $n = 0.5$.

$$\frac{B}{F} = \frac{NK}{1 + KF} + n. \tag{6}$$

At very high ligand concentrations the B/F ratio becomes equal to n and the line becomes parallel to the x-axis (see Fig. 3.2).

In a system which contains a heterogeneous population of binding sites (e.g., a solution of a polyclonal antibody), the Scatchard model groups the binding sites into m distinct classes. The class i contains a concentration N_i of individual sites that have the same affinity for the ligand. The site affinity constant K_i characterizes the sites of the ith class. The concentration of the ligand bound to the ith class is given by the equation:

$$B_i = \frac{N_i K_i F}{1 + K_i F}. \tag{7}$$

The total concentration of bound ligand is:

$$B = \sum_{i=1}^{m} \frac{N_i K_i F}{1 + K_i F}. \tag{8}$$

When the binding sites become saturated we have:

$$B = \sum_{i=1}^{m} N_i. \tag{9}$$

In the case of two classes of binding sites ($m = 2$), Eq. (8) becomes

$$B = \frac{N_1 K_1 F}{1 + K_1 F} + \frac{N_2 K_2 F}{1 + K_2 F}, \tag{10}$$

and the Scatchard plot is a hyperbola (Fig. 3.3). The asymptotes of the hyperbola

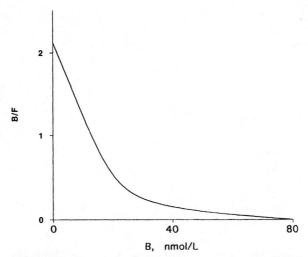

FIGURE 3.3 Scatchard plot representing the binding of a ligand to two groups of binding sites. $N_1 = 2 \times 10^{-8}\, M$, $K_1 = 10^8\, M^{-1}$, $N_2 = 6 \times 10^{-8}\, M$, and $K_2 = 2 \times 10^6\, M^{-1}$.

are defined by Eq. (11) and are useful in the graphical estimation of the binding parameters (3).

$$y = K_1 N_1 - K_1 X \qquad \text{and} \qquad y = K_2 N_2 - K_2 X \qquad (11)$$

The x-axis intercept of the plot gives the total concentration of binding sites, that is $N_1 + N_2$. In the presence of nonspecific binding, Eq. (10) becomes:

$$B = \frac{N_1 K_1 F}{1 + K_1 F} + \frac{N_2 K_2 F}{1 + K_2 F} + nF. \qquad (12)$$

Again, at high ligand concentrations $B/F = n$ and the line becomes parallel to the x-axis.

Calculation of the binding parameters by least-squares fitting is generally the recommended method (2). However, the choice of the dependent and independent variable is important for a statistically correct regression. The application of common least-squares programs (linear or nonlinear) directly to the Scatchard plot coordinate system often gives results which are inferior even to those obtained by graphical techniques. This is because the experimental errors affect both B/F and B and, also, are highly correlated and nonuniform. The total ligand concentration should be used as an independent variable whereas the raw, untransformed experimental data (e.g., counts, fluorescence) can serve as the dependent one. The nonspecific binding can be incorporated as an additional parameter in the model and allowed to take values that result in the best fitting (2).

2. EQUILIBRIA INVOLVING MANY LIGANDS AND A HETEROGENEOUS POPULATION OF BINDING SITES

The usefulness of this section becomes apparent when we have an immunoassay system containing the analyte and one or more crossreacting species (i.e., molecules which also bind to the antibody), along with a heterogeneous population of antibody binding sites (4, 5). Consider a system containing x number of ligands $L_1, L_2, \ldots, L_x$ and m groups of binding sites $s_1, s_2, \ldots, s_m$. Then, the binding of ligand L_i to sites s_j can be described by the reaction:

$$L_i + s_j \leftrightarrow L_i s_j. \tag{13}$$

The equilibrium constant K_{ij} is defined as:

$$K_{ij} = \frac{[L_i s_j]}{[L_i][s_j]}. \tag{14}$$

The mass conservation equations for ligand L_i and binding sites s_j are

$$T_i = [L_i] + \sum_{j=1}^{m} [L_i s_j] \tag{15}$$

$$N_j = [s_j] + \sum_{i=1}^{x} [L_i s_j], \tag{16}$$

for $j = 1, \ldots, m$ and $i = 1, \ldots, x$. T_i and $[L_i]$ represent the total and free concentrations of L_i, respectively, $[L_i s_j]$ is the concentration of L_i bound to s_j binding sites; N_j and $[s_j]$ are the total and free concentrations of the s_j binding sites, respectively. The second term of Eq. (15) represents the sum of the bound L_i to all m binding sites. The second term of Eq. (16) represents the sum of occupied binding sites, s_j, by all x ligands present. Substituting $[L_i s_j]$ from Eq. (14) into Eqs. (15) and (16) gives (4, 5):

$$T_i = [L_i]\left(1 + \sum_{j=1}^{m} K_{ij}[s_j]\right) \tag{17}$$

$$N_j = [s_j]\left(1 + \sum_{l=1}^{x} K_{lj}[L_l]\right). \tag{18}$$

Substituting $[s_j]$ from Eq. (18) in Eq. (17) yields:

$$T_i = [L_i]\left(1 + \sum_{j=1}^{m} \frac{K_{ij}N_j}{1 + \sum_{l=1}^{x} K_{lj}[L_l]}\right). \tag{19}$$

From the above general equation the bound fraction of L_i can be derived as $1 - [L_i]/T_i$. Alternatively, the bound/free ratio can be obtained as $T_i/[L_i] - 1$.

3. PRINCIPLES OF SATURATION ANALYSIS (6–12)

Assume that we have a system where the total analyte (ligand) concentration increases with a fixed antibody concentration. Then: (a) the concentration of bound ligand increases and the fraction of occupied binding sites, B/N, increases. (b) As the binding sites are gradually occupied, the concentration of the remaining unoccupied binding sites, $N - B$, decreases and the ratio B/F decreases (see Eq. (4)) or the ratio F/B increases. (c) The fraction of bound analyte is

$$B/T = (1 + F/B)^{-1}, \tag{20}$$

and decreases as the total ligand concentration increases. When half of the antibody binding sites are occupied, then $B = N/2$, $F = 1/K$ (from Eq. (4)), and Eq. (3) qives:

$$T = N/2 + 1/K. \tag{21}$$

In general, the distribution of an analyte between the bound and free forms (expressed by the ratios B/F, F/B, B/T, or B/N) is quantitatively related to the total analyte concentration. This simple observation forms the principle of immunological assays. Any binder (e.g., receptors, specific binding proteins) can be successfully used for the determination of an analyte–ligand. However, antibodies are the most widely employed binders because of their exceptional specificity. Moreover, antibodies for virtually any analyte can be raised and purified easily, giving stable preparations. On the other hand, receptors and circulating binding proteins can be applied only to a limited number of analytes and their preparations are usually unstable.

Assuming that there is only one class of homogeneous and noninteracting binding sites, we can derive the explicit equations which relate the fraction of bound ligand B/T (a commonly used response variable in immunoassay) to the total ligand concentration T as follows. If we designate by y the B/T ratio, then $B = yT$ and $F = T(1 - y)$. Substituting B and F in Eq. (2) gives

$$T = \frac{N}{y} - \frac{1}{K(1 - y)}, \tag{22}$$

and after rearrangement yields

$$TKy^2 - (TK + NK + 1)y + NK = 0. \tag{23}$$

Similarily, if $R = B/F$ then Eq. (24) holds:

$$R^2 + (TK - NK + 1) R - NK = 0. \tag{24}$$

Alternatively, from Eq. (7) (for $i = 1$) we have:

$$R = \frac{B}{F} = \frac{NK}{1 + KF}. \tag{25}$$

Substituting F with $T/(1 + R)$ in Eq. (25) gives (7):

$$R = \frac{N}{1/K + T/(1 + R)}. \tag{26}$$

Equation (26) is another form of Eq. (24) which becomes useful in the case of equilibria involving binding of an antigen to a heterogeneous antibody population. In this case, substitution of F in the general Eq. (8) yields:

$$R = \sum_{i=1}^{m} \frac{N_i}{1/K_i + T/(1 + R)}. \tag{27}$$

A constant term, which accounts for the nonspecific binding, may be added to the above equation (same as in Eq. (6)).

The distribution of the analyte between the bound and free forms can be monitored by adding a fixed, known concentration of radioactive analyte (tracer) in the reaction mixture, followed by separation of the bound from the free analyte and measurement of the radioactivity of the bound fraction. Analytes (or antibodies) labeled with radioisotopes were used as tracers at the first stages of immunoassay development. Nevertheless, the tracer can be labeled with an enzyme, a fluorescent, or chemiluminescent molecule, leading to the development of nonisotopic immunoassays. Moreover, sometimes the physicochemical properties of the tracer (e.g., fluorescence polarization) change upon its binding to antibody, thus allowing for a direct monitoring of the bound to total (or bound to free) ratio without prior separation of the bound from the free fraction (homogeneous immunoassays). In immunoassay literature, the total unlabeled analyte concentration is usually referred as "dose," the experimentally monitored quantity (or a transformation of it) is called "response," and the assay calibration curve is referred as a "dose–response" curve.

In a system containing analyte L, labeled analyte L*, and a homogeneous population of antibody binding sites s, the following reactions take place:

$$L + s \underset{k_2}{\overset{k_1}{\rightleftharpoons}} Ls \tag{28}$$

$$L* + s \underset{k_2^*}{\overset{k_1^*}{\rightleftharpoons}} L*s, \tag{29}$$

where k_1, k_1^* are the association rate constants and k_2, k_2^* the dissociation rate constants for the analyte and the tracer, respectively. If B^* and F^* are the concentrations of bound and free labeled analyte, respectively, then the concentration of unoccupied binding sites is $(N - B - B^*)$. The equilibrium constants K and K^* for Reactions (28) and (29) are defined by the equations:

$$K = \frac{B}{F(N - B - B*)} \tag{30}$$

$$K* = \frac{B*}{F*(N - B - B*)}. \tag{31}$$

By dividing Eq. (30) by Eq. (31), the B^*/F^* ratio can be obtained:

$$\frac{B*}{F*} = \frac{K*}{K}\frac{B}{F} \tag{32}$$

From Eq. (32) it follows that if labeled and unlabeled analyte have identical binding properties ($K = K^*$) then

$$R = \frac{B*}{F*} = \frac{B}{F} \quad \text{and} \quad y = \frac{B*}{T*} = \frac{B}{T}, \tag{33}$$

and from Eq. (22) the total analyte concentration can be obtained as

$$T = \frac{N}{y} - \frac{1}{K(1 - y)} - T*, \tag{34}$$

where T^* is the total labeled analyte concentration. If K^* is different than K, then a general expression can be formulated which relates y or R with T and T^* as follows:

$$B* = yT* \tag{35}$$

$$F* = (1 - y)T* \tag{36}$$

and

$$\frac{B^*}{F^*} = \frac{y}{1 - y}.$$

(37)

By combining Eqs. (32) and (37) we can obtain B as:

$$B = \frac{KyT}{K^*(1 - y) + Ky}.$$

(38)

After substituting B from Eq. (38) into Eq. (31) and performing the algebraic calculations we have:

$$T^*K^*y^2 - (T^*K^* + NK^* + 1)y + NK^* - \frac{TK^*Ky(1 - y)}{K^*(1 - y) + Ky} = 0,$$

(39)

and similarly,

$$R^2 + (T^*K^* - NK^* + 1)R - NK^* + \frac{TK^*KR(1 + R)}{K^* + KR} = 0.$$

(40)

When $K^* = K$, Eqs. (39) and (40) become identical to Eqs. (23) and (24), respectively. These equations essentially describe the dose–response curves in labeled-analyte (competitive) immunoassays. In these assays, the higher the concentration of analyte in the sample, the lower the B^*/T^* ratio.

In Fig. 3.4, simulated plots of the bound analyte fraction as a function of T, at two antibody concentrations (2×10^{-8} and $2 \times 10^{-7} M$), are shown. The theoretically predicted decrease of B/T with increasing analyte concentrations can be observed. As the antibody concentration increases the curve is shifted to higher B/T values, because a higher bound analyte concentration corresponds to each T value.

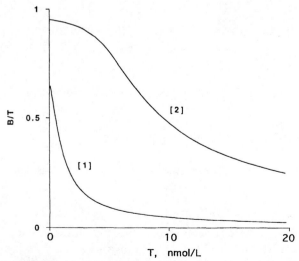

FIGURE 3.4 Plots of the bound/total analyte ratio with respect to the total analyte concentration, at two different concentrations of antibody binding sites: [1] $N = 2 \times 10^{-8} M$, [2] $N = 2 \times 10^{-7} M$.

Figure 3.5 presents simulated B/T vs T plots, where four different antibodies are employed. The concentration of antibody binding sites is fixed at $N = 2 \times 10^{-8}\,M$, but the affinity constants vary. In curve 1, an antibody with an infinitely high affinity constant is used and the binding reaction is irreversible. In this case, when $T \leq N$ all the analyte is bound to the antibody and $F = 0$, $B = T$, and $B/T = 1$. In consequence, this system cannot be used for the determination of analyte concentrations in the range from zero to N because the response B/T does not change with the dose in this range. When $T > N$, the antibody is saturated, $B = N =$ constant, and $B/T = N/T$, i.e., the response becomes inversely proportional to the dose and the system is now analytically useful. In curves 2, 3, and 4 the antibody affinity constants are 3.5×10^8, 6×10^7, and 2×10^7, respectively. Because in these curves the binding reaction is reversible, there is always a free analyte fraction, even when $T \leq N$. Therefore, $F > 0$, $B < T$, and $B/T < 1$, with B/T decreasing as T increases in the entire T range. As K decreases, the curve is shifted to the lower B/T values because a lower bound analyte concentration corresponds to each T.

The slope at any point indicates the expected change in the response caused by an infinitesimal increase in T at that point. The initial ($T = 0$) slope of the B/T vs T plot is an indicator of the detectability of the system. A steeper curve gives a lower detection limit, provided that the variance of the response remains unchanged (see last part of this chapter on detection limit). It can be seen in Fig. 3.5 that a high-affinity antibody gives a better curve (e.g., curve 2 vs 3 or 4) in terms of the overall change in response for the entire concentration range. However the initial slope is zero in curve 1, increases gradually in curves 2 and 3 (curve 3 has a higher initial slope), and then decreases rapidly (curve 4) as K becomes lower. Assume that we add a concentration T^* of a tracer which has identical binding properties with the analyte. Then, the shape of the response curve does not change, but for every T the observed B/T (B^*/T^*) is the one which corresponds to $T + T^*$ (the

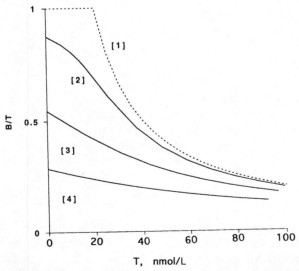

FIGURE 3.5   Graphical presentation of the bound/total analyte ratio vs total analyte concentration at a fixed concentration of binding sites ($N = 2 \times 10^{-8}\,M$) and different affinity constants: [1] K is infinitely high, [2] $K = 3.5 \times 10^8$, [3] $K = 6 \times 10^7$, [4] $K = 2 \times 10^7\,M^{-1}$.

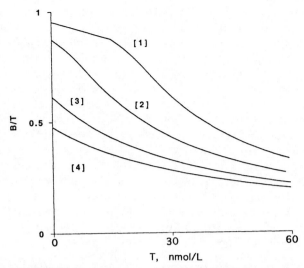

FIGURE 3.6 Plots of the bound/total analyte ratio vs total unlabeled analyte concentration at a fixed level of homogeneous binding sites ($N = 2 \times 10^{-8} M$, $K = 10^9 M^{-1}$) in the presence of varying concentrations of labeled ligand: [1] $T^* = 0$, [2] $T^* = 1.5 \times 10^{-8}$, [3] $T^* = 3 \times 10^{-8}$, [4] $T^* = 4 \times 10^{-8} M$.

real total concentration in the system). This is equivalent to a parallel shift of the vertical axis to the right by T^*. Thus, the B/T ratio and the initial slope at zero dose can be adjusted by changing T^*. For example if T^* is adjusted properly, then the low slope region at the beginning of curve 2 can be avoided. On the other hand, if T^* is too high, the initial slopes become very small. In Fig. 3.6 the effect of low and high T^* on B/T vs T plots is shown. The same antibody ($K = 10^9 M^{-1}$ and $N = 2 \times 10^{-8}$) is employed for all curves.

4. KINETICS OF IMMUNOASSAY (13, 14)

Study of the kinetics of an immunoassay system allows the derivation of equations which predict the concentrations of reactants and products at any time, even if the system has not yet reached equilibrium. The rate of the reaction between a ligand and a homogeneous population of identical binding sites (Eq. (28)) corresponds to the difference between the rates of immunocomplex formation and dissociation,

$$\frac{d[sL]}{dt} = k_1[s][L] - k_2[sL], \qquad (41)$$

where k_1 and k_2 are the association and dissociation rate constants, respectively, and t is the time. Figure 3.7 shows the time course of a binding reaction. Time 0 is when the antibody is mixed with the ligand. A plateau is reached at equilibrium. The reaction rate increases with increasing ligand concentration. The slope of the curve at $t = 0$ gives the initial reaction rate, v_0. At the beginning of the reaction [sL] is negligible and, practically, [s] = N and [L] = T. Thus, from Eq. (41) we have:

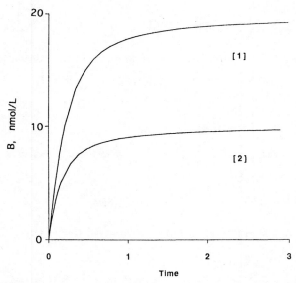

FIGURE 3.7   Time course of the binding reaction between an analyte and a homogeneous population of antibody binding sites: [1] high and [2] low total analyte concentration.

$$v_0 = k_1 NT \text{ and } k_1 = v_0/(NT). \tag{42}$$

Equation 42 gives an estimate of the association rate constant. Because this method utilizes only the initial part of the curve, it may introduce large errors in the estimated k_1 value. A more generalized and accurate approach is given later in this section. k_1 values are usually in the range of 10^7–10^8 M^{-1} sec^{-1}.

The dissociation reaction can be followed if the ligand is first allowed to react with the antibody until equilibrium is reached. Then the free ligand is removed (e.g., by washing the solid phase or by using an adsorbent) and the bound ligand concentration is measured as a function of time. An exponential decay curve can be obtained according to the equation

$$[sL] = [sL]_0 e^{-k_2 t}, \tag{43}$$

where $[sL]_0$ represents the bound ligand concentration at time 0. Taking the natural logarithms of both sides of Eq. (43) gives:

$$\ln[sL] = \ln[sL]_0 - k_2 t. \tag{44}$$

Therefore, $\ln[sL]$ is linearly related to the time and the dissociation constant k_2 is equal to the slope. The half-life ($t_{1/2}$) of the ligand–antibody complex can be obtained from Eq. (44) when $[sL]$ becomes equal to $[sL]_0/2$:

$$t_{1/2} = 0.693/k_2. \tag{45}$$

In the presence of a labeled ligand, Reactions (28) and (29) take place. We can designate by q the sum of bound analyte and tracer:

$$q = [sL] + [sL^*]. \tag{46}$$

If we assume that the analyte and tracer react with identical rate constants then the following differential equation can be written:

$$\frac{dq}{dt} = k_1[s]([L] + [L^*]) - k_2([sL] + [sL^*]). \tag{47}$$

The mass conservation equations for the antibody, analyte and tracer are as follows:

$$N = [s] + [sL] + [sL^*] \tag{48}$$

$$T = [L] + [sL] \tag{49}$$

$$T^* = [L^*] + [sL^*]. \tag{50}$$

Therefore, $[s] = N - q$ and $[L] + [L^*] = T + T^* - q$. Substituting these values in Eq. (47) gives

$$\frac{dq}{dt} = k_1(N - q)(T + T^* - q) - k_2 q, \tag{51}$$

which, after performing the calculations, obtains the general form (13)

$$\frac{dq}{dt} = fq^2 - gq + h, \tag{52}$$

where

$$f = k_1, \tag{53}$$

$$g = k_1(N + T + T^* + 1/K), \tag{54}$$

$$h = k_1 N (T + T^*), \tag{55}$$

and K is the equilibrium constant. The analytical solution of Eq. (52) is given by Eq. (56) (see Ref. 13),

$$q = \frac{q_1\left(\dfrac{q_2 - q_0}{q_1 - q_0}\right) - q_2 e^{-(q_2 - q_1)t}}{\left(\dfrac{q_2 - q_0}{q_1 - q_0}\right) - e^{-(q_2 - q_1)t}}, \tag{56}$$

where

$$q_1 = (g - \sqrt{g^2 - 4fh})/(2f), \tag{57}$$

$$q_2 = (g + \sqrt{g^2 - 4fh})/(2f), \tag{58}$$

and q_0 is the value of q at $t = 0$. Equation (56) is general and can be used for the nonlinear least squares fitting of association and dissociation curves simultaneously, for a more accurate description of the system.

If the analyte and the tracer are not added simultaneously in the reaction mixture, then the following equation (13, 14) describes the change of the bound tracer concentration with time:

$$\frac{dB^*}{dt} = k_1 (N - q)(T^* - B^*) - k_2 B^*. \tag{59}$$

The q value can be calculated from Eq. (56). The solution of Eq. (59) gives the bound tracer concentration in the reaction mixture at any time and includes the cases where analyte and tracer are not added simultaneously (13).

$$B^* = \frac{T^*q}{T^* + T} + \left[B_0^* - \left(\frac{T^*q_0}{T^* + T} \right) \right] \left(\frac{q_2 - q}{q_2 - q_0} \right) e^{-(k_1 N + k_2 - f q_1)t} \qquad (60)$$

Figure 3.8 demonstrates how the order in which reagents are added affects the dose (T)–response (B^*/T^*) curves. The curves are based on simulated data and the use of Eqs. (56) and (60). In curve 1, the analyte, tracer, and anibody are added simulataneously at Time 0. The system is not allowed to reach equilibrium and the response is measured at $t = t_1$. In this case, the bound tracer and analyte concentrations at Time 0 are zero, that is, $q_0 = B_0^* = 0$. In curve 2, the analyte is first incubated with the antibody until equilibrium is reached. Then, the tracer is added (at Time 0) and the response is measured at $t = t_1$. In this case, $B_0^* = 0$ and q_0 is equal to the bound analyte concentration derived by solving Eq. (23) with respect to y and then multiplying by T. Curve 2 has a greater slope than curve 1, thus leading to the conclusion that a delayed addition of the tracer results in higher sensitivity (13, 14). In curve 3, the tracer is first incubated with the antibody until equilibrium is reached. Then the analyte is added (at Time 0) and the response is measured at $t = t_1$. In this case, $q_0 = B_0^*$ and their value can be calculated from Eq. (23). It can be seen (curve 3) that a delayed addition of the analyte results in a lower sensitivity. At equilibrium (i.e., if t_1 is long enough), curves 1, 2, and 3 coincide.

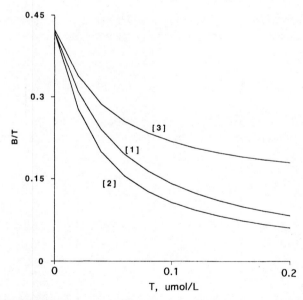

FIGURE 3.8 Simulated data showing the effect of the order in which the reagents are added on the dose–response curves. All the variables are given in arbitrary units. $k_1 = 10^8$, $k_2 = 1$, $T^* = 3 \times 10^{-8}$, $N = 2 \times 10^{-8}$, and $t_1 = 1.2$. Curve 1: Simultaneous addition of the tracer, analyte, and antibody at Time 0. Curve 2: The analyte is first incubated with the antibody until equilibrium is reached, then the tracer is added at Time 0. Curve 3: The tracer is first incubated with the antibody until equilibrium is reached, then the analyte is added at Time 0. In all cases, the response is measured at Time t_1.

5. THE THEORY OF TWO-SITE IMMUNOASSAYS (15–18)

A typical two-site (sandwich) immunoassay consists of the following steps:

(a) The capture antibody is immobilized on a solid phase (e.g., microtitration wells, test tubes, beads).

(b) The standard or sample is incubated with the solid-phase antibody, giving:

$$s_1 + L \underset{k_2}{\overset{k_1}{\leftrightarrow}} s_1L, \tag{61}$$

where s_1 represents the binding sites of the capture antibody and k_1 and k_2 are the association and dissociation rate constants, respectively.

(c) The solid phase is washed to remove the unbound analyte.

(d) A labeled antibody (detection antibody) is incubated with the solid phase. This antibody binds to a different antigenic site on the analyte molecule, giving

$$s_1L + s_2^* \underset{k_4}{\overset{k_3}{\leftrightarrow}} s_1Ls_2^*, \tag{62}$$

where s_2^* represents the binding sites of the labeled antibody and k_3, k_4 are the rate constants.

(e) The solid phase is washed to remove unbound labeled antibody.

(f) The labeled antibody bound to the solid phase ($s_1Ls_2^*$) is measured.

During the second incubation, there is always a degree of dissociation of the s_1L complex. The analyte released may subsequently react with the labeled antibody as follows:

$$L + s_2^* \underset{k_6}{\overset{k_5}{\leftrightarrow}} Ls_2^*. \tag{63}$$

The complex formed will be removed with the final wash, thus decreasing the observed signal. Alternatively, this complex may bind to the capture antibody as follows:

$$s_1 + Ls_2^* \underset{k_8}{\overset{k_7}{\leftrightarrow}} s_1Ls_2^*. \tag{64}$$

The relative magnitude of the rate constants k_5, k_6, k_7, and k_8 as well as the reactant concentrations determine which reaction will prevail at any time.

5.1. Kinetic Model

The rate of $s_1Ls_2^*$ production, at any time, is given by the difference between the rates of its formation and dissociation. Therefore, from Reactions (62) and (64) we have:

$$\frac{d[s_1Ls_2^*]}{dt} = k_3[s_1L][s_2^*] + k_7[s_1][Ls_2^*] - (k_4 + k_8)[s_1Ls_2^*]. \tag{65}$$

Similarly, from Reactions (61) and (62),

$$\frac{d[s_1L]}{dt} = k_1[s_1][L] + k_4[s_1Ls_2^*] - k_2[s_1L] - k_3[s_1L][s_2^*], \tag{66}$$

and from Reactions (63) and (64),

$$\frac{d[Ls_2^*]}{dt} = k_5[L][s_2^*] + k_8[s_1Ls_2^*] - k_6[Ls_2^*] - k_7[s_1][Ls_2^*]. \tag{67}$$

The concentrations refer to the species present in the reaction mixture at any moment. Applying the mass conservation law for the analyte and antibodies yields

$$T = [L] + [s_1L] + [Ls_2^*] + [s_1Ls_2^*] \tag{68}$$

$$N_1 = [s_1] + [s_1L] + [s_1Ls_2^*] \tag{69}$$

$$N_2 = [s_2^*] + [Ls_2^*] + [s_1Ls_2^*], \tag{70}$$

where N_1 and N_2 represent the total concentrations of binding sites of the capture and the detection antibody, respectively. Equations (65) to (70) represent a system of six equations with six unknowns. It can be solved numerically (15) and gives the composition of the assay mixture at any time.

The incubation time for the reaction between analyte and capture antibody (step b) should be long enough to reach equilibrium, otherwise the assay presents decreased slope, precision, and sensitivity. The ratio R of bound/free analyte at equilibrium is given by Eq. (71),

$$R^2 + R(1 + K_1T - K_1N_1) - K_1N_1 = 0, \tag{71}$$

where $K_1 = k_1/k_2$. Then, the concentration of bound analyte, B_1, before the washing step is

$$B_1 = \frac{R}{1 + R} T. \tag{72}$$

If the washing in step (c) is perfect (complete removal of free analyte without dissociation of the immunocomplex), then the initial concentration of bound analyte before the addition of detection antibody is $[s_1L]_0 = B_1$. The initial concentration of unoccupied capture antibody binding sites is $[s_1]_0 = N_1 - B_1$.

5.2. Equilibrium Model

The equilibrium model assumes that both Reactions (61) and (62) reach equilibrium. Furthermore, the model is simplified by assuming that there is no dissociation of the immunocomplexes during incubation. We designate $[s_1L]$ by B_1 and $[s_1Ls_2^*]$ by B_2. Also, $K_1 = k_1/k_2$ and $K_2 = k_3/k_4$ represent the affinity constants for the binding reactions of Eqs. (61) and (62), respectively. The following equation gives the concentration of analyte bound to the capture antibody after the first incubation,

$$B_1 = \frac{N_1K_1(T - B_1)}{1 + K_1(T - B_1)}, \tag{73}$$

where $(T_1 - B_1)$ corresponds to the concentration of unbound analyte. Equation (73) is identical to Eq. (5) (without the term accounting for the nonspecific binding). After a washing step, the detection antibody is allowed to react with the analyte. A similar equation can be written for this step,

$$B_2 = \frac{B_1 K_2 (N_2 - B_2)}{1 + K_2 (N_2 - B_2)} + n(N_2 - B_2), \tag{74}$$

where $(N_2 - B_2)$ represents the free labeled antibody concentration. The second term of this equation accounts for the nonspecific binding of the labeled antibody (18).

The dose–response curve in the two-site immunometric assay is sigmoidal, and the signal increases with the analyte concentration. A plateau is reached when the capture antibody becomes saturated. In some assays the dose–response curve shows the "high dose hook effect"; that is, the signal initially increases with the analyte concentration, reaches a peak, and subsequently decreases as the concentration becomes higher. In consequence, two samples, one with low analyte concentration and one with high analyte concentration, may give the same response value. This undesirable phenomenon has been attributed (16) to either a heterogeneity of the capture antibody or an inefficiency of the first washing step (step c above).

According to the first mechanism, the capture antibody is a heterogeneous population consisting of a low concentration of high-affinity binding sites and a high concentration of low-affinity binding sites. At high analyte levels a large percentage of the low-affinity binding sites are occupied. These relatively weak immunocomplexes have high dissociation rate constants and dissociate rapidly during the subsequent incubation with the detection antibody. The free analyte released reacts with the detection antibody, thus interfering with its binding to the solid-phase analyte. In this case the high-dose hook effect can be eliminated by increasing the concentration of the detection antibody.

According to the second mechanism, an inefficient washing step results in incomplete removal of the analyte from the reaction tube. The remaining analyte can react with the detection antibody and block its binding to the solid phase analyte (16). In this case, the extent of the hook effect depends on the initial concentration of the analyte, the percentage of the analyte left in the reaction tube after the first washing, and the concentration of the detection antibody.

6. GRAPHICAL PRESENTATATION OF IMMUNOASSAY DATA (12, 19)

Described in this section are the theoretical basis and the assumptions underlying the various techniques used for graphical presentation of immunoassay data. Some of the most widely used linearization methods for dose–response curves are presented.

Assume that the antibody is saturated (i.e., K is infinitely high and $T^* > N$). Then:

$$B + B^* = N. \tag{75}$$

Under this condition we have

$$y = \frac{B^*}{T^*} = \frac{B}{T} = \frac{B + B^*}{T + T^*} = \frac{N}{T + T^*}, \tag{76}$$

and the curve $y = f(T)$ is a hyperbola. Equation (76) gives:

$$\frac{1}{y} = \frac{T^*}{B^*} = \frac{T^*}{N} + \frac{T}{N}. \tag{77}$$

Equation (77) is also derived from Eq. (34) for an infinitely high K (the second term becomes equal to zero). When $T = 0$ (zero dose) then $B = 0$ and because $T^* > N$, we have $B_o^* = N$ and $y_o = N/T^*$, where B_o^* and y_o are the values of B^* and y at zero dose. Thus, Eq. (77) can be written as

$$\frac{1}{y} = \frac{1}{y_o} + \frac{T}{N}, \tag{78}$$

i.e., $1/y$ is a linear function with respect to the total analyte concentration. Dividing both sides of Eq. (77) by T^* yields:

$$\frac{1}{B^*} = \frac{1}{B_o^*} + \frac{T}{NT^*}. \tag{79}$$

Multiplying both sides of Eq. (79) by B_o^* gives:

$$\frac{B_o^*}{B^*} = 1 + \frac{T}{T^*}. \tag{80}$$

Substituting T^*/B^* with $(F^*/B + 1)$ into Eq. (77) and rearranging yields

$$\frac{F^*}{B^*} = \frac{F_o^*}{B_o^*} + \frac{T}{N}, \tag{81}$$

where F_o^* is the concentration of free tracer at zero dose ($F_o^* = T^* - N$). Multiplying both sides of Eq. (78) by y_o yields:

$$\frac{y_o}{y} = 1 + \frac{T}{T^*}. \tag{82}$$

Dividing both sides of Eq. (81) by F_o^*/B_o^* yields:

$$\frac{F^* B_o^*}{F_o^* B^*} = 1 + \frac{T}{F_o^*}. \tag{83}$$

Furthermore, Eqs. (80), (82), and (83) can be written in the general form

$$\frac{1}{r} = 1 + \frac{T}{c}, \tag{84}$$

where r is B^*/B_o^*, y/y_o, or $(B^*/F_o^*)/(B_o^*/F_o^*)$, and c is T^*, T^*, or F_o^*, respectively. Rearrangement of Eq. (84) gives

$$\frac{1 - r}{r} = \frac{T}{c}, \tag{85}$$

and taking the natural logarithms of both sides yields:

$$\ln \frac{r}{1 - r} = -\ln \frac{T}{c} \tag{86}$$

Because logit $r = \ln \dfrac{r}{1 - r}$, we have:

$$\text{logit } r = \ln c - \ln T. \tag{87}$$

The plot of logit r vs $\ln T$ is linear with a slope of -1. The logit transformation is probably the most widely used method for the graphical presentation of immunoassay data. Application of the logit transformation requires that B_o^* be known exactly, because it is required for the calculation of the ordinate values.

In conclusion, the plots $1/y$ vs T (Eq. (78)), $1/B^*$ vs T (Eq. (79)), B_o^*/B^* vs T (Eq. (80)), F^*/B^* vs T (Eq. (81)), y_o/y vs T (Eq. (82)), $(B^*/F^*)/(B_o^*/F_o^*)$ vs T (Eq. (83)), as well as the plot of logit r vs ln T (Eq. (87)) are linear, provided that the antibody is saturated (K is infinitely high and $T^* > N$). All of these plots have been used frequently for the graphical presentation of immunoassay dose–response curves. From the above equations, it can be seen that all of the plots are based on the same assumptions.

The corrected bound and total concentrations of the tracer, $(B^* - n)$, $(B_o^* - n)$, and $(T^* - n)$ (where n = nonspecific binding) must be used instead of B^*, B_o^*, and T^*, respectively, in all the expressions of the response variables. The nonspecific binding n represents the concentration of bound tracer in the absence of antibody or in the presence of a large excess of unlabeled analyte.

Because K is never infinitely high, there is always a degree of dissociation of the immunocomplex (existence of free unoccupied binding sites) which becomes significant at low concentrations of analyte. In this case, $B + B^* < N$ and y has a lower value than that expected from Eq. (76). In consequence, the plots described above deviate from linearity as the analyte concentration decreases.

7. CURVE FITTING OF IMMUNOASSAY DATA (20–27)

7.1. Model Based on the Mass-Action Law

This model is based on the quantitative description of the binding equilibria as it was presented in the beginning of this chapter. The model is theoretically sound and very useful in gaining insight into the behavior of the assay system. However, there are difficulties associated with its application which have resulted in the broad use of rather empirical models for fitting to the calibration data and calculating the concentrations of unknowns.

In a simple case involving one class of identical, independent, and noninteracting binding sites, the mass-action law model contains two parameters (K and N of Eq. (4)). Because the nonspecific binding of the tracer to reaction tubes is inevitable in every immunoassay, an additional parameter is incorporated to accommodate for the nonspecific binding (Eq. (5)). Moreover, in many immunoassay systems there is a heterogeneity of binding sites which calls for employment of the multiple binding site (Eq. (8)). The model with two classes of binding sites and nonspecific binding contains five parameters (K_1, K_2, N_1, N_2, and n; see Eq. (12)). Nonlinear least squares fitting of this model to experimental data converges slowly. In addition, the model requires accurate estimation of the concentration of labeled analyte and may fail when labeled and unlabeled analytes do not have the same affinities for the antibody, when the system was not allowed to reach equilibrium, or when the method used to separate bound and free analyte disturbs the chemical equilibrium. Attempts to accommodate for these effects result in very complicated models with too many parameters, which are not suitable for routine use.

7.2. **Linear Models**

In the previous section, it was shown that the variables y^{-1}, $(B^*)^{-1}$, $(B^*/B_o^*)^{-1}$, $(B^*/F^*)^{-1}$, and $[(B^*/F^*)/(B_o^*/F_o^*)]^{-1}$ are linear functions of T (Eqs. (78)–(83)) and that the logit r [where r is B^*/B_o^*, y/y_o, or $(B^*/F)/(B_o^*/F_o^*)$] is linearly related to ln T (Eq. (87)). All these relations rely on the assumption that the assay operates with an antibody which is 100% saturated by the tracer. Under these conditions, the equations are valid and linear regression analysis can be applied. However, a weighted linear least squares regression should be performed. This is because the inversion of variables introduces severe nonuniformity of variance. For instance, if the response variable is $y = B^*/T^*$ with a variance of $Var(y)$, then the variance of $1/y$ is (from the error propagation law):

$$Var\left(\frac{1}{y}\right) = \frac{1}{y^4}\,Var(y). \tag{88}$$

This means that in the $1/y$ vs T plot, the points corresponding to high analyte concentrations (low y values) have a large scatter which may affect the calculated regression parameters. Therefore, an appropriate weight, w_i, should be assigned to each $1/y_i$ value such that:

$$w_i = \frac{1}{Var\left(\dfrac{1}{y_i}\right)} = \frac{y_i^4}{Var(y_i)}. \tag{89}$$

The logit transformation also introduces a nonuniformity of variance. The variance of logit r, $Var(logit\ r)$, can be calculated by the following equation:

$$Var(logit\ r) = \frac{Var(r)}{r^2(1 - r)^2}. \tag{90}$$

In the next section, it will be shown that even the untransformed response variables present nonuniformity of variance, so that weighting is necessary in all cases.

The logit transformation is probably the most widely used linear model in immunoassay. This is because it linearizes the dose–response curves in some cases where the other linearization methods are unsatisfactory. These cases are described by Eq. (91):

$$\frac{1}{r} = 1 + \frac{T^b}{c}. \tag{91}$$

When $b = 1$, Eq. (91) becomes identical to Eq. (84). Logit transformation of Eq. (91) gives:

$$logit\ r = \ln c - b \ln T. \tag{92}$$

Equation (92) constitutes the generalized logit transformation. Although Eq. (91) is empirical it can successfully fit to the data in situations where some heterogeneity of binding sites exists. In these cases, Eq. (92) is still linear with a slope of b (different than unity), whereas Eqs. (78)–(83) deviate from linearity.

The log–logit transformation and the other linearization models fail to describe immunoassays with severe heterogeneity, allosteric effects, etc.

7.3. The Logistic Model

The four-parameter logistic model is given by the equation

$$Y = d + \frac{a - d}{1 + \left(\dfrac{T}{c}\right)^b},$$
(93)

where Y can be B^*, F^*, B^*/T^*, B^*/F^*, F^*/T^*, B^*/B_o^*, y/y_o. In this model, the values B^*, T^*, and B_o^* are used without correcting for the nonspecific binding. The parameter a represents the expected response Y at zero analyte concentration. The parameter b corresponds to the slope of the log–logit model. The parameter c corresponds to the analyte concentration, which gives $Y = (a + d)/2$, i.e., it determines the center of the curve. The parameter d corresponds to the expected response Y when T is infinitely high, i.e., represents the nonspecific binding n. In contrast to the log–logit model, which requires good estimates of both the response at zero dose and the nonspecific binding, the logistic model incorporates these quantities as parameters a and d, respectively, which are allowed to take values that ensure the best fit to the data.

Figures 3.9 and 3.10 present simulated y ($y = B^*/T^*$) vs log T plots based on the logistic model. It can be seen that, by changing the values of the parameters a and d, curves corresponding to a labeled analyte immunoassay (Fig. 3.9) or to a two-site immunometric assay (Fig. 3.10) are obtained.

The parameter b gives the slope of the Y vs ln T plot at its center. Indeed,

$$\text{slope} = \frac{dY}{d \ln T} = -\frac{b(a - d)}{[1 + (T/c)^b]^2} \left(\frac{T}{c}\right)^b.$$
(94)

When $T = c$, then slope $= -b(a - d)/4$, i.e., it is proportional to b. The following

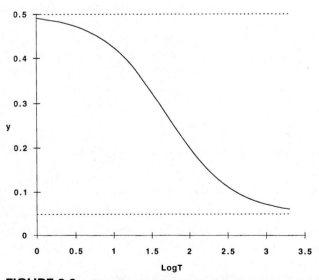

FIGURE 3.9 Graphical presentation of the logistic model for a labeled-analyte (competitive) immunoassay. $y = B^*/T^*$, $a = 0.5$, $b = 1$, $c = 50$, and $d = 0.05$. All the parameters are expressed in arbitrary units. The broken lines correspond to the values of the parameters a and d.

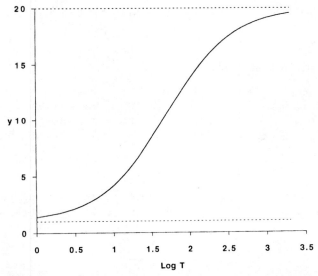

FIGURE 3.10   Graphical presentation of the logistic model for a "two-site" immunoassay; y represents the signal from the bound detection antibody, $a = 1$, $b = 1$, $c = 50$, and $d = 20$. All the parameters are expressed in arbitrary units. The broken lines correspond to the values of the parameters a and d.

equations show the relation between the logistic and the log–logit models. Rearrangement of Eq. (93) gives:

$$\frac{a - d}{Y - d} = 1 + \left(\frac{T}{c}\right)^{b}. \tag{95}$$

Equation (95) can be written as

$$\frac{1}{r} = 1 + \left(\frac{T}{c}\right)^{b}, \tag{96}$$

where $r = (Y - d)/(a - d)$. If $Y = B^*$ then r represents the B^*/B_o^* ratio corrected for the nonspecific binding. Equation (96) is a more general form of Eqs. (84) and (91). Logit transformation of Eq. (96) yields:

$$\text{logit } r = b \ln c - b \ln T. \tag{97}$$

Therefore, the parameter b of the logistic model corresponds to the slope of the log–logit curve and the parameter c corresponds to the analyte concentration which gives logit $r = 0$, i.e., $r = 0.5$. Indeed, if $Y = (a + d)/2$ then $r = 0.5$. Essentially c represents the x-axis intercept of the log–logit plot. The logistic model is considered to be the most useful and versatile one for fitting to dose–response (calibration) data in immunoassay (23). It can be used successfully in the labeled analyte immunoassay and in the two-site immunometric assay. However, a nonlinear least squares fitting is required for parameter estimation. The Gauss–Newton algorithm, as modified by Marquardt, performs well in fitting the model. The original (untransformed) raw data, i.e., signal vs total analyte concentration T, should be used as the dependent and independent variables, respectively. Initial estimates of the model parameters are required as starting points. Guess values for b and c can be obtained by using the log–logit plot.

7.4. Nonuniformity of Variance and Weighting

The model parameters and the analyte concentration T determine each time the expected (calculated) response variable Y_c. Because of the random errors that unequivocally accompany every analytical measurement, the observed Y differs from the theoretically calculated one (even if the model is correct) and the following equation holds,

$$Y_i = (Y_c)_i + e_i \tag{98}$$

where e_i is the experimental error associated with the ith measurement. The most probable values of the parameters are those that minimize the sum of the squares of residuals,

$$Q = \sum_{i=1}^{l} w_i[Y_i - (Y_c)_i]^2 = \sum_{i=1}^{l} w_i e_i^2, \tag{99}$$

where l is the number of standards used and w_i the statistical weight accompanying the ith measurement, $w_i = 1/\mathrm{Var}(Y_c)_i$. The function Q is minimized when its partial derivatives with respect to the parameters P become zero, i.e.,

$$\frac{\partial Q}{\partial P_j} = 0 \qquad \text{for } j = 1,2 \ldots , k, \tag{100}$$

where k is the number of the parameters depending on the model. Calculating the partial derivatives from Eq. (99) and introducing them in Eq. (100) gives:

$$\frac{\partial Q}{\partial P_j} = -2 \sum_{i=1}^{l} \frac{w_i e_i \partial (Y_c)_i}{\partial P_j} = 0 \qquad \text{for } j = 1,2 \ldots , k. \tag{101}$$

Relationship (101) is in fact a system of k equations with k unknowns. Solution of this system gives the parameter values which can be used subsequently in estimating the analyte concentration of the unknowns based on the observed responses and the model equation. It is also clear from the above equations that in order to derive statistically correct estimations of the parameters we must assign an appropriate weight factor to each experimental value of the response variable. This means that we have to know how the errors are distributed around the calibration curve, i.e., the way that $\mathrm{Var}(Y)$ changes with Y_c.

Random errors in immunoassays are due to:

(i) pipetting of standards/samples, tracer, and antibody
(ii) errors in separating or generally distinguishing the bound and free fractions (misclassification errors)
(iii) random variations of reaction time and temperature
(iv) random errors in measuring radioactivity, absorbance, fluorescence, etc.

It has been shown theoretically (21) and experimentally (25) that the response variable generally does not present a uniformity of variance. The response–error relation (RER) describes how variance of the response varies with the mean response level. The following empirical model has been recommended (23, 24),

$$\text{Var}(Y) = a_0 Y_c^J \tag{102}$$

where $J = 0$, 1, or 2. When $J = 0$, $\text{Var}(Y) = a_0 = \text{constant}$; when $J = 1$, $\text{Var}(Y)$ is proportional to the response, and when $J = 2$, the coefficient of variation of the response is constant. J remains constant from batch to batch analysis whereas a_0 changes. Another useful RER model is given by the equation:

$$\text{Var}(Y) = a_0 + a_1 Y + a_2 Y^2. \tag{103}$$

7.5. Spline Functions (26, 27)

While all of the above methods involve fitting of a well-defined model (theoretical or empirical) to the experimental data, smoothing by spline functions represents a different approach to immunoassay data reduction. Here the dose–response curve is first divided in segments. The points where the segments join are called knots. Subsequently, a linear least squares fitting of a cubic polynomial (given by Eq. (104)) to the data in each segment is performed.

$$Y = a_0 + a_1 T + a_2 T^2 + a_3 T^3 \tag{104}$$

Any response variable can be used as Y, whereas T is the independent variable. The parameters a_0, a_1, a_2, and a_3 are varied until the first and second derivatives of the curve segments on their knots are equal. This ensures that the entire curve is smooth.

A significant advantage of this method is that it is not dependent on any model and it does not fail in cases where antibody heterogeneity or allosteric effects are present. The spline function is just the best curve that fits the experimental points. Its precision increases with the number of experimental points. The number and location of the knots affect the performance of the fitting. For example, if there are too many knots, then the curve is forced to pass through every experimental point, including those with high experimental errors.

8. DETECTION LIMIT OF IMMUNOASSAYS (28, 29)

The lowest detectable analyte concentration or detection limit (DL) or sensitivity of an immunoassay is defined as the analyte concentration that gives a response which has a statistically significant difference from the response of the zero analyte sample.

Assume that the zero and the lowest detectable concentrations are analyzed with n_0 and n_1 replicates and give mean response values Y_0, Y_1 and variances s_0^2, s_1^2, respectively. Then $\text{Var}(Y_0) = s_0^2/n_0$, $\text{Var}(Y_1) = s_1^2/n_1$, and

$$\text{Var}(Y_1 - Y_0) = \frac{s_0^2}{n_0} + \frac{s_1^2}{n_1}. \tag{105}$$

We can perform the t test for the difference $Y_1 - Y_0$ (or $Y_0 - Y_1$) as follows (28):

$$t = \frac{Y_1 - Y_0}{\sqrt{(s_0^2/n_0) + (s_1^2/n_1)}}. \tag{106}$$

$(Y_1 - Y_0)$ is statistically different from zero when t is equal to or greater than the value of Student's t distribution for a certain probability level. The one-sided t test should be used because the detection limit cannot be lower than zero. From Eq. (106), the response that corresponds to the detection limit can be obtained:

$$Y_1 = Y_0 + t\sqrt{\frac{s_0^2}{n_0} + \frac{s_1^2}{n_1}}. \tag{107}$$

Furthermore, if we assume that the variances of the responses are constant over the region between Y_0 and Y, then $s_0^2 = s_1^2 = s^2$ and

$$Y_1 = Y_0 + ts\sqrt{\frac{1}{n_0} + \frac{1}{n_1}}. \tag{108}$$

The above relationships are valid only for responses which follow the Gaussian distribution, that is, for raw data (radioactivity, absorbance, fluorescence, chemiluminescence), B/T, B/B_0, or any linear transformation of them. The logit–log transformation distorts the original distributions. The response Y_1 from Eq. (107) or (108) is entered in the dose–response curve and the detection limit (DL) is calculated by interpolation. If the dose–response curve is linear between the zero dose and the detection limit, then

$$DL = \frac{Y_1 - Y_0}{(dY/dT)_0}, \tag{109}$$

where $(dY/dT)_0$ is the initial slope (at $T = 0$) of the dose–response curve. Combining Eqs. (108) and (109) yields:

$$DL = \frac{ts}{(dY/dT)_0}\sqrt{\frac{1}{n_0} + \frac{1}{n_1}}. \tag{110}$$

An important consequence of the above equation is that the detection limit becomes lower as the standard deviation of the response at zero dose decreases and the slope of the dose–response curve, at zero dose, increases. The slope alone is not an index of assay detectability. In some cases by simply transforming the data and changing the coordinate system, we may achieve higher slopes at zero dose but without any improvement in the detection limit because the standard deviation, s, of the response increases proportionally. A higher slope is desirable and gives lower detection limit only if s remains constant.

The factors that determine the ultimate sensitivity (lowest detection limit) of the analyte-labeled (competitive) immunoassays are the antibody affinity constant and the experimental errors, but not the detectability of the tracer (29). It has been calculated theoretically (29) that with $K = 10^{12} M^{-1}$ (the highest possible K for an antigen–antibody interaction) and a 1% coefficient of variation for the response at zero dose, the lowest detection limit possible for a competitive immunoassay would be $10^{-14} M$.

The factors limiting the ultimate sensitivity of two-site immunometric assays are the affinity constant of the antibody, the random experimental error, and the nonspecific binding of the labeled antibody, expressed as a percentage of the total labeled antibody. It has been estimated (see Ref. 29) that with $K = 10^{12} M^{-1}$, a 1% coefficient of variation of the response at zero dose, and a 1% nonspecific binding of the labeled antibody, the detection limit can be as low as $10^{-16} M$, i.e., two orders of magnitude lower than that of the competitive immunoassays. Moreover, the sensitivity of two-site immunometric assays can be increased further by using tracers with higher detectability and lower nonspecific binding. This is not feasible with the analyte-labeled immunoassays.

References

1. Scatchard G. The attraction of proteins for small molecules and ions. Ann NY Acad Sci 1949; 51:660–72.
2. Munson PJ, Rodbard D. Ligand: A versatile computerized approach for characterization of ligand-binding systems. Anal Biochem 1980; 107:220–39.
3. Feldman HA. Mathematical theory of complex ligand-binding systems at equilibrium: some methods of parameter fitting. Anal Biochem 1972; 48:317–38.
4. Rodbard D, Feldman HA. Theory of protein-ligand interaction. Methods Enzymol 1975; 36:3–16.
5. Feldman H, Rodbard D, Levine D. Mathematical theory of cross-reactive radioimmunoassay and ligand-binding systems at equilibrium. Anal Biochem 1972; 45:530–56.
6. Ekins R, Newman B, O'Riordan JLH. Theoretical aspects of 'saturation' and radioimmunoassay. In: Hayes RL, Goswitz FA, Murphy BEP, Eds. Radioisotopes in Medicine: In vitro Studies. Oak Ridge:US Atomic Energy Commission, 1968:59–100.
7. Ekins R, Newman GB, O'Riordan JLH. Saturation assays. In: McArthur JW, Colton T, Eds. Statistics in Endocrinology. Cambridge, MA:The MIT Press, 1970:345–78.
8. Ekins R, Newman B. Theoretical aspects of saturation analysis. In: Diczfalusy E, Diczfalusy A, Eds. Steroid Assay by Protein Binding. Karolinska Symposia on Research Methods in Reproductive Endocrinology. Stockholm:WHO/Karolinska Institut, 1970:11–30.
9. Ekins RP. General principles of hormone assay. In: Loraine JA, Bell I, Eds. Hormone Assays and Their Clinical Applications, IVth ed. Edinburgh:Churchill Livingstone, 1976:1–72.
10. Yalow RS, Berson SA. Introduction and general considerations. In: Odell WD, Daughaday WH, Eds. Principles of competitive protein-binding assays. Philadelphia:JB Lippincott, 1971:1–24.
11. Feldman H, Rodbard D. Mathematical theory of radioimmunoassay. In: Odell WD, Daughaday WH, eds. Principles of competitive protein-binding assays. Philadelphia:JB Lippincott, 1971:158–73.
12. Walker WHC. An approach to immunoassay. Clin Chem 1977; 23:384–402.
13. Rodbard D, Munson PJ, DeLean A. Improved curve-fitting, parallelism testing, characterisation of sensitivity and specificity, validation, and optimization for radioligand assays. In: Radioimmunoassay and Related Procedures in Medicine, Vol. I. Vienna:International Atomic Energy Agency, 1978:469–503.
14. Rodbard D, Ruder HJ, Vaitukaitis J, Jacobs HS. Mathematical analysis of kinetics of radioligand assays: Improved sensitivity obtained by delayed addition of labeled ligand. J Clin Endocrinol 1971; 33:343–55.
15. Rodbard D, Feldman Y. Kinetics of two-site immunoradiometric ("sandwich") assays. I. Immunochemistry 1978; 15:71–6.
16. Rodbard D, Feldman Y, Jaffe ML, Miles LEM. Kinetics of two-site immunoradiometric ("sandwich") assays. II. Immunochemistry 1978; 15:77–82.
17. Rodbard D, Weiss GH. Mathematical theory of immunoradiometric (labeled antibody) assays. Anal Biochem 1973; 52:10–44.
18. Jackson TM, Marshall NJ, Ekins RP. Optimization of immunoradiometric (labeled antibody) assays. In: Hunter WM, Corrie JET, Eds. Immunoassays for Clinical Chemistry, 2nd ed. Edinburg:Churchill Livingstone, 1983:557–75.
19. Rodbard D. Statistical quality control and routine data processing for radioimmunoassays and immunoradiometric assays. Clin Chem 1974; 20:1255–70.
20. Rodbard D, Tacey RL. Radioimmunoassay dose interpolation based on the mass action law with antibody heterogeneity. Anal Biochem 1978; 90:13–21.
21. Rodbard D. Statistical aspects of radioimmunoassays. In: Odell WD, Daughaday WH, Eds. Principles of Competitive Protein-Binding Assays. Philadelphia:JB Lippincott, 1971:204–16.
22. Rodbard D, Hutt DM. Statistical analysis of radioimmunoassays and immunoradiometric (labelled antibody) assays. A generalized weighted, iterative, least-squares method for logistic curve fitting. In: Radioimmunoassay and Related Procedures in Medicine. Vienna:International Atomic Energy Agency, 1974:165–92.

23. Dudley RA, Edwards P, Ekins RP, Finney DJ, McKenzie IGM, Raab GM, Rodbard D, Rodgers RPC. Guidelines for immunoassay data processing. Clin Chem 1985; 31:1264–71.
24. Finney DJ. Response curves for radioimmunoassay. Clin Chem 1983; 29:1762–6.
25. Sadler WA, Smith MH. Estimation of the response-error relationship in immunoassay. Clin Chem 1985; 31:1802–05.
26. Marschner I, Erhardt F, Scriba PC. Calculation of the radioimmunoassay standard curve by spline function. In: Radioimmunoassay and Related Procedures in Medicine. Vienna:International Atomic Energy Agency, 1974:111–21.
27. Malan PG, Cox MG, Long EM, Ekins RP. Curve fitting to radioimmunoassay standard curves: Spline and multiple binding site models. Ann Clin Biochem 1978; 15:132–4.
28. Rodbard D. Statistical estimation of the minimal detectable concentration ("sensitivity") for radioligand assays. Anal Biochem 1978; 90:1–12.
29. Jackson TM, Ekins RP. Theoretical limitations on immunoassay sensitivity. J Immunol Methods 1986; 87:13–20.

4 | DATA INTERPRETATION AND QUALITY CONTROL

H. EDWARD GROTJAN
Animal Science Department
University of Nebraska
Lincoln, Nebraska

BROOKS A. KEEL
Department of Obstetrics and
Gynecology
University of Kansas School of Medicine
Director, Womens Research Institute
Wichita, Kansas

1. INTRODUCTION

The overall objective in an immunoassay is to accurately determine the amount or concentration of an analyte. "Accurately determine" means to derive a true and correct estimate of the amount or concentration of analyte. In specific cases, such as tests for pregnancy, tumor markers, and antigens produced by viral infections, it is important to determine whether or not a given analyte is present. In any circumstance, it is desirable to develop objective criteria which can be used to determine whether the values obtained are meaningful. This chapter addresses two major topics: immunoassay validation and quality assessment. Mathematical and statistical concepts related to these topics are presented.

Immunoassay

1.1. Definitions

The term "potency estimate" is derived from bioassays and is another way of saying "estimated potency." For immunoassays, the potency estimate is usually the concentration of the analyte (for example, M, ng/ml, mIU/ml). Sensitivity is defined herein as the minimum amount of the analyte which can be accurately detected (1). Some definitions of sensitivity refer to the absolute position or the steepness of the dose–response curve rather than the lower limit of detection (1, 2). Specificity refers to the ability of the immunoassay to uniquely measure the analyte of interest. The degree to which other analytes cross react in the immunoassay affects specificity. Accuracy refers to the agreement between the true answer and the answer obtained in the immunoassay. Sometimes the term bias is substituted for inaccuracy. Precision refers to the agreement between replicate measurements. In immunoassays, precision usually is expressed as intra- and interassay variation calculated as a coefficient of variation.

1.2. Systematic versus Random Errors

There are two general types of errors in immunoassays: systematic and random (2). During immunoassay validation and quality assessment, attention must be paid to both types of errors. Systematic errors deflect repeated measures from the true or accurate value. Hence, a bias or consistent inaccuracy in the immunoassay results from systematic errors. Immunoassay validation is, in most respects, a thorough examination for potential systematic errors. Once recognized, systematic errors must be corrected or eliminated. Random errors are those which primarily affect precision. Random errors cannot be eliminated but can be minimized. The random errors accumulated during the course of an immunoassay can be quantitated statistically and used to assign confidence limits for potency estimates. Quality assessment involves determining whether a given immunoassay is free of systematic errors as well as continually assessing random errors.

1.3. Overview

Several years ago, a discussion of immunoassay validation and quality control was considerably more straightforward. Most immunoassays were performed as solution-phase, competitive systems and radiolabeled ligands served as the means of detection. In the last 15 years, the methodology and detection systems used in immunoassays have expanded significantly. Instead of being performed with solution-phase schemes, many modern immunoassays employ one or more components attached to a solid phase. Instead of using a single antibody, many contemporary immunoassays employ multiple antibodies.

Rather than dealing with the unique aspects of each system, we will attempt to develop a conceptual framework and thought process which can be applied to any type of immunoassay. Two types of immunoassays are taken as prototypic: classical solution-phase, competition-type immunoassays such as radioimmunoassays (RIAs), and solid-phase two-site immunochemical or immunometric assays (IMAs). Steroid and thyroid hormones are taken as prototypic analytes for substances which have a relatively low molecular weight and whose molecular structure is precisely defined. Protein hormones are used as a model system to discuss high-molecular-weight analytes whose molecular structure may not be fully characterized. Although most of the examples illustrate radioisotopic detection systems, the same principles apply to nonisotopic detection. RIA standard curves will be illustrated in linear response, log dose coordinate systems (3). Four-parameter logistic curve fitting (4, 5) is used as the primary method of RIA data reduction. IMA standard curves are illustrated in linear response, linear dose coordinate systems. Empirical curve fittings (6) of IMAs is illustrated.

Validation and quality assessment of immunoassays require an understanding of statistics. Readers are advised to consult a statistical text if they do not adequately understand statistical concepts and calculations.

2. ASSAY VALIDATION

The overall goal of assay validation is to determine whether the values obtained with the immunoassay are accurate and correct. Assay validation usually occurs in phases. The first phase is typically to evaluate sensitivity and specificity. The second phase is usually to examine the accuracy of the immunoassay via comparison with reference methods. A frequent goal in immunoassays is to obtain potency estimates for unknowns with minimal sample manipulation. Hence, assay validation also involves determining whether the sample matrix has a significant effect on the immunoassay and/or identifying which types of sample preparation are required to yield accurate potency estimates. The final phase of assay validation is limited clinical application of the immunoassay to determine whether useful information is obtained in the desired circumstances.

Although immunoassay validation is usually a time-consuming and tedious process, the effort expended returns dividends in the long run. Failure to properly or thoroughly validate an immunoassay can be disastrous.

The conceptual aspects of assay validation are discussed using a series of relevant questions. It is assumed that the reagents required to construct the immunoassay have been procured or produced, but otherwise the immunoassay is being built from the beginning.

2.1. What Is the Sensitivity of the Immunoassay?

When constructing an immunoassay, an early assessment of potential usefulness can be obtained by determining its sensitivity. Sensitivity is defined herein as the amount of analyte required to produce a change in the response which is significantly different from the response obtained in the absence of analyte (zero dose of analyte). Procedures for determining immunoassay sensitivity are presented subsequently. If the sensitivity is not low enough to be useful in the desired application, the production or procurement of alternate reagents should be considered.

2.2. How Specific Is the Immunoassay?

An extremely important consideration in any immunoassay is its specificity. That is, does the immunoassay uniquely measure the analyte of interest? Do other substances interfere with the immunoassay or cross react significantly? An initial screen is usually conducted by assaying a broad series of compounds at high dose levels, typically 1000 to 10,000 times the largest dose used to construct the standard curve. Substances which exhibit minimal inhibition of the binding of the analyte to the antibody or antibodies are considered not to cross react significantly. Compounds which inhibit binding of the analyte to the antibody at high doses should be examined in greater detail. The typical strategy is to construct dose–response curves for the test compounds and compare their dose–response curves to that of the analyte using a test of similarity ("parallelism"). The procedure determines whether the substance reacts in a manner similar to the analyte of interest, and its relative potency. For convenience, the cross reactivity of a particular substance in an immunoassay is frequently expressed as a percentage. Thus, a relative potency of 0.01 corresponds to 1% cross reactivity. An alternative way of saying the same thing is that a dose of test substance 100-fold greater than the dose of the reference analyte yields the same response in the immunoassay. Procedures for conducting tests of similarity are discussed in detail later.

An alternative strategy for assessing cross reactivity involves setting up a series of reactions which contain a fixed quantity of the analyte of interest (for example, a dose which is approximately equal to the midpoint of the dose–response curve). Increasing amounts of the test substance are added to this series of reactions. The dose of the test substance which does not cause a significant change in the response is taken as the maximum amount of the test substance which can be present in a sample and not interfere significantly with analyte antibody interactions.

When characterizing the specificity of an immunoassay, it is important to develop a rational strategy for assessing cross reactivity. To illustrate this point, consider the development of an immunoassay for testosterone. When constructing or utilizing an immunoassay for testosterone it is essential to know whether the assay cross reacts significantly with: other androgens such as 5α-dihydrotestosterone, androstenedione, dehydroepiandrosterone, and androstenediol; androgen metabolites such as the 5α-androstanediols, androsterone, and etiocholanolone; precursor steroids such as cholesterol, pregnenolone, progesterone, 17-hydroxypregnenolone, and 17-hydroxyprogesterone; and steroids in other classes which are likely to be present in body fluids such as estrogens, glucocorticoids, and mineralocorticoids. If the assay will be used to measure testosterone in patients who may be receiving synthetic steroids (such as contraceptive steroids and synthetic glucocorticoids) the cross reactivity of these substances should also be characterized. If the assay is to be utilized in a specific situation where certain compounds are present in high concentrations, it is desirable to demonstrate that these do not interfere. For example, when a testosterone RIA was used to assess the effect of prostaglandins on androgen production (7), it was essential to demonstrate that testosterone could be accurately measured in the presence of high concentrations of prostaglandins.

If an immunoassay to a small peptide is being developed, the cross reactivity of other peptides with similar structures should be examined. The specificity of immunoassays for small peptides can usually be clarified by generating fragments of the peptide synthetically and examining their cross reactivity.

The same concepts apply to the construction of immunoassays for protein hormones. Consider the development of an immunoassay for human chorionic gonadotropin (hCG). hCG is composed of two dissimilar subunits, designated alpha and beta. The alpha subunit of hCG is shared with the anterior pituitary hormones human luteinizing hormone (hLH), follicle-stimulating hormone (hFSH), and thyrotropin (hTSH). In addition, the beta subunit of hCG has an amino acid sequence which is very similar to that of hLH, except that hCG has an additional 24-amino-acid extension at the carboxyl terminus (8). A thorough characterization of an hCG immunoassay should include examining its cross reactivity with the full series of protein hormones produced in the anterior pituitary and placenta, the subunits of the anterior pituitary and placental hormones, as well as other protein hormones which may be present in body fluids. The ability of the immunoassay to distinguish hCG from hLH should be thoroughly characterized. If the distinguishing feature involves recognition of the unique carboxyl terminal peptide of hCG, examining the cross reactivity of a synthetic hCG carboxyl terminal peptide is warranted.

A question frequently asked by those validating an immunoassay is: At what percentage is cross reactivity significant? Cross reactivities of <0.001% (1 in 100,000) are usually not a major concern. Higher percentages must be appraised on a case by case basis. Again considering the testosterone example, a cross reaction of 5% for another androgen with a closely related structure such as 5α-dihydrotestosterone is not cause for alarm; in fact, an immunoassay which discriminates these two androgens at this level would be quite useful. However, 5% cross reactivity of testosterone in an immunoassay for 5α-dihydrotestosterone could be a cause for major concern if the intended application does not involve separation of the two steroids. A cross reaction of 1% for progesterone in any androgen immunoassay could be cause for major concern if the assay will be used to measure androgens during pregnancy without separation of the steroids. Ten percent cross reaction of hCG in an hLH immunoassay would probably not be a major concern if the assay was never to be used to measure samples from pregnant females. In contrast, 10% cross reaction of hLH in an hCG immunoassay would always be cause for concern. Thus, it is difficult to designate a specific percentage as "significant" cross reactivity. Rather, cross reactivities must be judged in the context of the intended application of an immunoassay.

One of the major advantages of IMAs using two antibodies is markedly increased specificity. It is possible to construct IMAs which are highly specific using one and sometimes two antibodies which by themselves would not be sufficiently specific to serve as the primary antibody in an RIA. The procedures outlined below for testing specificity can be used to characterize a single antibody or combination of antibodies; the principles are the same. However, in constructing and validating an IMA, an important consideration is identifying the epitope that each antibody recognizes. This topic is discussed in detail in other chapters. The epitope that each antibody recognizes is then considered in conjunction with the molecular structure of the analyte. Using this general strategy it is possible to build IMAs which are several orders of magnitude more specific than RIAs.

2.3. Are the Potency Estimates Obtained in the Immunoassay Accurate?

Another critical step in validation is to examine the accuracy of the immunoassay. The concept is to compare the values obtained in the immunoassay to those of a well-established and well-characterized reference method known to be accurate. The choice of using an immunoassay to measure a particular analyte is usually to facilitate sample throughput. Many reference methods are more complex and more time consuming, and may involve extensive sample manipulation. Their end points usually rely on measuring a chemical or biological response. Hence, specific recommendations applicable for all types of immunoassays cannot be made. However, a few comments are in order. For example, many early steroid immunoassays were validated against gas–liquid chromatography. Many immunoassays for proteins were validated against bioassays. When comparing the values obtained in the immunoassay to those of the reference method, one must be cognizant of the limitations, accuracy, and precision of the reference method.

2.4. Does the Sample Matrix Significantly Alter the Derived Potency Estimates?

In an immunoassay, everything in the sample other than the analyte constitutes its matrix. Common matrices for samples include serum, plasma, urine, saliva, and tissue extracts. Body fluids are complex mixtures of substances which can disrupt immunoassays in a variety of ways: by interfering with the binding of the analyte to a primary antibody, either via a competing compound or in a nonspecific manner, by providing a competing binder such as steroid or thyroid binding proteins, by interfering with the reagents used to separate free and bound forms, and/or by interfering with the detection system (quenching radioactivity, fluorescence, or enzymatic activity). Matrices which have a major influence on the immunoassay are usually apparent as inaccurate values. For example, the use of steroid immunoassays to directly measure concentrations in serum or plasma yields inaccurate values because the sample matrix contains high-affinity binding proteins for these hormones. Other types of matrix effects are more subtle. If present, these may be evident as dissimilar ("nonparallel") dose–response curves for analyte analyzed in a standard buffer mixture versus sample matrix. Conversely, demonstration that "similar" or "parallel" dose–response curves are obtained in a standard buffer mixture and sample matrix is not definitive proof that the immunoassay is devoid of matrix effects. Tests of similarity or parallelism must be interpreted in conjunction with tests of accuracy.

Three strategies for determining whether matrix effects are significant are: (i) comparing standard curves prepared in the diluent buffer to those prepared in the sample matrix known to be devoid of the analyte; (ii) determining whether increasing amounts of analyte added to a given amount of sample matrix can be quantitatively recovered (testing for additivity); and (iii) testing the effects of adding increasing amounts of the matrix. In the third case, the matrix represents a sample which contains an unknown amount of analyte. In the first and third cases, failure to generate curves of the same wave form (i.e., curves which are similar or parallel as defined below) is cause for concern. In order to make tests of similarity meaningful, they should be applied on multiple specimens which represent the diverse classes of samples that might be immunoassayed.

With the additivity approach, an unknown sample is assayed at a single dose level and aliquots of the sample are "spiked" with increasing amounts of the analyte. The amount of analyte in the spiked samples should equal the amount of analyte in the original sample plus the amount added. The additivity approach is a relatively weak test for matrix effects because the effects of sample matrix are usually assessed at a single level and the sample is usually spiked with purified analyte. Demonstration that increasing amounts of the sample matrix react similarly to the standard analyte is much more convincing.

If matrix effects are identified, a revision of the immunoassay protocol is usually required. This revision could include preparing the calibration curve in a matrix similar to that for unknowns but devoid of analyte, or could involve additional steps in sample preparation.

2.5. Does the Immunoassay Yield Useful Information?

The final phase of validation is to apply the immunoassay in the intended context using carefully chosen samples. For example, again assume that the task is development of an hCG immunoassay which is primarily designed to confirm pregnancy but also might be used in certain patients as a screen for hCG production by certain tumors. Obviously, samples from men and nonpregnant women should be nonreactive. Samples from females at various stages of pregnancy should be reactive and the concentrations obtained should correspond to those obtained using established reference methods. Samples from patients with tumors known to produce hCG should be reactive while samples from patients with tumors which do not produce hCG should not react. In this phase of immunoassay validation, the choice of reference samples is particularly important. Results from carefully chosen reference samples are then used to establish "normal values" for the immunoassay and limits of detectability.

3. DETERMINING IMMUNOASSAY SENSITIVITY

Immunoassay sensitivity refers to the minimum amount of analyte which can be accurately distinguished. This statement implies that it is more useful to express sensitivity in units of dose than in units of response. In practice, the response which is significantly different from that at zero dose is identified and converted to dose using the data reduction method employed in the immunoassay (for example, see Fig. 4.1). Sensitivity is frequently expressed as the Minimum Detectable Dose (MDD) (1). The MDD can then be extrapolated to the Minimal Detectable Concentration (MDC) if the immunoassay is to be used to measure the analyte in a specified volume of body fluids.

Two general approaches to defining sensitivity are to calculate confidence limits for the responses at zero dose and extrapolate the confidence limits to dose, and to designate a value empirically on the basis of experience and(or) doses used to construct the standard curve. Each approach has advantages and disadvantages. Methods for defining the MDD are illustrated using data obtained in RIAs and IMAs performed in the authors' laboratories.

3.1. Defining Sensitivity Using Statistical Approaches

Ekins (2) states that a simple and straightforward method to define assay sensitivity is to use the precision of the zero dose estimates. That concept forms the basis for all statistical definitions of immunoassay sensitivity. Nonetheless, there is not universal agreement regarding how the precision of the zero dose estimates (i.e., their variance) should be defined.

On the basis of Ekin's definition, a simple and straightforward method to estimate assay sensitivity is to calculate the mean and standard deviation of the zero dose

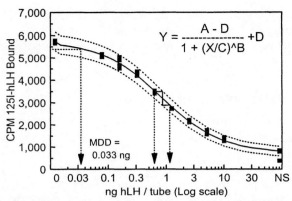

FIGURE 4.1 A standard curve obtained in the hLH RIA (9) analyzed by four-parameter logistic curve fitting (4–6). The variance in the responses of multiple assays was analyzed and used to derive an equation to predict the variance in responses. The predicted variances were converted to 95% confidence limits for responses which are illustrated by dashed lines. The lower 95% confidence limit at zero dose extrapolated to a MDD of 0.033 ng. Also illustrated is how the confidence limits in responses are extrapolated to confidence limits in dose. The confidence limits in response units are simply converted to dose using the data reduction scheme normally employed in the RIA or IMA.

standards. The mean and standard deviation would then be used to calculate confidence limits for the response at zero dose and extrapolated to dose to yield the MDD or MDC. This approach appears to be valid from both statistical and conceptual viewpoints. Nonetheless, it may be less than ideal depending on how the calculations are performed. For example, most immunoassays employ a relatively small number of samples (sometimes as few as two) to define the response at zero dose. Calculation of reliable confidence limits with small sample sizes is extremely difficult. An important consideration is the selection of a Student t statistic. Should confidence limits be calculated using a one- or two-tailed value for t? At what probability level should the confidence limits be calculated? Intuitively, it seems logical to use a one-tailed t value because immunoassay standard curves are monotonic (i.e., the dose–response curve only changes in one direction). Moreover, a one-tailed t value is the appropriate choice from a statistical perspective (1). The choice of a probability level is more difficult; it essentially represents a decision as to what chance of making a misclassification error is acceptable. The following examples illustrate 95% confidence limits (5% chance of making a misclassification error) recognizing that in certain circumstances, calculations at the more conservative 99 or even 99.9% probability levels might be appropriate (1).

Consider the hLH RIA and hCG IMA standard curves illustrated in Figs. 4.1 and 4.2, respectively. The hLH RIA (Fig. 4.1) utilized reagents obtained from the NIH Pituitary Hormone Distribution Program (9). The lower portion of a standard curve obtained with a Hybritech Tandem-β hCG immunometric assay (Hybritech Inc., San Diego, CA) is illustrated in Fig. 4.2. The zero dose standard in the hLH RIA yielded a response of 5726 ± 51 (SD; n = 4) counts per minute (cpm; Fig. 4.1). The 95% confidence limit in response units using a one-tailed t test was 5726 − (2.353 × 51) or 5606 cpm ($t_{\alpha = 0.05, 3\,df, 1\text{-tailed}}$ = 2.353). The 95% confidence limits using a two-tailed approach were 5726 ± (3.182 × 51) or 5563 and 5888 cpm

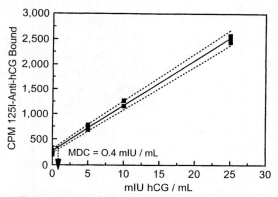

FIGURE 4.2 The lower portion of a standard curve obtained in a human chorionic gonadotropin (hCG) immunometric assay (Hybritech, Inc., San Diego, CA) analyzed by linear regression.
The variance in the responses of multiple assays was analyzed and used to derive an equation
to predict the variance in responses. The predicted variances were converted to 95% confidence
limits which are illustrated by dashed lines. The upper 95% confidence limit at zero dose
(303 cpm) extrapolated to a minimal detectable concentration (MDC) of 0.4 mIU/ml.

$(t_{\alpha = 0.05, \, 3 \, df, \, 2\text{-tailed}} = 3.182)$. Extrapolated to dose, 5606 and 5563 cpm yielded MDDs
of 0.013 and 0.017 ng, respectively. Similarly, the zero dose standard in the hCG
IMA yielded a response of 241 ± 30 (SD, $n = 4$) cpm (Fig. 4. 2). The 95% confidence
limits in response units using one- and two-tailed t tests were 312 and 336 cpm,
respectively. The extrapolated concentrations were 0.5 and 0.8 mIU hCG/ml, respectively. These simple definitions of sensitivity illustrate two major points: some
statistically valid definitions of assay sensitivity may not be informative in terms of
being able to distinguish the presence and absence of analyte, and one-tailed confidence limits, although more appropriate from a statistical perspective, yield the
more liberal (i.e., lower) estimates of MDD and MDC.

The major objection to using only the variation in responses for the zero standards
in a single assay to estimate sensitivity is that an extremely small amount of the
available information is taken into consideration. Thus, the derived estimates of
MDD or MDC are subject to large random errors. More appropriate estimates can
be derived by using the additional information available in a single assay and/or
information accumulated over multiple assays. A better strategy is to calculate the
variance of the zero standards in multiple assays and pool the variances (any good
statistical text describes how to pool variances). The pooled variance could then
be used to predict a variance for the zero standard in a particular assay. The
predicted variance could then be used to calculate confidence limits for the response
at zero dose in a particular assay and then be extrapolated to dose. Now let us
extend this concept one step further.

The random errors in RIA and IMA response variables are generally not constant
throughout the calibration curves (i.e., the variance is not homogeneous) and hence
a weighted regression analysis is preferable to an unweighted analysis (6, 10). One
powerful approach to performing a weighted regression analysis is to derive an
equation which predicts the variance for any response, including the response at
zero dose. Most of the computer programs developed by Drs. David Rodbard and
Peter Munson at the National Institutes of Health (NIH) in Bethesda, Maryland,
use a weighting or variance equation which has the general form:

$$\text{Predicted Variance, Response} = A0 + A1 * \text{Response}^{A2}. \tag{4.1}$$

Equation (4.1) is a composite of two separate equations: a linear relationship denoted by the A0 and A1 terms (A2 = 1), and a log–log or exponential relationship denoted by the A1 and A2 terms (A0 = 0). Note that A2 should be set to 1 for Eq. (4.1) to work in the linear mode. Older versions of the variance equation included a quadratic component (A2 × Response^2; A1 and A2 in Eq. (4.1) were denoted as A3 and A4, respectively, in previous versions of the equation). The exponential equation performs considerably better, so the quadratic portion of the equation is no longer used. In order to derive values for A0, A1, and A2, the variance in the responses for standards and unknowns assayed in replicate are used to fit linear or exponential equations (see Rodbard et al. (10) or Grotjan et al. (6) for a more detailed discussion). The derived equations can be used to predict the variance of each response, including the variance of the zero standard. When performing a weighted analysis, weights are assigned relative to the inverse of predicted variance. Note that this approach to portraying variances is somewhat empirical. Equation (4.1) describes the relationship between a response and its variance but does not consider the source of the variation.

Consider the hLH RIA and hCG IMA standard curves illustrated in Figs. 4.1 and 4.2, respectively. The IMA standard curve was truncated at an upper concentration of 25 mIU/ml to yield a segment which could be fit by standard linear regression techniques. The dashed lines depict the 95% confidence limits for the distribution of points around the fitted curve using four parameter logistic curve fitting (Fig 4.1) and linear regression (Fig. 4.2). Response variances in the hLH RIA were calculated with a linear equation where A0 = 3000, A1 = 3, and A2 = 1:

$$\text{Variance} = 3000 + 3 * \text{Response}. \tag{4.2}$$

Response variances in the hCG IMA were calculated with an exponential equation where A0 = 0, A1 = 0.22, and A2 = 1.28:

$$\text{Variance} = 0.22 * \text{Response}^{1.28}. \tag{4.3}$$

The derived confidence limits for the zero standard in response units for the RIA were 5340 and 6166 cpm while those for the IMA were 232 and 303 cpm. These responses extrapolated to a MDD of 0.033 ng for the hLH RIA and a MDC of 0.4 mIU/ml for the IMA. Estimates of immunoassay sensitivity calculated in this manner are robust because they are based on a relatively large body of information. Furthermore, they are appropriate from both statistical and conceptual perspectives. It would be reasonable to state that doses greater than 0.033 ng hLH are significantly different from zero in the RIA. However, in our judgement, it would be much harder to rationalize that a sample which contains 0.4 mIU hCG/ml is distinguishable from zero in the IMA.

Rodbard (1) presented an elegant and statistically rigorous method for calculating assay sensitivity. The essence of Rodbard's method is that the variance in the zero standards (calculated as outlined above) is considered in conjunction with the number of replicates assayed. The adjustment for replicates compensates for the greater statistical confidence associated with multiple determinations. Using Rodbard's method, estimated MDDs were 0.033, 0.024, 0.020, and 0.011 ng for single, duplicate, triplicate, and infinite determinations. Although this method is based on sound statistical theory and principles, MDDs derived by Rodbard's method can be considered to be somewhat liberal (in our opinion).

3.2. Designating Sensitivity Using Empirical Approaches

Consider the hLH RIA illustrated in Fig. 4.1. The standard curve was constructed using doses of 0.078 through 10 ng hLH. The cpm ^{125}I-hLH bound was used as the response variable. Figure 4.1 illustrates untransformed responses, but an equivalent method to graph the curve would have been to normalize the response at zero dose to 100% (or 1.0) and the response at infinite dose (nonspecific binding) to 0% (0.0). Two empirical definitions of sensitivity or MDD could be to designate the lowest dose used to construct the standard curve as the MDD, or a dose associated with a predetermined response as the MDD. For example, the dose associated with 90% binding in an RIA could be designated as the MDD if the responses are scaled to a range of 100 to 0%. The underlying rationale in both cases is equivalent to truncation of the standard curve (3). Both approaches are primarily based on experience. The experience could represent a general knowledge of immunoassays or could represent information obtained by assaying multiple curves with a particular immunoassay. A dose which consistently yields a response different from that obtained at zero dose (i.e., absence of analyte) should be chosen when using the "smallest dose used to construct the standard curve" method. It then becomes incumbent to select a dose which consistently provides a response distinguishable from the zero standard. The "predetermined response" approach is based primarily on general experience and knowledge of RIAs. Experience with a variety of RIAs suggests that 90% binding (10% displacement of the tracer) is usually distinguishable from the zero standard in a reasonably well behaved assay. The 90% binding point is somewhat arbitrary but not capricious—92, 94, or 88% binding could have been designated as the predetermined response on the basis of experience accumulated with a particular RIA. The definitions of MDD by the two empirical approaches for the curve illustrated in Fig. 4.1 give 0.078 (lowest dose used to construct the standard curve) and 0.060 ng (90% binding). Defining the MDD by one of these methods is simple and straightforward. The primary disadvantage of these methods is that they do not consider the statistical aspects of assay performance.

To demonstrate how empirical definitions of MDD can be applied in IMAs, consider Fig. 4.2. The directions supplied with the hCG IMA kit explicitly state that concentrations of less than 25 mIU hCG/ml should be considered "negative." The 25 mIU/ml concentration corresponds to the lowest standard used to construct the calibration curve. This designation of MDC was undoubtedly based on results with a large number of samples and was chosen to be conservative (i.e., having an extremely low probability of making a misclassification error). In terms of clinical utility, the patient, physician and clinical laboratory personnel prefer to know whether or not the patient is pregnant! Alternatively, the MDC could have been defined as the concentration associated with a response 2, 5, or 10 times the mean response obtained at zero dose. The increment over mean response at zero dose would be derived on the basis of experience with the IMA as well as degree of uncertainty which is acceptable.

3.3. Designating Sensitivity for a Particular Immunoassay

Several methods for defining or designating immunoassay sensitivity have been presented. The one thing that can be stated with certainty is that no method is ideal in all circumstances. The choice of a particular approach depends on what level of misclassification errors can be tolerated, the circumstances in which immuno-assay will be applied, and whether one chooses to be liberal or conservative. Empirical designations of MDD and MDC are useful in certain situations. If empirical designations of sensitivity are used, it is better to be conservative. In this context, conservative means that the definition of MDD or MDC should be slightly larger than the "true" value obtained by rigorous statistical tests. For any definition of sensitivity, it is important to understand how the estimate was derived, whether it yields a liberal or conservative estimate, and what are the possible limitations of the particular method used. As with any statistical analysis, estimates of immunoassay sensitivity should be interpreted with some common sense.

4. TESTS OF SIMILARITY (PARALLELISM)

When validating an immunoassay, it is essential to demonstrate that the analyte in the standards and unknowns reacts with the antibody (or antibodies, in the case of IMAs) in a similar manner. A detailed discussion of the condition of "similarity" is presented by Finney (11). Finney's discussion includes both conceptual and statistical definitions, particularly as they apply to *in vivo* bioassays. Nonetheless, concepts relevant in bioassays are directly applicable to immunoassays. Demonstration of similarity (in the statistical sense) is a necessary, but not sufficient, condition for establishing the validity of an immunoassay.

When there were only solution-phase RIAs to consider and linear regression was the primary method used for curve fitting, tests of similarity used to be called tests of "parallelism." The term parallelism is no longer appropriate considering how immunoassays have evolved and that nonlinear curve fitting methods are frequently used for data reduction. Other reasons for using "similarity" rather than parallelism will be apparent as the discussion focuses on IMAs.

As noted above, tests of similarity are usually conducted by assaying various amounts of an "unknown" sample and determining whether the dose–response relationship for the unknown is similar to that for the standard analyte. In the context of tests of similarity, the amount or volume of unknown sample assayed represents the "dose" unknown. Because the response in immunoassays is typically proportional to log dose (rather than a linear dose), the amounts of unknown assayed (volumes) should be chosen to cover as wide a range as is feasible. The amounts of unknown should chosen to be equidistant on a Log scale (i.e., 1, 2, 4, 8, 16, rather than 1, 2, 3, 4, 5). The larger the number of volumes, the better. Tests of similarity with only two volumes always leave a lot to be desired. In IMAs, the number of volumes required to perform an effective analysis is a function of the procedure used for the test of similarity.

In an ideal immunoassay, each unknown would be assayed at multiple volumes and tests of similarity would be performed as part of the calculations. Once the assay is thoroughly validated, this is usually not necessary. Nonetheless, it is prudent to assay each unknown at two volumes, particularly in IMAs which can give a "high dose hook effect" when large quantities of analyte are present.

The following section presents methods for conducting tests of similarity. In each case, the procedures for deriving a potency estimate or relative potency are presented. Relative potencies denote the dose of standard analyte and "dose" of unknown which yield the same response. It is convenient to express relative potencies as ratios where the dose of standard analyte is taken as the denominator. With this procedure, values greater than unity (1.0) denote substances more potent than the standard analyte. If the following analyses are applied in evaluating cross reactivities, relative potencies can be converted to percentages, if desired.

4.1. Simple Tests of Similarity

Simple tests of similarity are for the most part "quick" and sometimes "dirty." The underlying assumption is that the standard curve has been perfectly defined. The advantages of these tests are that they are simple to perform and that the calculations are straightforward. These tests can be applied easily with any data reduction scheme. Furthermore, they work equally well for RIA and IMA data. Although rigorous statistical tests for similarity are clearly more desirable, the following procedures usually work reasonably well. Simple tests of similarity ask one of two questions: Is the potency estimate independent of amount of sample assayed? Is the amount of analyte detected directly proportional to the amount of sample assayed?

For examples of simple tests of similarity, consider the data presented in Table 4.1. This data set was derived by analyzing a plasma sample containing hCG in a hLH RIA (9). The hLH RIA was known to react with hCG in a nonsimilar fashion and thus data were purposefully generated to illustrate what constitutes dissimilarity.

4.1.1. Simple Test for Similarity Using Analysis of Variance

The underlying assumptions are that the calculated potency estimates (concentrations) are independent of the amount (volume) of unknown assayed and the variance between potency estimates will not be significantly larger than the variance within replicate measurements. The basic approach is to perform a one-classification analy-

TABLE 4.1   **Data Used in Simple Tests of Similarity (Parallelism)**

Dose = volume (ml)[a]	Amount detected (ng hLH)	Potency estimate (ng/ml)	Log volume	Log amount detected	Log potency estimate
0.025	0.4832	19.33	−1.602	−0.3159	1.2862
0.025	0.4374	17.50	−1.602	−0.3591	1.2429
0.025	0.4587	18.35	−1.602	−0.3385	1.2636
0.025	0.4569	18.28	−1.602	−0.3402	1.2619
0.05	0.736	14.72	−1.301	−0.1331	1.1680
0.05	0.815	16.29	−1.301	−0.0890	1.2120
0.05	0.781	15.63	−1.301	−0.1071	1.1939
0.05	0.791	15.82	−1.301	−0.1018	1.1993
0.10	1.272	12.72	−1.000	0.1045	1.1045
0.10	1.265	12.65	−1.000	0.1020	1.1020
0.10	1.160	11.60	−1.000	0.0643	1.0643
0.10	1.341	13.41	−1.000	0.1276	1.1276
0.20	1.940	9.70	−0.699	0.2877	0.9867
0.20	2.073	10.36	−0.699	0.3165	1.0155
0.20	2.032	10.16	−0.699	0.3079	1.0069
0.20	2.147	10.74	−0.699	0.3319	1.0308

[a] In the context of tests of similarity, the "dose" for an unknown is typically the volume of sample assayed.

sis of variance (12) using the pooled variance in potency estimates within doses to calculate the error term. An F test is used to compare the variance in potency estimates between amounts assayed to the variance within replicates. If the F test is not significant, the potency estimates of the unknown are independent of dose and hence "similar" to the standard. The one-classification analysis of variance approach is used to analyze similarity for the hCG-containing sample in the hLH RIA (Table 4.1). The statistical calculations are presented in Table 4.2. The F test is highly significant and hence the analysis reveals that the unknown (i.e, the hCG-containing sample) and the hLH standard do not react similarly in the hLH immuno-assay.

An underlying assumption in an analysis of variance is that the variances are homogeneous. If the variances do not appear to be homogeneous, Bartlett's tests or F ratios (12) can be used to test for homogeneity of variances. If samples with nonhomogeneous variances are observed, the analysis of variance is performed using log transformed potency estimates which usually eliminates the nonhomogeneity.

From a statistical viewpoint, the analysis of variance approach is less than ideal because it does not consider the information associated with "doses" (volumes or amounts) of unknowns. Conceptually, it is better to use the dose information to examine the statistical relationship between dose and potency estimate. The following regression procedures are thus more desirable from a statistical perspective.

4.1.2. Simple Tests of Similarity Using Regression (13)

The simple tests of similarity presented below use standard statistical calculation procedures, primarily linear regression. Hence, minimal details of the calculations will be presented under the presumption that they can be performed, if the concept is understood. The statistical calculations for the examples illustrated in Figs. 4.3–4.6 were performed using a spreadsheet.

4.1.2.1. Linear Regression of Potency Estimate versus Amount of Sample Analyzed
Theoretically, potency estimates (concentrations) should be independent of the amount of unknown analyzed. Hence, a graph of potency estimates (Y) versus doses (X) should yield a flat line with a slope of zero. If the unknown reacts similar to the standard, the Y intercept equals the potency estimate. A t test is performed to determine if the observed slope is different from zero. The t value is calculated by dividing the observed slope minus zero (the slope anticipated if the unknown is similar) by the standard error of the slope (s_b):

$$t = (\text{Observed Slope} - 0)/s_b. \qquad (4.4)$$

TABLE 4.2 Test of Similarity Using a One-Classification Analysis of Variance[a]

Source	df	Sum of squares	Mean squares	F	p
Between doses	3	150.15	50.06	112.8	$4.5E - 08$
Error (within doses)	12	5.3235	0.4436		—
Total	15	155.4676			$P < 0.001$

[a] Comparison of the variance of potency estimates within replicates to the variance in potency estimates between doses (Is the potency estimate independent of dose?).

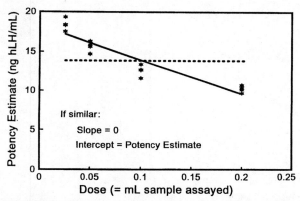

FIGURE 4.3   Simple test for similarity performed by regressing potency estimate on volume of sample assayed. If the standard analyte and unknown react similarly in the immunoassay, a line with a slope of zero should be apparent (denoted by a dashed line).

If the t value is significant at $n - 2$ degrees of freedom, the unknown does not react in a manner similar to the standard analyte. The data presented in Table 4.1 are analyzed using this procedure with the results presented graphically in Fig. 4.3. Note that the slope of the line illustrated in Fig. 4.3 (-43 ± 5) is significantly different from zero ($t = -9.63$, $P < 0.001$). Hence, the unknown does not react in the immunoassay in a manner similar to the standard analyte. Furthermore, the apparent potency estimate (18.27 ng/ml for the data illustrated in Fig. 4.3) for a dissimilar sample derived in this manner is not accurate.

4.1.2.2. Log–Log Regression of Potency Estimate versus Amount of Sample Analyzed   This approach is similar to the one illustrated previously except that the regression is performed after both the doses and the potency estimates have been log transformed. The log transformations provide a more robust analysis for potency estimates which have nonhomogeneous variances prior to transforma-

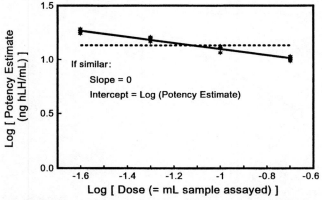

FIGURE 4.4   Simple test for similarity performed by regressing log (potency estimate) versus log (volume). If the standard analyte and unknown react similarly in the immunoassay, a line with a slope of zero should be apparent (denoted by a dashed line).

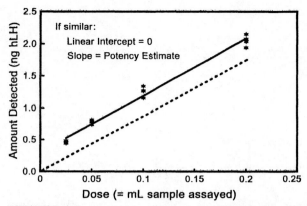

FIGURE 4.5 Simple test of similarity performed by regressing amount detected on volume of sample assayed. If the standard analyte and unknown react similarly in the immunoassay, the regression line should intersect the origin.

tion. Theoretically, the slope of the line should be zero. If the unknown and standard react similarly, the Y intercept equals the log of the potency estimate. The test for similarity is also performed by determining whether the observed slope is significantly different from zero. The data presented in Table 4.1 are analyzed by this approach and presented graphically in Fig. 4.4. In this example, the slope is significantly different from zero (-0.28 ± 0.01, $t = -19.18$, $P < 0.001$). Note that the nonparallelism in Fig. 4.4 is harder to appreciate by visual examination than that in Fig. 4.3. An inaccurate potency estimate (in this case, $10^{0.815} = 6.53$ ng/ml) is obtained if the unknown is dissimilar to the standard.

4.1.2.3. Regression of Amount Detected versus Amount of Sample Analyzed
The amount of unknown assayed (volume or "dose") is graphed on the X axis and the amount detected is graphed on the Y axis. If the standards and unknowns are similar, a straight line which intersects the origin is obtained. The

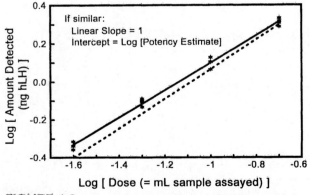

FIGURE 4.6 Simple test of similarity performed by regressing log (amount detected) versus log (volume). If the standard analyte and unknown react similarly in the immunoassay, the slope of the line should equal 1.0.

slope of the line defines the potency estimate (concentration). There are two ways to test for similarity in this system: calculate the confidence limits for the intercept and determine if the range includes zero, or use the extra sum of squares principle (11,12,14) where the first line is forced through the origin (the intercept is forced to equal zero) and the second line is described by fitting a line with an intercept. In the extra sum of squares procedure, the calculated residual variance of the two lines is compared. If forcing the line to have an intercept of zero significantly increases the residual variance, the intercept is significantly differently from zero. Of these two approaches, the second is better. Data presented in Table 4.1 are graphed as amount detected versus amount analyzed and are presented in Fig. 4.5. The F value calculated by the extra sum of squares test is highly significant ($F_{1,14} = 79.1$, $P < 0.001$). Note that the line in Fig. 4.5 does not intersect the origin and hence the unknowns do not react in a similar manner in the immunoassay to the standard analyte. The slope of the line fitted with an intercept is 8.9 ± 0.3 while the slope of the line forced through the origin is 11.0 ± 0.4. Thus, the line forced through the origin more closely describes the true potency estimate. Note that the observed (nonsimilar) line and the theoretical line of similarity appear to be parallel, which can be a source of confusion. Thus, it is particularly important to understand how to analyze for similarity and dissimilarity with this method.

4.1.2.4. Log–Log Regression of Amount Detected versus Amount of Sample Analyzed

A graph similar to Fig. 4.5 is constructed except that the dose and amount detected are log transformed. Log transformations are used to obviate nonhomogeneous variances, if present. The resultant graph should yield a straight line with a slope of unity (1.0). The Y intercept equals the log potency estimate, if the unknown and standard react similarly. Equation (4.4) is used to calculate a t value except that a 1.0 is substituted for the zero (0). A graphic illustration of the data presented in Table 4.1 is presented in Fig. 4.6. The unknowns illustrated in Fig. 4.6 are not similar to the standard (slope $= 0.72 \pm 0.01$, $t = 48.39$, $P < 0.001$). Although the calculations reveal that the unknown and the standard are not similar, the nonsimilarity is extremely difficult to discern visually. Furthermore, the apparent potency estimate ($10^{0.815} = 6.53$ ng/ml) for dissimilar samples is not accurate.

4.1.3. Which Simple Tests of Similarity Are Preferable?

Among simple tests for similarity, the graphic approaches illustrated in Figs. 4.3–4.6 are preferable to the analysis of variance method. Among the simple graphic analyses, dissimilarity or nonparallelism is much easier to visualize by plotting the potency estimates versus dose or log dose (Figs. 4.3 and 4.4). Nonparallelism is considerably harder to visualize when plotting the amount detected versus amount assayed (Fig. 4.5) or log amount detected versus log amount assayed (Fig. 4.6). Thus, statistical testing of the relevant regression parameters is more important than the construction of the graph. Precisely the same conclusions are evident with the four graphical procedures if they are used with appropriate statistical tests of similarity.

If one wants to increase the power of the simple graphic tests of similarity, a weighted regression analysis can be employed. The weights should be assigned relative to the inverse of the predicted error for the potency estimate or amount of ligand detected. If there is severe nonuniformity of variance (nonhomogeneous variances), the log transformed versions of the tests should be used because they are more appropriate from a statistical perspective (see Rodbard *et al.* (13) for a more detailed discussion).

4.2. Rigorous Tests of Similarity

Rigorous tests of similarity will be divided into four major groups corresponding to type of immunoassay under consideration (RIA or IMA) and the way in which the data are displayed or graphed (linear or nonlinear). This division is somewhat artificial but serves as a framework to build concepts one step at a time.

4.2.1. RIAs Analyzed by Linear Regression

Several data reduction schemes used in RIAs yield straight lines or large sections of the relationship which can be analyzed by linear regression if the ends are truncated (3): linear–log regression and logit–log regression of RIA curves, among others. Note that a log dose scale is used for both of these procedures. Tests of similarity using data expressed in linear coordinate systems employ classical bioassay statistical principles (11). Thus, these paradigms involve classical tests for parallelism. The methods used in the calculations are available in most standard statistical textbooks (11, 12) and will not be reiterated in detail here. Methods for comparison of regression lines are frequently found in the Analysis of Covariance section of standard statistical textbooks like Snedecor and Cochran (12). Tests for parallelism will be used to develop concepts. The concepts will then be extended to tests of similarity performed in nonlinear coordinate systems.

Tests for parallelism proceed in the following sequence. The parameters (slope and intercept) for each line are calculated independently. The residual variance for the two lines is compared using an F test to determine whether they are homogeneous. In ideal circumstances, the residual variances are homogeneous, indicating that the data from the two regression lines can be pooled. Nonhomogeneous variances are a cause for concern and are evidence that the standard and unknown do not react in the immunoassay in a completely analogous fashion. In order to perform the test of parallelism per se, the parameters for each regression line are recalculated, making the two lines share a common slope. The extra sum of squares principle (11, 12) is then used to determine if the sharing of slopes significantly increases the residual variance. If the extra sum of squares test is nonsignificant, the two lines are considered to be parallel. If the extra sum of squares test is significant, the two lines do not share a common slope and hence are not parallel. The final test is to determine whether the two lines share a common position. Conceptually, this can be viewed as the intercept, but the test is usually performed by comparing the midpoints of the lines. The test for position can also be made using the extra sum of squares principle, where the two lines are forced to share the same slope and intercept. If the extra sum of squares test is nonsignificant, the two lines share the same position. In the context of immunoassays, sharing the same position means that the unknown has a potency estimate equal to the standard. If the lines are parallel (have the same slope) but do not have the same position (as illustrated in Fig. 4.7), the difference in position of the two lines represents the potency estimate of the unknown. The pooled residual variance can then be used to calculate a confidence limit for the potency estimate. Tests of parallelism and calculation of potency estimates performed with these procedures are rigorous from a statistical

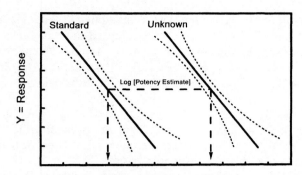

Log Dose (ng for standard; volume for unknown)

FIGURE 4.7 Test of parallelism for RIAs when the data are graphed in a linear–log or logit–log coordinate system. The log (potency estimate) is the distance between the parallel lines.

perspective. The information generated is therefore quite meaningful because they utilize information obtained with both the standard and the unknown.

The calculations used in tests of parallelism can be more involved depending on the coordinate system used to fit the regression lines and whether a weighted regression analysis is performed. Figure 4.7 could represent one of two popular approaches to RIA data reduction: data graphed in linear–log coordinates where the curves have been truncated to the "linear" portion, or data graphed in logit–log coordinates. In both cases, the abscissa is a log scale. Hence, the potency estimate in each case is returned in log units. A common practice is to calculate the potency estimate and confidence limits in log units and then convert the potency estimate as well as confidence limits by taking their antilogs. In both cases, it would be desirable to perform a weighted analysis, but this becomes particularly important with the logit–log coordinate system because the logit transformations acerbate any heteroscedasicity which is present (6).

The assignment of relative potencies or potency estimates is straightforward with parallel lines. The potency estimate (or relative potency) is simply the distance between the two lines, corrected by taking antilogs if a log dose scale has been used. When parallel, the distance between the two lines is equal (constant) at all points along the lines. However, when two lines are nonparallel, the assignment of a potency estimate is not straightforward. The potency estimate becomes a function of where one chooses to make the comparison. A common practice is to assign the potency estimate at the midpoint of the lines and use the residual variance of the lines forced to be parallel to assign confidence limits for the potency estimate. Sometimes this results in a particularly large confident limit. Thus, the calculation of potency estimates and confidence limits for lines which are nonparallel is frequently not very useful. The more important information in this case is that the lines are nonparallel and hence the standard and the unknown differ in the way they react in the immunoassay.

4.2.2. RIAs Analyzed by Nonlinear Curve Fitting

The availability of powerful computing resources, particularly microcomputers, provides the hardware resources required to perform nonlinear curve fitting and rigorous tests of similarity using nonlinear approaches in virtually every clinical and research laboratory. Rodbard and colleagues have developed excellent software for this purpose (ALLFIT and FLEXIFIT) and have adapted this software to run on most of the common operating systems used by microcomputers. The algorithms used to develop the programs have been presented (15–17). Rather than reiterating the algorithms, the following section will concentrate on strategies for using these programs.

To illustrate the principles, let us reconsider tests of parallelism. The lines are fit independently and then fit with a common slope. They are parallel if the shared slope does not significantly increase the residual variance. The same principle is used in tests of similarity in nonlinear coordinate systems. Essentially, the same series of questions is asked: What is the residual variance of the curves fit independently? If the curves are forced to be alike, is there a significant increase in the residual variance? If the residual variance increases significantly when the curves are forced to be alike, the standard and unknown do not react in the immunoassay in a similar fashion. To be more specific, what does "forcing the curves to be alike" mean? In the context of nonlinear curve fitting, it means to share common parameters, just as tests of parallelism and position of regression lines were performed by fitting the lines with shared parameters.

When performing tests of similarity in nonlinear coordinate systems, the major question that is asked is: Do the curves have the same wave form? If the curves have the same wave form or shape they are said to be congruent. An excellent way to analyze RIA data is the four-parameter logistic approach (4–6). This method of data analysis will be used to illustrate tests of similarity for RIAs analyzed by nonlinear curve fitting.

The four-parameter logistic equation used by Rodbard and colleagues is:

$$Y = (A - D)/(1 + (X/C)^B) + D, \tag{4.5}$$

where Y is the response variable, X is the dose, A is the response at zero dose, D is the response at infinite dose (typically the nonspecific binding), C is the midpoint dose (effective dose at 50% binding), and B is the slope or steepness factor. In some implementations of the four-parameter logistic, the meaning of parameters A and D is switched. Parameter D becomes the response at zero dose and parameter A becomes the response at infinite dose. The four-parameter logistic equation represents a semiempirical method for the analysis of RIA data and is the more general case of the logit–log method (4–6). Performing tests of similarity using the four-parameter logistic equation appears formidable, but actually is not too difficult if one understands the underlying principles and develops systematic strategies. When using four-parameter logistic curve fitting, tests of similarity can be performed with either ALLFIT (15) or FLEXIFIT (16,17). ALLFIT is the preferable program because it is designed specifically to analyze multiple four parameter logistic curves.

Data files for ALLFIT are constructed by listing the dose–response pairs for each curve, one per line. The data for each curve are preceded by one line of alphabetic (nonnumeric) information. The doses for each curve should be ordered smallest to largest. Rather than entering the full array of data points, the mean response for each dose is entered. The rationale for this tactic is that the resulting residual variance then reflects how well the curve fits the data rather than describing a combination of how well the curve fits the data plus the variation within replicates.

To illustrate strategies for using ALLFIT, consider the curves illustrated in Fig. 4.8. These curves were generated by assaying an unknown sample containing hCG and hCG standards in an hLH RIA. As above, this scenario was chosen specifically to illustrate dissimilarity. This data set also illustrates two separate cases: zero standard and nonspecific binding tubes were included with the hCG curve but were not available for the unknown. These two cases will be considered independently and then as a unit. When using ALLFIT, it is helpful first to construct a graph of the data which aids in the identification of parameters that may be shared among curves.

The general strategy for performing tests of similarity using ALLFIT is to first fit the curve with a minimum of parameter sharing. This forms a baseline for comparison with subsequent fits where specific parameters are shared. The strategy that works best is to first test whether the ends of the curves are similar (parameters A and D), then their slopes (parameter B), and lastly their positions (midpoints or parameter C). In order to present this discussion in a manner consistent with the nomenclature used in ALLFIT, the hLH curve 1 will be denoted as curve 1, the unknown will be designated as curve 2, and the hCG curve will be designated as curve 3. Thus, parameters A_1, B_1, C_1, and D_1 denote the parameters which describe curve 1, etc. Also note that parameters A_1 and A_2 (which describe parameter A for curves 1 and 2, respectively) are distinct from the "A1" and "A2" presented in Eq (4.1).

First let us consider the unknown. Because no data are available for the endpoints of the unknown curve (binding at zero and infinite doses), parameters A and D for the unknown curve are set equal to those observed for the hLH curve. That is, parameter A_2 is presumed to equal parameter A_1 and parameter D_2 is presumed to equal parameter D_1. This is a good assumption because the endpoints of all curves in an RIA should be equal. (This is not a good assumption when using ALLFIT to analyze bioassay data, though.) Also note that four is the absolute minimum number of points which should be submitted for analysis with the ends of a curve shared with the standard analyte. Theoretically, there are zero degrees of freedom if four parameters are fit to four data points. Thus, fitting two parameters

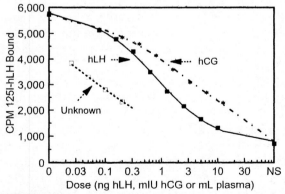

FIGURE 4.8   Tests of similarity (congruency) for RIAs analyzed by four parameter logistic curve fitting (4–6) and ALLFIT (15). In this example, hCG standards and an unknown sample containing hCG were analyzed in a hLH RIA (9). The endpoints of all three curves are statistically similar but the hCG standards and unknown have a different slope from the hLH standard.

to four data points with the endpoints shared with another curve leaves one degree of freedom according to the algorithm used by ALLFIT (see later comments regarding how the sharing of parameters affects the degrees of freedom assigned to each curve).

One cycle of curve fitting is executed. The resultant sum of squares serves as a basis for comparison with subsequent fits. Next, the two curves are fit with a shared slope (i.e., parameter B_2 is set to equal parameter B_1). Because the first cycle of curve fitting presumed equality in endpoints of the curves, parameter A_2 is shared with A_1 and parameter D_2 is shared with D_1 in the second cycle of curve fitting. In this particular case, the extra sum of squares test indicates that the sharing of slopes markedly increases the residual variance. The increase in residual variance must result from the sharing of slopes. Hence, the two curves are not congruent with regard to parameter B. If desired, a test for similarity of position could be performed (test whether $C_2 = C_1$) but a visual appraisal of the graph suggests that parameter C for each of the curves is significantly different. This could also be deduced from some of the intermediate data printed out by ALLFIT during each cycle of curve fitting, which includes the parameters for each curve and their standard errors.

Now consider the hCG curve. In the first cycle of curve fitting, parameters A_1, A_3, B_1, B_3, C_1, C_3, D_1, and D_3 are fit independently. The resulting sum of squares serves as the baseline for subsequent comparisons. Following the strategy outlined above, equality with regard to the ends of the curves is tested (Does $A_3 = A_1$? Does $D_3 = D_1$?). This could be performed by sharing one parameter at a time, or it could be performed in unison. A graphic examination of the data (Fig. 4.8) suggests that the endpoints of the two curves could be the same, so it is logical to test whether both endpoints are equal in one fit. In this particular case, the extra sum of squares test indicates no significant increase in the residual variance. Thus, we have established that $A_3 = A_1$ and $D_3 = D_1$. This equality is maintained in subsequent fits. Had the extra sum of squares test indicated that the two curves had different endpoints, it would be desirable to test each endpoint individually to determine if one but not the other should be shared. Now a test for equality of slopes is performed by having the two curves share parameter B (Does $B_3 = B_1$?) in addition to parameters A ($A_3 = A_1$) and D ($D_3 = D_1$). In this case, the sharing of parameter B significantly increases the residual variance by the extra sum of squares test, indicating that the curves do not share a common slope. If desired, the equality of parameter C could be tested but these two curves do not share a common position either.

One of the advantages of ALLFIT is that many curves can be fit simultaneously. Thus, the data illustrated in Fig. 4.8 can easily be analyzed simultaneously as one unit. When considered as a unit, the baseline fit (Fit 1) would be performed sharing parameters A and D for curves 1 and 2 ($A_1 = A_2$; $D_1 = D_2$). The best strategy would then be to test whether the endpoints for curve 3 (A_3 and D_3) equal the other two curves (Fit 2). In this case, all three curves have similar endpoints. The next fit asks the question: Do all three curves have similar slopes (Does $B_1 = B_2 = B_3$?; Fit 3)? In this case, the three slopes are not equal. A visual examination of the graph suggests that it is logical to test for equality in parameter B for curves 2 and 3 (Does $B_2 = B_3$?; Fit 4). This cycle establishes that parameter $B_2 = B_3 \neq B_1$. Although it is possible to test all possible combinations, a strategy which makes the most meaningful comparisons is most efficient. At this point, we have evaluated parameters A, B, and D for each curve. Thus, we could test whether $C_1 = C_2 = C_3$. However, a more efficient strategy is to test whether $C_2 = C_3$, because these are the closest graphically. In this case, when C_2 and C_3 are shared the residual variance increases significantly (Fit 5). Thus, the conclusion from this series of tests is: $A_1 = A_2 = A_3$, $B_1 \neq B_2 = B_3$ (curves 2 and 3 have similar slopes) $C_1 \neq C_2 \neq C_3$ (each curve has a unique position or potency), and $D_1 = D_2 = D_3$.

Each time ALLFIT performs a fit, the following data are written to a file: individual parameter estimates for each curve at multiple iterations until the residual variance changes by a minimal amount, the parameters for each curve and their standard errors, a table of relative potencies for each curve compared to curve 1 which is assumed to be the standard analyte, a covariance matrix (later versions only), a table of sum of squares plus results of the runs test, and a table of the extra sum of squares test for each fit.

In order to provide guidelines for interpretation of ALLFIT's output, the sum of squares table and the extra sum of squares test for Fits 4 and 5 above are illustrated in Table 4.3. The second column of the sum of squares table presents the sum of squares for each curve and its associated degrees of freedom. Note that

TABLE 4.3   Portions of the Data Output by ALLFIT

	Sum of squares	df	Mean square	F	Residuals (+)	(−)	Runs
				Fit No. 4			
Curve							
1	1.576946	7.33	0.215038	0.96 ($P = 0.944$)	5	5	5 (good)
2	0.186775	1.83	0.101877	0.43 ($P = 0.268$)	1	3	2 (good)
3	1.745821	6.83	0.255486	1.33 ($P = 0.674$)	5	4	6 (good)
Total	3.509543	16	0.219346		11	12	
Fit							
1	3.09591	13	0.238147	—			
2	3.33652	15	0.222435	0.51 ($P = 0.612$)			
3	37.56652	17	2.209795	36.19 ($P = 0$)			
4	3.50954	16	0.219346	0.58 ($P = 0.638$)			
				Fit No. 5			
Curve							
1	439.4024	7.83	56.0939	1.28 ($P = 0.716$)	6	4	3 (poor)
2	331.0431	2.33	141.8756	4.09 ($P = 0.080$)	0	4	1 (bad)
3	69.7910	6.83	10.2133	0.13 ($P = 0.004$)	9	0	1 (bad)
Total	849.2366	17	49.42568		15	8	
Fit							
1	3.09591	13	0.238147	—			
2	3.33652	15	0.222435	0.51 ($P = 0.612$)			
3	37.56652	17	2.209795	36.19 ($P = 0$)			
4	3.50954	16	0.219346	0.58 ($P = 0.638$)			
5	840.2366	17	49.42568	878.81 ($P = 0$)			

the degrees of freedom are not necessarily integers because parameters have been shared between curves; the degrees of freedom are divided according to the way parameters are shared. The fifth column illustrates F tests for the mean sum of squares (residual variance) for each curve. This F test is helpful in identifying curves which contribute disproportionally to the overall residual variance (i.e., are not ideally fit). The last two columns provide the output of the runs test and a statement concerning the goodness of fit. In Fit 4, each curve contributes about equally to the overall residual variance and each is adequately described by the shared parameters. The extra sum of squares test for each fit is also provided. For Fit 2 (Does $A_1 = A_2 = A_3$? Does $D_1 = D_2 = D_3$?), the F test has a low probability ($F = 0.51, P = 0.612$), indicating that the sharing of parameters did not significantly increase the residual variance. The residual variance was significantly increased in Fit 3 ($F = 36.19, P = 0$), denoting that all three curves did not have the same slope. In Fit 4, the residual variance was not increased significantly ($F = 0.58; P = 0.638$), indicating that curves 2 and 3 have similar slopes.

An examination of the same portions of ALLFIT's output for Fit 5 suggests that curves 2 and 3 contribute disproportionately to the residual variance. The runs test for curve 1 denotes a "poor" fit while the fits for curves 2 and 3 are "bad." Thus, the data in the sum of squares table are used to judge how well each curve is fit and the data in the extra sum of squares tests are used to judge whether specific parameters are statistically similar (i.e., can be shared) among curves.

ALLFIT also has several other features. Individual parameters can be set to specific values (i.e., "fixed" or held constant at a particular value). The program can accept initial estimates from the user for each parameter of each curve. ALLFIT is also designed to perform a weighted regression analysis using Eq. (4.1) to assign weights. In fact, the data analyzed in Fig. 4.8 and Table 4.3 were performed using Eq. (4.2) to predict variances.

As with tests of parallelism, curves which are congruent (have similar parameters A, B, and D) are equidistant. The assignment of a potency estimate or relative potency is straightforward. With curves which are not completely congruent, the assignment of a potency estimate or relative potency is more difficult. The procedure used by ALLFIT is to use parameter C (midpoint dose) of each curve and to calculate the standard error of each relative potency on the basis of shared parameters. Thus, one should be aware of this situation when examining the relative potencies provided by ALLFIT. The best estimates of relative potencies are usually obtained from the fit with maximum number of shared parameters which does not significantly increase the residual variance.

4.2.3. Tests of Similarity for RIAs Analyzed by Alternative Data Reduction Schemes

Tests of similarity for RIAs analyzed by other data reduction methods generally fall under the two classes listed above: those in which a large portion of the dose–response curve is linear, and those with nonlinear dose–response curves. For methods which can be truncated to linear segments, classical tests of parallelism are the preferred method. For RIAs analyzed by nonlinear methods other than four parameter logistic curve fitting, tests of similarity can be performed with FLEXIFIT (16, 17) (discussed in detail later). Theoretically, tests of similarity could be performed by Scatchard analysis (14). However, there are both theoretical and practical objections to performing these tests in Scatchard coordinates. Ideally, rigorous tests of cross reactivity should be performed using LIGAND (14) or a similar computer program. LIGAND fits data to binding isotherms using an algorithm similar to the four parameter logistic and then uses the curves to derive estimates for the affinity constant(s) and binding capacity(ies). Cross reactivities could then be assigned on the basis of affinity constants. From a practical perspective, it is more important to recognize which compounds cross react in the immunoassay, and to what degree, than it is to define precisely how they interact with the antibody. Although LIGAND could be used to characterize immunoassay cross reactivity, it would be difficult to assess matrix effects using this program.

4.2.4. What Constitutes Similarity and Dissimilarity in an IMA?

In order to delineate procedures for tests of similarity, it is important to define what similarity means in the case of an IMA. A brief history concerning the evolution of IMAs is in order. Most of the early IMAs (actually immunoradiometric assays) were not implemented with large excesses of antibodies. Hence, the curves generated were sigmoidal in nature. In fact, early IMAs stimulated the development of nonlinear algorithms for immunoassay data reduction (for example, see Rodbard and Hutt (4)). As the reagents used in IMAs have been improved and become more plentiful, the tendency has been to use a large excess of antibodies. Under these conditions, the low-dose region of the dose–response curve is nearly linear (3). Hence, the trend has been to use empirical methods for data reduction. Nonetheless, it is important to remember that an upward-sloping sigmoidal curve is obtained when the full range of doses is examined in an IMA (and the IMA is performed as a two-step procedure to prevent high-dose hook effects (18)).

To demonstrate what constitutes similarity and dissimilarity in an IMA, consider Fig. 4.9, which illustrates an hTSH IMA (Nichols Institute Diagnostics, San Juan Capistrano, CA). The product insert distributed with this kit recommends that the data be analyzed by linear regression in log–log coordinates. Hence, the standard curve has been graphed accordingly. The three dashed lines illustrate three unknown

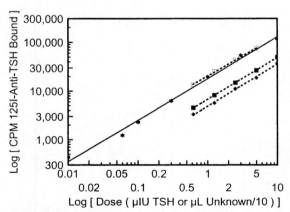

FIGURE 4.9 Definition of the condition of similarity when data from an IMA are graphed in a log–log coordinate system (i.e., fit to a power function). Three unknown samples were assayed at multiple volumes (dashed lines) in a human TSH IMA (Nichols Institute Diagnostics, San Juan Capistrano, CA). The volume of sample assayed was divided by 10 to facilitate illustration on the same dose scale.

samples which were assayed at multiple volumes to assess "parallelism." (Responses for unknowns were extrapolated on the basis of the concentrations provided in the product insert.) Note that all three samples yield dose–response curves parallel to the standard analyte with their positions determined by the amount of analyte present in the sample. Thus, one definition of similarity in an IMA is parallelism when the data are graphed in log–log coordinates.

Linear regression in log–log coordinates and using a power function (6) are exactly the same procedure. Although the dose–response relationship is adequately described by linear regression in log–log coordinates ($r^2 = 0.993$), evidence for a sigmoidal or logistic shape is still apparent after the transformations (carefully examine how the points are distributed around the line in Fig. 4.9).

A common practice is to graph data from an IMA in linear–linear coordinates. If the same data illustrated in Fig. 4.9 are regraphed in linear–linear coordinates (Fig. 4.10), the three lines for unknowns are not parallel to the standard; rather, an array of lines intersecting at the response of the zero standard is obtained. Obviously, one cannot test for similarity in an IMA analyzed in linear–linear coordinates using a test for parallelism. Thus, another definition of similarity is that an unknown should generate a curve or a line which intersects at the response of the zero standard. Note that the dose range in the Nichols' TSH IMA is sufficiently broad that there is a significant deviation from linearity above a dose of 3 μIU. This deviation from linearity would preclude statistical tests based on linear regression, if the data were extended beyond the 3 μIU dose,

As discussed in detail above, many RIA data reduction schemes use log transformation of the dose scale. If the same data illustrated in Figs. 4.9 and 4.10 are graphed in linear–log coordinates (Fig. 4.11), the resultant curves are upward-sloping rectangular hyperbolas. In fact, the resultant curves are the lower portions of sigmoidal or logistic curves. Thus, a third definition of similarity is that the unknown should generate a curve of the same wave form as the standard when graphed in linear–log coordinates.

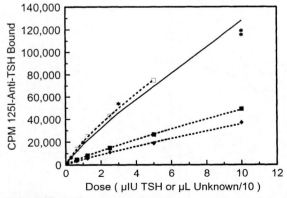

FIGURE 4.10 Definition of the condition of similarity when data from an IMA are graphed in a linear–linear coordinate system (same data as Fig. 4.9). Three unknown samples were assayed at multiple volumes (dashed lines). The volume of sample assayed was divided by 10 to facilitate illustration on the same dose scale. Note that the lines which describe the unknowns intersect with the standard curve at zero dose.

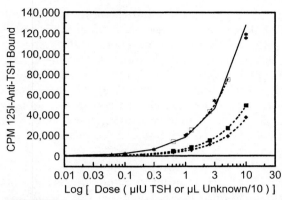

FIGURE 4.11 Definition of the condition of similarity when data from an IMA are graphed in a linear–log coordinate system (same data as Figs. 4.9 and 4.10). Three unknown samples were assayed at multiple volumes (dashed lines). The volume of sample assayed was divided by 10 to facilitate illustration on the same dose scale. Note that the lines which describe the unknowns are the lower portion of logistic curves.

What constitutes dissimilarity in an IMA? Unknowns which generate lines not parallel to the standard analyte, when graphed in a log–log coordinate system, exhibit dissimilarity. Unknowns which generate lines that do not intersect at the response at zero dose are dissimilar. Unknowns which do not generate a curve of the same shape when graphed in linear–log coordinates exhibit dissimilarity. It turns out that there is essentially no difference in the definitions of similarity and dissimilarity between IMAs and RIAs. The general definition of dissimilarity in both cases is failure to generate a curve of the same shape as (i.e., congruent) the standard analyte.

Nonetheless, tests for similarity in an IMA represent a special case because less than the full dose–response curve is typically available for analysis. The procedures for testing similarity in IMAs then become contingent upon the portion of the dose–response curve which is available for analysis, and the coordinate system used for data reduction. It is possible to perform tests for similarity in each of the coordinate systems illustrated in Figs. 4.9–4.11, if one understands what constitutes similarity and dissimilarity in that particular coordinate system.

4.2.5. IMAs Analyzed by Linear Regression

Intuitively, it would seem that tests of similarity for IMAs analyzed in linear–linear coordinate systems (for example, Fig. 4.10) would be straightforward. Depending on one's perspective, that is or is not the case. This section will cover both linear–linear and log–log coordinates because a portion of the resulting dose–response relationships in both cases can be truncated to a segment which can be analyzed by linear regression. First, consider log–log regression (i.e., fitting a power function). On first examination, it may seem rather strange to take the log of the responses. However, in the case of an IMA implemented with a large excess of detection antibody, the range of responses can extend over several orders of magnitude. Taking the logs of the responses obviates the nonhomogeneity of variances that is typically present in data which encompass broad ranges. A general strategy in statistics is to apply log transformations to eliminate nonhomogeneity of variances. Thus, analyzing log responses results in a more uniform response variable for statistical analyses. Nonetheless, this statement must be partially qualified—it applies in IMAs using radioisotopic, fluorescence, and chemiluminescence detection systems which, in essence, measure large numbers of discrete events. Log transformations of responses for enzyme-based detection systems are not recommended.

In RIAs, the conventional strategy for assessing similarity is to assay an unknown at various volumes. This strategy is also recommended for test of similarity in an IMA. Tests of similarity for an IMA analyzed in log–log coordinate systems are classical tests of parallelism (Figs. 4.7 and 4.9) and use the procedures previously outlined for tests of parallelism.

Now consider IMAs analyzed in linear–linear coordinates (Fig. 4.12). The hCG standard curve was truncated at 200 mIU in order to obtain a segment which could be analyzed by linear regression without a major deviation from linearity. As stated previously, the appropriate test of similarity in this context is intersection at zero dose. Theoretically, the two regression lines could be fit independently and examined for overlap at the Y intercept. From a statistical perspective, there is a much more powerful approach. The appropriate test of similarity for IMA data expressed in linear–linear coordinates is performed exactly as outlined by Finney for a Slope ratio bioassay (11).

The statistical model for a slope ratio assay is

$$Y = a + b_s * X + b_u * X, \qquad (4.6)$$

where Y is the response, X is the dose, and b_s and b_u are the slopes for the standard and unknown, respectively. The concept used in the analysis is similar to those presented previously. The two regression lines are fit simultaneously allowing each to have its own intercept. Then the two regression lines are fit simultaneously, forcing them to have a common intercept. An F test is used to determine if the difference in variances is significant. The relative potency in a slope ratio assay is the ratio of slopes (11):

$$\text{Relative Potency} = b_u/b_s. \qquad (4.7)$$

Equations for deriving the variance and confidence limits for the relative potency

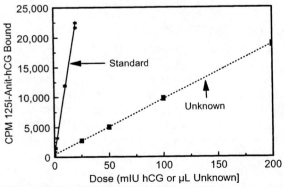

FIGURE 4.12   Definition of the condition of similarity for an IMA graphed in a linear–linear coordinate system and analyzed by linear regression. The statistical analysis for similarity is analogous to a slope ratio assay (11).

are also given by Finney (11). The calculations employ procedures used in multiple linear regression, as well as analysis of variance, and are rather involved for someone not familiar with these procedures. Unfortunately, Finney (11) does not provide a step by step protocol, The implicit assumption Finney makes is that the user thoroughly understands statistical calculations.

The end result of the analysis of the data in Fig. 4.12 as a slope ratio assay is presented in Table 4.4. The mean sums of squares (variances) for regressions and between doses are not calculated because they are assumed to be highly significant. The key points in the statistical analysis are F tests of whether the variances (mean sum of squares) for the zero standards, intersection, and curvature are significantly greater than variance within doses (i.e., the error term). In this case, none of the three F values reaches statistical significance at the 5% probability level. Thus, the conclusion is that the two lines have a common intersection and that the zero standards are an appropriate description of the point of intersection. Only the F test for curvature approaches statistical significance but, as discussed previously, the dose–response relationship in an IMA is not linear. For the data presented in Fig. 4.12, a relative potency of 0.0841 ± 0.0025 was obtained. This translates to a concentration of 0.0841 mIU/μl or 84.1 mIU/ml.

4.2.6. IMAs Analyzed by Nonlinear Curve Fitting

If the complete IMA dose–response curve is available, an analysis based on logistic curve fitting is recommended. Either ALLFIT (15) or FLEXIFIT (16, 17) could be used. FLEXIFIT would be the preferable program if there is asymmetry in the logistic curve. When less than the full dose–response curve is available (i.e., the typical situation; for example, see Fig. 4.13), the analysis is more challenging.

The original papers which describe FLEXIFIT (16, 17) state that it is "model-free" and can be used to fit curves of any shape. If this is true, FLEXIFIT should be ideally suited to perform tests of similarity for IMAs. The general philosophy used by FLEXIFIT is to use cubic spline fitting with some constraints. The constraints then allow estimates of residual variance to be calculated and for tests of goodness of fit (by testing for "runs") to be performed. The algorithm used by FLEXIFIT is to normalize the data to a user-specified template curve and then

TABLE 4.4 **Test of Similarity in an IMA Using Analysis of Variance of a Slope Ratio Assay**

Source of variation	df	Sum of squares	Mean squares	F
Regression	2	1091.4068		
Zero standards	1	0.0822	0.08220	1.781
Intersection	1	0.0063	0.00630	0.136
Curvature	6	0.7571	0.12618	2.734
Between doses	9	1092.2525		
Error (within doses)	10	0.4616	0.04616	
Total	19	1092.7141		

Note. All responses were divided by 1000 to facilitate the calculations.

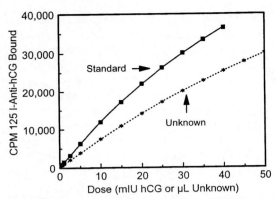

FIGURE 4.13 A test for similarity for an IMA graphed in linear–linear coordinates and analyzed by nonlinear curve fitting. The data for the standards are those obtained in an IMA but the line for the unknown is a hypothetical line which illustrates a relative potency of 0.6. Attempts to analyze these data with FLEXIFIT (16,17) without log transformation of doses were unsuccessful.

make judgments about the shape of the curves relative to the template. The program has a built-in template for logistic curve fitting. With some effort, the procedures for fitting a logistic curve can be gleaned from the documentation. Unfortunately, the documentation does not deal with curves of other shapes or provide any information about how to provide an appropriate template. In addition, there is the issue of "percent smoothing." The documentation states that the degree of smoothing must be set between 0 and 100%, and determines how closely the data are fit to the cubic splines. Minimal guidelines concerning what degree of smoothing should be specified for individual applications are provided. Initially, the one may assume that the statement "fit curves of any shape" means "in any coordinate system." On further examination, that does not appear to be the case. Either implicitly or explicitly, FLEXIFIT expects doses to be log transformed. The point is, if the documentation was more detailed and explicit and/or the program provided a large series of model templates, FLEXIFIT could be an extremely powerful tool. At present, these limitations impede its operation.

Nonetheless, FLEXIFIT can be used to perform tests of similarity for IMAs analyzed by nonlinear curve fitting. Consider the data illustrated in Fig. 4.13. The data are in part real and in part hypothetical. Additional points were added to the standard curve by fitting a parabolic relationship to the real data points and filling in intermediate values. The unknowns were derived assuming that an unknown with a concentration of 600 mIU/ml was assayed at various volumes. This is a high concentration but was chosen so the two curves could be illustrated on the same scale. This concentration translates to a relative potency of 0.6 if the volumes are entered in microliters. Responses for the hypothetical unknown curve were back-calculated by multiplying concentrations by volumes to obtain doses and converting doses to responses using the best fit parabolic regression equation. The combined real–hypothetical data set was constructed because none of the real data sets available had sufficient data points for an unknown to be fit by the methods outlined below. Thus, the first recommendation for using FLEXIFIT is to provide many data points. This is a circumstance where data points, distributed over a broad linear scale (in contrast to a strict Log scale), can be used.

The analysis of the data illustrated in Fig. 4.13 proceeded as follows. A data file was constructed as outlined for ALLFIT. In order to give the program minimal constraints, no restrictions and minimal suggestions were specified in initial attempts. This included not requesting log transformation of doses and specifying only 50% smoothing. With these inputs, either the program failed to reach a fit or the fit obtained was not very good. The parameter estimates were not very meaningful. The conclusion from these attempts was that log transformation of doses was obligatory. Hence, log transformation was specified in subsequent attempts. The shape of the curves, after log transformation of doses, is analogous to the bottom portion of a logistic curve (i.e., similar to the data illustrated in Fig. 4.11). Subsequent attempts to reach a fit after log transformation of doses was also unsuccessful unless the logistic template was specified. Thus, if the program was instructed to view the data as the bottom portion of a logistic curve, it could achieve an appropriate solution. The curves in Figs. 4.13 are the best fit lines provided by FLEXIFIT.

How was the fitting of curves accomplished? First, the dose scale was log transformed. Then, a logistic transformation formula was specified ("BLTIN3"). Finally, smoothing was set at 95% (whether this was optimal remains to be determined) during the analysis. FLEXIFIT uses four parameters (A, B, C, and D) to describe curves. These parameters have similar meanings to the four parameters used by ALLFIT except for parameter C. In FLEXIFIT, parameter C is the midpoint on a Log scale. A is the response at infinite dose, B is the slope factor, and D is the response at zero dose. Under these conditions, the template curve is set at $A = 3.6 \times 10^6$, $B = 1$, $C = 0$, and $D = 0$. This can be viewed as an upward sigmoidal curve whose asymptotes are 0 and 3.6×10^6, a slope of 1, and a position of 1 on a log scale ($\log 1 = 0$). Thus, FLEXIFIT fits each curve by normalizing the endpoints of each curve to these values. In the first fit (Fit 1), no sharing of parameters was specified. In subsequent fits, parameter sharing was specified in the sequence D, A, B, and C. Fit 2: $D_2 = D_1$; Fit 3: $D_2 = D_1$ and $A_2 = A_1$; Fit 4: $D_2 = D_1$, $A_2 = A_1$, and $B_2 = B_1$; Fit 5: $D_2 = D_1$, $A_2 = A_1$, $B_2 = B_1$ and $C_2 = C_1$. If FLEXIFIT works as it should, the sharing of parameters up to the last fit should not significantly increase the residual variance (because the curves were constructed to be identical except in potency). The relative potencies obtained were: Fit 1, 0.46 ± 0.04; Fit 2, 0.49 ± 0.04; Fit 3 = 0.60 ± 0.04; and Fit 4 = 0.60 ± 0.03. (Fit 5 was specified as 1.0.) Thus, the program ultimately achieved the correct solution. The version used (designated 2.1) did not perform the extra sum of squares test. However, the mean squares for an unweighted analysis was between 3.3 and 4.5×10^3 until Fit 5, when it reached a value of 1.4×10^7. Thus, a visual examination of these values suggests that there was no significant increase in residual variance until the curves were forced to share a common position. The alternative strategy of fixing parameter A (response at infinite dose) at the amount of detection antibody added did not aid FLEXIFIT in reaching a solution.

There are two major points to this discussion: First, FLEXIFIT can be used to analyze IMA analyzed by nonlinear curve fitting, provided the curves are viewed as the lower portion of logistic curves. Second, a more detailed documentation for FLEXIFIT would be helpful. Alternatively, new programs using the constrained cubic spline algorithm of FLEXIFIT but designed to handle data without Log transformation of doses could be developed. Thus, in the future it may be possible to perform tests of similarity using IMA data graphed in linear–linear coordinates (e.g., Fig. 4.13) using nonlinear curve fitting algorithms.

4.2.7. General Recommendations for Performing Tests of Similarity When Using IMAs

The previous section outlined several procedures for performing tests of similarity for IMAs. None of the tests is ideal for all circumstances. The test which should be used for any specified data set is dependent on how much of the dose–response relationship is available for analysis and how familiar one is with statistics and computing. For persons not familiar with computing and statistics, and in circumstances where IMAs are analyzed exclusively by empirical curve fitting routines, the simple tests for similarity using regression are recommended.

5. ALTERNATIVE METHODS FOR DEFINING CROSS REACTIVITY

Over the years a variety of alternative strategies for defining immunoassay cross reactivity have been proposed. Many of these strategies have been discussed by Miller and Valdes (19). Any of these methods can be used to characterize an immunoassay as long as one understands how to perform the calculations and how to interpret the data. Perhaps the most meaningful method of defining cross reactivity was put forth by de Lauzon et al. (20) in 1973. The concept used is relatively simple and straightforward. A standard curve is constructed. One dose on the standard curve is chosen. This dose of standard analyte and increasing amounts of the test substance are assayed. The maximum amount of test substance which does not cause significant displacement from the reference point on the standard curve, then, represents the maximum amount of the test substance which can be present in a sample without causing significant interference with the immunoassay. This concept is illustrated for RIAs in Fig. 4.14.

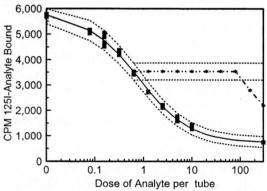

FIGURE 4.14 Alternative strategy for defining cross reactivity in an RIA (20). Increasing amounts of the test substance are assayed in the presence of one dose of the standard analyte (0.625 dose units in this case). The responses of test substances (spiked with the single dose of standard analyte) are graphed according to the dose of test substance. The maximum amount of test analyte (80 dose units in this case) which does not cause a significant decrease in the response is taken as the amount of test analyte which can be present and not interfere with the immunoassay.

6. QUALITY CONTROL

The overall objective of quality assessment procedures is to determine whether the data obtained in any given immunoassay are acceptable and meaningful. The specific objectives of quality control procedures are to recognize when a major systematic error has occurred (e.g., one of the reagents was incorrectly prepared), and to provide an estimate of the precision of the potency estimates for unknowns. Detailed strategies for quality assessment were published as immunoassays came into widespread use (21) and have since been refined (22–25). Quality control may be considered locally (within one assay, between multiple assays, between technicians), as well as globally (between laboratories). Irrespective, the principles remain the same. Information related to a single assay is typically termed intraassay variation, while information related to multiple assays for the same analyte, whether conducted in a single or multiple laboratories, is termed interassay variation.

6.1. Strategies for Quality Control Analyses

In this section we present a general or generic approach to quality control. This approach asks four basic questions: How does the standard curve compare to previous assays? What is the sensitivity of the assay (minimum amount of analyte which can be detected)? What is the precision of the potency estimates? And, How do the potency estimates of unknowns replicate between assays?

This may sound a bit archaic, but our recommendation is to record the quality control data by hand and then perform the statistical aspects of the analysis. Recording the data by hand ensures that someone has examined them and hopefully has thought about what they mean. It has been our experience that subtle changes in assay performance are immediately recognized by trained personnel. Admittedly, quality assessment data could easily be collected and judged by appropriate software. The problem with only using computers to track assay performance is that people have a tendency to accept information from a computer without question.

6.1.1. How Does the Standard Curve Compare to Previous Assays? What Is the Sensitivity of the Assay?

The specific data set used for assessing the reproducibility of standard curves is primarily a function of the type of immunoassay performed (RIA or IMA), as well as the procedures used for data reduction. In general terms, graphical and spline fitting routines, as well as some empirical data reduction schemes, provide relatively little statistical information (3, 6). Semiempirical, linear regression, and curve fitting procedures (3, 6) provide parameters which can be used to track the characteristics of the standard curve over time. Ideally, standard curve parameters should vary by a relatively small amount and should exhibit coefficients of variation of 5 to 10% or less (25). From a more practical perspective, the expected coefficients of variation may be higher if the detection reagent is subject to rapid degradation, such as those prepared with ^{131}I and ^{125}I. If a regression analysis is performed with appropriate weighting, the expected residual variance is unity (1.0). This can serve as another criterion for judging the quality of an assay. The sensitivity of each assay should also be noted. Causes for a marked change in sensitivity should be identified. Ideally, the software used for data reduction should provide a graph of the standard curve in the desired coordinates. If not, the standard curve should be graphed by hand.

In either case, a visual appraisal of the standard curve is recommended. This helps to immediately identify data points which are outliers or those which may have been entered into the calculator or computer erroneously.

As in previous sections, RIAs and IMAs will be taken as prototypic. For purposes of illustrating the extremes in data reduction procedures, RIA data have been analyzed by the four-parameter logistic curve fitting (4–6) while IMAs were analyzed by a simple point to point interpolation (6).

Data from six consecutive hLH RIAs are presented in Table 4.5 (upper portion). The first and second columns identify the particular assay and the amount of detection reagent added, respectively. The third through the eighth columns list the parameters A, B, C, and D from weighted four-parameter logistic curve fitting (4–6), the best fit residual variance, and the percentage of the detection reagent bound at zero dose (B_0/T). Note that the residual variances are near unity, which is what is expected when a weighted analysis is performed (4, 5). The final column in Table 4.5 is the sensitivity of each assay calculated as outlined by Rodbard (1). To track the performance of the assay over time, the mean and standard deviation for each column have been calculated and expressed as a coefficient of variation.

TABLE 4.5   Quality Assessment in Immunoassays: Standard Curve Metameters

Assay	Total cpm added	A (cpm)	B (slope)	C (ED$_{50}$) (ng hLH)	D (cpm)	Res. Var.	B0/T (%)	Sensitivity MDD2* (ng hLH)
				RIAs				
hLH01	16,852	9116	0.83	0.68	957	1.55	51.3	0.014
hLH02	22,076	8335	0.86	0.76	1141	0.94	34.4	0.014
hLH03	19,347	7946	0.81	0.68	959	1.06	38.0	0.011
hLH04	20,013	6999	0.85	0.81	1011	1.02	31.5	0.018
hLH05	14,190	5417	0.84	0.63	763	0.77	34.7	0.013
hLH06	19,892	5752	0.84	0.82	729	1.44	26.2	0.024
Mean	18,728	7261	0.838	0.730	927	1.13	36.0	0.0157
SD	2,782	1470	0.017	0.078	155	0.30	8.5	0.0047
CV(%)	14.9	20.3	2.1	10.7	16.8	26.7	23.5	29.8

Column span note: "Parameters from logistic curve fitting" spans A (cpm), B (slope), C (ED$_{50}$) (ng hLH), D (cpm), Res. Var.

Assay	Added	CV(%)	0	5	25	100	400
			IMAs				
hCG01	138,937	0.9	261	889	3220	11,943	36,517
hCG02	139,769	1.1	258	719	2511	9,545	27,551
hCG03	143,144	1.0	223	733	2519	8,853	27,280
hCG04	140,670	0.3	334	857	2938	10,852	32,838
hCG05	138,667	0.8	261	711	2582	9,519	30,615
hCG06	132,903	0.7	288	672	2410	9,120	25,264
Mean	139,015		271	763	2696	9,972	30,011
SD	3,401		37	88	314	1,185	4,165
CV(%)	2.4		13.7	11.5	11.7	11.9	13.9

Column span note: "Total cpm" spans Added, CV(%); "cpm bound at concentration (mIU/ml)" spans 0, 5, 25, 100, 400.

Note that the coefficients of variation for many of the columns in Table 4.5 are approximately 20% and thus exceed the ideal coefficients of variation of 10% or less (25). Table 4.5 represents assays conducted with a single iodination over about a 1-month period. Hence, the 20% values for the data expressed in cpm as well as the B_o/T (percentage of detection reagent bound) reflect, in part, variation associated with radioactive decay. Also note that parameters B and C (the slope factor and midpoint dose, respectively) have considerably smaller coefficients of variation. Parameters A and D are independent of radioactive decay and hence should exhibit lower coefficients of variation. Theoretically, the observed residual variance and sensitivity should also be independent of the detection reagent. From a more practical perspective, as the radioactivity in the detection reagent decays, the residual variance has a tendency to increase and the sensitivity has a tendency to decrease. Thus, the variation in residual variance and sensitivity also partially reflect degradation of the detection reagent. Nonetheless, the data illustrated in Table 4.5 reveal that the hLH RIA performed consistently over the period examined.

Table 4.5 also illustrates data from a series of hCG IMAs in which point to point interpolation was used for data reduction. This data reduction procedure provides no standard curve parameters which can be tracked over time. Nonetheless, the total cpm added (second column) and the observed coefficient of variation for total cpm (third column) provide important information about the particular assay, including an estimate of pipetting errors. The fourth through eighth columns list the cpm of ^{125}I-anti-hCG bound at various concentrations. An examination of the data presented in Table 4.5 also demonstrates that the hCG IMA is performing consistently over time. Even with the most empirical of data reduction methods, procedures to track reproducibility of the standard curve can be implemented with a little creativity.

If desired, the reproducibility of standard curves and assay sensitivity can be tracked graphically. One option is to construct Levey–Jennings plots (26, 27). For each metameter of standard curve performance, the mean and confidence limits from the previous 10 to 20 assays are calculated. Levey–Jennings plots are constructed by drawing graphs for each metameter with lines that represent the expected mean and its confidence limits. The values obtained in subsequent assays are graphed and values which fall outside the confidence limits are noted. The reference means and confidence limits are updated periodically. One of the primary advantages of Levey–Jennings plots is that they provide a means to recognize a sudden change in a particular characteristic of an immunoassay.

An alternative strategy is to construct cusum plots (26, 27). Cusum plots are particularly suited to identifying trends or changes in one direction. As with Levey–Jennings plots, the mean and standard deviation of previous assays are calculated and used to define target values. The term "cusum" denotes cumulative sum of the differences of serial values. Thus, the cusum is calculated as

$$\text{Cusum} = \sum_{i=1}^{n}(\text{metameter}_i - \text{metameter}_e), \qquad (4.8)$$

where metameter_i and metameter_e are the observed and expected values for a particular assay, respectively. When calculating cusums, it is important to accumulate algebraic sums (i.e., note both the sign and the absolute difference). The concept is that a stable assay will yield cumulative sums of zero—the cusum will fluctuate randomly above and below the line. If the assay is changing consistently in one direction, the line will progress upward or downward. An effective strategy is to use the standard deviation of the expected value to calculate confidence limits. When the cusum exceeds the confidence limits, the assay has changed significantly.

6.1.2. What Is the Estimated Precision of the Potency Estimates?

Two strategies for estimating the precision of the potency estimate for an unknown in a given assay are based on predicted variances in responses and observed precision from a series of quality control samples. Both tactics have desirable features. The ideal strategy is to use a combination of both approaches.

The basic concepts for accumulating information and fitting an equation (for example, Eq. (4.1)) or model (28) to predict the variance of any response have been previously discussed under "Defining Sensitivity Using Statistical Approaches." The predicted variance for any response can then be used to calculate confidence limits for that response and extrapolated to dose (for example, extrapolating the confidence limits for responses to doses in Fig. 4.1). Thus, it is possible to assign confidence limits in units of dose or concentration for any unknown. An excellent way to present this information is to calculate a predicted coefficient of variation for each unknown. Many of Rodbard's computer programs for immunoassay data reduction use this strategy (4, 5). Thus, an estimate of precision is provided for each unknown. If desired, the estimate of precision can be refined by taking into consideration the number of replicates assayed for a given unknown, using the same rationale as outlined in "Defining Sensitivity using Statistical Approaches." If this approach is used to predict confidence limits for unknowns, one aspect of quality control procedures becomes the collection of data which can be used to periodically update the equations used to predict variances in responses.

Intuitively, it might seem that a coefficient of variation of 4% for responses would translate to a coefficient of variation of 4% for doses. That, however, is not the case. Consider Fig. 4.1 which illustrates an RIA standard curve and the 95% confidence limits for responses around the best fit curve. An appropriate method to derive an estimate of precision in dose units is to convert the upper and lower confidence limits for responses by extrapolating them to doses. The predicted confidence limits for dose are partially dependent on the method used for data reduction. Nonetheless, this is appropriate from a statistical perspective. Figure 4.15 illustrates the observed coefficient of variation in responses, as well as the extrapolated confidence limits, in units of dose, for an RIA analyzed by four-parameter logistic curve fitting. The same data are presented as Table 4.6. In an RIA, the predicted coefficient of variation for doses increases markedly toward each end because of the sigmoidal shape of the standard curve. Predicted confidence limits in dose units for RIAs analyzed by the logit–log method (6) are even wider at the ends of the standard curve. The same phenomenon also occurs in IMAs (Table 4.6), except that the low-dose region is the primary concern. Also note that the predicted coefficients of variation in response and dose units are much more consistent for an IMA.

A second strategy is to incorporate a series of quality control samples into each assay and calculate an intraassay coefficient of variation. Details for performing the calculations are presented in the next section. The assumption, then, becomes that the observed coefficients of variation for the quality control samples and those for any given unknown are analogous.

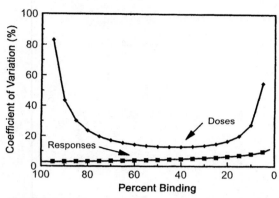

FIGURE 4.15   Relationship of the observed coefficient of variation in responses and predicted coefficient of variation in doses as a function of position on an RIA standard curve. Note that the coefficient of variation in response units increases slightly as the percentage binding decreases. However, the coefficient of variation of doses increases markedly at each end because of the sigmoidal shape of the RIA standard curve.

6.1.3. How Do the Potency Estimates of Unknowns Replicate between Assays?

A procedure for obtaining estimates of precision within and between assays was outlined by Rodbard (22) in 1968. The idea is to construct a series of quality control samples which are assayed in each assay. It is desirable to include multiple sets of quality control samples in large assays. The potency estimates for the quality control samples are then used to calculate intra- and interassay coefficients of variation. The observed intraassay coefficients of variation represent estimates of precision for a given assay, while the observed interassay coefficients of variation serve as estimates of precision between assays, between technicians, and between laboratories. This is one case in which the principles and calculations are the same for RIAs and IMAs.

The assessment of assay precision should be a continual process and should include data from each and every assay performed. Defining intra- and interassay coefficients of variation on the basis of a few carefully chosen (or performed) immunoassays simply will not provide reliable or meaningful estimates of precision.

Care should be exercised in selecting and constructing quality control samples or pools. At least three or four distinct samples should be included in each assay. Furthermore, these samples should be selected or constructed so that they represent different points on the standard curve. An alternative approach is to analyze one carefully chosen sample at three or four different amounts (volumes). For an RIA, these amounts (volumes) of quality control samples would typically be equally spaced on a Log scale. If the immunoassay is working as expected, the potency estimates should double with increasing amounts of sample assayed. Not only can the absolute potency be used as a measure of assay performance, but a quality control sample assayed at multiple volumes serves as an internal test for parallelism or similarity. A third strategy that is particularly popular among the manufacturers of immunoassay kits is to include quality control samples which have a known concentration of analyte. Comparison of the observed potency estimate to the

**TABLE 4.6   Relationship between the Variance in
Responses and Doses**

	RIAs			
	Response		**Dose**	
Percentage binding	**cpm bound**	**CV(%)**	**ng hLH**	**CV(%)**
95	5502	3.1	0.025	83.2
90	5251	3.1	0.060	43.5
85	4999	3.2	0.104	30.1
80	4748	3.3	0.158	23.5
75	4497	3.4	0.223	19.6
70	4245	3.6	0.300	17.1
65	3995	3.7	0.394	15.4
60	3744	3.8	0.508	14.2
55	3492	4.0	0.648	13.4
50	3241	4.2	0.823	12.9
45	2990	4.4	1.045	12.7
40	2739	4.7	1.334	12.7
35	2488	5.0	1.719	12.9
30	2237	5.3	2.256	13.5
25	1986	5.7	3.043	14.6
20	1734	6.3	4.285	16.4
15	1483	7.0	6.486	19.8
10	1232	8.0	11.250	27.2
5	980	9.5	27.376	55.0

	IMAs		
Response		**Dose**	
cpm bound	**CV(%)**	**mIU hCG**	**CV(%)**
261	6.5	0	
889	4.1	0.5	4.9
1,498	3.4	1.0	3.7
3,220	2.6	2.5	2.8
11,943	1.6	10.0	1.9
22,087	1.3	20.0	1.6
36,517	1.1	40.0	1.2

expected value provides a rapid and appropriate confirmation that the particular assay is performed as expected.

The strategy used in the authors' laboratories is to prepare sufficient quantities of quality control samples for 100 to 200 assays. The quality control pools consist of sets of multiple samples representing varying amounts of analyte. The samples are then aliquoted and frozen. A set of quality control samples is thawed, used in a single assay, and discarded. As one batch of quality control pools becomes depleted, a new batch is prepared. As the transition is made from one batch to the next, both sets of quality control samples are included in multiple assays so that they overlap. The matrix of quality control samples (serum, plasma, etc.) is chosen to correspond to the matrix of the unknowns. From a more general perspective, it is important that the analyte be stable under the conditions of storage. It is equally important that the quality control samples not be given preferential treatment so that they indeed are representative of a typical unknown. However, if quality control samples are to be distributed among multiple laboratories, it may be desirable to lyophilize them so that they are as stable as possible with minimal requirements for shipping and storage.

Calculation of an intraassay coefficient of variation can be accomplished using only the data from the series of quality control samples, or by including data from all unknowns assayed in replicate. The only proviso is that the variances must be homogeneous for them to be pooled. As noted above, the predicted coefficient of variation for doses (and hence concentrations) is related to the position on the standard curve (Fig. 4.15). However, most laboratories prefer to report a single intraassay coefficient of variation to keep things simple. In practical terms, this can be accomplished if samples which fall at the extremes of the standard curve are excluded (for example, greater than 80% binding and less than 20% binding in Fig. 4.15). However, all who are provided with this single estimate of intraassay precision should be made aware that it only applies over a specific range of doses or concentrations. A better option is to calculate the observed coefficient of variation for different regions on the curve.

In recent years, computer resources have become plentiful in clinical and research laboratories. Although computer programs specifically designed to calculate intra- and interassay coefficients of variation are available (25), all of the required calculations can be performed using a spreadsheet computer program such as Lotus 1-2-3 or Excel. The subsequent calculations were performed using Lotus 1-2-3. A word of caution: It is important to understand how to use the functions and which functions to use with any specific spreadsheet. For example, Lotus 1-2-3 provides two functions to calculate variances, one for populations and one for samples. The variance function for samples is the appropriate one.

To illustrate the principles used in the calculation of an intraassay coefficient of variation, data from four quality control pools assayed in quadruplicate in a single hLH RIA (hLH01 in Table 4.5) will be used. The mean and variance for each quality control pool or unknown are calculated (Table 4.7). If the variances are homogeneous, they can be pooled over samples. A pooled variance (s_p^2) is calculated as the weighted average of the individual variances (s^2), where the weights are the degrees of freedom (df) associated with each variance:

$$s_p^2 = (\sum_{i=1}^{n}(\mathrm{df}_i * s_i^2))/\sum_{i=1}^{n} \mathrm{df}_i). \tag{4.9}$$

The pooled standard deviation is then calculated by taking the square root of the pooled variance. The pooled mean is calculated by substituting individual means for variances in Eq. (4.9). The intraassay coefficient of variation for a single assay (pooled over samples) is then calculated by dividing the pooled standard deviation by the pooled mean and multiplying the result by 100 (to convert it to a percentage). Using this procedure, a pooled intraassay coefficient of variation of 4.65% was derived for the quality control pools assayed in the RIA designated hLH01.

This same procedure can be extended one step further to calculate a coefficient of variation pooled over samples and pooled over multiple assays (Table 4.8). The

TABLE 4.7 Calculation of the Intraassay Coefficient of Variation for One Assay Pooled over Samples

	Potency estimates: quality control samples			
	1	2	3	4
Mean	10.24	12.59	15.62	18.36
n	4	4	4	4
Variance	0.187	0.562	0.433	0.566
df	3	3	3	3
SD	0.43	0.75	0.66	0.75
CV(%)	4.22	5.95	4.21	4.10

Note. Calculate the pooled variance (S_p^2) using Eq. (4.9). Take the square root to obtain the pooled standard deviation (SD_p): $S_p^2 = 0.437$ (pooled variance); $SD_p = 0.661$ (pooled standard deviation). Calculate the pooled mean (X_p) using Eq. (4.9), substituting individual means for variances: $X_p = 14.20$ (pooled mean). Calculate the pooled coefficient of variation (CV_p) by dividing the pooled SD by the pooled mean ($\times 100$ for percent): $CV_p = 4.65\%$.

variance from each assay, pooled over samples, is pooled over assays (if homogeneous). As above, the pooled variance is calculated and converted to a pooled standard deviation by taking its square root. The pooled mean and coefficient of variation are calculated as outlined previously. The resultant intraassay coefficient of variation, pooled over samples and pooled over assays, for the six hLH RIAs illustrated in Table 4.5 was 8.33%. This means that, on the average, the actual concentration for an unknown sample in a single assay has a 95% probability of

TABLE 4.8 Calculation of the Intraassay Coefficient of Variation Pooled over Multiple Assays

Assay	Pooled variance (S_p^2)	df	Pooled mean (X_p)	Assay CV(%)
hLH01	0.661	12	14.2	5.7
hLH02	2.772	12	13.1	12.7
hLH03	0.812	12	11.7	7.7
hLH04	1.843	12	13.3	10.2
hLH05	0.621	12	12.2	6.5
hLH06	0.437	12	14.2	4.7

Note. Calculate the pooled variance (S_p^2) using Eq. (4.9). In this case, the pooled variance from each assay (calculated as outlined in Table 4.7) is pooled over assays. Take the square root to obtain the pooled standard deviation (SD_p): $S_p^2 = 1.191$ (pooled variance); $SD_p = 1.091$ (pooled standard deviation). Calculate the pooled mean using Eq. (4.9) but substitute individual means for variances: $X_p = 13.10$ (pooled mean). Calculate the intraassay coefficient of variation (CV_p) pooled over assays by dividing the pooled SD by the pooled mean ($\times 100$ for percent): $CV_p = 8.33\%$.

falling within the confidence limits defined on the basis of the observed concentration and a standard deviation of 8.3% of the observed value.

The principles used in calculating interassay coefficients of variation are analogous. The typical strategy is to use the best estimate obtained in each assay for each quality control sample. The best estimate could be the mean of replicate determinations or it could be a weighted average of replicate determinations. The variance between assays for each quality control sample is calculated first (Table 4.9). If the variances are homogeneous, they can be pooled over samples using Eq. (4.9). The pooled mean and coefficient of variation are calculated. When these calculations were performed for the six hLH RIA listed in Table 4.5, a pooled interassay coefficient of variation of 8.5% was obtained (Table 4.9). This means that, on the average, the actual concentration for an unknown sample in any assay has a 95% probability of falling within the confidence limits defined on the basis of the observed concentration and a standard deviation of 8.5% of the observed value.

Excellent target values for intra- and interassay coefficients of variation are 5 and 10%, respectively (26). For assays conducted over long periods of time, intra- and interassay coefficients of variation of 7 and 15% are typical. When intraassay coefficients of variation exceed 10% and interassay coefficients of variation exceed 20%, it is time to identify the source of the variation. As with other aspects of quality assessment, the potency estimates for individual quality control samples can be tracked graphically with Levey–Jennings graphs or cusum plots.

TABLE 4.9 Calculation of the Interassay Coefficient of Variation Pooled over Samples

| | Best potency estimate: quality control sample | | | |
	1	2	3	4
Assay				
hLH01	10.24	12.59	15.62	18.36
hLH02	9.08	11.46	15.59	16.15
hLH03	8.30	10.90	13.05	14.64
hLH04	10.09	11.93	14.75	16.42
hLH05	8.83	11.05	13.43	15.31
hLH06	10.23	12.59	15.60	18.34
Mean	9.5	11.8	14.7	16.5
n	6	6	6	6
Variance	0.70	0.55	1.36	2.37
df	5	5	5	5
SD	0.83	0.74	1.16	1.54
CV(%)	8.81	6.30	7.94	9.31

Note. Calculate the mean and variance for each sample using the best estimate of potency in each assay. Calculate the variance pooled over samples (S_p^2) using Eq. (4.9). Take the square root to obtain the pooled standard deviation (SD$_p$): S_p^2 = 1.24 (pooled variance); SD$_p$ = 1.11 (pooled standard deviation). Calculate the pooled mean (X_p) using Eq. (4.9) but substitute individual means for variances: X_p = 13.11 (pooled mean). Calculate the pooled interassay coefficient of variation (CV$_p$) by dividing the pooled SD by the pooled mean ($\times$100 for percent): CV$_p$ = 8.50%.

7. SUMMARY

This chapter has reviewed procedures for immunoassay validation and quality control. The philosophy we have taken is to present relevant questions and then discuss detailed mathematical and statistical procedures for answering them. The goal is that readers will be able to apply these questions and obtain answers in their specific situation or application. Our perspective has not been to provide a highly theoretical discussion but to present the underlying theory in a manner useful to any person performing immunoassays.

Acknowledgments

We thank Robin Hopper and Rhonda Greiss for their help in preparing this chapter, Drs. David Rodbard and Peter Munson for providing software and helpful discussions, and Dr. Merlyn Nielsen for assistance with the statistical analysis of slope ratio assays.

References

1. Rodbard D. Statistical estimation of the minimal detectable concentration ("sensitivity") for radioligand assays. Anal Biochem 1978; 90:1–12.
2. Ekins R. Immunoassay design and optimisation. In: Price CP, Newman DJ, Eds. Principles and Practice of Immunoassay. New York: Stockton Press, 1991.
3. Grotjan HE, Keel BA. Immunoassay data reduction: Part 1. Basic concepts. In Service Training and Continuing Education, Endo, Am Assoc Clin Chem 1991; 10:7–20.
4. Rodbard D, Hutt DM. Statistical analysis of radioimmunoassays and immunoradiometric (labelled antibody) assays. A generalized weighted, iterative, least-squares method for logistic curve fitting. In: Radioimmunoassay and Related Procedures in Medicine, Vol. I. Vienna: International Atomic Energy Agency, 1974.
5. Grotjan HE Jr, Steinberger E. Radioimmunoassay and bioassay data processing using a logistic curve fitting routing adapted to a desk top computer. Comput Biol Med 1977; 7:159–63
6. Grotjan HE, Keel BA. Immunoassay data reduction: Part 2. Approaches to fitting the standard curve. In Service Training and Continuing Education, Endo, Am Assoc Clin Chem 1991; 10:7–22.
7. Grotjan HE Jr, Heindel JJ, Steinberger E. Prostaglandin inhibition of testosterone production induced by luteinizing hormone, dibutyryl cyclic AMP or 3-isobutyl-1-methyl xanthine in dispersed rat testicular interstitial cells. Steroids 1987; 32:307–22.
8. Stockell-Hartree A, Renwick ACG. Molecular structures of glycoprotein hormones and functions of their carbohydrate components. Biochem J 1992; 287:665–79.
9. Grotjan HE, DesJarials SE, Rand SE. Characterization of human LH isohormones using chromatofocusing. In: Chen WW, Boime I, Eds. Glycoprotein Hormones: Structure, Synthesis and Biologic Function. Norwell, MA: Serono Symposium, 1990.
10. Rodbard D, Lenox RH, Wray LH, Ramseth D. Statistical characterization of the random errors in the radioimmunoassay dose-response variable. Clin Chem 1976; 22:350–358.
11. Finney DJ. Statistical Method in Biological Assay, 3rd ed. New York: Macmillan, 1978.
12. Snedecor GW, Cochran WG. Statistical Methods, 8th ed. Ames: Iowa State University Press, 1989.
13. Rodbard D, Munson PJ, De Lean A. Improved curve-fitting, parallelism testing, characterization of sensitivity and specificity, validation and optimization for radioligand assays. In: Radioimmunoassay and Related Procedures in Medicine, Vol. I. Vienna: International Atomic Energy Agency, 1978.
14. Rodbard D, Munson PJ. LIGAND: A versatile computerized approach for characterization of ligand-binding systems. Anal Biochem 1980; 107:220–39.
15. De Lean A, Munson PJ, Rodbard D. Simultaneous analysis of families of sigmoidal curves: Application to bioassay, radioligand assay and physiological dose-response curves. Am J Physiol 1978; 235:E97–102.
16. Guardabasso V, Rodbard D, Munson PJ. A model-free approach to estimation of relative potency in dose-response curve analysis. Am J Physiol 1987; 252:E357–64.
17. Guardabasso V, Munson PJ, Rodbard D. A versatile method for simultaneous analysis of families of curves. FASEB J 1988; 2:209–15.

18. Zweig MH, Csako G. High-dose hook effect in a two-site IRMA for measuring thyrotropin. Ann Clin Biochem 1990; 27:494–5.
19. Miller JJ, Valdes R. Methods for calculating crossreactivity in immunoassays. J Clin Immunoassay 1992; 15:97–107.
20. de Lauzon S, Cittanova N, Desfosses B, Jayle MF. A new approach for quantitative evaluation of cross-reactivity of steroids with an antiserum by radioimmunoassay: Application to a high specific antiestriol. Steroids 1973; 22:747–61.
21. Rodbard D, Rayford PL, Cooper JA, Ross GT. Statistical quality control of radioimmunoassay. J Clin Endocrinol Metab 1978; 28:1412–8.
22. Rodbard D. Statistical quality control and routine data processing for radioimmunoassays and immunoradiometric assays. Clin Chem 1974; 20:1255–70.
23. McDonagh BF, Munson PJ, Rodbard D. A computerized approach to statistical quality control for radioimmunoassays in the clinical chemistry laboratory. Comput Prog Biomed 1977; 7:179–90.
24. Munson PJ, Rodbard D. An elementary components of variance analysis for multi-centre quality control. In: Radioimmunoassay and Related Procedures in Medicine, Vol. II. Vienna: International Atomic Energy Agency, 1978.
25. Thakur AK. Statistical methods for serum hormone assays. In: Keel BA, Webster BW, Eds. CRC Handbook of the Laboratory Diagnosis and Treatment of Infertility. Boca Raton, FL: CRC Press, 1990.
26. Mosley J. Quality control in hormonal assays. In: Penningtion GW, Naik S, Eds. Hormone Analysis: Methodology and Clinical Interpretation, Vol I. Boca Raton, FL: CRC Press, 1981.
27. Chard T. An Introduction to Radioimmunoassay and Related Techniques, Amsterdam/New York: Elsevier, 1987.
28. Sadler WA, Smith MH. Use and abuse of imprecision profiles: Some pitfalls illustrated by computing and plotting confidence intervals. Clin Chem 1990; 36:1346–50.

5 | PRODUCTION AND PURIFICATION OF ANTIBODIES

AILSA M. CAMPBELL
University of Glasgow
United Kingdom

Immunoassay

1. INTRODUCTION

The main requirement for immunoassays is an antibody preparation that has a standard, reproducible, specific, and high-affinity interaction with the analyte under assay. Additional desirable qualities include stability in storage and the capacity for production in large amounts. Finally, because many immunoassays require that the antibody be labeled, it should be possible to readily purify it of all contaminating material in a small number of simple steps. In this chapter, strategies designed to achieve these goals are discussed.

2. POLYCLONAL VERSUS MONOCLONAL ANTIBODIES

Polyclonal antibody production results from the classical immune response of an animal to an injected antigen. The animal is immunized and bled and the resultant antiserum is used as a reagent. The antiserum can be absorbed to remove antibodies that react with irrelevant material, and its IgG fraction can be purified. Even then, a pure preparation of IgG made from antiserum carries a mixture of several hundred different antibodies.

In monoclonal antibody (MAB) production, the short-lived B lymphocytes from the spleen are individually immortalized by fusion with an immortal myeloma cell line to give a range of clones of B lymphocytes (hybridomas), each producing its own antibody. The most appropriate clones are then selected and expanded in tissue culture (1). A comparison is shown in Fig. 5.1.

Polyclonal antiserum reacts with several epitopes on the antigen and includes antibodies with the capacity to make high- and low-affinity contacts. The antibodies themselves will be of various classes and subclasses and will include a substantial amount of the IgM class. Each time the animal is exposed to the antigen, it makes a variety of antibodies, some useful and some less so. In addition, unless the animal is kept under sterile conditions, its immune response is frequently diverted by routine infections, so that any preparation of antiserum contains a wide variety of irrelevant antibodies. In monoclonal antibody production, the lymphocyte producing a single antibody that reacts with a single epitope and is of a defined class (IgG) and subclass is selected, immortalized, and expanded in tissue culture.

The cooperative effects of two monoclonal antibodies on different epitopes is illustrated in Fig. 5.2. The differences in the properties of monoclonal and polyclonal antibodies are given in Table 5.1.

It is evident from Table 5.1 that a monoclonal antibody, properly selected, is the preferable reagent since it is standard and eternal. However, its development cost is always greater than that of the polyclonal. In an established laboratory, the cost of developing a MAB to a simple antigen can be quite low. However, the development of one to a complex antigen—for example, one requiring human monoclonal antibody technology—requires salaries and consumables for two highly trained technicians over a period of 12—18 months. The production costs of monoclonals are also higher, in that large-scale sterile tissue culture is required.

In consequence, the usual approach is to test the immunoassay system for any new animal on a polyclonal system using a few rabbits. Only when this has shown potential is it advisable to move to the monoclonal system. Monoclonal systems are inherently different in that they are an artifact created by the scientist and do

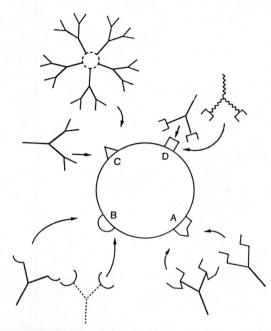

FIGURE 5.1   The reaction of polyclonal antiserum with antigen. At epitope A are two antibodies of the same class but different specificities and affinities. At epitope B are two antibodies of different subclass, specificity, and affinity. At epitope C are two antibodies of different class, one being an IgM, but of the same specificity and affinity (this is rare: IgM antibodies are usually of lower affinity). At determinant D are two antibodies of different subclass but of the same specificity and affinity. In polyclonal serum, the proportions of all these antibodies will vary with each animal and bleed. In monoclonal antibody technology, each can be independently immortalized (Reprinted from A. M. Campbell, Monoclonal antibody and immunoassay technology, 1991, with kind permission from Elsevier Science—NL, Sara Burgerhartstraat 25, 1055 KV Amsterdam, The Netherlands.)

not represent the normal immune response. Thus, they do not precipitate the antigen unless it carries multiple identical epitopes. They also lack the additivity of binding affinity conferred by two different antibodies creating a higher affinity bond than any one alone. This is known as the "bonus effect." Therefore, for small molecules in particular, the primary advantages of moving to monoclonal reagents are that they are standard and eternal.

Monoclonal antibodies can also be overspecific and not detect variants, particularly in viral infections (see Fig. 5.3). All of these defects can be corrected by the creation of a panel of monoclonal antibodies which, intelligently combined, give the required equivalent to a polyclonal response and at the same time are under the control of the clinical scientist and not subject to the vagaries of the immune system of the experimental animal.

3. CHOICE OF ANIMAL

3.1. Ethical and Legal Considerations

The production of antiserum or antibodies is generally classified as an experiment on an animal, and such work is tightly controlled in all developed countries. Animals

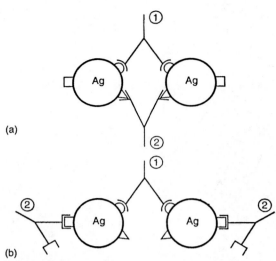

(a)

(b)

FIGURE 5.2   Cooperative effects of two monoclonal antibodies to different epitopes. This occurs particularly in solution type assays. In (a) the geometry of each MAB–antigen complex is such that the two MABs can act cooperatively, stabilizing the binding of each other. As a result, the two MABs together have a higher affinity than would be expected from a mixture. In (b) the position of the epitopes is such that cooperative binding does not occur (Reprinted from A. M. Campbell, Monoclonal antibody and immunoassay technology, 1991, with kind permission from Elsevier Science—NL, Sara Burgerhartstraat 25, 1055 KV Amsterdam, The Netherlands.)

must be housed in specified areas with precise conditions of space, warmth, and light, and each "experiment" on each animal must be documented in detail from first immunization to final bleed (2). Any incoming animals must be quarantined. Most large institutions have a veterinary adviser who monitors the animals' welfare and provides advice on the acceptability of the procedures involved in the production of any new antibody. Information on more precise animal handling can be found in detailed texts (3, 4).

In many countries where public concern about animal rights is increasing and groups campaigning against research on animals are active, strict licensing requirements have been imposed for laboratory workers who use animals. In the United

TABLE 5.1   Comparison of the Main Features of Polyclonal and Monoclonal Antibodies

	Polyclonal antiserum	Monoclonal antibody
How standard?	Variable with animal and bleed	Standard
How specific?	Variable	Specific if selected to be so
What affinity?	Variable	High affinity if selected to be so
How reproducible	Variable	Reproducible
How much available?	Depends on size of animal and its lifetime	As much as is required for as long as it is required
What development cost?	Purchase of animal plus antigen	$1000–50,000
What production cost for 1000 assays?	Maintenance of animal	$1000–2000

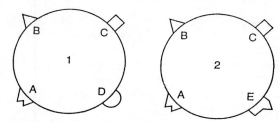

FIGURE 5.3   A single monoclonal antibody may be too specific. Antigens 1 and 2 are largely similar but differ in epitopes D and E. Polyclonal serum will crossreact extensively between the two, and MABs to A, B, and C will crossreact 100%. However, MABs to D and E will not recognize both antigens (Reprinted from A. M. Campbell, Monoclonal antibody and immunoassay technology, 1991, with kind permission from Elsevier Science—NL, Sara Burgerhartstraat 25, 1055 KV Amsterdam, The Netherlands.)

Kingdom, for example, under the Animals (Scientific Procedures) Act of 1986, each person who handles animals must have both a personal license and a series of project licenses covering the procedures to be undertaken. The animal, route of injection, method of killing, and so on must be specified in detail. Legislation varies among countries. For example, in Germany the production of ascites fluid is generally not permitted.

3.2. The Use of Humans

Almost all immunoassays involve material taken from human subjects. In addition, sometimes immunoassays (such as those for HIV) involve the measurement not of the antigen, but of the antibody response to it. As with animals, research with human subjects is subject to ethical and legal guidelines—particularly in the handling of material—which are designed to protect both the patient and the laboratory scientist. These should be consulted before any new procedure is initiated (5, 6).

3.3. Sex and Age of Animal

The sex of the animal is irrelevant except in the case of animals that share cages, usually mice. Male mice are more aggressive and tend to injure one another, which can lead to opportunistic infections that divert the immune response. Older animals generally have a poorer response to injected antigens because their immune system has been engaged by so many other environmental antigens that their capacity to respond to new ones is limited. Thus, in the case of rabbits, it is preferable to start with healthy ones under 6 months of age, and in the case of mice, to start with females or single caged males under 3 months of age.

3.4. Animals Suitable for the Generation of Polyclonal Antiserum

Suitable animals generally are rabbits, sheep, goats, and donkeys, the most common by far being rabbits due to the simplicity and low cost of their maintenance. Because of the complexity and expense of housing large experimental animals, they generally are used only for production of secondary antibodies (e.g., donkey anti-rabbit IgG and sheep anti-mouse IgG) that can be used for a variety of analytes. Large animals are seldom used to generate antiserum directed solely to the precise analyte under test.

All of these animals, including rabbits, are genetically outbred with respect to their major histocompatibility (MHC) antigens and other immune response genes. This means that any two rabbits, albeit from the same strain and same colony, are likely to respond differently to the same antigen. In essence, the amount of essential "help" given by the CD4 T helper cells of the animal will depend on its capacity to "present" peptides derived from the foreign antigen (or the carrier) in the groove of its Class II MHC molecules to such cells (7) (see Fig. 5.4.). Consequently, it is advisable to use a minimum of two and preferably four animals for each antigen. In addition, because the background response of each animal is highly variable, it is necessary to take a bleed of preimmune serum from each animal before proceeding with immunization.

3.5. Animals Suitable for the Generation of Monoclonal Antibodies

There are only three main systems used for classical monoclonal antibody production: mouse, rat, and human (1). It is not possible to make hybridomas from outbred animals such as rabbits, sheep, and goats, as suitable myeloma lines are not readily generated in these animals. Human hybridomas can be further subdivided into chimeric ones reconstructed to humanize the immune responses of rodent MABs by the use of recombinant DNA technology, and "genuine" human MABs which immortalize the natural human immune response. (See Chapter 6.)

The original mouse system developed by Kohler and Milstein (8) is the most widely used since it yields more clones. It also carries no patent restrictions, which is a relevant consideration of most laboratories with restricted budgets. The Balb/c mouse is the animal of choice since it is the only strain compatible with the myeloma lines available for fusion. Unlike outbred animals, all Balb/c mice respond identically to antigen (provided it is administered identically). If this strain is a poor responder to the antigen under test, it is possible to use other strains of mice since these fuse well with the myeloma strains derived from Balb/c. If rat fusions are essential, the most appropriate host is the Lou rat (named for Louvain, a city in Belgium). Technically, the cell lines of the mouse, but not the rat, will also fuse

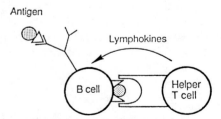

Antigen

Lymphokines

B cell

Helper T cell

FIGURE 5.4 An antigen-presenting cell. A B cell recognizes one epitope on antigen, internalizes it, and "presents" another epitope to T cells in the groove of MHC class II molecules. In this case, a B lymphocyte presents different peptide sequences from those recognized by antibodies to acquire essential T cell help (Reprinted from A. M. Campbell, Monoclonal antibody and immunoassay technology, 1991, with kind permission from Elsevier Science—NL, Sara Burgerhartstraat 25, 1055 KV Amsterdam, The Netherlands.)

productively with B lymphocytes from the Syrian (also called Armenian) hamster or the guinea pig; however, such a strategy adds considerably to production costs.

4. IMMUNIZATION PROCEDURES

4.1. The Natural B Cell Response

The natural B cell response is generated by regular challenge with diverse extracellular antigens in the environment. These invade nonsterile areas such as the gastrointestinal tract and occasionally, by tissue damage, the bloodstream. Each new challenge generates a new low-affinity IgM response. This will only mature to a high-affinity IgG response on continued challenge. This maturation is essential to create memory. If the animal subsequently encounters the same antigen, mature memory B lymphocytes will be stimulated to much faster action. To mimic this, it is therefore necessary to give the animal a minimum of two injections of antigen separated in time by at least 10 days. If the response is suitable, the immunological memory of the animal can be called up thereafter by a small amount of antigen (see Fig. 5.5).

4.2. The Size of the Antigen

All natural B cell antigens are large, and therefore the antigen should always be presented to the immune system in that context. Thus, small molecules must be presented as haptens cross-linked to a foreign carrier protein. The carrier is usually an inexpensive protein available in large amounts, such as bovine serum albumin (except for use in cattle), ovalbumin, or keyhole limpet hemocyanin (KLH), which is large and very foreign to all species used for antibody production. Cross-linking can be done by use of the amino, carboxyl, hydroxyl, or sulfydryl groups, the operative rule being that the part of the molecule that is regarded as unique for the assay is not involved. Classical methods of cross-linking work well for most antigens (9), but newer methods that have the antigen chemically linked to the carrier by heterobifunctional reagents have also been developed (10).

4.3. The Chemical Nature of the Antigen

The natural B cell response has evolved to deal with bacteria whose cell surface is largely carbohydrate. With the exception of the standard structures which are present on N- and O-linked glycoproteins, carbohydrates elicit a massive B-cell response. Protein responses are highly variable and depend on the degree of homology of the protein to the "self" protein in the experimental animal. Thus, for example, highly conserved proteins such as histones are seldom foreign across mammalian species, whereas most blood proteins are clearly foreign even when the species difference is small, such as rat in mouse. This must again be seen in context of the T helper cell response (see Fig. 5.4), as the altered peptide sequence must not only appear foreign to B cells but also be able to elicit T helper cell response in the groove of the animal's MHC antigens.

A protein antigen that is different in one amino acid between mouse or rabbit and man may elicit a poor response. It is, however, possible to make protein appear

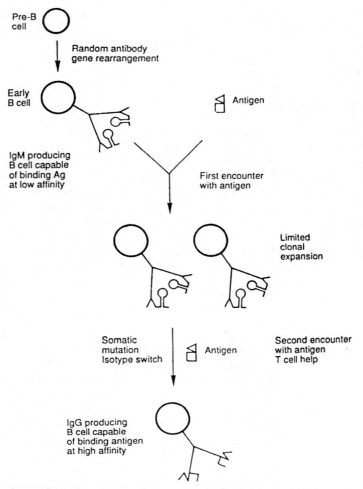

FIGURE 5.5 Low-affinity antibodies and high-affinity antibodies. Low-affinity antibodies are produced by first encounter with antigen. High-affinity antibodies generally occur only after somatic mutation during isotype switch (Reprinted from A. M. Campbell, Monoclonal antibody and immunoassay technology, 1991, with kind permission from Elsevier Science—NL, Sara Burgerhartstraat 25, 1055 KV Amsterdam, The Netherlands.)

more foreign by chemically cross-linking it to a clearly foreign protein such as KLH, which carries peptide sequences able to generate T cell help in almost all species and strains. The disadvantage of using it is that a substantial part of the B cell response is diverted to KLH peptides, so that only a small amount is bound to epitopes on the protein under study.

Nucleic acids are extremely poor antigens, and antisera to them are usually generated only from individuals with systemic lupus erythematosus or inbred strains of mice such as *lpr*, in which antibodies to DNA are part of the pathological condition. Lipids such as phospholipids and triglycerides are also very poor antigens. Glycolipids such as human ABO blood group substances are very dominant antigens, but this relates largely to the carbohydrate portion of the molecule. Lipid-soluble drugs or steroids can be made antigenic by presentation on covalent linkage to a foreign molecule.

4.4. Adjuvants

The purpose of adjuvant is to slow the release of antigen into the body, thus maximizing the immune response. A foreign protein injected in saline will be quickly removed, but a foreign protein as an emulsion or solid complex will leach out slowly, mimicking the natural antigen and eliciting a greater immune response. The addition of killed bacteria to such adjuvants was originally thought to enhance the response. The best known adjuvant is Complete Freund's Adjuvant (CFA), a suspension of killed mycobacteria in mineral oil which was first described over 50 years ago. Incomplete Freund's Adjuvant (IFA) is mineral oil without the killed mycobacteria. Currently, IFA alone is used successfully since the mineral oil emulsion gives the required slow release and the mycobacteria in CFA can divert the immune response. Mixing antigen in aqueous solution with either CFA or IFA is very similar to making mayonnaise, which is also an oil–water emulsion. Original methods involved injecting the aqueous solution from the barrel of one syringe across into the barrel of a second "head-to-head" linked syringe containing the oil. Nowadays, many laboratories mix the two with antigen in aqueous solution being added in small (10 μl) aliquots to IFA with repeated vortexing. The final emulsion should be thick and creamy and should not separate after standing for some hours.

Another less toxic adjuvant is aluminum hydroxide. The antigen is either trapped onto the surface of the aluminum hydroxide as it is precipitated from solution or adsorbed onto the preformed aluminum hydroxide. This is less toxic than Freund's adjuvant but is less convenient to prepare.

It is relevant to note that any animal immunized with adjuvant alone will show a low-affinity titre to the antigen under study. This is generally due to low-affinity IgM antibodies produced as a result of interaction with the adjuvant. Such antibodies have the capacity to cross-react with a wide variety of antigens, including the antigen under test. They are, however, too low in affinity to be suitable diagnostic reagents.

The possibility of *in vitro* immunization was extensively investigated in the 1980s, and some early protocols based on this possibility were published. The rationale was that this would circumvent the obvious problem of immunizing humans with unacceptable pathogens. However, such procedures have never yielded a useful antibody, and since they are in conflict with modern knowledge about antibody maturation in germinal centers, they are not advised (4).

4.5. Route of Immunization

The usual routes of injection are subcutaneous (sc), intraperitoneal (ip), and intravenous (iv). The intravenous route is used only for the final boost via either the ear vein of the rabbit or the tail vein of the mouse. More complex and traumatic methods of injection such as intradermal or footpad were originally thought to give a better response by direct access to the lymphatic circulation, but again, these have been overtaken by modern immunological knowledge, modern experience, and tighter legislative controls on animal experiments. Most soluble antigens emulsified with CFA or IFA are injected subcutaneously. Cellular antigens are usually injected intraperitoneally in mice and subcutaneously in rabbits.

4.6. Amount of Antigen

The immune system does not respond on a quantitative basis. If the antigen is foreign, or has been made to appear foreign, a small amount will have the desired effect. Larger amounts of antigen do not give a better response. Generally around 40 μg of protein is quite sufficient, and 400 or 4000 μg will not improve results. Large amounts are often deleterious to the response, since small quantities of contaminating antigenic material can sidetrack the animal's immune response.

4.7. Immunization Schedules

As described above, it is essential to immunize the animal twice, with the first and second injections being a minimum of 10 days apart (preferably longer). A test bleed should be taken 2–4 weeks after the second injection to measure the animal's titre, the dilution of serum at which the result is positive with respect to a prebleed from the same rabbit or mouse at the same dilution. If titre is poor, it is possible to reimmunize the animal; however, if the first and second injections have been executed correctly, a third is unlikely to improve results since the problem is probably due to the nature of the injected antigen.

The final boost is essential in monoclonal antibody production and is useful for polyclonal antibody production. As with the main immunization, it should be small—in this case, very small. The reason is that a small amount of antigen will only activate the high-affinity memory B cell clones (see Fig. 5.5). Thus, the resultant antiserum (or B lymphocyte population) will be of the highest quality. Generally, the final boost is one-tenth of the original, administered intravenously in saline 4 days before fusion for monoclonals (when the B cells are responding maximally), or 7 days before bleeding for polyclonals (when the antibody produced by the responding B cells starts to appear in the blood).

5. OBTAINING AND PROCESSING BLOOD AND LYMPHOCYTES

5.1. Bleeding a Rabbit

The rabbit is usually bled with a diagonal cut across the ear vein which opens but does not sever the vein. The ear is then stroked gently and the blood collected in a 20-ml container. Various chemicals such as xylene or benzene that increase the blood flow can cause subsequent irritation to the animal and are generally unnecessary. The blood flows better from a warm ear, and an infrared lamp is often used to achieve this. Since a nervous animal usually yields blood poorly due to peripheral vasoconstriction, the animal is kept relaxed by stroking and soothing. The amount of blood that can be obtained depends on the legal restrictions imposed by a particular country, but generally 40 ml a month is sufficient to leave the rabbit healthy.

Cardiac puncture is used for animals which for some reason must be put down, and this can yield around 100 ml. The animal is first anesthetized and blood is withdrawn from the heart into a 100-ml syringe through a 21G needle.

5.2. Bleeding Rats and Mice

Obviously, rats and mice are not used for large-volume production, and the usual requirement is to perform a test bleed to ascertain that the serum titre is suitable for monoclonal antibody production. This requires only 50–100 μl of blood, which is most readily achieved by cutting off the very tip of the tail and collecting the small volume in a 1-ml conical centrifuge tube.

If the animal is being sacrificed (usually at the time of removing the spleen for a fusion), cardiac puncture can yield around 0.5 ml of blood.

5.3. Bleeding Larger Animals

Sheep, goats, and donkeys are usually bled from the jugular vein collecting through a 21G needle into a 500-ml bottle.

5.4. Bleeding Humans

This should not be attempted without first ensuring that the appropriate legal requirements have been met. Human blood is generally withdrawn from the median cephalic vein in the arm. In general, anticoagulants are used and the sample provided is plasma rather than serum (i.e., it contains fibrinogen).

5.5. Recovery of Serum, Plasma, or Lymphocytes from Blood

Samples obtained from experimental animals are usually allowed to clot. Clotting is a biochemical process, as is clot retraction. The clotted blood sample will therefore yield the most serum if incubated at room temperature or 37°C and shaken to allow the fibrinolytic enzymes to loosen the clot, thereby yielding the maximal amount of serum. The residual clot can then be centrifuged and the serum withdrawn.

In the case of human samples for which an anticoagulant has been used, serum can readily be aspirated from the erythrocytes that settle naturally or can be centrifuged. If human lymphocytes are required for human monoclonal antibody production, the blood is gently layered over an equal volume of Ficoll and centrifuged at 600g for 15 min. The erythrocytes sediment to the pellet and the population at the interface between the Ficoll and plasma contains lymphocytes together with few monocytes. This is harvested and washed. Of the 10^7 lymphocytes yielded by 10 ml of blood, 20% will be B cells.

5.6. Obtaining Lymphocytes from Other Tissues

Solid tissues such as spleen, thymus, tonsil, and lymph node are used more frequently in human work than in animal work. This tissue is generally spilled by stabbing with a needle while cutting finely with a scalpel blade. It is also possible to extrude the material through a sterile wire mesh or tea strainer.

5.7. Purifying Human B Lymphocytes

Human T lymphocytes have a molecule called CD2 which gives them chance high affinity for sheep red blood cells (SRBCs). They are readily removed from a human (but not mouse) mixed lymphocyte sample by binding to SRBCs to leave a cell population enriched in B cells and monocytes. SRBCs alone are not an ideal reagent, as the ability to bind T cells is widely variable. The affinity for SRBCs is increased by pretreatment with enzymes such as neuraminidase or with sulfydryl reagents (11), and separation on Ficoll as described earlier. The human T cells bind to the SRBCs and centrifuge with the dense erythrocyte layer, leaving the B lymphocytes at the interface.

5.8. Storage of Serum, Plasma, and Lymphocytes

IgG antibodies are very stable molecules held together by several disulfide bonds. As a pure, sterile solution, they will maintain activity for several weeks at room temperature and several months at 40°C. However, antibodies obtained as serum (polyclonal) or as tissue culture supernatant (monoclonal) are contaminated with proteases and serum samples are generally collected under conditions that render them nonsterile. This can be circumvented by employing the following procedures:

1. The sample can be heated to 60°C for 5–10 min with little loss in antibody binding capacity. This destroys most but not all proteolytic activity.
2. Before or after heating, the sample can be frozen (in aliquots) at −70°C. This minimizes proteolytic activity.
3. Chemicals such as sodium azide or sodium fluoride can be added. This stops bacterial growth but has little effect on proteolytic activity. In addition, it may affect assays involving oxidative enzymes.

Lymphocytes are stored in a solution containing 90% fetal calf serum (FCS) and 10% dimethylsulfoxide (DMSO). The DMSO is essential as it minimizes the size of water crystals formed. The ampules are then encased in a liquid nitrogen vat which, if properly maintained, keeps them below −170°C. While some lymphocytes die, the majority remain viable for several months under these conditions.

6. MONOCLONAL ANTIBODY PRODUCTION

6.1. Animals and Tissues

The general procedure for monoclonal antibody production in rodents is illustrated in Fig. 5.6. As described above, the usual animal is the Balb/c mouse, which is readily available from any laboratory supplier and routinely bred on all large university campuses. The usual tissue is the spleen, which is located on the right of the animal's body when it is viewed lying on its back. The spleen is dark red like the liver, but is grainier and elongated in appearance. It contains approximately 10^8 cells of which one-third are T cells, one-third are B cells, and the rest are cells of supporting tissues (fibroblasts, endothelial cells, etc.). The mouse is immunized as described above and then boosted 4 days before fusion so that the B cells making the required antibodies have been stimulated into growth. This is vital because only growing cells fuse well.

In the case of humans, spleens from suitably immunized people are not available and it is usually necessary to use blood lymphocytes. As these are not actively replicating, blood is a comparatively poor source.

6.2. Cell Lines Required for Fusion

The cell line used for fusion must be an immortal (i.e., tumor) line. It must also be a myeloma (or plasmacytoma) line, that is, a B lymphocyte well down the

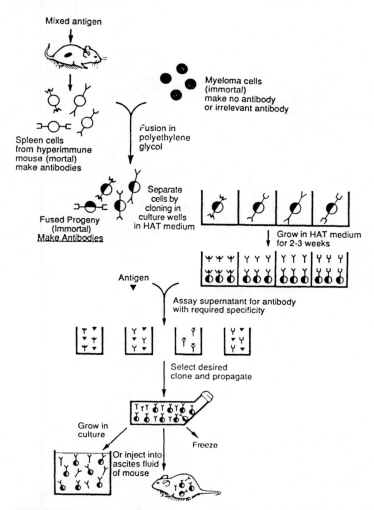

FIGURE 5.6   The general procedure for monoclonal antibody production in rodents (Reprinted from A. M. Campbell, Monoclonal antibody and immunoassay technology, 1991, with kind permission from Elsevier Science—NL, Sara Burgerhartstraat 25, 1055 KV Amsterdam, The Netherlands.)

developmental lineage that has acquired an established endoplasmic reticulum, enabling it to secrete large amounts of antibody. Yet it should not secrete its endogenous irrelevant antibody, although it should possess the apparatus to do so. Thus, after fusion, the hybrid of antibody and immune lymphocyte should only secrete the required antibody (see Fig. 5.7). Finally, it must lack some essential gene so that it dies in selective medium unless it fuses with a lymphocyte carrying not only this lost gene, but also the genes encoding the desired antibody. Thus, when myeloma cells, lymphocytes, and their hybrid progeny are grown together in tissue culture, the only viable progeny are antibody-producing hybrids.

All the available mouse fusion partners that have these necessary properties have their origins in the Balb/c mouse, which is susceptible to the induction of IgA-producing plasmacytomas upon intraperitoneal injection with mineral oil. Consequently, most of the cell lines are prefixed with the letters MOPC for Mineral

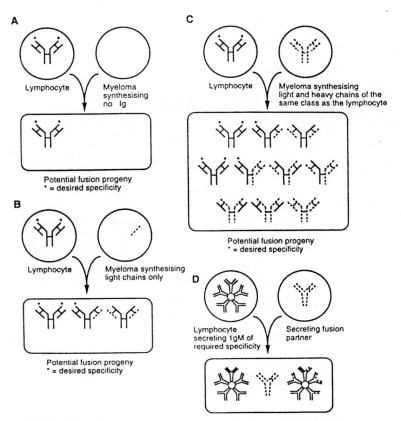

FIGURE 5.7   The importance of having a nonsecreting fusion partner. View A is the ideal situation that can be achieved in the mouse system. View B is an acceptable situation, common to most rat systems. Views C and D reflect the human system (Reprinted from A. M. Campbell, Monoclonal antibody and immunoassay technology, 1991, with kind permission from Elsevier Science—NL, Sara Burgerhartstraat 25, 1055 KV Amsterdam, The Netherlands.)

Oil Induced PlasmaCytoma and contain the letters Ag for azaguanine resistance (indicative of susceptibility to the hypoxanthine, aminopterin, and thymidine selective medium), along with a multiplicity of other letters that simply relate to clone identification. Most of the commonly used ones originate from a single cell line, P3K, and its sub-line P3-X63-Ag8, which secretes antibody but lacks the enzyme hypoxanthine phosphoribosyl transferase (HPRT). There are only three major lines used throughout the world, all developed from P3K and all readily available without patent restrictions. These are P3-X63-Ag8-653, which has the normal mouse DNA content; SP2/0-Agl4, selected from P3-X63-Ag8 by fusion with nonimmunized mouse spleen cells; and NS0/1. While all three lines work well in fusion, the first two are the more widely used, and SP2/0 cells have a particular advantage in that they are slightly adherent and tend to stick to plastic, making feeding simple. The cells are grown up until they occupy two medium-sized (80 cm^2) plastic flasks (around 10^7 cells). As with the splenic lymphocytes, it is important that they be actively dividing at the time of fusion, and the myeloma cells should always be subcultured the day before fusion.

6.3. Chemicals Required for Fusion and Selection

The chemical used to induce fusion is polyethylene glycol (PEG),

$$HO(CH_2CH_2O)_nCH_2CH_2OH,$$

with n being 6–60 and the concentration being 50% (w/v). This can be purchased in sterile aliquots at low cost, but it is also readily prepared in the laboratory. The mode of action is thought be that PEG sequesters water, thus allowing cells to approach closer to one another than is normally permitted by the charges on their membranes. Thereafter, membrane fusion occurs naturally.

The chemicals required for selection are hypoxanthine, aminopterin, and thymidine (HAT). Most parent myeloma lines have been selected for their lack of HPRT. In effect, this means that they cannot grow in the presence of the one carbon unit inhibitor, aminopterin. Since aminopterin also blocks thymidine synthesis, thymidine must also be included (see Fig. 5.8). The consequence is that:

1. Normal B lymphocytes secreting the desired antibody are mortal and die within 7–10 days, regardless of the culture medium.

2. Myeloma cells are normally immortal in culture, but myeloma cells which are HPRT negative die in the HAT medium.

3. The fused cells obtain the immortal characteristics of the myeloma parent, the HPRT gene, and its encoded enzyme function, and the antibody-secreting capacity of the immunized B lymphocyte parent.

Thus, only the small percentage (around 0.001%) of the cells that are fusion products of the two types survive in culture. The HAT medium is normally 0.1 mM

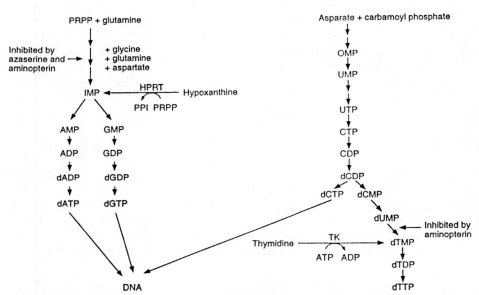

FIGURE 5.8 The main pathways of purine and pyrimidine biosynthesis and major sites of aminopterin and azaserine blockage. Azaserine may also inhibit pyrimidine biosynthesis but at comparatively higher concentrations (Reprinted from A. M. Campbell, Monoclonal antibody and immunoassay technology, 1991, with kind permission from Elsevier Science—NL, Sara Burgerhartstraat 25, 1055 KV Amsterdam, The Netherlands.)

hypoxanthine (nontoxic), 0.4 mM aminopterin(toxic), and 0.016 mM Thymidine (not toxic but can inhibit DNA synthesis if used in greater amounts). It is made up as a hundred-fold concentrate and added as 1 ml to every 100 ml of tissue culture medium.

6.4. Fusion Procedures

The fusion of the two cell types is very simple and takes less than 5 min. The dispersed cells from a single mouse spleen are mixed with myeloma cells from two medium sized (80 cm^2) plastic flasks (see discussion above). The mixture of cells is centrifuged and the pellet is then suspended in 2 ml PEG for 1–2 min with gentle mixing. It is then slowly diluted out with serum-free tissue culture medium and the cells are centrifuged free of PEG and resuspended in HAT medium containing 20% FCS. They are then plated out on 8–10 96-well tissue culture plates at 200 μl per well (10^5 cells per well). If the fusion is successful, this should produce about one single clone in each well.

6.5. Screening and Subcloning

The day after a fusion, the tissue culture plates look like Armageddon: over 99% of the cells are dead or dying. One week after fusion, however, the clear clusters of emerging hybridoma clones can be seen. When they have reached 60–80 cells in size, they are ready to have 100 μl supernatant removed for assay, with fresh medium being added to replace it. The most convenient assay is ELISA (see Chapter 13), since it is also carried out in 96-well plates and is readily adapted to multiple assays for up to 1000 clones. However, if the final intended use of the antibody is not for ELISA, it is better to screen by the projected application. A good compromise is to screen by ELISA and then do a second screen of the 20 best ELISA positives using the immunoassay system to be developed.

Screening must be carried out within 4–5 days. Mouse clones are initially unstable and cells tend to lose their ability to secrete antibody. Cells that lose this ability usually grow faster and outgrow any cells in the same well that are still secreting antibody. Hence, it is necessary to isolate the slow-growing clones that still make antibody. This is performed by breaking up the original colony (by now numbering about 200 cells) and cloning it at 1 cell per well. Since B lymphocytes require lymphokines produced by other B lymphocytes and do not readily grow alone, they are given "feeders" of Balb/c spleen cells from a young, nonimmunized mouse. A single mouse spleen, dispersed in the same manner as the original immune spleen, gives 10 $\times$ 96 wells of feeders, and the hybridomas are then plated out at 1 cell per well, 2 each of the best 20 original clones to each plate. The plates are then reassayed after the clones emerge, and by this time they are stable.

6.6. Expansion of Cells Making the Required Antibodies

After a clone has been selected, it is expanded and the several pots of the cells in logarithmic growth are frozen for safe storage. A separate aliquot is then grown in large (175 cm^2) plastic culture flasks to exhaustion; this is important because the cells make the most antibody while they are dying. The dead cells are then centrifuged and discarded and the supernatant is used for purification or more detailed work. This yields up to 100 μg/ml antibody contaminated with 7 mg/ml serum protein from the FCS essential for the tissue culture medium.

The most economical method for expanding clones is *in vivo*. Around 10^6 hybridoma cells are injected into Balb/c mice which have been primed 7–10 days earlier with pristane (2,6,10,14-tetramethyl pentadecane). Pristane has been shown to operate by depressing the normal immune function of the mouse so that internally produced or injected myeloma cells are able to grow without rejection (12). Ascites fluid obtained from the peritoneal cavity of tumor-cell-injected mice or rats is generally very like serum in that it has irrelevant immunoglobulins, complement components, albumin, and all the enzymes of the blood-clotting cascade. Hence, if the cells are required, it must be collected, like blood, in anticoagulants. While the fluid can furnish very large amounts of specific antibody (10–20 mg/ml) with little effort and cost as compared to tissue culture systems, this antibody is contaminated with irrelevant mouse IgG, which is difficult to remove without antigen-based affinity purification. Therefore, ascites fluid is seldom used for commercially produced antibodies that require good quality control.

If, at a later stage, the antibody has proven potential and larger-scale culture is appropriate, hollow fiber reactors (13), large fermenters (14), or microencapsulation (15) may be used.

While there are claims that antibodies may be produced in the high-yield baculovirus system (16,17) or in plants (18), these are seldom as cost effective as larger-scale tissue culture.

6.7. Human Monoclonal Antibody Production

Human monoclonal antibodies are projected to have considerable potential in therapy since they avoid the rejection problems experienced by animal antibodies and the dangers of HIV or hepatitis B transmission in the use of human polyclonal preparations. Thus, considerable effort has been devoted to their production, although the clinical results to date have been disappointing.

The strategies used to make humanized monoclonal antibodies from monoclonal antibodies produced in mice using recombinant DNA technology are described in Chapter 6. This section deals with the production of genuine human antibodies. It is a difficult procedure but occasionally is required to immortalize the natural human response (see Fig. 5.9). The best known situation to date in which this is required is in the production of antibodies to rhesus antigens, in which the human response in mice is eclipsed by the larger response to erythrocyte glycolipid ABO antigens. In ABO-matched humans who are rhesus negative, however, rhesus antigens elicit a strong response that can be fatal to the newborn. Anti-rhesus antibodies given to the mother can remove this danger, and consequently there is a substantial clinical demand for this procedure.

Genuine human MABs are made by transformation with Epstein Barr Virus (EBV), which has its target human (but not mouse) B lymphocytes bearing the CD21 [also called Complement Receptor 2 (CR2)] molecule on their surface. CD21 is generally present only on comparatively early B cells, most before commitment to isotype switch and memory cell production. As a result, EBV-transformed cells are generally polyspecific IgM secretors. However, a small population of EBV-transformed cells are IgG or IgA secretors, and these can be expanded into potentially useful reagents. The usual source is the B95-8 line of Miller and Lippman

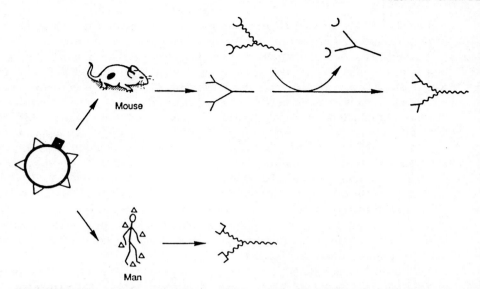

FIGURE 5.9 The two strategies for human MAB production yield different MABs. On the top line is the strategy for "humanizing" mouse MABs using recombinant DNA technology. The mouse has responded to a major foreign human antigen which may not be the antigen to which a human MAB is required. On the bottom line is a human, in whom the major antigen (triangle) is seen as self so that the response is only to the minor antigen, thus giving a "genuine human" MAB to this minor antigen. It is this second strategy that is required for production of antihuman rhesus antibodies since the murine response is dominated by reactivity to human ABO antigens (Reprinted from A. M. Campbell, Monoclonal antibody and immunoassay technology, 1991, with kind permission from Elsevier Science—NL, Sara Burgerhartstraat 25, 1055 KV Amsterdam, The Netherlands.)

(19), which is a marmoset line; the basic transformation method is not patented. The B95-8 line is very widely used to produce EBV. The lines are unstable and require repeated cloning. Consequently, the production of such antibodies can take many months.

There are two basic strategies. The first is to remove the T cells by rosetting (see earlier discussion of purifying human B lymphocytes) and transform the resultant B cell population (20, 21). The second is to retain the T cells and treat with T cell mitogens to allow T-derived lymphokines to encourage CD21 expression and/or isotype switching to high-affinity clones(22, 23). Both methods have now yielded useful anti-rhesus antibodies.

7. ANTIBODY PURIFICATION

7.1. Final Use of Antibody

If the antibody is to be used unlabeled in an immunoassay, then limited purification is required (though protein A is recommended; see later discussion). If it is to be labeled, then it should be more than 80% pure or the label will be wasted. If it is to have any *in vivo* application, then it must be demonstrably pure and free of any trace toxins (pyrogens).

7.2. Main Contaminants of Antibody Preparations

Serum is 70 mg/ml protein of which 40 mg ml is albumin, approximately 12 mg/ml IgG, and 5–6 mg/ml IgA plus IgM. Only a small amount of the IgG (1–10%)

will be reactive with the analyte under test—the greater amount will relate to the animals immunological history. The other serum proteins are complement components, notably C3 and C5 and other transport proteins such as transferrin and lipoproteins. Thus, the specific IgG in serum is 0.1–1.5% of the total serum protein. Ascites fluid is similar to serum.

Hybridoma supernatants contain 10% fetal calf serum and thus have 7 mg/ml irrelevant protein, of which over half is bovine albumin. The important difference is that FCS contains very little nonspecific IgG. Thus a typical hybridoma supernatant will have 5–100 μg/ml IgG as 5–10% of the total protein.

7.3. Ammonium Sulfate Precipitation

Ammonium sulfate precipitation is a classic method for subfractionating serum proteins. While it may give some purification, it is mainly a method for concentrating antibody. High Grade Analar ammonium sulfate should be used, as the lower-grade material is frequently contaminated with heavy metal ions which can affect subsequent assays.

The simplest method is to prepare a 100% saturated (>770 g/l) ammonium sulfate solution at pH 7 and mix this with the serum or hybridoma supernatant at 40% ammonium sulfate to 60% antibody. The pellet contains the antibody. It should then be redissolved in phosphate buffered saline and dialyzed before any further manipulations are made, since the excess ammonium sulfate will interfere with most of these further procedures.

7.4. DEAE and QEAE Sepharose

These are positively charged matrices designed to remove negatively charged albumin, which is the major contaminant of antibody preparations. DEAE and QEAE are available attached to fast-flow matrices such as sephadex, sepharose, or acrylamide bead. In addition, FPLC columns containing similar matrices (Mono Q columns) are now available. IgG molecules bind poorly to such matrices and elute first in a gentle salt gradient while negatively charged albumin stays on the column. The advantage of this step is low-cost removal of the bulk of the albumin without exposing the antibody to extremes of pH.

7.5. Protein A and Protein G

Protein A is the method that has found widest acceptance in antibody purification. In most cases, other steps such as ammonium sulfate or DEAE are unnecessary. It is a 42-kDa protein found on the cell walls of *Staphylococcus aureus,* which binds to the Fc region of a wide range of antibody subclasses from many species (24, 25).

While crude preparations of *S. aureus* may be used, protein A is generally coupled to various matrices such as sepharose, since column chromatography is more convenient than centrifugation. Protein A binds to all the main antibodies that the clinical scientist is likely to generate in the laboratory (see Table 5.2). However, it binds poorly to the mouse IgG1 subclass, the human IgG3 subclass, and most rat MABs. For this reason, a second, more expensive product, Protein G (60 kDa mol wt), was recently developed to attempt to fill these small gaps in the repertoire of protein A. IgM and IgA antibodies, albumin, and other serum

**TABLE 5.2   Binding of Various IgG
Subclasses to Protein A and Protein G**

	Protein A	Protein G
Rabbit IgG	Strong	Strong
Mouse IgG1	Medium	Strong
Mouse IgG2a	Medium	Strong
Mouse IgG2b	Strong	Medium
Mouse IgG3	Weak	Medium
Rat IgG1	Weak	Weak
Rat IgG2a	Weak	Strong
Rat IgG2b	Weak	Weak
Rat IgG2c	Medium	Medium
Human IgG1	Strong	Strong
Human IgG2	Medium	Strong
Human IgG3	Weak	Strong
Human IgG4	Strong	Strong

proteins do not bind protein G. It was designed by evolution to be specific for IgG and is so.

The procedure is very simple. The protein A gel is suspended in the barrel of a small laboratory syringe plugged with glass wool. The serum, monoclonal supernatant, or dialyzed ammonium sulfate precipitate at pH 7–8 are applied and washed through. The eluate is albumin and other proteins. The bound protein A can then be eluted with 0.1 M sodium citrate (pH 3.5) into tubes containing 1 M Tris/HCl (pH 8) so that the antibody is at low pH for the minimum time. A small amount of gel has substantial capacity and can absorb the IgG from a substantial amount of hybridoma supernatant.

7.6. Affinity Chromatography

Affinity chromatography is generally used only for polyclonal antibodies. There are two basic types, positive and negative; negative is the more common. The usual requirement is in situations in which a foreign protein has been used as a carrier of a hapten, particularly a peptide hapten. The carrier is immobilized on a gel matrix and antibodies in the serum sample that are reactive with it are removed. The eluate contains only antibodies that are reactive with the analyte under assay.

Positive selection is more rigorous. The analyte itself is bound to the solid matrix and irrelevant antibody is removed in the eluate. Antibodies specific to the analyte are then eluted. It is this elution which is difficult. A truly high-affinity antibody, which is required for a good immunoassay, is extremely difficult to elute without destruction of activity. The classical coupling matrix has been cyanogen bromide-activated sepharose, but it should be noted that many other coupling methods are available, and particularly that the length of the "arms" of the cross-linking molecules may alter the ability of the matrix to bind the selected protein. Cyanogen bromide reacts with amino groups and most proteins, including antibodies, have a high proportion of these. However, if selection by antigen is required and the antigen has a small number of amino groups, then other types of activated sepharose which will bind to acidic or cysteinyl(-SH) groups may be more effective.

References

1. Campbell AM. Monoclonal antibody and immunosensor technology. Amsterdam: Elsevier, 1991.
2. Bruin H. Publications for the Society for Laboratory Animal Science No 1. The planning and structure of animal facilities for institutes performing laboratory experiments, 2nd English ed. GV-SOLAS Biberach a.d. Riss, 1989.
3. Williams CA, Chase MW. Methods in Immunology and Immunochemistry, Vol. 1. New York: Academic Press, 1967.
4. Herbert WJ, Kristensen F, Aitken RM, Eslami MB, Ferguson A, Gray KG, Penhale WJ. Laboratory animal techniques for immunologists. In: Weir DM, Herzenberg C, Herzenberg LA, Eds. Handbook of Experimental Immunology, Vol. 3, 3rd ed. Oxford: Blackwell, 1986:133.1–133.6.
5. World Health Organization. WHO Technical Report Series No. 786. Requirements for the collection, processing and quality control of blood, blood components and plasma derivatives. 1989.
6. The Council of Europe. Guide for the preparation, use, and quality assurance of blood components. 1992.
7. Brown JH, Jardetzky TS, Gorga JC, Stern LJ, Urban RG, Strominger JL, Wiley DC. Three dimensional structure of human class II histocompatibility antigen HLA DR1. Nature 1993; 364:33–9.
8. Kohler G, Milstein C. Continuous culture of fused cells secreting antibody of predefined specificity. Nature 1975; 256:495.
9. Erlanger BF. The preparation of antigenic hapten-carrier conjugates: a survey. In: Van Vanukis H, Langone JJ, Eds. Methods in Enzymology, Vol. 70. New York: Academic Press, 1980:85–104.
10. Tramontano A, Schoeder D. Production of antibodies that mimic enzyme catalytic activity. In: Van Vanukis H, Langone JJ, Eds. Methods in Enzymology, Vol. 178. New York: Academic Press, 1989:531.
11. Kaplan ME, Clark C. An improved rosetting assay for the detection of human T lymphocytes. J Immunol Methods 1974; 5:131.
12. Freund YR, Blair PB. Depression of natural killer activity and mitogen responsiveness in mice treated with pristane. J Immunol 1982; 29:2826.
13. Altschuler GL, Dziewulski DM, Sowek J, Befort G. Biotechnol Bioeng 1986; 28:646.
14. Birch JR, Boraston R, Wood L. Bulk production of antibody in fermenters. Trends Biotechnol 1985; 3:162.
15. Duff RG. Microencapsulation techniques: a novel method for monoclonal antibody production. Trends Biotechnol 1989; 3:167.
16. Zu Pulitz JZ, Kubasek WL, Duchene M, Marget M, Specht BVS, Domday H. Antibody production in baculovirus infected insect cells. Biotechnology 1990; 8:651.
17. Haseman CA, Capra JD. High level production of a functional immunoglobulin heterodimer in a baculovirus expression system. Proc Natl Acad Sci US 1990; 87:3942.
18. Hiatt A, Cafferkey R, Bowdish K. Production of antibodies in transgenic plants. Nature 1989; 342:76.
19. Miller G, Lippman M. Release of infectious Epstein Barr virus by transformed marmoset leukocytes. Proc Natl Acad Sci USA 1973; 70:190.
20. Foung SKH, Blunt JA, Wu PS, Ahearn P, Winn LC, Engleman EG, Grumet FC. Human monoclonal antibodies to Rhesus D. Vox Sang 1987; 53:44–7.
21. Goosens D, Champonier F, Rouger P, Salmon C. Human Mabs against blood group antigens. J Immunol Methods 1987; 101:193.
22. Kumpel, BM, Wiener E, Urbaniak SJ, Bradley BA. Human monoclonal anti-D antibodies. Br J Haematol 1989; 71:415.
23. Melamed MD, Thompson JM, Gibson T, Hughes-Jones MC. J Immunol Methods 1987; 104:245.
24. Langone JJ. The use of labelled Protein A in quantitative immunochemical analysis of antigens and antibodies. J Immunol Methods 1982; 51:3.
25. Langone JJ. Applications of immobilized Protein A in immunochemical techniques. J Immunol Methods 1982; 55:277.

6 | ANTIBODY ENGINEERING

PAUL R. HINTON
Protein Design Labs
Mountain View, California

BOB SHOPES
Tera Biotechnology Corporation
La Jolla, California

1. INTRODUCTION

The medical importance of antibodies has been realized since the turn of the century. The goal of using antibodies in the treatment of human disease has remained elusive, however, despite many important discoveries during the succeeding decades. The application of antibody engineering during the past 10 years has resulted in substantial progress toward this end and is the subject of this review.

Studies in the early 1960s began to reveal the first structural details of immunoglobulins. These studies showed that an antibody molecule consists of two Fab fragments that are responsible for antigen binding and an Fc fragment that mediates biological effector functions. Each Ig molecule is a four-chain heterodimer composed of two identical heavy and two identical light chains. The primary sequence of an entire immunoglobulin was determined by the late 1960s. During the early 1970s, the first three-dimensional structures of antibody combining sites were determined by x-ray crystallography, both for a light-chain dimer and for several Fab fragments.

Two important new technologies emerged during the 1970s that together launched the field of antibody engineering. One was the development of recombinant DNA technology, which has revolutionized nearly every aspect of biology and medicine. The other was the invention in 1975 of hybridoma technology by Kohler and Milstein (1). This technology made possible the continuous production of antibodies of predefined specificity and has had a significant impact on biological research. The combination of these two technologies, along with advances in gene expression technology made during the 1980s, has enabled scientists to manipulate the structure and activity of antibodies at will. The first decade of antibody engineering has been very promising; the next decade is likely to bring to fruition the hope of using monoclonal antibodies to treat human disease.

2. CLONING ANTIBODY VARIABLE REGION GENES

By the early 1980s, the majority of the immunoglobulin heavy- and light-chain constant region genes of rodent and human origin had been cloned and sequenced. Given the availability of these genes, it is now only necessary to clone and sequence the variable region genes of an antibody of interest to do antibody engineering experiments. Although the methodology for cloning constant and variable region genes is essentially the same, only techniques for cloning V-genes are presented below.

2.1. Genomic and cDNA Cloning

Two methods were initially used to isolate immunoglobulin variable region genes, namely, genomic cloning and cDNA cloning. Genomic cloning (Fig. 6.1A) involves fragmenting genomic DNA into ~20-kb fragments, usually by partial digestion with restriction enzymes, and ligating the resulting fragments into modified bacteriophage lambda vectors. The ligated DNA is packaged *in vitro* such that each phage particle contains a single, contiguous fragment of genomic DNA. This collection of phage clones is called a genomic library.

Since immunoglobulin genes are highly expressed in antibody-producing cells, it is also possible to clone Ig genes starting with mRNA rather than genomic DNA. Construction of a so-called cDNA library begins with the isolation of RNA which is usually followed by enrichment for mRNA and sometimes by size fractionation for species of the expected size. Because single-stranded RNA cannot be cloned directly, it is converted to a double-stranded DNA form called a complementary DNA or cDNA by a series of enzymatic steps (Fig. 6.1B). These cDNA fragments are ligated into a bacteriophage lambda vector and packaged *in vitro,* yielding a cDNA library. The choice between genomic and cDNA library construction depends on the starting materials available, one's expertise in the respective methods, and the intended use of the resulting V-genes.

Screening either a genomic or a cDNA library follows the same series of steps (Fig. 6.1C). The library is plated at high plaque density on a lawn of bacteria on agar plates which results in the formation of cleared areas called plaques. Every plaque is clonal, containing identical phage particles each carrying the same piece of DNA. Phage particles are transferred to nitrocellulose filters, immobilized, and denatured to expose their DNA. Identifying the plaque(s) corresponding to the

A

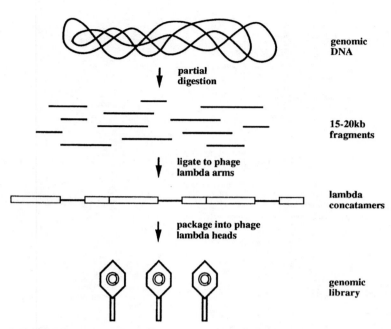

genomic
DNA

partial
digestion

15-20kb
fragments

ligate to phage
lambda arms

lambda
concatamers

package into phage
lambda heads

genomic
library

FIGURE 6.1   (A) Construction of genomic library. Genomic DNA is partially digested with a restriction enzyme (e.g., *Mbo*I) into fragments ~15–20 kb in length. Phage lambda arms are prepared by digestion with a compatible restriction enzyme (e.g., *Bam*HI). The genomic restriction fragments are ligated into the phage lambda arms, forming concatamers. The lambda concatamers are then packaged *in vitro,* resulting in a genomic library. (B) Construction of cDNA library. Total cellular RNA is isolated followed by enrichment for messenger RNA. A first strand complementary DNA copy is made using reverse transcriptase by priming with oligo dT. The mRNA template is nicked using RNase H, converted to a double-stranded DNA form by nick translation using DNA polymerase I, and blunt-ended using the exonuclease activity of T4 DNA polymerase. Restriction enzyme adaptors (e.g., *Eco*RI) are ligated to the flush ends of the cDNA. The modified cDNA is ligated into phage lambda arms that have been prepared by digestion with an appropriate restriction enzyme (e.g., *Eco*RI), resulting in concatamers. The concatamers are packaged *in vitro,* yielding a cDNA library. (C) Screening genomic or cDNA libraries. Phage are plated at high density on a lawn of bacteria on agar plates. Phage particles are transferred to nitrocellulose filters, immobilized, and denatured to expose their DNA. The filters are hybridized with a radiolabeled probe that is homologous to the target gene. After extensive washing to reduce nonspecific binding, the filters are exposed to x-ray film. Dark spots on the film identify corresponding plaques containing the gene of interest. The screening process is repeated several times at lower plaque density until individual plaques can be identified. Phage DNA is isolated from positive plaques, subcloned into a plasmid, and sequenced.

gene(s) of interest usually involves using nucleic acid probes, either cloned DNA fragments or synthetic oligonucleotides. Probes are chosen on the basis of expected homology to the target gene and contain a region that is shared between the target gene and previously cloned genes, such as the enhancer region, the J region, or the constant region. Radiolabeled probes are hybridized with the immobilized targets on nitrocellulose filters under conditions that favor the formation of heteroduplexes between the probe and homologous sequences. Following a series of washes to

B

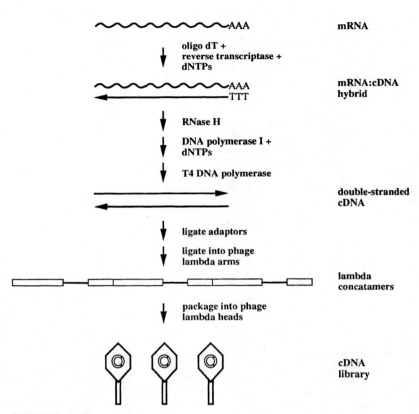

mRNA

oligo dT +
reverse transcriptase +
dNTPs

mRNA:cDNA
hybrid

RNase H

DNA polymerase I +
dNTPs

T4 DNA polymerase

double-stranded
cDNA

ligate adaptors

ligate into phage
lambda arms

lambda
concatamers

package into phage
lambda heads

cDNA
library

FIGURE 6.1   (*Continued*)

reduce nonspecific binding, the filters are exposed to x-ray film. By carefully aligning the spots on the film with the plates, plaques containing DNA sequences homologous to the probe can be identified. Individual phage plaques can usually be isolated after several rounds of screening at lower plaque density. These phages can be amplified and grown in large quantities to produce DNA corresponding to the identified gene. The gene is then excised from the bacteriophage lambda cloning vector and subcloned into a smaller vector where it can more easily be manipulated, mapped, and sequenced.

2.2. Polymerase Chain Reaction (PCR)

While both genomic and cDNA cloning methods are still in use, they are relatively laborious and have been largely supplanted by the polymerase chain reaction (PCR) (2). This method is based on enzymatic, primer-directed amplification of a target sequence (Fig. 6.2A). The template, which may be cDNA or genomic DNA, is first denatured by heating to disrupt base-pair interactions. It is then cooled and annealed to an excess of primers which hybridize to the regions immediately flanking the target sequence. Finally, the template–primer complex is extended with a DNA

C

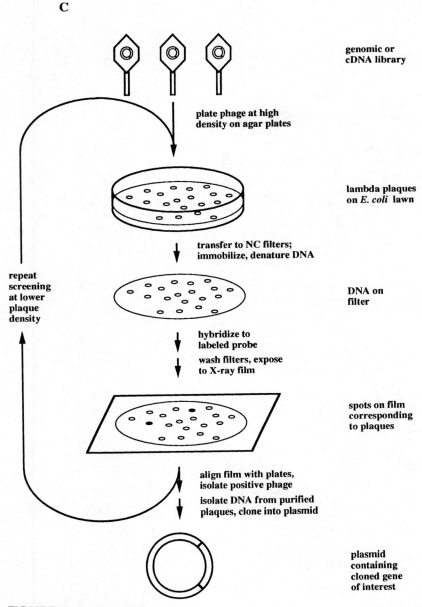

genomic or
cDNA library

plate phage at high
density on agar plates

lambda plaques
on *E. coli* lawn

transfer to NC filters;
immobilize, denature DNA

DNA on
filter

repeat
screening
at lower
plaque
density

hybridize to
labeled probe

wash filters, expose
to X-ray film

spots on film
corresponding
to plaques

align film with plates,
isolate positive phage

isolate DNA from purified
plaques, clone into plasmid

plasmid
containing
cloned gene
of interest

FIGURE 6.1 (*Continued*)

polymerase, usually the thermostable *Taq* polymerase. This cycle of denaturation, annealing, and extension is repeated 30 to 40 times. Because the product of each cycle serves as a template for each subsequent cycle, this process results in a doubling of the target sequence after each cycle and an exponential accumulation of the product. Since nonhomologous nucleotide sequences at the 5′ ends of PCR primers do not interfere with hybridization, the primers are usually designed with restriction sites to facilitate subsequent cloning of the PCR product.

A

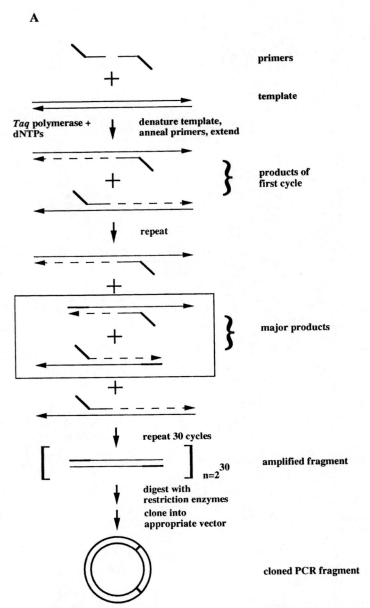

primers

template

Taq polymerase +
dNTPs

denature template,
anneal primers, extend

products of
first cycle

repeat

major products

repeat 30 cycles

amplified fragment

digest with
restriction enzymes

clone into
appropriate vector

cloned PCR fragment

FIGURE 6.2   (A) Polymerase chain reaction. Template DNA is denatured by heating, annealed
to an excess of primers, and extended with *Taq* polymerase. The process is repeated for 30–40
cycles, resulting in an exponential accumulation of the product. Since restriction enzyme sites
can be incorporated at the 5′ ends of primers without affecting hybridization to the target, the
amplified fragment can be digested with restriction enzymes and cloned into a plasmid. (B) PCR
cloning strategy. Primers are chosen which hybridize at the 5′ end of the V-gene and the 3′ end
of the C-gene. PCR of a cDNA using such primers will result in amplification of the entire V–J–C
coding region. When the DNA sequence of the 5′ end of the V-gene is unknown, degenerate
primers are often used (see text). A similar strategy can be used to clone heavy-chain V-genes.

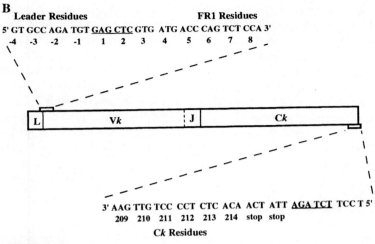

B

Leader Residues   FR1 Residues

5' GT GCC AGA TGT <u>GAG CTC</u> GTG ATG ACC CAG TCT CCA 3'
-4   -3   -2   -1   1   2   3   4   5   6   7   8

| L | Vk | J | Ck |

3' AAG TTG TCC CCT CTC ACA ACT ATT <u>AGA TCT</u> TCC T 5'
   209 210 211 212 213 214 stop stop

Ck Residues

FIGURE 6.2   (*Continued*)

Although there is a finite error rate associated with DNA amplification by PCR, variable region genes are well within the size range that can be accommodated by the technique. When high fidelity is required—for example, when cloning the variable region genes of a hybridoma—it is often necessary to examine several clones (ideally from two separate PCR amplifications) to determine the correct sequence. Authenticity can then be verified by expressing a recombinant form of the antibody (see Section 3.1.1) and comparing its binding activity with that of the original antibody.

Since PCR involves primer-directed DNA synthesis, some prior knowledge of the target sequence is required. Initial experiments relied on N-terminal amino acid sequence information from purified immunoglobulin heavy and light chains (3). While this approach is adequate for cloning antibody V-genes from clonal sources such as hybridoma cell lines (Fig. 6.2B), it is impractical for cloning variable region genes from heterogeneous sources such as spleen cells. A more general approach takes advantage of the many known sequences of rodent and human variable regions as well as the high level of sequence homology within the Ig gene family. By definition, the constant regions are much less heterogeneous than the variable regions: there are only five heavy-chain classes (as well as several subclasses) and two light-chain types in both rodents and humans. Likewise, there are only four to six J regions in the heavy and light chain loci in these species. These observations make the design of 3' primers very straightforward. Careful alignment of Ig variable region sequences shows that there are two conserved regions at the 5' end of V-genes, namely the sequences corresponding to the leader regions and to the amino termini of the mature heavy- and light-chain polypeptides. Based on this principle, both degenerate "universal" primers (4) and multiple unique primers (5) have been designed and used successfully.

An alternative method called anchored PCR (6) bypasses the need to have upstream sequence information by joining a fixed "anchor" sequence at the 5' end of the target and using a primer complementary to the anchor sequence to amplify the target. Specificity is provided by the use of an appropriate 3′ primer. This approach is particularly suited to cloning V-genes from hybridomas.

PCR is now fully automated and can be completed in a few hours. This reduces cloning time from weeks, using conventional genomic or cDNA library methods, to days using PCR. Moreover, this technique allows not only the heavy- and light-chain variable region genes of a given cell line but also V-gene repertoires to be cloned. Furthermore, once V-genes of interest have been cloned, PCR itself offers a rapid, convenient, and general means of introducing mutations within the coding regions of the cloned genes. Thus, libraries representing the entire humoral immune response of an animal can be captured, manipulated, and expressed outside the host immune system (see Section 5.3.1).

3. EXPRESSION OF RECOMBINANT ANTIBODIES

During the past dozen years, methods have been developed for expression of recombinant immunoglobulin genes in mammalian cells, bacteria, yeast, insect cells, and even plants. Most attention has focused on expression systems in mammalian cells and in *Escherichia coli.*

3.1. Mammalian Expression

3.1.1. Transfection

Successful gene transfer of immunoglobulins was first reported in mouse lymphoid cells (7–10). Since lymphoid cells normally express antibodies, recombinant heavy and light chains are correctly processed, glycosylated, and assembled in transfectomas. These are the principle advantages of mammalian expression systems. Unfortunately, recombinant immunoglobulins are typically produced in lesser amounts in transfectomas than in the corresponding parental hybridomas.

Transient transfection of mammalian cells can be used to study gene regulatory mechanisms and to generate small amounts of antibody for initial characterization, but production of large amounts of engineered antibody requires stable expression techniques. Stable transformants are rare—only 1 in 10^3 to 1 in 10^6—so powerful selection schemes are necessary to recover transformed cells. A number of dominant selectable markers have been used including *gpt, dhfr, neo, hyg,* and glutamine synthetase. Since these markers rely on different mechanisms of action, they can be combined to select for heavy and light chains that have been introduced either sequentially or simultaneously into recipient cells. Many cell types are compatible with these markers, though the heavy- and light-chain nonproducing myeloma cell lines SP2/0 and P3X63.Ag8.653 are most commonly used. Nonlymphoid recipients such as Chinese hamster ovary (CHO) cells have also been used (11).

The most frequently used expression system for lymphoid cell gene transfer is based on the pSV2 vector series (12). A typical mammalian expression vector (Fig. 6.3A) contains an SV40 replication origin which permits replication of the plasmid in mammalian cells, a selectable marker (such as *Ecogpt*) under control of the SV40 promoter, and a prokaryotic replication origin and antibiotic resistance gene which allow maintenance of the plasmid in a bacterial host. Under appropriate selection conditions, the vector becomes randomly integrated into the genome of the recipient cell. Immunoglobulin genes inserted into this vector will be expressed, provided

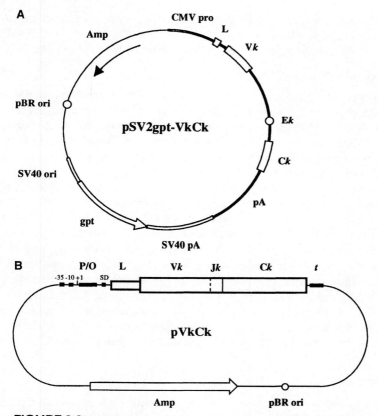

FIGURE 6.3 (A) Mammalian expression vector. The pSV2gpt-VkCk expression vector consists of the following elements (arranged clockwise): human CMV promoter; kappa leader sequence, and intron; kappa variable region gene; kappa intron containing the kappa transcriptional enhancer element; kappa constant region gene; kappa 3' untranslated region containing the polyadenylation signal; SV40 polyadenylation signal; *gpt* dominant selectable marker; SV40 early promoter and replication origin; and bacterial pBR322 DNA containing the replication origin and ampicillin resistance gene. A similar vector can be used to express heavy-chain genes. (B) Bacterial expression vector. The pVkCk expression vector consists of the following elements (arranged clockwise): *lac* promotor (−35 and −10 elements); *lac* operator (i.e., repressor binding site); ribosome binding site (i.e., Shine–Dalgarno sequence); *ompA* leader sequence; kappa V–J–C coding sequence; *trpA* transcriptional terminator; and pBR322 DNA containing the origin of replication and ampicillin resistance gene. The heavy-chain gene can be expressed on the same vector in the form of a bicistronic operon, or on a separate vector.

that the construct contains appropriate promoter and enhancer sequences. Expression levels vary among individual clones, but primary transfectants producing 1–5 μg/ml/24 hr/10^6 cells are typical. Amplification of the gene copy number is possible with some vectors, such as those containing the *dhfr* or glutamine synthetase modules, and this can result in expression levels of >20 μg/ml/24 hr/10^6 cells. In practice, amplification of the heavy-chain vector suffices because it results in concomitant amplification of the light-chain vector. Higher expression levels have been reported under fermentation conditions.

A number of transfection methods have been devised for transfer of expression vectors into mammalian cells, including DEAE–dextran precipitation, calcium phosphate precipitation, protoplast fusion, and more recently electroporation. The latter approach is the method of choice since it typically results in equivalent or higher transfection efficiencies than the other methods and is more reproducible.

3.1.2. Transgenic Animals

Transgenic animal technology is a useful complement to transfection of mammalian cells. Injection of cloned genes into fertilized mouse embryos followed by implantation of the embryos into a surrogate mother gives rise to a small percentage of transgenic offspring. The foreign DNA usually becomes integrated into the genome at a presumably random location on the chromosome in a tandem array of 20 to 100 copies. If integration occurs at the single-cell stage, all cells of the transgenic offspring will carry the foreign gene which will be transmitted to progeny according to Mendelian rules of inheritance; otherwise, the animal will be a mosaic and germline cells may or may not carry the foreign gene.

Expression of functional, rearranged kappa and mu transgenes in mice was reported by several groups (13–15). These studies showed that expression of the Ig transgenes was restricted to lymphoid tissues and that functional antibodies could be produced. These results were subsequently extended by others to show that germline Ig transgenes could undergo rearrangement and expression to yield functional antibodies. Transgenic technology provides a means of studying fundamental aspects of immunology, such as allelic exclusion, and represents a potentially powerful approach to antibody engineering and production (see Section 5.3.3).

3.2. Bacterial Expression

The demonstration of functional immunoglobulin gene expression in *E. coli* represented a milestone in molecular immunology. Although bacteria are incapable of glycosylation or splicing, *E. coli* is easily manipulated, grows to high cell densities in inexpensive media, and can be induced to produce large amounts of foreign proteins. Bacterial expression of Ig genes has thus brought the full power of molecular biology to bear on the field of antibody engineering.

3.2.1. Secretion

Many early attempts succeeded in expressing heavy- and light-chain polypeptides, or their fragments, in the cytoplasm of *E. coli*, but functional assembly of active binding fragments was problematic (16, 17). These polypeptides were often found as insoluble aggregates in inclusion bodies and required extensive *in vitro* resolubilization and refolding, under redox conditions, to reform disulfide bonds. Though the refolded material was antigenically and functionally active, these procedures were inefficient and impractical for routine use.

The breakthrough in functional bacterial assembly of Ig fragments was the development of expression systems that directed the transport of the heavy- and light-chain polypeptides into the more oxidizing environment of the periplasm (18, 19). Periplasmic transport mimics the transport of eukaryotic proteins from the cytoplasm to the lumen of the endoplasmic reticulum and is likewise dependent on the presence of an amino terminal leader sequence or signal peptide. This approach evidently facilitates the many steps which are necessary for functional expression of an antibody fragment in *E. coli*, including: coordinated and stoichiometric synthesis of heavy- and light-chain polypeptides; transport to the periplasm; correct processing (i.e., cleavage of the signal peptide); proper folding of the domains; hetero-dimer assembly; and disulfide bond formation (four intrachain and one interchain in the case of an Fab fragment). A typical bacterial secretion vector (Fig. 6.3B) consists of: a bacterial promoter, such as the inducible *lac* promoter-operator; a ribosome-binding site (i.e., Shine–Dalgarno sequence); a leader sequence, such as the *ompA* signal peptide; the V–J–C coding unit; a transcription terminator, such as the *trpA* terminator; an antibiotic resistance gene, such as ampicillin; and a replication origin, such as the pBR origin.

Another approach to the expression of antibody combining site fragments in *E. coli* is based on the use of single-chain Fv (scFv) analogs (20, 21). These novel fragments consist of a VL domain linked to a VH domain by a flexible linker between the carboxy terminus of one domain and the amino terminus of the other domain. Though these fragments were originally expressed as cytoplasmic proteins which required *in vitro* renaturation, this technology has now been adapted to periplasmic secretion and phage display technologies (see below). Because of their small size and lack of constant regions, the use of scFv fragments may be advantageous in certain applications. However, a substantial loss of binding affinity (approximately four- to eightfold) was observed for several recombinant scFv fragments compared to enzymatically prepared Fab fragments (20, 21).

3.2.2. Filamentous Phage Display

Within the past several years, many groups have tried to directly clone antibodies using molecular biology techniques. While functional expression of Ab combining sites in *E. coli* can be considered the *sine qua non* for capturing immunological repertoires in bacteria, it is equally important to develop efficient screening techniques. Initially, lambda phage library cloning methods were used to identify mouse and human antibodies of predetermined specificity (see Section 5.3.1). More recently, phage display of Ab combining sites using M13 phage or phagemid cloning systems has become the preferred method. Following the pioneering work of Smith and co-workers (22), several groups demonstrated that random peptide libraries could be displayed on the surface of filamentous phage. Shortly thereafter, this approach was extended to the display of single-domain proteins and then to scFv or Fab fragments (23–26). Recently, a cloning vector was developed which combines the ease of creating libraries in a lambda phage vector with the power of screening libraries using an M13 phagemid display system (27).

The coliphage fd, f1, and M13 are filamentous, single-stranded DNA phages that infect male *E. coli* via the F pilus. Phage adsorption is mediated by the minor coat protein (gpIII). Approximately three to five molecules of gpIII are displayed at one end of the phage particle: the amino terminal region recognizes the F pilus, while the carboxy terminal region anchors the protein to the phage particle. The major coat protein (gpVIII) mainly serves a structural role in the assembly of phage particles and is present in several thousand copies per particle. Fusion of peptides or protein domains (such as antibody fragments) to a small fraction of these coat proteins can be tolerated provided that wild-type copies of the coat proteins are also present. This permits construction of recombinant phage expressing scFv or Fab fragments fused to either the gpIII or gpVIII coat proteins. Such phage bear the binding activity conferred by displaying the scFv or Fab fragments on their surface and contain a DNA insert which encodes that binding activity (Fig. 6.4). Thus, genotype and phenotype are physically linked. Both phage (which are capable

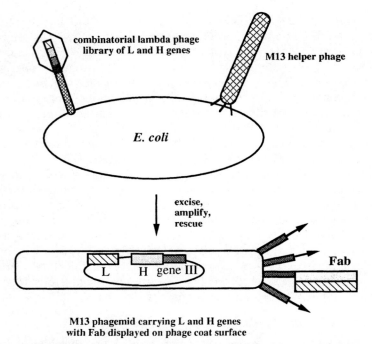

FIGURE 6.4   M13 phagemid display. Infection of *E. coli* with a combinatorial lambda phage library followed by rescue with M13 helper phage yields a collection of M13 phagemid particles displaying an Fab fragment on their surface which is encoded by the phage genome inside the particle. This physical linkage between phenotype and genotype allows phagemid particles to be selected on the basis of binding properties and characterized by DNA sequencing.

of self-replication) and phagemid (which require helper phage for replication) genomes have been used in conjunction with this system. However, phagemids are generally preferred for library construction since they provide higher transduction efficiencies (two to three orders of magnitude) than recombinant phage. With a phagemid display library it is possible to enrich for and identify clones of interest on the basis of a binding activity given judicious use of selection pressure (see Section 5.3.1).

3.2.3. Bacterial Surface Expression

An alternative approach to phage display systems is based on *E. coli* surface expression of Ab combining sites. Several recent reports have described surface display systems based on fusion of scFv fragments either to the peptidoglycan associated lipoprotein (28) or to an *lpp–ompA* hybrid (29). In one system the scFv is linked to the anchoring protein through its carboxy terminus (28), while in the other system the scFv is linked through its amino terminus (29). The accessibility of the combining site to antigen was verified in both systems by fluorescence microscopy using fluorescently labeled antigen or hapten. A 10^5-fold enrichment was obtained after two rounds of fluorescence-activated cell sorting (FACS) when cells displaying scFv fragments were mixed with cells not displaying a combining site (29). Due to the high number of scFv fragments displayed on the surface of *E. coli*, identification of low-affinity binding sites in large libraries may be possible using bacterial surface expression systems.

3.3. Yeast Expression

The yeast *Saccharomyces cerevisiae* has also been adapted as a host organism for expression of recombinant immunoglobulins. Several reports (30, 31) have documented the successful expression, processing, glycosylation, and secretion of heavy- and light-chain polypeptides in yeast. Although hapten- or antigen-binding properties were retained, overall expression levels were low and *in vivo* assembly into functional antibodies was minimal. Notably, a chimeric whole IgG from yeast failed to mediate complement-dependent cytotoxicity (CDC), though it was equivalent in antibody-dependent cell-mediated cytotoxicity (ADCC) activity to material produced in mammalian cells (31). The authors attributed this functional deficiency to glycosylation differences between yeast and mammalian cells. While both yeast and mammalian cells recognize the same target for N-linked glycosylation and add the same core oligosaccharide, processing differences result in high-mannose glycoproteins in yeast while mammalian cells add complex terminal carbohydrate groups. Although yeast shares many advantages with *E. coli* as an experimental organism, its transformation efficiency is several orders of magnitude lower, which may preclude its use in cloning applications.

Yeast expression systems based on cytoplasmic expression of heavy- and light-chain genes have also been reported (32). Low but significant levels of intracellular assembly of functional whole IgG or Fab fragment were reported with these systems, although *in vivo* disulfide bond formation would not be expected to occur in the reducing environment of the cytoplasm. Also, the amino termini of the expressed polypeptide chains would necessarily initiate with a novel Met residue. Despite these shortcomings, sufficient intracellular activity was observed to partially neutralize the activity of a target enzyme *in vivo* (32).

3.4. Other Expression Systems

Other expression systems have been developed with the aim of high-level production of fully functional, glycosylated whole antibodies. One such system is based on infection of cultured insect cells with baculovirus transfer vectors. With other foreign proteins, very high expression levels (50–75% of total cellular protein) have been observed using this system. Successful expression and assembly of a fully functional whole IgG was recently reported (33). The recombinant protein retained hapten-binding and idiotypic characteristics, and was found to be glycosylated. However, because of processing differences between insect and mammalian cells, it is unlikely that the carbohydrate moieties will be identical. The consequences of these differences on antibody function remain to be determined for this system.

Expression and functional assembly of antibodies in transgenic tobacco plants have also been reported recently (34). Because the glycosylation pattern of plants differs from that of mammalian cells, "plantibodies" may not be suitable for *in vivo* therapeutic uses due to immunogenicity or loss of functional properties. However, transgenic plants may offer an inexpensive method for large-scale production of engineered antibodies for other purposes (such as oral immunization), as well as a means of controlling infection of plants by bacterial, viral, or fungal pathogens.

4. ANTIBODY STRUCTURE–FUNCTION STUDIES

For structural studies, myelomas have provided an abundant source of particular immunoglobulin molecules, although such proteins rarely have known or desired antigenic specificity and cannot be easily altered. Somatic cell genetics provides a method of generating either point mutants or isotype-switch variants of a particular hybridoma protein, but is both tedious and limited to naturally occurring variants. The development of technologies for cloning, manipulating, and expressing recombinant immunoglobulins has advanced our knowledge of antibody structure–function relationships by extending the scope of previous methods.

Transfection of cloned Ig genes provides an immortal, clonal source of antibodies of predefined specificity which can be thoroughly manipulated and produced in abundant quantities. Rare Ig classes (e.g., IgE) can be produced in sufficient quantities for structure–function studies. Matched sets of chimeric antibodies with the same variable domains, but different constant regions, can easily be generated. These molecules can be modified at will either by introducing specific point mutations or by site-directed randomization of a particular residue or residues. Moreover, completely unnatural variants resulting from "domain swapping," other novel combinations of Ig domains (e.g., bifunctional Abs), or genetic fusions to enzymes or other non-Ig domains can be produced. These techniques not only allow antibodies themselves to be thoroughly dissected, but could potentially yield valuable diagnostic and therapeutic agents (see Sections 5 and 6).

4.1. Combining Site Engineering

4.1.1. Antigen Binding

Proteolytic studies have shown that antigen binding is mediated by the Fab fragment of the antibody, specifically by the Fv fragment. Genetic studies have confirmed this observation. Thus, genetic engineering of antibody combining sites involves the manipulation of cloned heavy- and light-chain V-genes and their expression as Fab or Fv fragments, or as whole antibody molecules.

Prior to the development of systems for recombinant antibody expression, information about antigen-binding specificity was often inferred from the study of large collections of hybridoma proteins directed against simple organic haptens. Another approach is based on the identification of rare spontaneous variants. These have been found in myeloma cells and by FACS cloning of hybridoma cells. Studies using these approaches have been limited to rodent antibodies that recognize haptens.

Specific hypotheses concerning antigen recognition can be efficiently and directly tested by systematic mutagenesis of the combining site. Mutagenesis can be guided by primary amino acid sequence analysis, molecular modeling, or three-dimensional structural information from x-ray or NMR studies. Depending on the quality of the information available, mutations can be made rationally, semirationally, or randomly, although the latter approach requires powerful screening methods.

Since the amino acid sequence is readily determined from the DNA sequence of cloned V-genes, this information is most often used as a basis for antibody engineering experiments. Sequence comparison of a family of antibodies raised against an experimental hapten may allow correlations to be made between the primary sequence and hapten binding. For example (35), analysis of a family of antibodies specific for the hapten p-azobenzenearsonate (Ars) showed an invariant Ser residue at the variable-diversity junction of the heavy chain. A conservative

Ser to Thr mutation which preserves the hydroxyl group retained Ars-binding activity, while a Ser to Ala mutant had no detectable activity.

In another study with a family of 4-hydroxy-3-nitrophenylacetyl (NP)-binding antibodies (36), a single somatic mutation in an H2 residue (Trp33Leu) was proposed to be responsible for a 10-fold increase in affinity among secondary-response antibodies, despite the presence of numerous other somatic mutations in these antibodies. This hypothesis was confirmed by engineering a single amino acid change into an otherwise germline VH gene and showing that this mutation was sufficient to account for the affinity difference between primary- and secondary-response antibodies.

In one exceptional example, sequence information alone was used to deduce the structural basis for a 200-fold affinity difference between two hybridoma antibodies specific for the hapten Ars (37). Although 19 amino acid differences existed between the high- and low-affinity antibodies (11 light-chain and 8 heavy-chain differences), chain shuffling experiments suggested that the affinity difference between the antibodies was dependent mainly on the heavy chain. By systematically replacing each of the 8 amino acids in the low-affinity heavy chain with the corresponding amino acids from the high-affinity heavy chain, residues critical for binding were identified. Finally, combining three of these substitutions in the low-affinity heavy chain was sufficient to reproduce high-affinity binding.

Molecular modeling has also been used as a basis for antibody engineering experiments. In one study (38), site-directed mutagenesis was used to confirm a model of an antibody originally raised against a peptide from hen egg-white lysozyme (HEL) which also binds the native protein. A prediction of the model was that alteration of two "key" charged residues in the periphery of the proposed combining site would substantially reduce antigen binding. Quite unexpectedly, simultaneous substitution of these charged residues with noncharged polar residues (VK-Glu28Ser, VH-Lys56Gln) resulted in an apparent eightfold increase in affinity for HEL. This affinity increase was accompanied by a decrease in the cross-reactivity of the mutant with variant lysozymes from other species. In this case, modeling based on primary sequence alone was not a good predictor of antigen–antibody interactions.

The combination of molecular modeling with structural data from NMR or x-ray crystallography has been somewhat more successful in increasing our understanding of antigen binding. For example, a structural model of an antibody Fv fragment specific for the hapten 2-phenyloxazol-5-one (phOx) was built from canonical hypervariable loops, and the hapten was "docked" into the model using a combination of NMR and site-directed mutagenesis data. On the basis of this model, a predicted "bad contact" was removed by mutagenesis, resulting in a modest threefold improvement in affinity (39). In a follow-up study (40), semirational design was used to further improve hapten affinity by phage display of mutants in which key residues were randomized by site-directed mutagenesis. Mutants recovered after several rounds of selection, and containing a single mutation in either L3 or H3, showed a 3- to 5-fold improvement in affinity. When heavy- and light-chain point mutants were combined, an overall affinity improvement of 11- to 14-fold was observed compared to wild-type. Since the wild-type genes are germline, this affinity increase may be reminiscent of the process of affinity maturation observed during a secondary immune response.

In another example, site-directed mutagenesis was used to confirm the general features of a molecular model of an anti-digoxin antibody combining site (41). The model was based on a conformational search algorithm starting with the x-ray crystal structure of an unrelated phosphorylcholine (PC)-binding immunoglobulin, McPC603. This model was used to identify residues that might participate in binding. Semiconservative changes in the putative combining site generally resulted in only modest binding changes, although a few mutants had significantly lower binding affinity (100- to 200-fold) compared to wild-type. Specificity changes were also observed in some of the mutants. This information was used to infer an approximate binding mode for digoxin. The general features of this model concur with recently available x-ray structural data, although the fine details differ.

A successful example of affinity improvement guided by structure-based modeling was recently reported (42). A molecular model of an anti-phosphotyrosine antibody Fv fragment was developed using the conformational search algorithm. The model was based on the x-ray crystal structure of an unrelated Fab fragment (R19.9) directed against the hapten Ars. The resulting model was tested by mutational analysis of 12 heavy- and light-chain residues postulated to be near the proposed hapten-binding pocket. Most of the mutations tested had, as expected, either a negative or a neutral effect on binding. Surprisingly, two independent mutations in H3 (Tyr105Ala, Tyr106Ala) each resulted in an apparent 10-fold increase in affinity (although changing both residues simultaneously had a detrimental effect on binding). These results confirmed certain aspects of the model, although the effects of specific mutations on binding were unpredictable.

In a few cases, site-directed mutagenesis has been used as an adjunct to x-ray crystallography to interpret antigen–antibody binding. The contributions of particular amino acids to hapten binding in the anti-PC antibody McPC603 were studied in this way (43). Many observed features of the binding interaction in the crystal were confirmed by mutagenesis. Surprisingly, no increase in binding was observed when a hydrophobic H1 residue (Tyr33), which forms a hydrogen bond with the negatively charged phosphate group of the hapten, was replaced with any of the positively charged amino acids (His, Arg, or Lys). In fact, the Tyr33Arg and Tyr33Lys mutants failed to bind to a phosphorylcholine affinity column.

Similarly, alanine-scanning mutagenesis was used to study the role of six contact residues in the crystal structure of the anti-fluorescein monoclonal antibody 4-4-20 (44). Several of these contact residues were found to be critical for binding since substitution with Ala reduced the affinity for fluorescein by 1000-fold. However, when an L1 residue (Arg34) believed to be critical for high-affinity binding was substituted into three idiotypically related low-affinity antibodies, the binding affinities of these antibodies were not improved.

Crystal structures of antigen–antibody complexes involving protein antigens have also been probed by site-directed mutagenesis. Three different antibody co-complexes with HEL have been described, and two of these have been the focus of mutagenesis studies. Replacing a somatically mutated H3 residue in the HyHel-10 antibody with the corresponding germline residue (Asp101Ala) reduced antigen binding by ~10^4-fold, while replacing an adjacent somatically altered residue with its germline counterpart (Asp100Thr) had little effect on affinity, but altered the fine specificity of the antibody (45).

A second anti-lysozyme antibody, D1.3, has been studied by several groups. Following the surprising discovery that the isolated VH domain from this antibody had an affinity for HEL only 10-fold lower than that of the Fv fragment, PCR mutagenesis of H3 was used to generate several thousand mutants, one of which had an approximately 3-fold higher affinity than that of the isolated VH domain

(46). In a separate study of the Fv fragment of this antibody (47), conservative changes in seven contact (plus two additional) residues resulted in a library of about 500 mutants. Due to differential production levels in *E. coli,* 19 mutants were chosen for further study and, of these, 13 were analyzed for binding. Eleven of these mutants had about the same affinity as the wild-type, while only two suffered drastic affinity losses. The authors speculated that changes in entropy compensate for changes in enthalpy such that better binders are rarely found. A temperature-dependence analysis of binding affinity would confirm this hypothesis. An alternative hypothesis is that the contact residues inferred from the static x-ray data do not reflect the actual contact between antigen and antibody as two dynamic interlocking objects.

Another thermodynamic analysis of an antigen–antibody interaction resulted in a different interpretation (48). In this study of an anti-p185^{HER2} antibody, alanine-scanning mutagenesis identified 4 residues (out of a total of 22 in the CDRs) which made a large contribution to binding, although many more residues were implicated in binding. Binding was shown to be primarily entropy driven and appeared to be dominated by the hydrophobic effect.

Specificity of antigen binding has also been studied by site-directed mutagenesis (49). Using anti-idiotypic antibodies as a model for soluble protein antigens and an efficient codon-based mutagenesis procedure, the specificity of an anti-tumor antibody was altered (i.e., binding to one anti-Id was retained, while binding to another anti-Id was eliminated).

In summary, mutagenesis studies of antibody combining sites have been successful in many instances to confirm the effects of somatic mutations, to verify molecular models, and to support NMR and x-ray structural data. While mutations expected to improve affinity sometimes appear obvious on the basis of structural data, the consequences of rational mutagenesis of antibody combining sites have rarely been predictable. The success of antibody combining site engineering is likely to improve as the speed of x-ray structure determination increases, as the quality of computer models improves, and as powerful new genetic techniques to study these structures continue to be developed.

4.1.2. Catalytic Antibodies

Pauling proposed more than 45 years ago that transition state stabilization is the basis for enzymatic catalysis. More than 25 years ago, Jencks advanced the notion that antibodies raised against transition state analogs might mimic natural enzymes. Indeed, these hypotheses not only have had a profound influence on enzymology over the succeeding decades, but have spawned the discovery of catalytic antibodies in 1986 by groups led by Lerner, Benkovic, and Schultz (see Ref. 50 for review). Many antibodies to transition state analogs with catalytic activity (abzymes) have now been described, although other strategies have also been tried. Modest progress through antibody engineering has been achieved by site-directed mutagenesis to add reactive side chains, by engineering metal coordination sites into the binding pocket, and by the application of repertoire cloning, phage display, and transgenic animal technologies.

Several site-directed mutagenesis studies have been attempted with the aim of improving the catalytic activity of anti-PC binding antibodies. This family is particularly suited to such efforts for several reasons. The anti-PC family consists of a large number of members that have been well characterized in terms of both binding properties and amino acid sequence. The crystal structure of a prototypical member of this family, McPC603, has been determined. Finally, expression systems have been developed both for whole anti-PC antibody in transfected eukaryotic cells and for Fab fragments in *E. coli*.

In one mutagenesis study (51), a myeloma protein with PC-binding activity but no intrinsic catalytic activity, MOPC315, was chosen as a starting point. Although a detailed structure of this antibody was unavailable, affinity labeling data as well as amino acid sequence analysis suggested that VL-Tyr34 and VH-Lys52 are in proximity to the binding site for PC and might therefore represent reasonable targets for the introduction of catalytic residues. Substitution of the VL-Tyr34 residue with Phe did not diminish PC binding, implying that this residue is not in contact with the hapten. A VL-Tyr34His mutant, however, had significant catalytic activity with a catalytic rate constant (k_{cat}) that was 45-fold higher than that of the wild-type antibody, despite a 6-fold reduction in binding affinity.

In another mutagenesis study with a PC-binding antibody (52), two conserved heavy-chain residues of the myeloma protein S107 thought to be important in binding and hydrolysis were systematically mutated. Substitution of VH-Arg52 with Cys or Gln caused a significant reduction in both k_{cat} and K_m while a VH-Arg52Lys mutant had values very similar to those of the wild-type antibody. These results suggest that electrostatic interactions play a key role in the catalytic mechanism of this antibody. Substitution of VH-Tyr33 with Phe had little effect on the catalytic activity of S107, while substitution of this residue with Glu or Asp caused a reduction in the catalytic activity of the antibody. A VH-Tyr33His mutation resulted in an eightfold increase in k_{cat} compared to the wild-type. Although only a modest increase in catalytic efficiency could be achieved despite the detailed preexisting body of knowledge regarding this antibody family, the results of these two studies are promising.

Another antibody engineering strategy to improve the catalytic efficiency of antibodies has been the introduction of metal coordination sites near the binding pocket of the antibody. In principle, the presence of a metal ion in proximity to the substrate could significantly enhance the catalytic potential of abzymes as mimics of natural metalloenzymes. Furthermore, the combination of a light chain that complexes a metal ion or other cofactors with a library of substrate-binding heavy chains potentially represents a powerful genetic approach to creating catalytic antibodies at will.

By comparing the architecture of catalytic metal-binding sites in metalloenzymes with the CDRs in antibody light chains of known structure, a zinc-binding site was engineered into the light-chain CDRs of a fluorescein-binding antibody, 4-4-20, by introducing three His residues (53). The mutant was found to bind zinc with high affinity. Based on the known structure of 4-4-20, the bound zinc ion was predicted to occupy a solvent-exposed pocket at the bottom of the binding site in good position to interact with bound hapten.

A more general approach to generating antibodies that coordinate metals involves screening semisynthetic combinatorial libraries (54) (see Section 5.3.1). In this case, mutagenesis of VH-CDR3 yielded antibodies capable of binding a variety of metals. Diversification of the library by chain shuffling or mutagenesis of other CDRs may allow selection of metalloantibodies of the desired specificity. To date, however, the only report describing the successful generation of a catalytic metalloantibody is based on immunization with a hapten that is itself capable of coordinating metals (55).

A third approach to improving the catalytic efficiency of abzymes involves the use of classical biological selections or screening techniques in conjunction with modern molecular biology methods. One approach involves the use of substrates that, upon hydrolysis by the abzyme, release either biotin or a thiamine precursor (56). The use of such substrates in auxotrophic *E. coli* strains should confer a growth advantage to antibody mutants with enhanced catalytic activity. Although unproven, it seems likely that such genetic selection schemes will ultimately provide a powerful method of improving catalytic antibodies.

Thus, as in the case of engineering the combining site to approve affinity, attempts to improve the catalytic efficiency of abzymes have been limited to a few rare successes. The success rate will probably rise, however, as new genetic engineering techniques continue to be developed and applied to these exciting and important targets of antibody engineering.

4.2. Constant Region Engineering

Modifications to the constant regions of immunoglobulins by genetic engineering have focused on structure–function relationships in the triggering and control of antibody effector functions. Previously, knowledge of the properties of human Igs was based on the study of myeloma proteins which differed not only in their heavy-chain constant regions, but also in binding specificity and light-chain type. One of the first applications of the genetic engineering approach was the generation of matched sets of chimeric antibodies sharing the same variable domains and light-chain constant regions, but differing in their heavy-chain constant regions (57, 58). Comparison of C1q-binding and ADCC activities among these chimeric antibody families showed, for example, that the human IgG1 and IgG3 subclasses have the most potent complement fixation activities.

The binding site for C1q and the role of the Ig hinge in complement activation have been studied by genetic engineering. Site-directed mutagenesis studies pinpointed several residues in the CH2 domain of mouse IgG that were essential for C1q binding and, presumably, complement fixation (59). However, because these residues are conserved among human IgG subclasses which differ in their ability to activate complement, there must be additional structural features involved in C1q binding and activation. A study using domain-switched mouse–human chimeric antibodies showed that additional residues in the carboxy terminus of CH2 are responsible for human IgG subclass-specific differences in complement activation (60). A recent site-directed mutagenesis study has specifically identified polymorphic residues in the CH2 domain of human IgG which account for subclass-specific differences in complement activation (61).

Previous studies using isotype-switched or genetically engineered antibodies demonstrated a correlation between segmental flexibility and effector function, and further suggested that the Ig hinge region might play an important role in complement activation. Because the human IgG hinge regions are far more diverse in length and sequence than the constant regions, it has been proposed that these hinge differences might provide a structural basis for the differential ability of the various subclasses to activate complement. Analysis of a set of genetically engineered chimeric antibodies with different hinge lengths and compositions showed, however, that while hinge length indeed correlated with segmental flexibility, both C1q binding and complement fixation were nearly independent of the hinge domain (62). For example, replacing the hinge of a human IgG3 antibody with the IgG4 hinge did not significantly reduce the complement activation ability of the mutant, while an IgG4 antibody containing the IgG3 hinge displayed no complement activity. Thus, the hinge alone does not seem to be responsible for subclass-specific differences in complement activation. Furthermore, subsequent work showed that engineering the hinge or CH1 domains, so as to hinder the movement of the Fab arms, did not impair complement-mediated cytotoxicity (63). From these data it appears that complement is likely activated by multivalent binding of C1q to the CH2 domains of several clustered IgG molecules. This genetic dissection of the molecular interactions involved in C1q binding and activation has led to the engineering of a mutant human IgG1 that forms tail-to-tail homodimers (64). The dimeric IgG1 molecule is several hundred-fold more efficient at cytolysis than monomeric IgG1 (64, 65). This observation may lead to highly effective engineered antibodies for therapeutic modalities where cytolysis is important.

Other major immune system defenses, phagocytosis and type I hypersensitivity, are mediated by the binding of antibodies to membrane-bound Fc receptors of leukocytes. IgG typically directs the clearance of pathogens through the interaction of immune complexes with phagocytes bearing either a high-affinity Fc receptor (FcγRI) or a low-affinity Fc receptor (FcγRII or FcγRIII). Binding of IgE to mast cells or basophils potentiates an allergic response and may be important in the immune response to parasites. Site-directed mutagenesis has provided insight into the varied interactions of these antibodies with their receptors.

A site-directed mutagenesis study showed that binding of mouse IgG2b to human high-affinity FcγRI could be improved 100-fold with a Glu235Leu mutation (66). This result indicates that the upper portion of the CH2 domain or the lower hinge domain is important for binding to human FcγRI. The relative importance of each domain in this interaction was determined with a set of antibodies created by exchanging constant region domains between mouse IgE (which normally does not bind the human Fc receptor) and human IgG1 (67). This study concluded that the CH2 domain of human IgG1 contributes about 75% of the binding energy with the CH3 domain contributing the rest. A combination of domain-swapping and site-directed mutagenesis confirmed that multiple amino acids in the CH2 domain of human IgG are important in FcγRI binding and further indicated that the hinge influences this binding interaction (67, 68). Similarly, the binding of human IgG to FcγRII seems to require both the CH2 and CH3 domains (67) and appears to involve multiple points of interaction on the CH2 domain.

Using small fragments of the human epsilon constant domains synthesized in *E. coli,* the binding site of human IgE to FCεRI was mapped to a region of 76 residues at the junction between the CH2 and CH3 domains of IgE (69). While the CH4 domain of IgE does not appear to be directly involved in binding, it is likely that this domain serves to hold the other domains in the proper conformation for binding. Direct support for this hypothesis came from domain-swapping experiments which showed that substitution of the CH4 domain of mouse IgE with the CH3 domain of human IgG did not affect binding to FcεRI (70).

In summary, the ability to engineer novel immunoglobulins at will by genetic manipulation has yielded significant, though not always simple, information on the relationship between structure and function in the triggering and control of effector functions in the immune system. This information not only may explain basic biological functions in molecular detail but also may directly lead to better antibodies for human therapy.

4.3. Glycosylation

The importance of glycosylation in both the constant and variable domains of immunoglobulins has also been probed by antibody engineering. Glycosylation of Ig molecules can be either N-linked or O-linked, but only N-linked glycosylation can be altered by mutagenesis. N-linked (or Asn-linked) glycosylation may occur at the target sequence Asn–X–Ser/Thr, although not all targets are actually glycosylated. Studies in which N-linked glycosylation targets have been added or removed by site-directed mutagenesis have been informative.

The role of the carbohydrate moiety linked to the CH2 domain of IgG in effector functions has been studied by mutagenesis. Removal of the N-linked carbohydrate attachment site by site-directed mutagenesis in human IgG1 and IgG3 completely ablated complement fixation in both mutants (71). One of the modified IgGs had slightly altered pharmacokinetics but the other did not. In another study, a human IgG1 with a deleted carbohydrate attachment site in the CH2 domain retained a significant, albeit lower, level of CDC, but was incapable of ADCC (72).

While the functional importance of carbohydrate in the constant regions of immunoglobulins is well documented, its presence and importance in variable domains have only recently been explored by genetic engineering. According to one estimate, about 30% of human heavy-chain variable domains contain carbohydrate. The functional importance of heavy-chain variable region glycosylation in a series of anti-dextran antibodies was demonstrated by creating novel glycosylation sites by site-directed mutagenesis (73). The position of these carbohydrate moieties within CDR2 of the heavy-chain variable regions not only affected the affinity of the antibodies for antigen, but also influenced the structure of the attached carbohydrate groups.

In a recent study of a mosaic (see Section 5.2.2) anti-CD33 antibody (74), the CDR-grafted antibody displayed a binding affinity for antigen that was several-fold higher than that of the original mouse antibody. Site-directed mutagenesis confirmed that a carbohydrate group originally present in the mouse antibody, but eliminated in the mosaic version, was responsible for the increase in binding: restoring the glycosylation site in the mosaic antibody reduced its affinity to that of the mouse antibody, while removing the glycosylation site from the original mouse antibody increased its affinity. These two studies demonstrate that the presence of carbohydrate in the variable region can either enhance or attenuate antigen binding.

5. THERAPEUTIC ANTIBODIES

One of the few disappointments of hybridoma technology has been the inability to routinely produce human monoclonal antibodies using this technique. Human antibodies of predefined specificity would be invaluable in therapeutic applications. Within 10 years of the seminal work of Kohler and Milstein, it became possible to express recombinant antibodies, thus making antibody engineering possible. *In vitro* manipulation of Ig V-genes has yielded "humanized" versions of rodent monoclonal antibodies directed against many useful therapeutic targets. This technique is only useful for antibodies that are not subject to the limitations of tolerance. Raising antibodies to certain highly conserved "self" antigens, for example, has been extremely difficult. New and powerful genetic technologies, such as repertoire cloning, have emerged in recent years which offer the prospect of directly accessing the genes of the immune system without the limitations of tolerance. Another approach involves establishing a functional humoral immune system in experimental animals such as mice. In principle, this approach may allow human antibodies to be generated routinely following immunization. These technologies will undoubtedly contribute to the growing number of human monoclonal antibodies with therapeutic potential.

5.1. Human Antibodies

Despite the efforts of many labs to produce human monoclonal antibodies using hybridoma technology, there has been only limited success with this approach. Techniques used to immortalize antigen-specific human B cells include both mouse × human and human × human somatic cell fusions, as well as Epstein–Barr virus (EBV) transformation. These techniques generally suffer from several shortcomings, namely: (i) mouse × human hybridomas are unstable, preferentially segregating human chromosomes (especially chromosome 2, which contains the kappa locus); (ii) although genetically stable, human myeloma cell lines suitable for producing intraspecies hybrids can rarely be maintained in culture; and (iii) EBV-transformed cell lines are genetically unstable, produce low amounts of Ab, and usually produce Abs of the IgM class. In addition, ethical and technical considerations limit the source of immune B cells to special situations, such as viral infections or cancer.

Many of the problems of genetic instability associated with somatic cell fusions have been overcome by the development of trioma (human × mouse × human) technology (75, 76). This approach has been used to isolate human antibodies against cytomegalovirus, gp120 of human immunodeficiency virus type 1, hepatitis B surface antigen, tetanus toxin, and other viral antigens. As with other somatic cell fusion techniques, trioma technology is limited to those situations in which immune human B cells can be ethically obtained, and is probably most appropriate for generating antibodies against viral, cancer, or transplantation antigens. Since triomas are stable and produce adequate amounts of antibody, this approach should find increasing use in generating human antibodies against these important classes of antigen.

5.2. Humanized Antibodies

5.2.1. Chimeric Antibodies

Rodent antibodies are problematic in therapeutic applications primarily due to their immunogenicity. Chimeric antibodies, consisting of rodent variable regions and human constant regions, were first described in 1984 with the expectation that they would be less immunogenic, more efficacious, and have a longer half-life than their rodent counterparts (77, 78). In the 10 years since this technology was introduced, chimeric antibodies against many therapeutic targets have been developed (see Ref. 79 for review). These targets include many cancer-associated antigens, viruses, and cell-surface receptors. Expectations concerning immunogenicity, efficacy, and pharmacokinetics have generally been met.

One particularly well-characterized chimeric antibody is derived from the mouse hybridoma 17-1A which recognizes a cancer-associated surface antigen found on colorectal carcinoma cells. Chimeric antibodies representing all four human IgG subclasses have been made (80, 81). The chimeric antibodies have binding properties identical to those of the mouse monoclonal antibody from which they were derived. *In vitro* comparison of the biological effector functions of the four human IgG subclasses showed that the IgG1 antibody was comparable to the parental mouse antibody and superior to the other human IgG chimeras in its antitumor activity. When the chimeric IgG1(κ) antibody was infused into 10 patients with metastatic colorectal adenocarcinoma (82), the half-life was improved sixfold compared to the mouse antibody and the chimeric was indeed less immunogenic (although one patient did develop a modest anti-idiotypic response). No allergic or other toxic side effects were observed in any of the patients. Unfortunately, 7 patients had objective evidence of tumor progression 6 weeks after antibody administration, while 3 patients stabilized.

A preliminary clinical trial of a chimeric anti-CD4 antibody (Leu3a) in seven patients with mycosis fungoides showed that the chimeric had improved pharmacokinetics, reduced immunogenicity, and minimal toxic side-effects compared to the mouse antibody, but displayed only modest clinical efficacy (83). Several other phase I clinical trials with chimeric antibodies have given similar results. These early data suggest that chimeric antibodies may indeed be effective therapeutics, especially when single or limited doses are sufficient to produce clinical benefit.

5.2.2. Mosaic Antibodies

Chimeric antibodies, consisting of four rodent variable domains and, typically, eight human constant domains, are two-thirds human (Fig. 6.5). While chimeric antibodies are expected to be less immunogenic than rodent antibodies, it is possible that the rodent variable domains may remain immunogenic in the context of the human constant domains, giving rise to an anti-idiotypic immune response. Indeed, a modest anti-idiotypic response has been observed in several clinical trials with chimeric antibodies (82, 83) which may limit repeated long-term administration of these antibodies. To reduce this possibility, Winter and colleagues pioneered a genetic engineering approach designed to "humanize" the variable domains themselves (84–86). This technique involves replacing variable region residues not directly involved in binding with corresponding residues from appropriate human variable domains. Since only about one-fourth of the residues in the variable domains—specifically the complementarity determining regions (CDRs)—are involved in antigen binding, the resulting antibodies would be greater than 90% human (Fig. 6.5). Due to the patchwork alternation of rodent and human residues in these engineered variable domains, we propose calling such molecules mosaic antibodies.

The structural basis for this approach depends on the conserved architecture of the antibody combining site (see Chapter 2). A typical variable domain consists of two antiparallel β sheets, pinned together by a conserved disulfide, forming a β-sheet sandwich. Each variable domain has a four-stranded sheet which is solvent-exposed and a five-stranded sheet which forms the VH–VL interface. There are

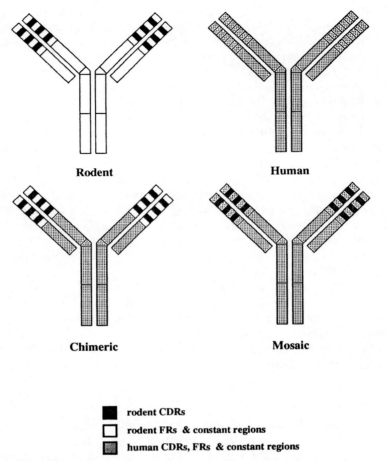

FIGURE 6.5   Chimeric vs mosaic antibodies. Chimeric antibodies consist of rodent variable regions and human constant regions. Mosaic antibodies are composed of humanized variable regions (i.e., rodent CDRs grafted onto human frameworks) and human constant regions.

four loops connecting the β strands of the variable domain, three of which are structurally equivalent to the CDRs. Though separated in the primary sequence, the six CDRs (three each from the heavy and light chains) come together in the tertiary structure to form the antigen combining site. In the half-dozen antigen–antibody structures that have been examined by x-ray crystallography (see Ref. 87 for review), all six CDRs appear to be involved in antigen binding. An antibody engineering study confirmed this finding (88), but also showed that some CDRs are critical for binding while others are less important.

While the three-dimensional structure of the framework residues is highly conserved among variable domains, until recently the CDRs were presumed to have no structural constraints due to the sequence hypervariability of these regions. However, theoretical studies suggest that the CDRs themselves are relatively conserved in structure, falling into several canonical classes (89, 90). This observation partly underlies the success of CDR grafting. In addition, the CDR grafting method depends on three critical assumptions: (i) antigen binding is solely mediated by

CDR residues, or by conserved framework residues; (ii) the conformations of the CDRs are independent of the framework to which they are attached; (iii) the VH–VL domain interface is highly conserved between rodent and human antibodies.

The simplest embodiment of the approach outlined by Winter would be to replace the framework residues of the rodent variable domains with the corresponding framework residues from human variable domains. While this approach was successful for simple haptens (84), subsequent studies showed it probably would not be universally successful (85, 86). For example, a 10-fold loss of binding affinity was observed following simple CDR grafting of the heavy chain of an anti-lysozyme antibody (86). This antibody suffered a 100-fold affinity loss following simultaneous CDR grafting of both heavy and light chains (91). These affinity differences were attributed to two main causes: the loss of critical, nonconserved framework residues important for binding which fell just outside the classical definition of H1 (violating assumption (i)), and the loss of key framework residues, not directly involved in antigen binding, but important in maintaining the structures of the CDRs (violating assumption (ii); see also Refs. 89, 90). When these human framework residues were replaced with the original mouse sequences, near wild-type affinity for lysozyme was restored (91). The importance of key framework residues in preserving the antigen-binding characteristics of the original rodent antibody in the mosaic version has been verified in several other studies.

Queen and co-workers developed an improved method of variable-region humanization, initially applied to an antibody (anti-Tac) recognizing the IL-2 receptor (92), that has proved to be quite general. This approach depends on careful selection of human framework donors bearing the highest overall sequence homology to the rodent variable domains, followed by molecular modeling to assess the importance of framework residues in either influencing the conformation of the CDRs or directly interacting with antigen. Framework residues meeting these criteria, as well as residues found to be atypical of related human V regions, are retained as their rodent counterparts. While the resulting humanized antibodies may be slightly less "human" than antibodies designed by simple CDR grafting, this study and many subsequent studies with other antibodies humanized by this approach have shown that this method produces antibodies which retain binding affinities at or very near wild-type levels. A variation of this approach involves the use of consensus human framework sequences rather than homologous individual human sequences (93, 94). These studies also relied on molecular modeling to identify important framework contacts. In one case (94), direct comparison of these methods showed that both were capable of producing high-affinity mosaic antibodies.

A third approach to V-region humanization was outlined by Padlan (95). According to this approach, only solvent-exposed residues in the frameworks which differed from those normally found in the parental rodent antibody would be replaced with human residues. This "veneering" approach has not yet been subjected to experimental verification.

Mosaic antibodies against a wide variety of antigens, reflecting the diversity of available rodent monoclonal antibodies, have now been produced (see Ref. 96 for review). The ultimate success of mosaic antibodies will depend not on the theoretical approach used to design them, but rather on their degree of immunogenicity compared to rodent (or chimeric) antibodies. This raises important questions about this approach: Is the ability to build mouse CDR residues into a human framework merely a nifty feat of protein engineering, or does this method really yield a molecule that will appear to be human to the human immune system? In essence, will the immune system "see" the conserved variable region residues as human in the context of the human frameworks, or as mouse in the context of the mouse CDRs? Early clinical results with one mosaic antibody against the human anti-lymphocyte antigen CAMPATH-1 appear promising in this regard (97). Only the results of the many clinical trials now underway will resolve these questions.

5.3. *In Vitro* Antibodies

5.3.1. *Repertoire Cloning*

The development of repertoire cloning (see Section 2.2) and filamentous phage display (see Section 3.2.2) technologies has ushered in a new era of man-made antibodies which may ultimately obviate the need to immunize animals to obtain antibodies against virtually any target (see Ref. 98 for review). At the very least, these technologies should enable genetic immortalization of Fab fragments from man and other species where traditional hybridoma technology has failed.

Two groups, led by Winter (99) and Lerner (100), were the first to demonstrate the feasibility of recovering functional antibody fragments from combinatorial libraries. Winter's group at Cambridge showed that antigen-specific clones with dissociation constants in the nanomolar range could be obtained when rearranged VH genes from the spleen of mice immunized with lysozyme were cloned by PCR and expressed in *E. coli* as isolated VH domains. Lerner and co-workers in La Jolla extended this result by generating a combinatorial library of immunoglobulin heavy-chain Fd fragments and light chains derived from a mouse immunized with the hapten *p*-nitrophenylphosphonamidate (NPN) and expressing the cloned Fab fragments in a bacteriophage lambda system. Because the heavy- and light-chain combinations generated by this approach are random, they do not necessarily reflect the original combinations present in individual B cells. Nevertheless, mouse Fab fragments capable of binding the hapten NPN were recovered from the combinatorial library.

The hypothesis that random combinations of heavy and light chains could produce specific antibodies was confirmed when antibodies recognizing influenza virus hemagglutinin (HA) were recovered from a combinatorial library generated from the mRNA of an immunized mouse (101). Sequence analysis of the resulting hemagglutinin-specific Fab fragments showed that the heavy chains were distinct, yet highly related, members of a gene family likely derived from a single B cell clone. This resemblance to the pattern of clonally related antibodies isolated by hybridoma technology led the authors to conclude that antibodies isolated from the combinatorial library were closely related to the immune response of the donor mouse.

Using tetanus toxoid (TT) as a model system, the isolation of human Fab clones from combinatorial libraries derived from peripheral blood lymphocytes (PBLs) of an immunized donor was reported (102). Antibody fragments with high affinity and specificity, characteristic of a secondary immune response, were obtained. Sequence analysis indicated greater sequence diversity than had been previously observed in the mouse HA-specific fragments.

Another group used this technology to isolate human autoantibody Fab fragments against human thyroid peroxidase (TPO) from B cells infiltrating the thyroid of patients with Graves' disease (103). These antibodies had very high affinities

($K_d \sim 10^{-10}M$) characteristic of serum autoantibodies. Like serum autoantibodies, these Fab fragments recognized two closely associated immunodominant regions on TPO. Sequence analysis of a panel of 30 Fabs revealed only five heavy- and light-chain combinations derived from four heavy- and three light-chain germline genes. Further, identical heavy–light combinations were found in more than one patient.

One limitation of the original repertoire cloning technology is that the number of clones expressing soluble antibody fragments produced in *E. coli* that can be examined at one time, even in phage lambda systems, is only about 10^6–10^7. Moreover, screening more than several hundred thousand lambda plaques is laborious. Although the immune repertoire is estimated to be on the order of 10^7–10^9, the loss of the original heavy–light pairings in the combinatorial process, as well as the variable production levels of antibody fragments expressed in *E. coli,* requires generating much larger libraries and, hence, demands more efficient screening methods. The application of phage display technology to antibody combining site fragments (23–27) has provided an elegant solution to this problem.

Phagemid display libraries can be enriched for binding clones by biopanning on polystyrene wells or dishes (23, 26) or by biochromatography (27). In biopanning (Fig. 6.6), an amplified M13 phagemid display library is loaded onto a well coated with antigen as in a conventional ELISA. The nonspecific phage are removed by copious washing and the bound phage are eluted by disrupting the "foreign domain"–ligand interaction. The elution of phage or phagemid particles can be accomplished with low or high pH (23), chaotropic agents, or free ligand or antigen (23, 27). The eluted phage constitute an enriched library. The enriched library can be amplified and another biopanning cycle performed if desired. Typically, enrichments of 10-fold to several thousand-fold are observed during each cycle, but this depends greatly on the particular system being studied. Isolated single clones can be obtained from the enriched library by infecting *E. coli* and selecting colonies that bear the antibiotic resistance marker carried by the plasmid. When sufficient enrichment has occurred, usually in three to six cycles, the binding specificity of isolated clones can be determined by an appropriate binding assay. In addition, the gene sequence encoding the Fab or Fv can be readily obtained from the plasmid contained within the phage.

One of the first applications of combinatorial libraries displayed on phage was the generation of human antibodies against the surface glycoprotein gp120 of human immunodeficiency virus type 1 (104). In theory, neutralizing human antibodies against this target could prove extremely valuable in passive immunotherapy of AIDS patients. A relatively restricted IgG1(κ) library was prepared from the bone marrow of an asymptomatic human immunodeficiency virus (HIV)-seropositive individual and a panel of high-affinity antibodies specific for gp120 from the IIIB strain of HIV-1 was recovered. Some of these Fab fragments were found to have neutralizing activity against both the IIIB and MN strains. Sequence analysis showed that the heavy chains appeared to have undergone somatic mutation characteristic of an antigen-driven immune response. Chain shuffling (see below) failed to improve the affinity of the binders, although differences in fine specificity were not examined in this study.

Libraries from two other asymptomatic carriers of HIV-1 yielded Fab fragments against several other viruses including cytomegalovirus, herpesvirus, varicella-zoster virus, and rubella (105). Recovery of these binding activities was correlated with the presence of high virus titers in the sera of these donors. Combining the variable

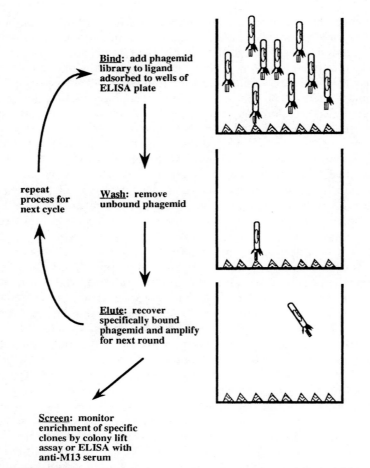

Bind: add phagemid
library to ligand
adsorbed to wells of
ELISA plate

repeat
process for
next cycle

Wash: remove
unbound phagemid

Elute: recover
specifically bound
phagemid and amplify
for next round

Screen: monitor
enrichment of specific
clones by colony lift
assay or ELISA with
anti-M13 serum

FIGURE 6.6   Screening phagemid libraries. A phagemid library is panned against a ligand that has been adsorbed to the wells of a conventional ELISA plate. Following washes to remove nonspecific phage, bound phage are eluted using either acid or excess free ligand. The process is repeated as necessary until the phagemid population is enriched for binders. Individual binders can be assayed for binding specificity and characterized by DNA sequencing.

domains from these anti-viral Fab fragments with the appropriate human constant region genes by standard chimeric antibody technology should yield recombinant human antibodies of vast therapeutic potential.

Since PBLs are a relatively poor source of blast cells that are actively involved in the immune response—and because consenting immunized human spleen donors can rarely be found—several investigators have begun to investigate the feasibility of recovering antigen-specific antibody fragments from combinatorial libraries derived from nonimmune donors. Though such libraries are not likely to be truly "naive," in principle it should be possible to recover low-affinity binders against a variety of antigens from a single large library. Secondary phage libraries in which V-genes recovered from the primary library are further modified might yield antibody fragments with improved affinities. Methods to increase diversity in the primary library include random point mutagenesis, chain shuffling, and the construction of semisynthetic libraries.

The construction of diverse libraries containing mu and gamma heavy chains as well as kappa and lambda light chains from the PBLs of unimmunized donors represented the first test of these ideas (106). From relatively large combinatorial libraries (10^7–10^8 clones) a few binders were identified with specificity for the "hapten" phOx or the "antigen" turkey egg-white lysozyme. These binders were mostly derived from mu-expressing B cells and had low affinities ($K_a \sim 10^6$–$10^7\ M^{-1}$), characteristics of antibodies resulting from a primary immune response. This result represents the first demonstration that antibodies of defined specificity can be obtained without the need for immunization. Further analysis of these libraries (containing mu, kappa, and lambda chains only) yielded a collection of low-affinity ($K_a \sim 10^6\ M^{-1}$) binders with specificity for various human self-antigens (107). These antibody fragments appeared to be derived from both germline and somatically mutated V genes. In several cases where more than one binder recognized the same protein, these appeared to recognize different epitopes.

Another group attempted to recover Fabs specific for progesterone from a combinatorial library consisting of mu and kappa chains derived from the bone marrow of unimmunized mice (108). A few binders of very low affinity ($K_a \sim 10^4$–$10^5\ M^{-1}$) that were cross-reactive with an unrelated protein antigen were recovered from the library. This disappointing result was perhaps due to the modest size of the library (5×10^6 clones), the use of a multivalent gpVIII phagemid display system rather than the monovalent gpIII system used by Marks *et al.* (106), and the choice of PCR primers which probably excluded a rare VH family that is associated with high-affinity anti-progesterone hybridoma antibodies. Despite these shortcomings, affinity maturation was mimicked by mutagenesis of the heavy- and light-chain V-genes using error-prone PCR, followed by phage display in a monovalent gpIII phagemid system. After several rounds of enrichment, clones with an approximately 10- to 30-fold increase in apparent affinity were identified. The clone with the highest affinity also had the lowest cross-reactivity to an irrelevant protein antigen.

Error-prone PCR was combined with an improved method for distinguishing antibodies of similar affinities to screen a small library of mutants derived from a mouse anti-4-hydroxy-5-iodo-3-nitrophenylacetyl (NIP) hybridoma antibody (109). A mutant with a fourfold increase in affinity (from $K_d = 4.2 \times 10^{-8}$ to $9.4 \times 10^{-9}\ M$) for the NIP hapten was recovered from the library. This modest affinity increase is typical of that observed for secondary response hybridomas.

Chain shuffling has also been suggested as a method to increase the diversity of initial binders with the goal of improving their affinity. An initial series of experiments with a panel of anti-phOx binding clones provided the groundwork for this approach (25). From a relatively small combinatorial library (2×10^5 clones) derived from the spleen of an immunized mouse, 23 phOx binders, composed of eight different VH genes and seven different VK genes, were recovered from a hapten affinity column. The best binder had an affinity typical of an antibody resulting from a secondary immune response ($K_d = 1 \times 10^{-8}\ M$). The heavy- and light-chain genes from this clone were recombined with the complementary light- or heavy-chain repertoires from the original immunized mice. The resulting "hierarchical" libraries, each consisting of 4×10^7 clones, yielded many strong binders after a single pass over an affinity column. Sequence analysis of a portion of these secondary clones identified many new partners for the original heavy and light chains, none of which had been recovered in the original library. Most of these differed from each other by small differences in the CDRs, although the affinities of these new binders were not reported.

Another series of experiments with NPN-binding clones provided further support for this approach (110). When several individual heavy or light chains from hapten-binding clones were recombined with complementary chains from the original immune NPN library, NPN binders were regenerated at a surprisingly high frequency. Unfortunately, the affinities of the new binders derived from these chain-shuffled libraries were not measured. By contrast, when this chain-shuffling experiment was repeated with complementary chains derived from a nonimmune mouse, human bone marrow, or human PBLs, no NPN-binding clones were found. Thus, while functional hapten-binding chains appear largely interchangeable in this system, this seems to be very dependent on prior antigenic stimulation.

Chain shuffling was applied to one of the weak anti-phOx binders (K_d = 3.2 × 10^{-7} M) from the naive human library of Marks et $al.$ (106) to dramatically increase its affinity (111). Shuffling the VH gene of this clone with a library of kappa and lambda light chains from the same unimmunized donor used to prepare the original library yielded almost 60 clones which appeared to have increased affinity for phOx. The best of these had an affinity (K_d = 1.5 × 10^{-8} M) that was 20-fold higher than that of the original clone. This new lambda light-chain gene was shuffled with a library of human VH1-family heavy-chain genes in which the original sequence of CDR3 was held constant to maintain hapten binding. Ninety new clones with higher apparent affinities were recovered. The affinities of 3 of the 5 mutants with the highest binding constants (K_d = 2.6 × 10^{-8} to 1.1 × 10^{-9} M) were higher than that of the intermediate binder from which they were derived, representing an overall increase of 12- to 320-fold compared to the original clone. Sequence analysis of heavy and light chains indicated in both cases that they were derived from the same germline genes found in the original clone and differed from those genes only by point mutations.

Chain shuffling has also been applied to antibody combining sites recognizing protein antigens. The panel of human anti-gp120 Fab fragments produced by Barbas et $al.$ (104) was used in an initial series of experiments (112). Heavy and light chains of 21 representative clones from the panel were recombined with each other using a binary plasmid system to generate about 400 new heavy–light pairings. A surprisingly high fraction of these combinations regenerated binding activity against gp120, with many having no significant loss in apparent binding affinity. When these heavy chains were combined with the light chain from an anti-tetanus toxoid clone, most of the recombinants retained anti-gp120 binding activity and had affinities (K_a ~ 10^7 M^{-1}) only about 5-fold below that of the parent. Similarly, when anti-gp120 light chains were paired with an anti-tetanus toxoid heavy chain, TT-binding activity was retained although the affinities of the recombinants were lowered 10- to 100-fold compared to that of the original tetanus toxoid Fab fragment. The dominance of the heavy chain in the antigen–antibody interaction has given rise to the term "chain promiscuity" and probably occurs naturally in hybridoma and myeloma antibodies.

Recently, a chain-shuffling experiment with a human autoantibody Fab fragment specific for human TPO was reported (113). Shuffling the heavy- and light-chain genes from a high-affinity parental Fab fragment (K_d = 8 × 10^{-9} M) with the parental light- and heavy-chain libraries yielded secondary libraries each consisting of ~10^7 clones. The frequency of TPO-binding clones in the secondary libraries was 10- or 100-fold higher than that in the parental library. Sequence analysis of 17 new clones showed they were identical or nearly identical to the parental clone, although one divergent heavy chain was found. The affinities of two of these clones for TPO (including the clone with the divergent heavy chain) were very similar to that of the parental clone ($K_d = 1.0 \times 10^{-10}$, 1.4×10^{-10} M) and both clones appeared to recognize an epitope that was the same or similar to that recognized by the parent.

From these studies, it is difficult to make generalizations about whether chain shuffling will be useful in improving the affinity of Fabs recognizing protein antigens. In some cases it is successful, while in others it is not. This may be a function of the particular antigen–antibody interaction involved, or a reflection of the limited size of reshuffled libraries used to date. Chain shuffling might also be useful for altering the fine specificity of antibody combining sites derived from repertoire cloning or for reducing the immunogenicity of human antibodies, though these ideas remain to be tested.

A third method of creating diversity in naive libraries involves combining cloned V-genes with synthetic CDRs, resulting in semisynthetic combinatorial libraries. This approach was used to create a fluorescein binding site in an antibody that originally had no affinity for this ligand (114). A human Fab fragment specific for tetanus toxoid was assumed to be "naive" with respect to fluorescein. Its heavy-chain CDR3 was randomized by PCR using synthetic oligonucleotides and combined with the light chain from the original clone. This method could potentially generate $\sim 10^{20}$ clones, but only a subset of 5×10^7 random clones was represented in the library. Phagemids were screened by panning and eluted either with acid or fluorescein. Acid-eluted clones had lower affinities for fluorescein ($K_d \sim 1 \times 10^{-6}$ M), were more cross-reactive, and displayed no consensus sequences within the synthetic CDR3. By contrast, fluorescein-eluted clones had higher affinities ($K_d \sim 1 \times 10^{-7} M$), were less cross-reactive, and showed strong conservation of several sequence motifs in CDR3. The affinities of the best binders obtained in this study were similar to the average affinities of hybridoma antibodies resulting from a secondary immune response in immunized mice.

A slightly different approach was used to create a semisynthetic library from which several clones that recognized the haptens phOx or NIP were recovered (115). A collection of about 50 human heavy-chain germline genes was cloned by PCR. These genes were modified to contain a synthetic CDR3 consisting of five or eight randomized residues and combined with a single germline lambda light-chain gene derived from an anti-BSA clone. Screening of these two libraries, each consisting of $\sim 10^7$ clones, yielded many binders for each hapten. The best of these binders had dissociation constants in the micromolar range, similar to those of hybridoma antibodies resulting from a primary immune response to these haptens. Sequencing revealed that most of the clones were unique, although many were derived from a single VH gene family. Limited chain shuffling with a few light chains generally abolished binding, indicating that the light chain is indirectly, or perhaps directly, involved in hapten binding. When the semisynthetic library was panned against several protein antigens, a single clone specific for human tumor necrosis factor was identified, but no binders were identified which recognized either turkey egg-white lysozyme or human thyroglobulin. Thus, the utility of this method in generating even low-affinity clones which recognize protein antigens has not been firmly established.

A naive human semisynthetic combinatorial library in which the CDR3 segments of both heavy and light chains were synthetic was shown to contain several clones specific for concanavalin A (Con A) (116). In this case, the CDRs were not completely random, but rather were biased toward the most common naturally occurring human amino acids at each position. This strategy reduced the potential number of clones in the library while presumably minimizing the possibility of introducing amino acids having deleterious structural consequences. Moreover, this consideration may also have important implications for the immunogenicity of the variable domains selected from such a library. A second major difference between this study and previous studies was the use of heavy- and kappa-chain gene segments resulting from PCR amplification of human genomic DNA rather than one or a restricted set of germline V-genes. Although only a small percentage of potential sequences was accessible due to limitations of library size, a number of clones with low affinity, but high specificity, for Con A were identified and six of these were further characterized. Sequence analysis showed that while several amino acids in the CDR3s were conserved, an expected Con A-binding tripeptide core sequence was not observed in these V-genes.

Recently, two groups have reported panning phage display libraries using whole cells rather than purified antigen (117, 118). One group used transfected CHO cells displaying TPO on their surface to recover six new human Fab autoantibodies for TPO from a library derived from patients with Graves' disease (117). These clones had high affinities for TPO ($K_d \sim 10^{-10}$ M) and consisted of heavy- and light-chain sequences that were similar, but not identical, to those of Fab fragments previously isolated by screening a bacteriophage lambda form of the same library with purified antigen. Another group used human red blood cells to recover antibody fragments specific for blood group antigens of the ABO, Rh, and Kell systems from a phage display library derived from two unimmunized donors (118). This strategy provides a new approach to cloning antibody fragments which recognize cell surface antigens, including human antibodies to self antigens.

5.3.2. Metaphoric Antibodies

The metaphoric process harnesses the power of phagemid display selection to evolve mouse antibodies into fully human antibodies. The basis of the metaphoric process is the promiscuous pairing of antibody heavy and light chains. Promiscuity refers to the ability of a given heavy chain to combine with many different light chains (or vice versa) to create a binding site for antigen. This phenomenon has been observed in chain shuffling, where a cloned chain is paired with a library of matching chains and typically many different combinations are found to form functional combining sites (25, 104, 110–113). Chain shuffling has been done successfully within the boundaries of a single species—for example, by combining a human heavy chain with a library of human light chains—for the modification of affinity. The metaphoric process is simply chain shuffling across species borders. Mouse antibody light chains, derived from clones that bind cognate antigen (27), have been used to identify active human heavy chains (119). The second half of the metaphoric process is the substitution of mouse light chains with human light chains. By the metaphoric process, a panel of mouse antibody clones was transformed into a panel of fully human antibody clones that bound the same antigen. This method may be useful in generating human anti-self antibodies that otherwise would be very difficult to obtain. In general, it may be possible to convert previously identified mouse antibodies with desirable binding characteristics into human antibodies with similar binding properties.

5.3.3. Humanized Mice

In addition to repertoire cloning, several new approaches have emerged in recent years aimed at generating human antibodies by genetic engineering. These approaches could perhaps best be characterized as trying to build a better mouse.

One approach is based on the development of so-called SCID-Hu mice (120, 121). Severe combined immunodeficiency (SCID) mice suffer from a complete lack of B and T cells and are therefore rendered completely immunodeficient. However, immunocompetence can be restored by transplanting either human PBLs (120) or human fetal liver stem cells (121). The presence of a functional human immune system in SCID recipients raises the possibility that immunization of these mice might give rise to human antibodies which could be immortalized by hybridoma technology or repertoire cloning. Though the hybridoma approach has had little success, repertoire cloning was used in one case to rescue human Fab fragments from SCID-Hu mice immunized with hepatitis B core antigen (122).

Another approach is based on replacing the Ig locus of the mouse with the human Ig locus at the gene level. In principle, such engineered mouse strains might be capable of mounting an immune response to an immunogen, rearranging their human Ig genes, undergoing affinity maturation in the context of an immune system, and producing authentic human antibodies. Recent efforts with transgenic mice have supported the feasibility of several aspects of this approach. Transgenic mouse strains have been constructed that are capable of rearranging human heavy- (123, 124) and light- (124) chain genes, and of producing antibodies containing human sequences. Sequence analysis of rearranged heavy chains in the transgenic mice showed that most of the major mechanisms that contribute to antibody diversity appear to be active for the transgenes. Although no evidence of somatic mutation was observed in this study, the authors attributed this to a lack of antigenic stimulation due to the sterile environment in which the mice were maintained. Methods of introducing large (~100 kb) genomic segments of the human Ig locus into transgenic mice have recently been described (123). If these mice are capable of responding to antigenic stimulation and undergoing affinity maturation, hybridomas derived from such animals may represent a useful source of human monoclonal antibodies.

Instead of replacing the entire mouse Ig locus with human Ig genes, a slightly less ambitious approach involves replacing only the mouse constant regions with their human counterparts in transgenic mouse strains. Immunization of such mice should yield chimeric mouse–human antibodies without the need of further *in vitro* manipulation. Progress toward this goal was made recently when a mouse strain was described that produces kappa chains with human constant regions (125). This strain was capable of producing antigen-specific antibodies, following immunization with various haptens, and appeared to undergo affinity maturation via somatic hypermutation.

Finally, when rodent hybridomas producing antibodies of desirable specificity are already available, homologous recombination can be used to replace the rodent constant regions with human constant regions, yielding hybridoma cell lines which produce chimeric rodent–human antibodies (126). The potential advantages of this method compared to traditional recombinant DNA methods include expediency and the possibility of creating stable cell lines producing wild-type (i.e., hybridoma) levels of chimeric antibody.

6. DESIGNER ANTIBODIES

The globular structure and functional independence of immunoglobulin domains not only underlie the successful construction of chimeric antibodies, but also provide the basis for a variety of fusion proteins containing immunoglobulin domains. These fusions are generally of two types. In one type of Ig fusion protein, the antigen-binding specificity of the variable domains is retained while the Ig constant regions are replaced with some other activity (e.g., enzyme, toxin, growth factor). Such fusion proteins find applications as *in vitro* and *in vivo* diagnostics and as therapeutics. The other main type of Ig fusion protein consists of an amino terminal fusion of non-Ig domains to the Ig constant regions. This strategy has been successfully used to create soluble forms of several cell-surface receptors (e.g., TCR, MHC) for structure–function studies, as well as to produce several potential therapeutics.

6.1. *In Vitro* Diagnostics

The first reported designer antibody (127) consisted of an (Fab')$_2$-like molecule in which the CH2 and CH3 domains of a mouse anti-hapten antibody were replaced with the nuclease from *S. aureus*. The resulting fusion protein retained both hapten-binding specificity and nuclease activity and was active in an ELISA-type assay. These results have provided the basis for subsequent fusions of this type which have potential as *in vitro* diagnostic reagents.

A potentially useful immunofusion protein was generated by replacing the Fc region of an anti-hapten antibody with the photoprotein aequorin from *Aequorea victoria* (128). Aequorin is capable of generating bioluminescence upon oxidation of luciferin in the presence of Ca^{2+}. The resulting Fab'-like molecule was purified by hapten affinity chromatography and retained essentially wild-type aequorin activity. The utility of the fusion protein in a solid-phase ELISA format was demonstrated. Substitution of other antigen-binding activities could result in a highly sensitive bioluminescent assay for hormones, peptides, or proteins.

Another application of this technology is to genetically fuse the Fab or (Fab')$_2$ portion of an antibody to an enzyme that is traditionally used in immunoassays. To demonstrate this principle, the Fab' portion of an antibody against a neurotoxin was fused to alkaline phosphatase (PhoA) of *E. coli* (129). Since PhoA is active only as a dimer, the fusion protein was secreted to the periplasm of *E. coli* where it formed an (Fab')$_2$-like molecule. The immunofusion protein retained wild-type affinity for the neurotoxin and retained at least 50% of the enzymatic activity of purified PhoA.

Though most immunofusions which retain antigen-binding activity involve a carboxy terminal fusion of a non-Ig domain to the Fv or Fab fragments of an antibody, there is one example of a fusion to the amino terminus of a variable domain (130). In this case, the B fragment of staphylococcal protein A was fused to the amino terminus of a hapten-specific single-chain Fv. Following *E. coli* expression, renaturation, and purification, the fusion protein retained wild-type affinity both for hapten and for immunoglobulin Fc domains through its protein A moiety.

6.2. *In Vivo* Diagnostics

For certain *in vivo* applications such as tumor imaging, the use of Fab or (Fab')$_2$ fragments is preferred over whole Ig due to the greater tissue penetration, more rapid clearance, and lack of effector functions (e.g., Fc receptor binding) of these fragments. However, these fragments are not always easily prepared by conventional proteolytic digests due to low yield, degradation of the products, or difficulties in purification. A clever solution to these problems was to engineer a mutant lacking the CH2 domains (131). This mutant assembled correctly and appeared to have enhanced antigen-binding properties, but lost the abilities to mediate ADCC and CDC. The mutant had pharmacokinetic properties similar to an authentic human (Fab')$_2$ and localized to tumors more rapidly than the parental chimeric antibody. These properties could make this engineered deletion mutant an excellent vehicle for radioimaging of tumors.

Another aspect of radioimaging that has been addressed by recombinant DNA techniques is the conjugation of metallic radionuclides to the targeting antibody. Chemical coupling of metal chelators to antibodies yields a heterogeneous product, often leads to aggregation, and can give rise to an immune response. Genetic fusion of the ubiquitous, metal-binding protein metallothionein to an (Fab')$_2$ fragment, which circumvents these problems, was recently reported (132). The resulting molecule could be labeled to high specific activity and localized to artificial targets in mice. An Fv-like version of this antibody–metallothionein fusion protein with similar properties was produced in *E. coli.* Chimeric or mosaic versions of such fusion proteins could be useful in radioimaging of human tumors.

6.3. Therapeutics

6.3.1. Immunotoxins

In some therapeutic applications, it will be appropriate to use "naked" chimeric, mosaic, or recombinant human antibodies, with heavy-chain constant regions chosen to elicit certain desirable effector functions. In other applications, such as cancer therapy, it may be more desirable to use the targeting properties of the antibody to deliver a toxin directly to the target cells. Such toxins, generally derived from bacterial or plant sources, are quite potent and must be directly conjugated to the antibody to avoid nonspecific cell killing. Chemical conjugation has several drawbacks, including heterogeneity of the product and low yield. Genetic methods have therefore been applied to produce recombinant immunotoxins linked to *Pseudomonas* exotoxin (PE) or a modified form with lower cytotoxicity (PE40), diphtheria toxin (DT), ricin, and other toxins (see Ref. 133 for review). Since these toxins are harmless to bacteria, recombinant immunotoxins can be produced in *E. coli.*

The first recombinant immunotoxin consisted of a single-chain Fv specific for the interleukin-2 receptor (anti-Tac) linked to PE40 and was produced in *E. coli* (134). The affinity of the immunotoxin was about threefold lower than that of intact anti-Tac, which is not unprecedented for scFv constructs (see Section 3.2.1). However, the recombinant version was significantly more potent *in vitro* than the chemically conjugated molecule. The scFv-immunotoxin was cytotoxic to cells expressing the IL-2 receptor on their surface including T-cell leukemia cell lines, activated human lymphocytes, and cells from patients with adult T-cell leukemia and chronic lymphocytic leukemia, but was not cytotoxic to cells lacking this marker.

Recombinant immunotoxins have also been made using diphtheria toxin. A single-chain Fv (anti-Tac) was linked to a truncated form of diphtheria toxin and expressed in *E. coli* (135). Unlike the PE40 immunotoxins which had the toxin fused at the carboxyl end of the Fv, the DT immunotoxin was constructed with the toxin fused at the amino terminus. This molecule was very cytotoxic to cell lines bearing the IL-2 receptor but not to cells lacking the receptor.

Potent anti-CD5 immunoconjugates were produced using chimeric Fab' or (Fab')$_2$ fragments that were synthesized in *E. coli* and chemically conjugated to a truncated form of the plant toxin ricin A (136). The Fab' conjugate had a fourfold loss of affinity compared to the conjugated whole antibody, while the (Fab')$_2$ conjugate had no affinity loss. The Fab' conjugate was slightly less cytotoxic than either the (Fab')$_2$ or whole antibody immunoconjugates.

For therapeutic applications using immunotoxins, it is desirable to minimize immunogenicity. However, the toxins most commonly used in the construction of immunotoxins are themselves highly immunogenic. An alternative approach is to use toxin moieties of human origin, rather than toxins derived from bacteria or plants, and to couple these toxins to chimeric, mosaic, or human variable regions. An example of this approach is the production of a chimeric antibody fragment directed against the human transferrin receptor in which the CH2 and CH3 domains were replaced with human angiogenin, a cytotoxic inhibitor of protein synthesis (137). This immunotoxin retained the antigen specificity of the original antibody and was moderately effective in inhibiting protein synthesis in cells expressing the receptor. The recombinant molecule was significantly more potent than chemically linked versions.

A novel approach to antibody-mediated tumor therapy is to target an enzymatic activity to tumor areas using an antibody–enzyme fusion, which then converts a nontoxic prodrug into an active chemotherapeutic agent. Though not strictly immunotoxins, the use of such fusions is exemplified by a single-chain anti-carcinoma antibody fused to β-lactamase (138). This molecule was produced in *E. coli*, was capable of binding to tumor cells, and rendered antigen-bearing tumor cells sensitive to the effects of a prodrug in a dose-dependent manner.

6.3.2. Bifunctional Antibodies

Antibodies normally combine target specificity with the ability to mediate effector functions through their constant regions. Bifunctional (or bispecific) antibodies represent another approach to antibody-based therapy (see Ref. 139 for review). In bifunctional antibodies, target specificity is combined with effector cell specificity. Generally, effector cells are targeted either through the T cell receptor/CD3 complex on cytotoxic T cells or through Fc receptors for IgG on various myeloid cells.

Several methods of producing bifunctional antibodies are commonly used. Fusion of two hybridoma cell lines with desired specificities to create a hybrid hybridoma (or quadroma) is the classical approach. A major drawback of this method is that such cell lines produce a mixture of many different heavy–light combinations (up to 10), which results not only in a low yield of the desired combination but also in a challenging purification problem. Moreover, this method is limited to production of whole Ig molecules which are more likely to be immunogenic than smaller Ig fragments. This approach can, however, be easily adapted to the use of chimeric or mosaic antibodies by fusing transfectomas, although the problems of yield and purification remain.

Another widely used approach is chemical cross-linking of antibody Fab or Fab' fragments. Coupling strategies have been devised which ensure that only heteroconjugates are formed, although the yields are often low due to difficulties in producing the enzymatic fragments. Direct expression of Fab' fragments in *E. coli* followed by chemical coupling was shown to be a relatively efficient method of producing a bivalent (Fab')$_2$ fragment (140). This technology was used to produce a mosaic bispecific (Fab')$_2$ fragment with specificity for both tumor cells and CD3-expressing effector cells. Further engineering of the Fab' fragments permitted direct assembly in *E. coli* of bivalent (though not bispecific) (Fab')$_2$ fragments.

Another recombinant solution to the problem of efficiently producing bifunctional antibodies involves the use of leucine zippers to guide heterodimer formation (141, 142). Leucine zippers are short amphipathic helices with leucine occurring every seventh residue. One group used this approach (among others) to produce bivalent Fv fragments in *E. coli* (141). Another group exploited the propensity of the leucine zippers of Jun and Fos to preferentially form heterodimers in order to produce a bispecific (Fab')$_2$-like fragment which binds both the IL-2R and CD3 (142).

Recently, a new method of producing bivalent or bispecific antibody fragments in *E. coli* was described (143). This method uses single-chain VH–VL polypeptides connected with a linker that is too short to allow the domains to pair with each other. This forces the domains on one chain to pair with the complementary domains on another chain, forming a bivalent dimeric antibody fragment, or "diabody," with antigen-binding sites oriented in opposite directions. Bispecific diabodies can also be produced by mixing heavy- and light-chain variable domains from two antibodies on complementary chains.

6.3.3. Other Antibody Fusions

One of the first recombinant antibody fusions with therapeutic potential consisted of a monoclonal antibody, specific for the fibrin β-chain, in which the Fc portion was replaced with an engineered version of the β-chain of tissue-type plasminogen activator (t-PA) (144). The resulting (Fab')$_2$-like fusion protein retained fibrin-binding activity within 10-fold of the wild-type whole Ig and possessed at least 70% of the activity of native t-PA. This recombinant represents a thrombolytic agent that is more specific and more potent than t-PA alone which could provide increased clot dissolution with less systemic fibrinogenolysis.

Another class of antibody fusions termed "immunoadhesins" consists of various domains of CD4 fused to Ig heavy- (145, 146) or light-chain (146, 147) constant regions. The resulting molecules are analogous to anti-gp120 antibodies with the CD4 portion substituting for the variable domains. Since CD4 is the cellular receptor for gp120, it is conceivable that a soluble form of the receptor might block HIV-1 infectivity. Two immunoadhesins were constructed in which the first two or first four Ig-like domains of CD4 were fused to the human IgG1 heavy chain. These immunoadhesins had many features expected for a human anti-gp120 antibody, including wild-type gp120-binding affinity, longer *in vivo* half-life than recombinant soluble CD4 alone, Fc receptor binding (but unfortunately no detectable C1q binding), and the ability to protect against HIV-1 infection *in vitro* (145).

Similarly, molecules in which the first two CD4 domains were fused to the mouse kappa constant region or the CH2 and CH3 domains of mouse IgM or IgG2a constant regions were also capable of inhibiting syncytium formation (146). These heavy-chain fusion proteins retained binding to both FcR and C1q. A chimeric light chain consisting of the amino terminal domain of CD4 fused to the mouse kappa constant region suggested that the first domain of CD4 has an Ig variable region-like character which allows these chimeric light chains to form covalent dimers (147). However, this conclusion is difficult to reconcile with the recent crystal structure of CD4. Moreover, it is unlikely that CD4 acts as a dimer *in vivo*.

Fusions of antibodies to growth factors have also been described. For example, the Fc region of a chimeric anti-dansyl human IgG3 antibody was replaced with insulin-like growth factor 1 (148). The resulting $(Fab')_2$-like molecule bound the dansyl hapten but only weakly bound the growth factor receptor, although the latter result may be explained by the use of rat rather than human IGF1. Similarly, epidermal growth factor was genetically fused to the CH3 domain of a chimeric anti-CD3 human IgG1 antibody (149). This molecule recognized both CD3 and the EGF receptor and was capable of targeting human cytotoxic T cells to lyse EGF receptor-bearing tumor cells.

Two types of fusions between IL-2 and antibody have been described (150, 151). Human IL-2 was fused to the human IgG1 constant region so as to replace the heavy-chain variable domain (150). The resulting "immunoligand" was secreted in the form of a covalent heavy-chain homodimer, displayed the ability to bind the IL-2 receptor, retained the proliferation-inducing activity of authentic IL-2, and had both CDC and modest ADCC activity. Another Fab'-like antibody–IL-2 fusion was produced by replacing the Fc region of a chimeric anti-tumor human IgG1 antibody with human IL-2 (151). Both tumor and IL-2R binding activities were retained in the fusion protein, although its ability to support tumor cell destruction using low-affinity IL-2R-bearing effector cells from resting human PBLs was substantially less than that of rIL-2.

6.4. Cell-Surface Receptor–Antibody Fusions

Producing recombinant, soluble cell-surface receptors for structure–function analyses has been problematic. One successful approach involves genetic fusion of the extracellular domains of the receptor to Ig constant region domains which enables secretion of the fusion protein. Alternatively, Ig variable domains can be fused to cell-surface receptors to create cells with predefined specificity.

In an attempt to solubilize the T cell receptor, several TCR–Ig fusions were made (152). When a TCR Vα domain was fused to an Ig heavy-chain constant region, pairing occurred with the endogenous light chain of the transfected cells, forming an Ig-like tetramer which retained both TCR and Ig antigenic determinants. However, when a TCR Vβ domain was fused to the same constant region, this fusion protein neither was secreted nor did it assemble with light chain. In addition, a light chain consisting of the Vβ domain fused to Cκ did not assemble with the chimeric Vα heavy chain. Thus, the TCR Vα domain has Ig-like character, while the Vβ domain apparently does not.

To create a population of T cells with MHC-independent specificity, an Ig VH region gene was fused to a TCR Cα constant region gene to make a line of transgenic mice (153). T cells expressing the chimeric α-chain in association with an endogenous β-chain formed a functional receptor that retained an idiotope characteristic of the Ig. Further, these cells were activated by the hapten recognized by the original antibody, demonstrating that the hybrid TCR was functional. Along similar lines, a functional non-MHC-restricted TCR was produced by fusing the heavy- and light-chain variable domains of an anti-hapten antibody to the α- and β-chain constant domains of the TCR (154). Cells transfected with these genes produced a surface receptor that exhibited an idiotope characteristic of the antibody, and responded to hapten in a non-MHC-restricted manner, as evidenced by either IL-2 production or cytolytic activity. Fusion of an anti-hapten heavy chain to either Cα or Cβ was sufficient to produce a functional TCR (154).

Ig–MHC fusion molecules involving either class I or class II molecules have also been described. For example, substitution of the amino terminal domains of the α- and β-chains of an MHC class II molecule with the heavy- and light-chain variable domains, respectively, of an anti-CD4 antibody resulted in a hybrid cell-surface receptor that retained both idiotypic and antigen-binding characteristics of the original antibody (155). This highly specific, non-MHC-restricted class II molecule should facilitate studies of class II-mediated effector functions.

A soluble, divalent MHC class I–Ig fusion protein was also recently described (156). This molecule was produced by fusing the three extracellular domains of the class I molecule to an intact Ig heavy chain upstream of the variable domain. Cotransfection of this chimeric heavy chain with β2-microglobulin into a light chain producing cell line yielded an Ig-like complex composed of chimeric heavy chains, light chains, and β2-microglobulin. This molecule had serological and biochemical features of both the Ig and MHC molecules. In addition, it inhibited lysis of target cells by alloreactive T cells at low concentrations and bound to these cells with high affinity.

7. FUTURE DIRECTIONS

In view of the tremendous progress that has been made in the past several years in repertoire cloning and phage display technologies, it appears likely that continued efforts in these areas will be productive. This progress has led to speculation that a functional immune system could be recapitulated in a bacterium (157). Many aspects of the immune system have already been mimicked in *E. coli* using molecular biology techniques, including combinatorial association of heavy and light chains, clonal selection, somatic mutation, and repertoire shift (i.e., chain shuffling).

One mechanism of generating antibody diversity that has not yet been demonstrated in bacteria is gene conversion. This mechanism plays an important role in avian immune systems, and has also been shown to contribute to Ig diversity in mammalian systems. This process could be mimicked in *E. coli* either by PCR recombination *in vitro* (158), or by *in vivo* transfer of V-gene "donors" using either F factors or P1 transducing phage. Fortunately, the majority of human germline kappa-, lambda-, and heavy-chain genomic V-genes have already been cloned and sequenced.

A further aspect of Ig diversity that has not yet been attempted in bacteria is active *in vivo* VJ or VDJ recombination. Several mammalian enzymes responsible for this process have been cloned, sequenced, and expressed in transfected mammalian cells (159). If these genes can be functionally expressed in *E. coli,* perhaps recombination of genomic V-gene segments can also be achieved in bacteria.

Another area of future research is to more accurately mimic somatic mutation of V-genes in *E. coli.* Though this process has been imitated by randomizing CDR residues (see Section 4.1.1), the number of potential mutants that can be generated by this approach exceeds the number of molecules in the universe. Evidently the immune system is far more efficient than this since productive mutants can be generated and selected *in vivo* within a period of weeks. Therefore, an understanding of the mechanism of somatic mutation might lead to more purposeful *in vitro* or *in vivo* mutagenesis of recombinant antibodies. Alternatively, perhaps a "somatic mutase" activity will someday be cloned from the mammalian immune system and transplanted into *E. coli.*

Rather than attempting to reproduce the mammalian humoral immune repertoire in *E. coli,* perhaps it may be possible to produce diverse repertoires in bacteria that greatly exceed the capabilities of the mammalian immune system. The probability of finding binding clones of arbitrarily high affinity is a steep function of the number of clones in the library. With new technologies in development, it may become feasible to create libraries of 10^{12} members nearly as easily as libraries of 10^8 members are created today (160).

The availability of very large libraries would undoubtedly require more efficient screening techniques. The use of biological selection schemes, rather than screening techniques, would provide a more powerful approach to identifying binders (see Section 4.1.2). One idea is to display target antigens on the surface of *E. coli* such that recognition of antigen by antibody-displaying phage is required for infection (161). In this way, populations of phage with affinity for the target could be quickly enriched after several rounds of infection.

Considering the challenges that remain to reproducing a fully functional immune system in bacteria, others have chosen to reproduce a functional human immune system in mice. This goal appears tenable on the basis of progress that has already been made (see Section 5.3.3), although the construction of mouse strains is quite time-consuming. Whether the objective is to reproduce an immune system in *E. coli* or a human immune system in mice, the ability to routinely produce useful antibodies will determine the ultimate utility of these methods.

Just as the combination of recombinant DNA and hybridoma technologies in the 1970s gave rise to the field of antibody engineering, it seems likely that the merger of structure determination and computer modeling technologies will stimulate new advances in the antibody field in the 1990s and beyond. The number of x-ray structures of antibody combining sites has risen from a handful in the 1970s to almost 50 today. About half of these are antigen–antibody co-complexes. This increase is due to the advent of recombinant DNA technology, improvements in techniques for growing crystals, the use of more powerful x-ray sources (i.e., synchrotrons) to generate data, and advances in computer technology. Recently, NMR has emerged as a powerful adjunct method of generating partial structural information about antibody combining sites, although crystallography remains the method of choice. Together, these two methods of structure determination will continue to add to the existing database of three-dimensional structures of antibody combining sites.

In lieu of a high-resolution crystal structure, which typically requires several years to complete, several groups have relied on computer modeling to guide antibody engineering experiments. To date, this approach has been particularly helpful in designing mosaic antibodies (see Section 5.2.2). Its application to improving antibody affinity, even when accurate structural information is available, has had limited success (see Section 4.1.1). Advances in structure modeling algorithms as well as continual improvements in the speed and power of computers will likely result in significant progress in antibody modeling in the next decade. Moreover, since many modeling techniques are based on the structural database, the accuracy of computer models will undoubtedly improve as the number of three-dimensional structures increases.

An area likely to benefit from advances in structure-based modeling is the design of antibody mimetics, small peptide analogs or organic molecules that can mimic the binding properties of antibodies. For many therapeutic applications, small molecule mimetics would be preferable to whole antibodies, antibody fragments, or peptides due to their lack of immunogenicity, greater tissue penetration, solubility (compared to peptide mimics), resistance to proteolysis, oral availability, lower cost of production, and potential to cross the blood–brain barrier. But toxicity and mutagenicity are potential problems. Molecular modeling might aid the production of antibody-based mimetics not only in pharmacophore identification, but also in the design of organic analogs of antibody CDR loops. Modest success in this approach has already been achieved (162).

A frontier area in the biological application of computer modeling is the *ab initio* design of binding sites with properties and activities similar to those of naturally occurring antibodies and enzymes. While this goal remains beyond both the computing capabilities of today's computers and our current level of biochemical understanding, perhaps the next century will bear witness to its achievement.

Acknowledgments

P.R.H. acknowledges the invaluable contributions of Ed Snate in the preparation of this manuscript. B.S. thanks the N.I.H. (AI-32822, AI-33250, AI-34203, CA-59077) for its generous support.

References

1. Kohler G, Milstein C. Continuous cultures of fused cells secreting antibody of predefined specificity. Nature 1975; 256:495–7.
2. Mullis KB, Faloona FA. Specific synthesis of DNA *in vitro* via a polymerase-catalyzed chain reaction. Methods Enzymol 1989; 155:335–50.
3. Chiang YL, Sheng-Dong R, Brow MA, Larrick JW. Direct cDNA cloning of the rearranged immunoglobulin variable region. BioTechniques 1989; 7:360–6.
4. Orlandi R, Gussow DH, Jones PT, Winter G. Cloning immunoglobulin variable domains for expression by the polymerase chain reaction. Proc Natl Acad Sci USA 1989; 86:3833–7.
5. Sastry L, Alting-Mees M, Huse WD, Short JM, Sorge JA, Hay BN, Janda KD, Benkovic SJ, Lerner RA. Cloning of the immunological repertoire in *Escherichia coli* for generation of monoclonal catalytic antibodies: Construction of a heavy chain variable region-specific cDNA library. Proc Natl Acad Sci USA 1989; 86:5728–32.
6. Loh EY, Elliott JF, Cwirla S, Lanier LL, Davis MM. Polymerase chain reaction with single-sided specificity: Analysis of T cell receptor delta chain. Science 1989; 243:217–20.
7. Rice D, Baltimore D. Regulated expression of an immunoglobulin kappa gene introduced into a mouse lymphoid cell line. Proc Natl Acad Sci USA 1982; 79:7862–5.
8. Oi VT, Morrison SL, Herzenberg LA, Berg P. Immunoglobulin gene expression in transformed lymphoid cells. Proc Natl Acad Sci USA 1983; 80:825–9.
9. Ochi A, Hawley RG, Shulman MJ, Hozumi N. Transfer of a cloned immunoglobulin light-chain gene to mutant hybridoma cells restores specific antibody production. Nature 1983; 302:340–2.
10. Neuberger M. Expression and regulation of immunoglobulin heavy chain gene transfected into lymphoid cells. EMBO J 1983; 2:1373–8.
11. Wood CR, Dorner AJ, Morris GE, Alderman EM, Wilson D, O'Hara Jr RM, Kaufman RJ. High level synthesis of immunoglobulins in Chinese hamster ovary cells. J Immunol 1990; 145:3011–6.

12. Mulligan RC, Berg P. Expression of a bacterial gene in mammalian cells. Science 1980; 209:1422–7.
13. Brinster RL, Ritchie KA, Hammer RE, O'Brien RL, Arp B, Storb U. Expression of a microinjected immunoglobulin gene in the spleen of transgenic mice. Nature 1983; 306:332–6.
14. Grosschedl R, Weaver D, Baltimore D, Constantini F. Introduction of a mu immunoglobulin gene into the mouse germ line: Specific expression in lymphoid cells and synthesis of functional antibody. Cell 1984; 38:647–58.
15. Rusconi S, Kohler G. Transmission and expression of a specific pair of rearranged immunoglobulin mu and kappa genes in a transgenic mouse line. Nature, 1985; 314:330–4.
16. Boss MA, Kenten JH, Wood CR, Entage JS. Assembly of functional antibodies from immunoglobulin heavy and light chains synthesized in *E. coli*. Nucleic Acids Res 1984; 12:3791–805.
17. Cabilly S, Riggs AD, Pande H, Shively JE, Holmes WE, Rey M, Perry LJ, Wetzel R, Heyneker HL. Generation of antibody activity from immunoglobulin polypeptide chains produced in *Escherichia coli*. Proc Natl Acad Sci USA 1984; 81:3273–7.
18. Skerra A, Pluckthun A. Assembly of a functional immunoglobulin Fv fragment in *Escherichia coli*. Science 1988; 240:1038–41.
19. Better M, Chang CP, Robinson RR, Horwitz AH. *Escherichia coli* secretion of an active chimeric antibody fragment. Science 1988; 240:1041–3.
20. Huston JS, Levinson D, Mudgett-Hunter M, Tai M-S, Novotny J, Margolies MN, Ridge RJ, Bruccoleri RE, Haber E, Crea R, Oppermann H. Protein engineering of antibody binding sites: Recovery of specific activity in an anti-digoxin single-chain Fv analogue produced in *Escherichia coli*. Proc Natl Acad Sci USA 1988; 85:5879–83.
21. Bird RE, Hardman KD, Jacobson JW, Johnson S, Kaufman BM, Lee S-M, Lee T, Pope SH, Riordan GS, Whitlow M. Single-chain antigen-binding proteins. Science 1988; 242:423–6.
22. Smith GP. Filamentous fusion phage: Novel expression vectors that display cloned antigens on the virion surface. Science 1985; 228:1315–7.
23. McCafferty J, Griffiths AD, Winter G, Chiswell DJ. Phage antibodies: Filamentous phage displaying antibody variable domains. Nature 1990; 348:552–4.
24. Kang AS, Barbas CF, Janda KD, Benkovic SJ, Lerner RA. Linkage of recognition and replication functions by assembling combinatorial antibody Fab libraries along phage surfaces. Proc Natl Acad Sci USA 1991; 88:4363–6.
25. Clackson T, Hoogenboom HR, Griffiths AD, Winter G. Making antibody fragments using phage display libraries. Nature 1991; 352:624–8.
26. Barbas CF, Kang AS, Lerner RA, Benkovic SJ. Assembly of combinatorial antibody libraries on phage surfaces: The gene III site. Proc Natl Acad Sci USA 1991; 88:7978–82.
27. Hogrefe HH, Amberg JR, Hay BN, Sorge JA, Shopes B. Cloning in a bacteriophage lambda vector for the display of binding proteins on filamentous phage. Gene 1993; 137:85–91.
28. Fuchs P, Breitling F, Dubel S, Seehaus T, Little M. Targeting recombinant antibodies to the surface of *Escherichia coli*: Fusion to a peptidoglycan associated lipoprotein. Bio/Technology 1991; 9:1369–72.
29. Francisco JA, Campbell R, Iverson BL, Georgiou G. Production and fluorescence-activated cell sorting of *Escherichia coli* expressing a functional antibody fragment on the external surface. Proc Natl Acad Sci USA 1993; 90:10444–8.
30. Wood CR, Boss MA, Kenten JH, Calvert JE, Roberts NA, Emtage JS. The synthesis and *in vivo* assembly of functional antibodies in yeast. Nature 1985; 314:446–9.
31. Horwitz AH, Chang CP, Better M, Hellstrom KE, Robinson RR. Secretion of functional antibody and Fab fragment from yeast cells. Proc Natl Acad Sci USA 1988; 85:8678–82.
32. Carlson JR. A new means of inducibly inactivating a cellular protein. Mol Cell Biol 1988; 8:2638–46.
33. Hasemann CA, Capra JD. High-level production of a functional immunoglobulin heterodimer in a baculovirus expression system. Proc Natl Acad Sci USA 1990; 87:3942–6.
34. Hiatt A, Cafferkey R, Bowdish K. Production of antibodies in transgenic plants. Nature 1989; 342:76–8.
35. Sharon J, Gefter ML, Manser T, Ptashne M. Site-directed mutagenesis of an invariant amino acid residue at the variable-diversity segments junction of an antibody. Proc Natl Acad Sci USA 1986; 83:2628–31.
36. Allen D, Simon T, Sablitzky F, Rajewsky K, Cumano A. Antibody engineering for the analysis of affinity maturation of an anti-hapten response. EMBO J 1988; 7:1995–2001.
37. Sharon J. Structural correlates of high antibody affinity: Three engineered amino acid substitutions can increase the affinity of an anti-p-azophenylarsonate antibody 200-fold. Proc Natl Acad Sci USA 1990; 87:4814–7.

38. Roberts S, Cheetham JC, Rees AR. Generation of an antibody with enhanced affinity and specificity for its antigen by protein engineering. Nature 1987; 328:731–4.
39. Riechmann L, Weill M, Cavanagh J. Improving the antigen affinity of an antibody Fv-fragment by protein design. J Mol Biol 1992; 224:913–8.
40. Riechmann L, Weill M. Phage display and selection of a site-directed randomized single-chain antibody Fv fragment for its affinity improvement. Biochemistry 1993; 32:8848–55.
41. Near RI, Mudgett-Hunter M, Novotny J, Bruccoleri R, Ng SC. Characterization of an anti-digoxin antibody binding site by site-directed in vitro mutagenesis. Mol Immunol 1993; 30:369–77.
42. Ruff-Jamison S, Glenney Jr JR. Molecular modeling and site-directed mutagenesis of an anti-phosphotyrosine antibody predicts the combining site and allows the detection of higher affinity interactions. Prot Eng 1993; 6:661–8.
43. Glockshuber R, Stadlmuller J, Pluckthun A. Mapping and modification of an antibody hapten binding site: A site-directed mutagenesis study of McPC603. Biochemistry 1991; 30:3049–54.
44. Denzin LK, Voss Jr EW. Construction, characterization, and mutagenesis of an anti-fluorescein single chain antibody idiotype family. J Biol Chem 1992; 267:8925–31.
45. Lavoie TB, Drohan WN, Smith-Gill SJ. Experimental analysis by site-directed mutagenesis of somatic mutation effects on affinity and fine specificity in antibodies specific for lysozyme. J Immunol 1992; 148:503–13.
46. Ward ES, Gussow DH, Griffiths A, Jones PT, Winter GP. Expression and secretion of repertoires of VH domains in Escherichia coli: Isolation of antigen binding activities. Prog Immunol 1989; 7:1144–51.
47. Ito W, Iba Y, Kurosawa Y. Effects of substitutions of closely related amino acids at the contact surface in an antigen-antibody complex on thermodynamic parameters. J Biol Chem 1993; 268:16639–47.
48. Kelley RF, O'Connell MP. Thermodynamic analysis of an antibody functional epitope. Biochemistry 1993; 32:6828–35.
49. Glaser SM, Yelton DE, Huse WD. Antibody engineering by codon-based mutagenesis in a filamentous phage vector system. J Immunol 1993; 149:3903–13.
50. Lerner RA, Benkovic SJ, Schultz PG. At the crossroads of chemistry and immunology: Catalytic antibodies. Science 1991; 252:659–67.
51. Baldwin E, Schultz PG. Generation of a catalytic antibody by site-directed mutagenesis. Science 1989; 245:1104–7.
52. Jackson DY, Prudent JR, Baldwin EP, Schultz PG. A mutagenesis study of a catalytic antibody. Proc Natl Acad Sci USA 1991; 88:58–62.
53. Iverson BL, Iverson SA, Roberts VA, Getzoff ED, Tainer JA, Benkovic SJ, Lerner RA. Metalloantibodies. Science 1990; 249:659–62.
54. Barbas III CF, Rosenblum JS, Lerner RA. Direct selection of antibodies that coordinate metals from semisynthetic combinatorial libraries. Proc Natl Acad Sci USA 1993; 90:6385–9.
55. Wade WS, Ashley JA, Jahangiri GK, McElhaney G, Janda KD, Lerner RA. A highly specific metal-activated catalytic antibody. J Am Chem Soc 1993; 115:4906–7.
56. Lesley SA, Patten PA, Schultz PG. A genetic approach to the generation of antibodies with enhanced catalytic activities. Proc Natl Acad Sci USA 1993; 90:1160–5.
57. Bruggemann M, Williams GT, Bindon CI, Clark MR, Walker MR, Jefferis R, Waldmann H, Neuberger MS. Comparison of the effector functions of human immunoglobulins using a matched set of chimeric antibodies. J Exp Med 1987; 166:1351–61.
58. Dangl JL, Wensel TG, Morrison SL, Stryer L, Herzenberg LA, Oi VT. Segmental flexibility and complement fixation of genetically engineered chimeric human, rabbit and mouse antibodies. EMBO J 1988; 7:1989–94.
59. Duncan AR, Winter G. The binding site for C1q on IgG. Nature 1988; 332:738–40.
60. Tao M-H, Canfield SM, Morrison SL. The differential ability of human IgG1 and IgG4 to activate complement is determined by the COOH-terminal sequence of the CH2 domain. J Exp Med 1991; 173:1025–8.
61. Tao M-H, Smith RIF, Morrison SL. Structural features of human immunoglobulin G that determine isotype-specific differences in complement activation. J Exp Med 1993; 178:661–7.
62. Tan LK, Shopes RJ, Oi VT, Morrison SL. Influence of the hinge region on complement activation, C1q binding, and segmental flexibility in chimeric human immunoglobulins. Proc Natl Acad Sci USA 1990; 87:162–6.
63. Shopes B. A genetically engineered human IgG with limited flexibility fully initiates cytolysis via complement. Mol Immunol 1993; 30:603–9.

64. Shopes B. A genetically engineered human IgG mutant with enhanced cytolytic activity. J Immunol 1992; 148:2918–22.
65. Caron PC, Laird W, Co MS, Avdalovic NM, Queen C, Scheinberg DA. Engineered humanized dimeric forms of IgG are more effective antibodies. J Exp Med 1992; 176:1191–5.
66. Duncan AR, Woof JM, Partridge LJ, Burton DR, Winter G. Localization of the binding site for the human high-affinity Fc receptor on IgG. Nature 1988; 332:563–4.
67. Shopes B, Weetall M, Holowka D, Baird B. Recombinant human IgG1-murine IgE chimeric Ig: Construction, expression, and binding to human Fc-gamma receptors. J Immunol 1990; 145:3842–8.
68. Canfield SM, Morrison SL. The binding affinity of human IgG for its high affinity Fc receptor is determined by multiple amino acids in the CH2 domain and is modulated by the hinge region. J Exp Med 1991; 173:1483–91.
69. Helm B, Marsh P, Vercelli D, Padlan E, Gould H, Geha R. The mast cell binding site on human immunoglobulin E. Nature 1988; 331:180–3.
70. Weetall M, Shopes B, Holowka D, Baird B. Mapping the site of interaction between murine IgE and its high affinity receptor with chimeric Ig. J Immunol 1990; 145:3849–54.
71. Tao M-H, Morrison SL. Studies of aglycosylated chimeric mouse-human IgG. Role of carbohydrate in the structure and effector functions mediated by the human IgG constant region. J Immunol 1989; 143:2595–601.
72. Dorai H, Mueller BM, Reisfeld RA, Gillies SD. A glycosylated chimeric mouse/human IgG1 antibody retains some effector functions. Hybridoma 1991; 10:211–7.
73. Wright A, Tao M-H, Kabat EA, Morrison SL. Antibody variable region glycosylation: Position effects on antigen binding and carbohydrate structure. EMBO J 1991; 10:2717–23.
74. Co MS, Scheinberg DA, Avdalovic NM, McGraw K, Vasquez M, Caron PC, Queen C. Genetically engineered deglycosylation of the variable domain increases the affinity of an anti-CD33 monoclonal antibody. Mol Immunol 1993; 30:1361–7.
75. Ostberg L, Pursch E. Human × (mouse × human) hybridomas stably producing human antibodies. Hybridoma 1983; 2:361–7.
76. Teng NNH, Lam KS, Riera RC, Kaplan HS. Construction and testing of mouse-human heteromyelomas for human monoclonal antibody production. Proc Natl Acad Sci USA 1983; 80:7308–12.
77. Morrison SL, Johnson MJ, Herzenberg LA, Oi VT. Chimeric human antibody molecules: Mouse antigen-binding domains with human constant region domains. Proc Natl Acad Sci USA 1984; 81:6851–5.
78. Boulianne GL, Hozumi N, Shulman MJ. Production of functional chimaeric mouse/human antibody. Nature 1984; 312:643–6.
79. Morrison SL. In vitro antibodies: Strategies for production and application. Annu Rev Immunol 1992; 10:239–65.
80. Sun LK, Curtis P, Rakowicz-Szulczynska E, Ghrayeb J, Chang N, Morrison SL, Koprowski H. Chimeric antibody with human constant regions and mouse variable regions directed against carcinoma-associated antigen 17-1A. Proc Natl Acad Sci USA 1987; 84:214–8.
81. Steplewski Z, Sun LK, Shearman CW, Ghrayeb J, Daddona P, Koprowski H. Biological activity of human-mouse IgG1, IgG2, IgG3, and IgG4 chimeric monoclonal antibodies with antitumor specificity. Proc Natl Acad Sci USA 1988; 85:4852–6.
82. LoBuglio AF, Wheeler RH, Trang J, Haynes A, Rogers K, Harvey EB, Sun L, Ghrayeb J, Khazaeli MB. Mouse/human chimeric monoclonal antibody in man: Kinetics and immune response. Proc Natl Acad Sci USA 1989; 86:4220–4.
83. Knox SJ, Levy R, Hodgkinson S, Bell R, Brown S, Wood GS, Hoppe R, Abel EA, Steinman L, Berger RG, Gaiser C, Young G, Bindl J, Hanham A, Reichert T. Observations on the effect of chimeric anti-CD4 monoclonal antibody in patients with mycosis fungoides. Blood 1991; 77:20–30.
84. Jones PT, Dear PH, Foote J, Neuberger M, Winter G. Replacing the complementarity-determining regions in a human antibody with those from a mouse. Nature 1986; 321:522–5.
85. Riechmann L, Clark M, Waldmann H, Winter G. Reshaping human antibodies for therapy. Nature 1988; 332:323–7.
86. Verhoeyen M, Milstein C, Winter G. Reshaping human antibodies: Grafting an antilysozyme activity. Science 1988; 239:1534–6.
87. Davies DR, Sheriff S, Padlan EA. Antibody-antigen complexes. J Biol Chem 1988; 263:10541–4.
88. Glaser SM, Vasquez M, Payne PW, Schneider WP. Dissection of the combining site in a humanized anti-Tac antibody. J Immunol 1992; 149:2607–14.
89. Chothia C, Lesk AM. Canonical structures for the hypervariable regions of immunoglobulins. J Mol Biol 1987; 196:901–17.

90. Chothia C, Lesk AM, Tramontano A, Levitt M, Smith-Gill SJ, Air G, Sheriff S, Padlan EA, Davies D, Tulip WR, Colman PM, Spinelli S, Alzari PM, Poljak RJ. Conformations of immunoglobulin hypervariable regions. Nature 1989; 342:877–83.

91. Foote J, Winter G. Antibody framework residues affecting the conformation of the hypervariable loops. J Mol Biol 1992; 224:487–99.

92. Queen C, Schneider WP, Selick HE, Payne PW, Landolfi NF, Duncan JF, Avdalovic NM, Levitt M, Junghans RP, Waldmann TA. A humanized antibody that binds to the interleukin 2 receptor. Proc Natl Acad Sci USA 1989; 86:10029–33.

93. Carter P, Presta L, Gorman CM, Ridgway JBB, Henner D, Wong WLT, Rowland AM, Kotts C, Carver ME, Shepard HM. Humanization of an anti-p185^{HER2} antibody for human cancer therapy. Proc Natl Acad Sci USA 1992; 89:4285–9.

94. Kolbinger F, Saldanha J, Hardman N, Bendig MM. Humanization of a mouse anti-human IgE antibody: A potential therapeutic for IgE-mediated allergies. Prot Eng 1993; 6:971–80.

95. Padlan EA. A possible procedure for reducing the immunogenicity of antibody variable domains while preserving their ligand-binding properties. Mol Immunol 1991; 28:489–98.

96. Winter G, Harris WJ. Humanized antibodies. Immunol Today 1993; 14:243–6.

97. Hale G, Dyer MJS, Clark MR, Phillips JM, Marcus R, Riechmann L, Winter G, Waldmann T. Remission induction in non-Hodgkin lymphoma with reshaped human monoclonal antibody CAMPATH-1H. Lancet 1988; 2:1394–9.

98. Winter G, Milstein C. Man-made antibodies. Nature 1991; 349:293–9.

99. Ward ES, Gussow D, Griffiths AD, Jones PT, Winter G. Binding activities of a repertoire of single immunoglobulin variable domains secreted from *Escherichia coli*. Nature 1989; 341:544–6.

100. Huse WD, Sastry L, Iverson SA, Kang AS, Alting-Mees M, Burton DR, Benkovic SJ, Lerner RA. Generation of a large combinatorial library of the immunoglobulin repertoire in phage lambda. Science 1989; 246:1275–81.

101. Caton AJ, Koprowski H. Influenza virus hemagglutinin-specific antibodies isolated from a combinatorial expression library are closely related to the immune response of the donor. Proc Natl Acad Sci USA 1990: 87:6450–4.

102. Mullinax RL, Gross EA, Amberg JR, Hay BN, Hogrefe HH, Kubitz MM, Greener A, Alting-Mees M, Ardourel D, Short JM, Sorge JA, Shopes B. Identification of human antibody fragment clones specific for tetanus toxoid in a bacteriophage lambda immunoexpression library. Proc Natl Acad Sci USA 1990; 87:8095–9.

103. Chazenbalk GD, Portolano S, Russo D, Hutchison JS, Rapoport B, McLachlan SM. Human organ-specific autoimmune disease: Molecular cloning and expression of an autoantibody gene repertoire for a major autoantigen reveals an antigenic immunodominant region and restricted immunoglobulin gene usage in the target organ. J Clin Invest 1993; 92:62–74.

104. Barbas III CF, Collet TA, Amberg W, Roben P, Binley JM, Hoekstra D, Cababa D, Jones TM, Williamson RA, Pilkington GR, Haigwood NL, Cabezas E, Satterthwait AC, Sanz I, Burton DR. Molecular profile of an antibody response to HIV-1 as probed by combinatorial libraries. J Mol Biol 1993; 230:812–23.

105. Williamson RA, Burioni R, Sanna PP, Partridge LJ, Barbas III CF, Burton DR. Human monoclonal antibodies against a plethora of viral pathogens from single combinatorial libraries. Proc Natl Acad Sci USA 1993; 90:4141–5.

106. Marks JD, Hoogenboom HR, Bonnert TP, McCafferty J, Griffiths AD, Winter G. By-passing immunization: Human antibodies from V-gene libraries displayed on phage. J Mol Biol 1991; 222:581–7.

107. Griffiths AD, Malmqvist M, Marks JD, Bye JM, Embleton MJ, McCafferty J, Baier M, Holliger KP, Gorick BD, Hughes-Jones NC, Hoogenboom HR, Winter G. Human anti-self antibodies with high specificity from phage display libraries. EMBO J 1993; 12:725–34.

108. Gram H, Marconi L-A, Barbas III CF, Collet TA, Lerner RA, Kang AS. *In vitro* selection and affinity maturation of antibodies from a naive combinatorial immunoglobulin library. Proc Natl Acad Sci USA 1992; 89:3576–80.

109. Hawkins RE, Russell SJ, Winter G. Selection of phage antibodies by binding affinity: Mimicking affinity maturation. J Mol Biol 1992; 226:889–96.

110. Kang AS, Jones TM, Burton DR. Antibody redesign by chain shuffling from random combinatorial immunoglobulin libraries. Proc Natl Acad Sci USA 1991; 88:11120–3.

111. Marks JD, Griffiths AD, Malmqvist M, Clackson TP, Bye JM, Winter G. By-passing immunization: Building high affinity human antibodies by chain shuffling. Bio/Technology 1992; 10:779–83.

112. Collet TA, Roben P, O'Kennedy R, Barbas III CF, Burton DR, Lerner RA. A binary plasmid system for shuffling combinatorial antibody libraries. Proc Natl Acad Sci USA 1992; 89:10026–30.
113. Portolano S, Chazenbalk GD, Hutchison JS, McLachlan SM, Rapoport B. Lack of promiscuity in autoantigen-specific H and L chain combinations as revealed by human H and L chain 'roulette.' J Immunol 1993; 150:880–7.
114. Barbas III CF, Bain JD, Hoekstra DM, Lerner RA. Semisynthetic combinatorial antibody libraries: A chemical solution to the diversity problem. Proc Natl Acad Sci USA 1992; 89:4457–61.
115. Hoogenboom HR, Winter G. By-passing immunisation: Human antibodies from synthetic repertoires of germline VH gene segments rearranged in vitro. J Mol Biol 1992; 227:381–88.
116. Akamatsu Y, Cole MS, Tso JY, Tsurushita N. Construction of a human Ig combinatorial library from genomic V segments and synthetic CDR3 fragments. J Immunol 1993; 151:4651–9.
117. Portolano S, McLachlan SM, Rapoport B. High affinity, thyroid-specific human autoantibodies displayed on the surface of filamentous phage use V genes similar to other autoantibodies. J Immunol 1993; 151:2839–51.
118. Marks JD, Ouwehand WH, Bye JM, Finnern R, Gorick BD, Voak D, Thorpe SJ, Hughes-Jones NC, Winter G. Human antibody fragments specific for human blood group antigens from a phage display library. Bio/Technology 1993; 11:1145–9.
119. Shopes B. Human antibodies from a phagemid library. In: Borrebaeck CAK, Ed. Antibody Engineering, 2nd ed., Oxford: Oxford University Press 1995; 133–57.
120. Mosier DE, Gulizia RJ, Baird SM, Wilson DB. Transfer of a functional human immune system to mice with severe combined immunodeficiency. Nature 1988; 335:256–9.
121. McCune JM, Namikawa R, Kaneshima H, Shultz LD, Lieberman M, Weissman IL. The SCID-hu mouse: Murine model for the analysis of human hematolymphoid differentiation and function. Science 1988; 241:1632–9.
122. Duchosal MA, Eming SA, Fischer P, Leturcq D, Barbas III CF, McConahey PJ, Caothien RH, Thornton GB, Dixon FJ, Burton DR. Immunization of hu-PBL-SCID mice and the rescue of human monoclonal Fab fragments through combinatorial libraries. Nature 1992; 355:258–62.
123. Bruggemann M, Spicer C, Buluwela L, Rosewell I, Barton S, Surani MA, Rabbitts TH. Human antibody production in transgenic mice: Expression from 100kb of the human IgH locus. Eur J Immunol 1991; 21:1323–6.
124. Taylor LD, Carmack CE, Schramm SR, Mashayekh R, Higgins KM, Kuo CC, Woodhouse C, Kay RM, Lonberg N. A transgenic mouse that expresses a diversity of human sequence heavy and light chain immunoglobulins. Nucleic Acids Res 1992; 20:6287–95.
125. Zou Y-R, Gu H, Rajewsky K. Generation of a mouse strain that produces immunoglobulin kappa chains with human constant regions. Science 1993; 262:1271–4.
126. Fell HP, Yarnold S, Hellstrom I, Hellstrom KE, Folger KR. Homologous recombination in hybridoma cells: Heavy chain chimeric antibody produced by gene targeting. Proc Natl Acad Sci USA 1989; 86:8507–11.
127. Neuberger MS, Williams GT, Fox RO. Recombinant antibodies possessing novel effector functions. Nature 1984; 312:604–8.
128. Casadei J, Powell MJ, Kenten JH. Expression and secretion of aequorin as a chimeric antibody by means of a mammalian expression vector. Proc Natl Acad Sci USA 1990; 87:2047–51.
129. Ducancel R, Gillet D, Carrier A, Lajeunesse E, Menez A, Boulain J-C. Recombinant colorimetric antibodies: Construction and characterization of a bifunctional F(ab)$_2$/alkaline phosphatase conjugate produced in Escherichia coli. Bio/Technology 1993; 11:601–5.
130. Tai M-S, Mudgett-Hunter M, Levinson D, Wu G-M, Haber E, Oppermann H, Huston JS. A bifunctional fusion protein containing Fc-binding fragment B of staphylococcal protein A amino terminal to antidigoxin single-chain Fv. Biochemistry 1990; 29:8024–30.
131. Mueller BM, Reisfeld RA, Gillies SD. Serum half-life and tumor localization of a chimeric antibody deleted of the CH2 domain and directed against the disialoganglioside GD2. Proc Natl Acad Sci USA 1990; 87:5702–5.
132. Das C, Kulkarni PV, Constantinescu A, Antich P, Blattner FR, Tucker PW. Recombinant antibody-metallothionein: Design and evaluation for radioimmunoimaging. Proc Natl Acad Sci USA 1992; 89:9749–53.
133. Pastan I, Chaudhary V, FitzGerald DJ. Recombinant toxins as novel therapeutic agents. Annu Rev Biochem 1992; 61:331–54.
134. Chaudhary VK, Queen C, Junghans RP, Waldmann TA, FitzGerald DJ, Pastan I. A recombinant immunotoxin consisting of two antibody variable domains fused to Pseudomonas exotoxin. Nature 1989; 339:394–7.

135. Chaudhary VK, Gallo MG, FitzGerald DJ, Pastan I. A recombinant single-chain immunotoxin composed of anti-Tac variable regions and a truncated diptheria toxin. Proc Natl Acad Sci USA 1990; 87:9491–4.

136. Better M, Bernhard SL, Lei S-P, Fishwild DM, Lane JA, Carroll SF, Horwitz AH. Potent anti-CD5 ricin A chain immunoconjugates from bacterially produced Fab' and F(ab')₂. Proc Natl Acad Sci USA 1993; 90:457–61.

137. Rybak SM, Hoogenboom HR, Meade HM, Raus JCM, Schwartz D, Youle RJ. Humanization of immunotoxins. Proc Natl Acad Sci USA 1992; 89:3165–9.

138. Goshorn SC, Svensson HP, Kerr DE, Somerville JE, Senter PD, Fell HP. Genetic construction, expression, and characterization of a single chain anti-carcinoma antibody fused to beta-lactamase. Cancer Res 1993; 53:2123–7.

139. Fanger MW, Segal DM, Wunderlich JR. Going both ways: Bispecific antibodies and targeted cellular cytotoxicity. FASEB J 1990; 4:2846–9.

140. Carter P, Kelley RF, Rodrigues ML, Snedecor B, Covarrubias M, Velligan MD, Wong WLT, Rowland AM, Kotts CE, Carver ME, Yang M, Bourell JH, Shepard HM, Henner D. High level *Escherichia coli* expression and production of a bivalent humanized antibody fragment. Bio/Technology 1992; 10:163–7.

141. Pack P, Pluckthun A. Miniantibodies: Use of amphipathic helices to produce functional, flexibly linked dimeric Fv fragments with high avidity in *Escherichia coli*. Biochemistry 1992; 31:1579–84.

142. Kostelny SA, Cole MS, Tso JY. Formation of a bispecific antibody by the use of leucine zippers. J Immunol 1992; 148:1547–53.

143. Holliger P, Prospero T, Winter G. 'Diabodies': Small bivalent and bispecific antibody fragments. Proc Natl Acad Sci USA 1993; 90:6444–8.

144. Schnee JM, Runge MS, Matsueda GR, Hudson NW, Seidman JG, Haber E, Quertermous T. Construction and expression of a recombinant antibody-targeted plasminogen activator. Proc Natl Acad Sci USA 1987; 84:6904–8.

145. Capon DJ, Chamow SM, Mordenti J, Marsters SA, Gregory T, Mitsuya H, Byrn RA, Lucas C, Wurm FM, Groopman JE, Broder S, Smith DH. Designing CD4 immunoadhesins for AIDS therapy. Nature 1989; 337:525–31.

146. Traunecker A, Schneider J, Kiefer H, Karjalainen K. Highly efficient neutralization of HIV with recombinant CD4-immunoglobulin molecules. Nature 1989; 339:68–70.

147. Frey T, Estess P, Oi VT. Dimerization of CD4-CK chimeric molecules leads to loss of CD4 epitopes. Mol Immunol, 1993; 30:797–804.

148. Shin S-U, Morrison SL. Expression and characterization of an antibody binding specificity joined to insulin-like growth factor 1: Potential applications for cellular targeting. Proc Natl Acad Sci USA 1990; 87:5322–6.

149. Gillies SD, Wesolowski JS, Lo K-M. Targeting human cytotoxic T lymphocytes to kill heterologous epidermal growth factor receptor-bearing tumor cells. J Immunol 1991; 146:1067–71.

150. Landolfi NF. A chimeric IL-2/Ig molecule possesses the functional activity of both proteins. J Immunol 1991; 146:915–9.

151. Fell HP, Gayle MA, Grosmaire L, Ledbetter JA. Genetic construction and characterization of a fusion protein consisting of a chimeric F(ab') with specificity for carcinomas and human IL-2. J Immunol 1991; 146:2446–52.

152. Gascoigne NRJ, Goodnow CC, Dudzik KI, Oi VT, Davis MM. Secretion of a chimeric T-cell receptor-immunoglobulin protein. Proc Natl Acad Sci 1987; 84:2936–40.

153. Becker MLB, Near R, Mudgett-Hunter M, Margolies MN, Kubo RT, Kaye J, Hedrick SM. Expression of a hybrid immunoglobulin-T cell receptor protein in transgenic mice. Cell 1989; 58:911–21.

154. Gross G, Waks T, Eshhar Z. Expression of immunoglobulin-T-cell receptor chimeric molecules as functional receptors with antibody-type specificity. Proc Natl Acad Sci USA 1989; 86:10024–8.

155. Zwirner J, Weissenhorn W, Karlsson L, Becker A, Rieber EP, Riethmuller G, Weiss EH, Peterson PA, Widera G. Expression of a functional chimeric Ig-MHC class II protein. J Immunol 1992; 148:272–6.

156. Dal Porto J, Johansen TE, Catipovic B, Parfiit DJ, Tuveson D, Gether U, Kozlowski S, Fearon DT, Schneck JP. A soluble divalent class I major histocompatibility complex molecule inhibits alloreactive T cells at nanomolar concentrations. Proc Natl Acad Sci USA 1993; 90:6671–5.

157. Marx J. Learning how to bottle the immune system. Science 1989; 246:1250–1.

158. Near RI. Gene conversion of immunoglobulin variable regions in mutagenesis cassettes by replacement PCR mutagenesis. BioTechniques 1992; 12:88–97.

159. Oettinger MA, Schatz DG, Gorka C, Baltimore D. RAG-1 and RAG-2, adjacent genes that synergistically activate V(D)J recombination. Science 1990; 248:1517–23.
160. Hogrefe HH, Shopes B. Construction of phagemid display libraries with PCR amplified immunoglobulin sequences. PCR Meth Appl 1994; 4:S109–22.
161. Little M, Fuchs P, Breitling F, Dubel S. Bacterial surface presentation of proteins and peptides: An alternative to phage technology? Trends Biotechnol 1993; 11:3–5.
162. Saragovi HU, Fitzpatrick D, Raktabutr A, Nakanishi H, Kahn M, Greene MI. Design and synthesis of a mimetic from an antibody complementarity-determining region. Science 1991; 253:792–5.

7 | INTERFERENCES IN IMMUNOASSAYS

JAMES J. MILLER
Department of Pathology
University of Louisville School
of Medicine
Louisville, Kentucky

STANLEY S. LEVINSON
Department of Veterans Affairs Medical Center
Louisville, Kentucky

1. INTRODUCTION

The accuracy of immunoassays may be compromised by a variety of interfering substances. The interference may be positive or negative and may vary in magnitude depending on the concentration of the interfering substance in the sample. The purpose of this chapter is to discuss the sources of these interferences that are specific to immunoassays and their detection mechanisms. These sources include cross-reactivity, endogenous interfering antibodies, masked antigens, interferences with the indicator mechanism (e.g., enzyme inhibitors in enzyme immunoassays), and matrix effects. The examples will be predominantly for quantitative assays, but the same sources and mechanisms also apply to qualitative immunoassays. In addition, examples will include a variety of assay formats including two-site "sandwich" assays, competitive binding (CB) assays, and nephelometric assays, but the principles also apply to other types of immunoassays, such as radial immunodiffusion and agglutination techniques.

We will discuss general techniques for detecting the presence of interfering substances, sources, and mechanisms of the major types of interferences in immunoassays and specific approaches for identifying and eliminating or reducing these interferences. Depending on the magnitude and frequency of the interference, the remedy may be built into an improved assay or applied to individual samples when they occur. Some remedies may be complex and require the resources of a research and development laboratory while others may be easily implemented in a clinical laboratory. In some cases, it may not be possible to eliminate the interference; however, knowledge of the sources and mechanisms of interference may help to confirm the inaccuracy, choose an alternate assay known to be unaffected by the interference, or suggest appropriate annotation of the reported result.

In recent years there have been many methodological advances in immunoassays, including monoclonal antibody technology, nonisotopic detection systems, and two-site sandwich assays. These advances have allowed great improvements in sensitivity, convenience in terms of automation and rapid turn-around times, and development of immunoassays for many "new" analytes. However, these improvements have been accompanied by some new types of interference. It is likely that future developments will also uncover novel mechanisms of interference. An understanding of the known sources and mechanisms of interference should be helpful for recognizing and eliminating interferences in the future.

2. DETECTING INTERFERENCES

Detection of interference can be very difficult. As defined above interferences cause inaccurate results. However, we rarely know the true concentration of the analyte and, therefore, have no basis on which to judge the accuracy of a result. The best opportunity to detect and characterize interferences is during the evaluation of an assay. If the evaluation of interference is thorough, troubleshooting possible aberrant results during routine use will be facilitated.

2.1 Detecting Interferences during Evaluation

Several of the routine analyses performed during evaluation of an assay allow detection of interference. The strategy is to identify samples with apparent interference present and then to characterize the interference or at least to determine the conditions under which one might suspect the interference to be present in the future. In method comparison studies, samples giving unexpected results, i.e., outliers, are likely to contain an interferent. To increase the chances of finding these samples, they should include samples from patients with liver and kidney disease, and from patients with potentially interfering antibodies such as rheumatoid factor (RF), anti-nuclear antibodies (ANA), and human anti-mouse antibodies (HAMA). After identifying obvious outliers for further study and removing those points from the statistical analysis, a low correlation coefficient may indicate that interference is contributing to the scatter. Samples may be put in two groups, those with the most positive bias and those with the most negative bias, to identify samples with possible interferences present. It is important to keep in mind: (i) that the interference may be in the comparison method and not in the new method; and (ii) if the interference affects both assays equally, it will not be detected by the comparison study.

In linearity studies, often referred to as tests of parallelism in the case of immunoassays, nonlinearity upon dilution usually indicates the presence of some type of interference, the effect of which is diminished by dilution. Often one (or more) sample with a high analyte concentration is diluted with the recommended diluent or a sample with a low concentration of the analyte. In addition, those samples identified in the method comparison study as possibly containing an interferent should be retested after dilution. It is important to keep in mind that although nonlinearity implies inaccuracy due to interfering substances, linearity does not guarantee accuracy.

In recovery studies, a known amount of pure analyte, if available, or a small volume of a sample with a very high analyte concentration is spiked into samples and analyzed for the expected increase in concentration. Results significantly different than 100% recovery may indicate incorrect assignment of the calibrator values or the presence of an interfering substance in the samples to which the analyte is added. As with linearity studies, recovery studies should be done on those samples identified in the method comparison study as possibly containing an interferent.

Of course, the commonly tested interferents, lipemia, icterus, and hemolysis, may also be included. Sometimes the effects of these potential interferences can be appreciated by including samples containing them in the method comparison studies. If these samples are outliers, one of the assays is subject to interference. However, if these samples are not outliers, it is possible that there is no interference or that both assays have a similar degree of interference.

Whenever specimens with interfering substances are identified, other laboratory data and clinical information on the patient, especially any acute and chronic diseases and medications, should be obtained. This information may provide clues to the cause of the interference and samples can be obtained from other patients based on these clues. Information from several such patients may allow identification of the interfering substance. Changes in the degree of interference in a series of samples from the same patient can be compared with the clinical course of the patient and with the dosing of medication, which may give clues to the cause of the interference. Finally, attempts to separate the analyte from the interfering substance or to separate heterogeneous forms of the analyte may be pursued by various extraction, chromatographic, or electrophoretic techniques.

2.2. Detecting Interferences during Routine Use

In routine use there may be no indication that an interfering substance is causing inaccurate results. Usually the only clue is a result that does not fit the clinical picture. It is important to remember that an interfering substance may cause results to be falsely normal whether the true result is abnormally low or high. The initial evaluation of interferences may have identified certain clinical conditions or drug therapies in which interference is common. Results from patients in these categories may be scrutinized more thoroughly. Sometimes automated immunoassay instruments report a blank reading which, if atypical, may be a clue to the presence of an interferent. In assays that have a high frequency of anomalous results, extreme measures to test for interferences may be necessary, such as testing nonspecific binding or two dilutions on all samples.

3. CROSS-REACTIVITY AND HETEROGENEOUS ANALYTES

The power of immunoassays is derived from their analytical sensitivity and specificity of the antigen–antibody reaction for the ligand of interest (analyte). In many cases, however, this specificity is compromised by the ability of other molecules with structurally similar or identical epitopes to bind to the antibody. This competition is commonly referred to as cross-reactivity. The problems and solutions to interferences associated with multiple forms of the analyte (e.g., isoforms and partially degraded forms of proteins) are often similar to those of cross-reactivity and will be included in this section. The subject of antibody specificity and cross-reactivity have been discussed in numerous book chapters and reviews (1–4). In this section we will discuss some general concepts related to cross-reactivity. Various approaches for decreasing cross-reactive interference will be discussed in a later section.

3.1. Sources of Cross-Reactivity

Reports of cross-reactive interferences are so numerous as to prohibit a comprehensive listing. We will describe, however, examples of some commonly encountered sources of cross-reactivity, as well as examples of some subtle or unusual sources. Hopefully, this selection of examples will allow the reader to anticipate problems of cross-reactivity in the future.

3.1.1. Large Analytes

For large analytes such as proteins, cross-reactive interference is due predominantly to the presence of multiple similar proteins or to heterogeneity of the analyte. A classic example is the similarity in structure of the glycoprotein hormones, e.g., human chorionic gonadotropin (hCG), luteinizing hormone (LH), and follicle stimulating hormone (FSH) due to their common α-subunit. The antisera used in the original assays for these proteins had significant cross-reactivity with the other members of this group. Although these cross-reactions were eliminated by the development of antisera specific for the β-subunits (5), further improvements in specificity and sensitivity have led to the recognition of multiple molecular forms of these glycoprotein hormones. For example, besides intact hCG, other recognized forms include free β-subunits (6), carbohydrate variants (7), and several partially degraded forms (8, 9). In addition, peptide hormones may exist in serum along with precursor forms, for example, insulin, proinsulin, and C-peptide (10). And, finally, for any protein antigen, genetic variants may exist. Some epitopes of genetic variants may have altered immunoreactivity due to conformation changes, and some epitopes may be absent. This latter situation is suspected to be the cause of discrepancy in two reported cases in which LH was not detectable by some assays (11, 12).

The heterogeneity of protein antigens and variations of the relative distribution of the different forms in different patient samples and in the same patient at different times (see Section 3.2) can cause marked differences in immunoreactivity, resulting in inaccurate results. This problem is magnified by the fact that the analyte in the calibrators often is not identical to the analyte in specimens. If this is the case, the sample will not dilute in parallel with the calibrators, resulting in variable error throughout the analytical range. This type of interference is well illustrated by the analysis of monoclonal free light chains of immunoglobulins (Bence–Jones proteins). These are immunologically different from normal intact light chains used to calibrate assays and from one another. As illustrated in Fig. 7.1, they show nonparallel behavior as compared to the calibrator and to one another (13).

3.1.2. Small Analytes

Many sources of cross-reactivity in immunoassays for small molecules such as nonprotein hormones, vitamins, and drugs, are similar to those in assays for proteins. For example, there is a large number of steroid hormones of very similar structure, each usually having multiple metabolites also with similar structures. This can be particularly problematic for urinary steroid assays due to the presence of metabolites. In

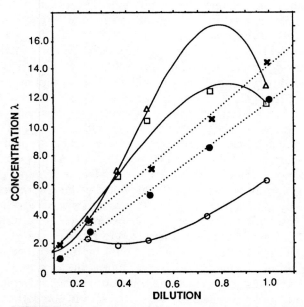

FIGURE 7.1 Nonparallel behavior of Bence–Jones proteins. The measured concentration of λ- chains in mg/liter is plotted against the dilution of the samples. Three different Bence–Jones proteins in urine (open triangles, squares, and circles); intact immunoglobulin in urine (X); intact immunoglobulin calibrator (filled circles). This figure is reprinted from S. S. Levison, Studies of Bence Jones proteins by immunonephelometry, Annals of Clinical and Laboratory Science, 1992, 22:100–9, with the permission of the publisher (Copyright 1992 by the Institute for Clinical Science, Inc.).

assays for drugs, the most common source of cross-reactive interference is from metabolites of the drug. Cyclosporin A, for example, has a large number of metabolites,
some of which cross-react to some extent in the newer monoclonal assays (14).

In drug assays for the purpose of therapeutic drug monitoring, cross-reactivity
with other drugs can occasionally be a problem. Examples include the measurement
of pentobarbital in the presence of phenobarbital (15) and the measurement of
digoxin in the presence of spironolactone (16). On the other hand, cross-reactivity
with other drugs is a common problem when screening for drugs of abuse. The
cross-reactivity of many nonprescription cold medications in amphetamine assays
is well known; however, some unexpected cases of cross-reactivity have also been
reported, e.g., metabolites of chlorpromazine and brompheniramine (17) and a
metabolite of the synthetic sweetener cyclamate (18).

Some additional examples of cross-reactivity will be given in the following sections of this chapter; however, we believe the examples above give a good overview
of the problem and will serve as a guide to recognizing and anticipating cross-
reactive interference.

3.2. Variations in Cross-Reactive Molecules in Disease States

In the previous section we reviewed some sources of cross-reactive molecules.
The concentrations of various cross-reactive molecules may increase dramatically
in disease states, especially in renal insufficiency and liver disease. This is because
cross-reactants are often metabolites of the analyte and because of the roles of the
liver and kidney in formation and excretion of metabolites. The effects of liver and
kidney disease are especially important in contributing to interferences in drug
assays. Positive interferences in the assays for theophylline (19, 20) and phenytoin
(21) have been reported in patients with kidney failure. A particularly interesting
interferent in digoxin assays is digoxin-like immunoreactive factor (DLIF) which
is increased in the serum of patients with liver or kidney disease, and in pregnant
and neonatal individuals (22). Due to the importance of digoxin assays and the
marked interference by DLIF in some digoxin assays, many strategies have been
developed for reducing the cross-reactive interference by DLIF.

There are many other examples of variations in the concentration of cross-
reactive molecules in disease states. For example, parathyrin (PTH) is cleaved in
the circulation into N-terminal and C-terminal fragments. The N-terminal portion
is further degraded and generally causes no problem, whereas the C-terminal fragment is usually removed by glomerular filtration; therefore, its concentration can
increase dramatically in renal failure. This increase can cause positive interference
in older, less specific PTH assays and has been reported to cause negative interference in some two-site intact PTH assays using C-terminal capture antibodies (23).
With glycoprotein antigens the changes in disease are often due to changes in the
carbohydrate moieties. For example, carcinoembryonic antigen (CEA) concentration can increase due to colorectal cancer or liver disease and the carbohydrate
moieties are different in these two diseases (24). Sometimes disease related changes
in the carbohydrate moieties of glycoproteins can be used for diagnosis or differential diagnosis. For example, carbohydrate-deficient transferrin can be used to detect
alcohol abuse (25) and the extent of concanavalin A-binding of prostate-specific
antigen may be able to differentiate patients with prostate cancer from those with
benign prostatic hyperplasia (26).

3.3. Cross-Reactivity with Monoclonal Antibodies

A common misconception is that MAb are absolutely specific; often this is not the case. Since a Mab is directed against a single epitope, it may be referred to as monospecific. However, all considerations regarding cross-reactivity also apply to the binding to that epitope. That is, molecules having structural similarity to the epitope may compete for binding and the identical epitope may be present in many different molecules. For example, the cross-reactivity of cyclosporin metabolites is reduced, but not eliminated, in monoclonal cyclosporin assays (27). Cross-reactivity may even be greater in a monoclonal assay than in a polyclonal assay (17). These examples indicate the necessity for thorough screening of MAb to select those with minimal cross-reactivity.

3.4. Relevance of Cross-Reactivity

Obviously the cross-reactivity of a particular compound is only a problem if that compound is present in the samples being analyzed at a concentration high enough to significantly elevate the apparent concentration of the analyte of interest. If this is not the case, a relatively nonspecific assay may give acceptable performance. For example, cross-reactivity of tri-iodothyronine (T3) in thyroxine (T4) assays is unlikely to be a problem because of the much lower serum concentration of T3 compared to T4; however, for the same reason, even slight cross-reactivity of T4 in a T3 assay could be a serious problem. This example demonstrates that the presence of cross-reactivity is not always a problem. A certain degree of cross-reactivity may be desirable. In many cases, one or more of the metabolites of a drug may have some therapeutic activity. In such cases, an assay of optimum specificity would be such that the metabolites cross-react in proportion to their therapeutic activity (28). Finally, in some cases cross-reactivity may be put to good use. Examples include the measurement of caffeine using a theophylline assay (29) and the measurement of cyclosporin G with a cyclosporin A assay (30).

4. REDUCING CROSS-REACTIVE INTERFERENCES

The accuracy of immunoassays depends on eliminating or at least minimizing the effect of cross-reactive components in the sample. MAb have greatly increased the specificity of immunoassays; however, cross-reactivity can still be a problem. Similarly, the use of two-site assays, which require two distinct epitopes on the antigen to be recognized by the capture and detection antibodies, greatly decreases, but does not eliminate, cross-reactive interference. In addition, two-site assays are only applicable to the measurement of analytes large enough to simultaneously bind to two antibodies. For small molecules such as steroids, small peptides, and drugs, other solutions to achieve immunoassay specificity have been found to be useful. The following approaches will deal primarily with assays for small molecules. In recent years, much creativity and work have been applied to decreasing the cross-reactive interference from endogenous DLIF in digoxin assays. Therefore, many of the approaches cited pertain to DLIF. However, the concepts and approaches discussed here are general and apply to minimizing interference caused by a wide variety of cross-reacting molecules.

4.1. Separation of Ligands Prior to Immunoassay

A commonly used approach for eliminating interference from cross-reacting molecules is to separate these molecules from the analyte prior to analysis. The type and efficiency of the separation will depend on differences in the physicochemical properties of the molecules in question. Differences in size, charge, solubility, and protein binding are important criteria for selecting a mode of separation. The mode of separation may be relatively simple, as in the organic extraction of cortisol from cross-reactive metabolites in urine (31), or sophisticated, as in the combined solid-phase extraction, reversed-phase high-performance liquid chromatography (HPLC) separation of digoxin from its metabolites and DLIF, followed by radioimmunoassay (RIA) of collected fractions (32).

If there are differences in size between the cross-reactant and analyte, methods based on size, such as gel filtration or ultrafiltration, may be useful. This may be an actual difference in size or a difference based on differential binding to serum proteins. The use of gel filtration is exemplified by the separation of free α-subunits of glycoprotein hormones (e.g., hCG, LH, FSH) from the intact hormones (33). Digoxin and DLIF are of similarly small size, but differ significantly in their degree of protein binding. Based on this difference Graves *et al.* (34) were able to separate digoxin and DLIF by centrifugal ultrafiltration.

4.2. Chemical Destruction of the Cross-Reactant

Occasionally a cross-reactant and the analyte will differ in their susceptibility to chemical reaction such that the cross-reactant can be converted to a less cross-reactive species without affecting the analyte. For example, testosterone can be destroyed by oxidation eliminating its extraction along with dihydrotestosterone (35) and pentobarbital can be measured when phenobarbital is also present by destruction of the latter with NaOH (15).

4.3. Adjusting the Incubation Time

The kinetics of antigen–antibody reactions is such that, in most cases, cross-reactivity decreases with incubation time and is minimal when equilibrium is reached. Vining *et al.* (36) showed that decreasing the incubation times of steroid assays increases the degree of cross-reaction with structurally similar compounds. The time necessary to reach equilibrium varies considerably depending on reaction conditions, but for most CB immunoassays it is typically in the range of hours to days. In addition, it is important to note that the presence of cross-reacting compounds in the sample will increase the time necessary to reach equilibrium (36). Therefore, the desire for rapid assays to reduce turn-around times and increase productivity must be carefully weighed against the possibility of decreased specificity.

4.4. Adjusting the Incubation Temperature

Cross-reactivity may vary with temperature for two reasons. First, as explained above, cross-reactivity decreases with incubation time to a minimum at equilibrium. Since reaction rates increase with temperature, equilibrium is achieved more quickly at higher temperatures. Therefore, increasing the incubation temperature may decrease cross-reactivity. The second reason is that the equilibrium constant may vary with temperature. If the change in equilibrium constant is different for the analyte and the cross-reactant, then the cross-reactivity will vary with temperature. Although the overall effect of temperature on cross-reactivity is not predictable, improvements in specificity can often be demonstrated empirically.

4.5. Use of More Specific Antibodies

Another obvious approach to reducing cross-reaction in immunoassays is to develop more specific antibodies. As discussed in Section 3.3, all antibodies, including MAb, have some cross-reactivity. However, several approaches can be used to decrease cross-reactivity to levels that may rarely be a problem. These approaches include insightful selection of the immunogen, affinity purification of antibodies, use of MAb, and use of two-site assays. In addition, the cross-reactivity of the antiserum or MAb may be modulated by addition of excess cross-reactant or anti-cross-reactant antibody.

4.5.1. Selection of Immunogen

Small molecules not large enough to be immunogenic themselves (haptens) must be covalently conjugated to a carrier protein. Antibodies generated against the hapten will be directed toward epitopes distal to the protein attachment site. In an excellent review of steroid immunoassays, Pratt (37) discussed the effect of the position of attachment of the hapten to the protein immunogen on antibody specificity. Comparison of the structures of the analyte and potential cross-reactants, such as metabolites, may provide clues to the best attachment site for minimizing cross-reactivity.

4.5.2. Affinity Purification of Antibodies

In polyclonal antisera, much of the cross-reactivity is attributable to heterogeneous populations of antibodies with different specificities. Specificity may be improved by using affinity binding techniques to absorb specific antibodies. Either the analyte or the cross-reactant may be covalently bound to a solid support. As discussed in Section 4.5.1, the attachment site of haptens to carrier proteins is important in determining the antibody specificity. Likewise the attachment site of haptens to affinity column support material is important in determining the specificity of affinity-purified antibodies.

4.5.3. Use of Monoclonal Antibodies

The goal in obtaining antibodies with maximum specificity is essentially to eliminate antibody populations with low specificity. The ultimate approach for achieving this goal is the use of MAb. Typically with this technique, several MAb are obtained with differing specificities which can be screened to select the most specific clone(s). Two recent studies have used this approach in developing antibodies to steroid hormones (38, 39).

4.6. Use of Two-Site Assays

For analytes large enough to simultaneously bind two antibodies, two-site immunoassays can greatly increase the specificity. The use of two antibodies with specificity for two distinct epitopes on the analyte, if appropriately chosen, can increase the probability of detecting little else but the ligand of interest. Some examples of this approach are found in assays for LH, FSH, and hCG in which homology between the polypeptide subunits has traditionally made it difficult to achieve specificity.

4.7. Blocking of Cross-Reactivity

Two interesting approaches for increasing the specificity of antisera involve blocking of cross-reactivity. In one, the less specific antibodies are saturated by the addition of the cross-reactant to the antiserum (2). This approach is based on the assumption that the least specific antibodies will preferentially bind the cross-reactant, leaving the more specific antibodies to bind the analyte or the tracer. In the other approach, antibodies raised against the cross-reactant are added to the antiserum. These bind the cross-reactant, making it unavailable to compete with the analyte and tracer. This technique was first described by Pratt *et al.* (3). They demonstrated reduced cross-reactivity of cortisone and cortisol in assays for cortisol and cortisone, respectively.

5. HETEROPHILE AND ANTI-ANIMAL ANTIBODIES

Heterophilic antibodies are a group of antibodies that are poorly defined and react with a wide spectrum of antigens. Historically, heterophile antibodies were defined as a group of IgM antibodies associated with mononucleosis that bind to sheep erythrocytes and can be removed from serum by absorption with beef red blood cells, but not with guinea pig kidney. About 90% of adolescents and young adults with mononucleosis can be shown to have heterophile antibodies.

More recently, antibodies that interfere with immunoassays have been called heterophile and, more commonly, heterophilic antibodies, or more appropriately heteroantibodies (40). These antibodies are a group of poorly defined antibodies that react with a wide spectrum of antigens. Heteroantibodies include idiotypic antibodies, RF, and multispecific antibodies. Although the mechanism of interference by heteroantibodies is well understood, information regarding the nature of the antibodies themselves continues to evolve and will be discussed below. The mechanism of interference by heteroantibodies is the same as interferences caused by anti-animal antibodies, such as HAMA. Anti-animal antibodies may develop as a result of treatment with animal immunoglobulins for the purpose of immunotherapy or immunodiagnosis, or in persons who have continued, close occupational exposure to animals, such as animal handlers. The two types of antibodies should be distinguished from one another, at least theoretically, because anti-animal antibodies are specific antibodies produced against a defined immunogen, and are removed by absorption when the antigen is known (41). On the other hand, heteroantibodies are directed against ill-defined antigens and may be more difficult to identify and to remove. These antibodies mainly interfere with two-site immunometric assays, and assays that use cells as the solid-phase binder such as Raji cells, and only to a lesser extent with CB and light scatter assays (turbidimetric, nephelometric).

5.1. The Nature of Heteroantibodies

Heteroantibodies are endogenous polyreactive antibodies that are produced against no clear immunogen. An understanding of the nature and mode of production of these antibodies is important for recognizing conditions for attributing interference to them, determining how to best avoid these interferences, and deciding how to reduce the interference when possible.

5.1.1. Polyspecific Antibodies

These antibodies include those with a single antigen combining site that cross-react with a wide variety of antigens that may be similar in chemical composition, shape, or charge, or antibodies that have multiple combining sites per variable region and can bind to several very different types of antigens (41).

Figure 7.2 illustrates the concepts of polyspecificity and cross-reaction. When the antigens have similar epitopes, theoretically, immunological behavior will follow the same mechanisms as for cross-reactivity (see Section 3). This type of cross-reaction differs from the usual concept because: (i) the immunizing antigen is not well defined, and, as will be discussed below, may not even exist since the conformation of the paratope may have been directed by the genome prior to exposure to the antigen; and (ii) it is usually not possible to distinguish this type of cross-reaction from that of other types of binding interactions of multispecific antibodies where similarities in epitope structure do not exist.

Polyspecific anti-DNA antibodies with an affinity for phosphodiesters in DNA that cross-react with phosphodiesters in membranes are an example of cross-reaction (41), while antibodies that bind to tetanus toxoid antigen and DNA are an example of polyspecific antibodies reacting with very different epitopes (41). Polyspecific antibodies have an immunological affinity for binding to cell components similar to those constituting membranes, cytoplasmic, and nuclear structures.

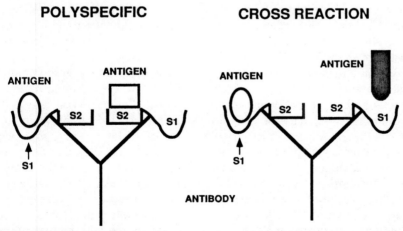

FIGURE 7.2 Illustration of polyspecific binding to antigens of different structures and cross-reactive binding to antigens of similar structures. Left, multiple binding to antibody with different paratopes binding to rectangular and circular antigens. Right, cross-reaction, where both paratopes bind to epitopes with circular structure on different molecules. S1 is binding site 1 and S2 is binding site 2.

Mouse monoclonal anti-DNA antibodies were shown to bind to a variety of polynucleotides and phosholipids, including cardiolipin (41). Human monoclonal and polyclonal anti-DNA antibodies were also shown to bind to proteoglycans (i.e., hyaluronic acid and chondroitin sulfate), the cytoskeletal protein vimentin, polypeptides called lupus-associated membrane proteins, trinitrophenyl derivatives, glycolipids from mycobacterial cell walls, and membranes that contain a hydrophobic–aromatic structure located near a negatively charged structure (41). Many other antibodies have been shown to be polyspecific, including: monoclonal anti-tuberculosis IgG antibodies, which have been shown to combine with single stranded (ss) DNA, double stranded (ds) DNA, polynucleotides, and cardiolipin; cytoskeletal antibodies that combine with dsDNA; monoclonal IgM RF, which combine with ssDNA, thyroglobulin, insulin, tetanus toxoid, and lipopolysaccharide; monoclonal anti-Mycobacterium leprae, which reacts with mitochondria, ssDNA, cytoskeletal proteins, and acetylcholine. Many of these antibodies also bind to DNA and, therefore, may be classified as anti-DNA antibodies (41).

The basis for polyspecific binding may be due to the antigen combining site being much larger than that needed to bind to a single epitope, and, therefore, allowing binding to other ligands as well (41). Conformational epitopes, hydrogen bonding, hydrophobic interactions, and charge interactions may all be important in this binding.

5.1.2. Idiotypes on Antibodies

Besides an antigen combining site, the Fab portion of immunoglobulins is itself composed of antigenic determinants, each referred to as an idiotope (Id), or collectively as idiotype. Some idiotopes lie within the antigen combining site or paratope, while others are outside this region. Antibodies that bind to Id are called anti-idiotypic antibodies (anti-Id). Two types of Id have been recognized: private Id and cross-reactive Id (CRI), the latter sometimes being called public or common idiotopes. Private idiotopes are clonally unique, being different from all other Id, and are found on antibodies with similar antigen combining sites. CRI are found on antibodies originating from different clones of lymphocytes that bind to different antigens, but contain similar antigenic properties within the idiotype. These concepts are illustrated in Fig. 7.3. The same CRI have been identified on diverse antibodies within the same person, in different people, and in different species of animals (41).

Jerne reasoned that there should be antibodies whose variable region should have a lock and key complementarity to the three-dimensional structure of other immunoglobulins (42). Thus, if antibody 1 (Ab1) is directed against an immunogen, and Ab2 is directed against the variable region of Ab1 (Ab1 is serving as an Id), then Ab2 will have a similar three-dimensional structure to the original immunogen. Ab2 may be called an auto-anti-idiotypic antibody. Ab3, with activity against Ab2, is an auto-anti-anti-idiotypic antibody. The structure of Ab3 is the same as that of Ab1, so these antibodies cannot be distinguished. In most cases these interactions would be expected to be much weaker and the complex more easily dissociated than binding of antigens to antibodies produced by specific immunization. As a result, anti-Id would be expected to cause more interference with assays where noncompetitive binding mechanisms are responsible, such as in two-site assays, and less interference in assays where the interference involves competition between a specific antigen and anti-Id, such as CB assays.

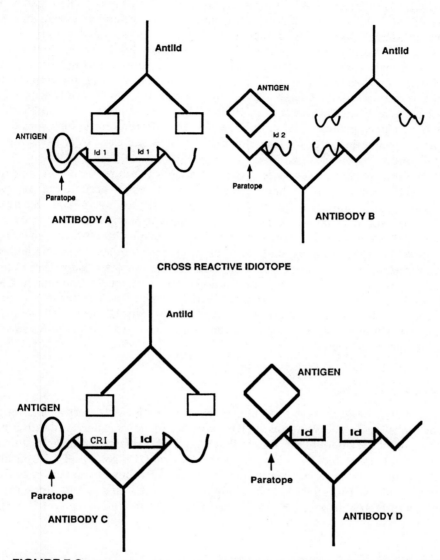

FIGURE 7.3 Illustration of common or cross-reactive idiotope (CRI) and private idiotope (Id). Top, antibody A and antibody B exhibit different antigen binding sites (circular and V shaped) and different Id (square and squiggle shaped). Bottom, antibody C and antibody D exhibit different paratopes (circular and V) but the same rectangular Id (common). The same anti-idiotypic antibody (AntiId) will bind antibodies C and D, but different AntiId bind antibodies A and B.

5.1.3. Mechanisms That Produce Heteroantibodies

Much of the antibody diversity can be explained on a genetic basis. The heavy-chain variable region is coded for by three separate genes: V, D, and J, and the light chain by two genes, V and J. The heavy-chain genes are on chromosome 14, κ-light chain on chromosome 2, and λ-light chain on chromosome 22. There are about 1000 different V, 10 different D, and 4 different J heavy-chain genes. There are about 200 V and 6 J light-chain genes. Each gene family consists of multiple DNA coding sequences (exons) separated by noncoding sequences (introns). Before transcription, the genes are randomly rearranged on the chromosome with a set of variable region genes being translocated to form a continuous functional gene (i.e., VDJ for the heavy chains and VJ for the light). During this rearrangement the introns are extruded. This process is illustrated in Fig. 7.4. These functional genes direct the synthesis of the protein chains. This process allows for combinations of gene products giving rise to more than 5×10^7 different antibodies with different antigen combining sites (43). In this way, the genome can direct the synthesis of rudimentary forms of all antibodies.

As antigenically driven cells divide, somatic mutations occur at a surprisingly high rate. B-cells that contain surface receptors which best fit the antigen are encouraged to multiply, while those with a lesser fit are not (43). As illustrated in Fig. 7.5, it follows that antibodies generated early in this process may show a large degree of multispecificity with broad reactivity for many different types of molecules.

Since both the paratope and the idiotype may encompass the same amino acid sequences of the variable region, both will deviate more and more from the germ cell as somatic mutations proceed. It follows that polyspecific binding and CRI will be more common in more primordial earlier antibodies, i.e., those produced by clones which have not deviated far from the primordial germ cell, while those antibodies undergoing somatic mutation as a result of continued antigen exposure will show more specificity.

5.2. Rheumatoid Factors

RF are autoantibodies that bind to multiple antigenic determinants on the Fc portion of IgG. The synthesis of RF, like that of polyspecific antibodies, may be directed by a segment of the V gene that is not highly diversified from the primordial germline (41). It has been suggested that RF may be generated as anti-idiotype antibodies. Like other autoantibodies, subsets of RF have been shown to be polyspecific, binding to ssDNA, thyroglobulin, insulin, tetanus toxoid, lipopolysaccharide, and DNA histone. RF also appear to be rich in CRI.

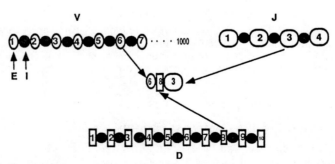

FIGURE 7.4 Illustration of rearrangement of a heavy-chain genome. The exons (numbered segments) are the coding regions. The introns (filled circles) are not included in the final gene. V, J, and D represent, respectively, the variable, joining, and diversity genes which are randomly rearranged into a unique heavy chain gene.

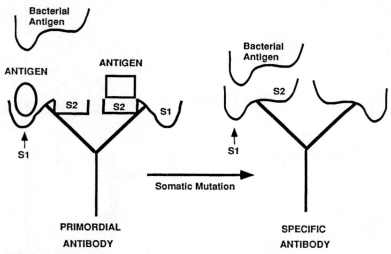

FIGURE 7.5 Evolution due to somatic mutation from multispecificity to monospecificity. Sites S1 and S2 evolve to exactly fit the bacterial antigen.

5.3. Mechanism of Interference by Heteroantibodies and Anti-Animal Antibodies

Heteroantibodies can cause interferences by the following three mechanisms and anti-animal antibodies by the first two: (i) Immunoglobulin aggregation. With two-site immunometric assays, the interfering antibody cross-links the capture antibody to the detection antibody in the absence of the analyte (see Section 5.3.1). With light scatter assays, the interfering antibody adds to the size of the precipitating immune complex (see Section 5.3.3). These types of interferences lead to falsely elevated levels of analyte. (ii) Blocking the binding site. This most commonly occurs with CB assays leading to falsely increased levels of analyte (see Section 5.3.2). The binding sites of two-site assays may also be blocked. If there is not an excess of the capture antibody, this may cause falsely decreased results. (iii) Polyspecific binding to a capture antigen. This may occur in assays designed to measure endogenous antibody levels, and could cause either false decreases or increases in the measured antibody (see Section 5.3.4).

5.3.1. Two-Site Immunometric Assays

As illustrated in Fig. 7.6, the most common type of antibody interference occurs with two-site sandwich type assays where the capture antibody is coupled to the detection antibody by the interfering antibody. The aggregation may occur as a result of Fab–Fab binding or as a result of binding to the Fc portion. RF causes Fab–Fc reactions (40, 41), and idiotypic antibodies Fab–Fab interferences (41). Both anti-animal antibodies and heteroantibodies may cause aggregation by both mechanisms. When the interference occurs in the absence of an analyte, false-positives occur. If the interference occurs when the analyte is present, the analyte appears artificially elevated.

5.3.2. CB Assays

Solid-phase CB assays may be affected by interfering antibodies due to the interfering antibody blocking the binding site of the capture antibody. CB assays

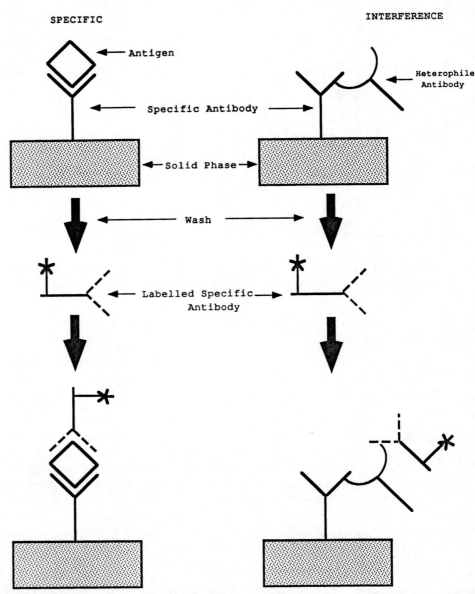

FIGURE 7.6 Interference with two-site immunoassay by endogenous antibodies. Left shows specific assay without interference. Right shows nonspecific assay with interference by heterophile (or anti-animal) antibody. Antibody attached to the rectangle is the capture antibody (specific antibody). Label attached to the signal antibody (labeled specific antibody) is represented by *.

are less affected than two-site binding assays, because of the greater affinity (binding energy) of the labeled and unlabeled antigen for the binding site as compared to the blocking antibody. Usually, a great deal of interfering antibody must be present to cause significant interference. This can happen if a large amount of sample is used. For example, a sensitive RIA for α-fetoprotein that used 50% patient serum and a long incubation period showed false-positive interference when a serum with very high titer of heterophilic antibody was assayed (44). It might be expected that anti-animal antibody would interfere more than true heteroantibodies because of the greater specificity of the former causing a high binding energy. A negative interference with a liquid-phase CB assay has also been described (44). Very high titer of heterophilic antibodies caused a reduced recovery when double-antibody techniques were used to separate the free and bound fractions. This interference was postulated to occur by the production of an antibody (immune) complex prior to the addition of the second antibody, causing an enhanced precipitation in affected samples.

5.3.3. Light Scatter Assays

Interferences with light scatter techniques have not been as widely reported in the literature as have interferences with two-site immunometric assays. There seem to be two reasons: (i) Polymeric forms of antigens often cause minimal variation in light scatter techniques. (ii) Generally, light scatter has been used for assaying substances which are present in fairly large amounts (milligram quantities) as compared to much smaller quantities measured by CB and two-site immunometric techniques.

Nevertheless, sera with very elevated titers of RF have been reported to interfere with light scatter assays (45, 46). Generally, the interference appears to be due to IgM-RF complexing with animal anti-human antibody used for detection. Also, sera containing IgG and IgM-RF in concentrations high enough to form circulating immune complexes (CIC) (47) and cryoglobulins (48) have been shown to interfere with light scatter assays. In the former case, CIC are precipitated in the assay by polyethylene glycol (PEG) which is used to facilitate the antigen–antibody reaction.

5.3.4. Assays Using Solid-Phase Antigen to Measure Antibody Titer

Many assays, such as assays for anti-nuclear antibodies (ANA) and anti-thyroid antibodies, use antigens to capture the specific antibodies in conjunction with an anti-human detection antibody to identify the presence of (or to measure levels of) the specific antibody. Polyspecific antibodies can interfere with immunoassays for these antibodies by competing with a specific antibody for the capture antigen, or by binding to a component other than the capture antigen (neighboring antigen). The latter mechanism is especially applicable when cells or cell fractions are used as a solid phase to capture antibodies because polyspecific antibodies have a great affinity for binding to components similar to those constituting membranes and cell structures. Polyspecific antibodies which are not major contributors to the disease process, with minor affinity for the antigen of interest and stronger affinities for other antigens, may appear concurrently and in varying concentrations along with the punitive antibodies. Since the labeled detection antibody cannot differentiate between them, a false-positive can result. For example, in Graves disease the poor correlation between disease activity and thyrotropin-receptor antibody titer may be due to the presence of antibodies with varying affinities and varying pathological capabilities in different stages of the disease (49).

6. RECOGNIZING AND REDUCING INTERFERENCE FROM ENDOGENOUS ANTIBODIES

In the following discussion, we will make a distinction between antigen assays and specific antibody assays. Assays used to measure endogenous molecules which are not antibodies such as thyrotropin or prolactin will be referred to as antigen assays. Assays used to measure the presence or titer of specific endogenous antibodies, such as assays for ANA or antithyroid antibodies in which various antigens are used to capture antibodies with activity directed against them, will be referred to as antibody assays.

6.1. Recognizing Interference from Endogenous Antibodies

6.1.1. Techniques for Identifying Suspect Sera

Since CB assays are minimally affected by cross-linking, suspected interferences may be identified by comparing a CB assay with a two-site immunometric assay. A significantly higher result from the two-site immunometric assay may indicate an interference.

Certain patient populations may exhibit heterophile-type interference more frequently than others. These include patients with chronic and acute diseases such as mycobacterial infections, bacterial endocarditis, autoimmune disease, and Klebsiella infections, and patients who show elevated levels of RF and ANA.

6.1.2. Detecting the Presence of HAMA

HAMA may reduce the efficacy of immunotherapy by forming CIC or may cause false-positive or false-negative results with various immunoassays. Analytical methods have been developed to measure HAMA. These consist of ELISA in which mouse monoclonal or polyclonal capture and detection antibodies are incubated with suspect sera. Positives are obtained when HAMA in the sera cross-link the detection antibody to the capture antibody. Alternatively, cross-linking can be directly identified without ELISA by using high-performance liquid chromatography or other techniques to directly measure the formation of immune complexes in a reaction mixture containing mouse immunoglobulins incubated with suspect sera containing HAMA.

Most laboratories have developed their own assays, but some commercial assays are also available (50, 51). An interlaboratory study indicated that although there was a general conformity among laboratories in identification of HAMA, as would be expected, RF interfered with most assays and false-positives and false-negatives occurred, presumably as a result of idiotype and epitope differences (50). The use of antigen (immunoglobulin), which is the same as the specific immunoglobulin used for immunotherapy, to block the HAMA may reduce nonspecific interferences (51).

6.1.3. Antibody Neutralization for Antigen Assays

In certain testing, where a positive result inflicts an undesirable stigma or a requirement for potentially toxic drugs or life-long treatment, such as testing for viral hepatitis or human immunodeficiency virus (HIV), it is necessary to include an antibody neutralization step with the assay as well as a mechanism for reducing interferences. Figure 7.7 illustrates the principles underlying this additional step. After the initial assay for antigen which gives a positive result, the assay is repeated with the sera being preincubated with exogenous antibody against the antigen (usually a virus). The assay is then repeated. The exogenous antibody binds to the

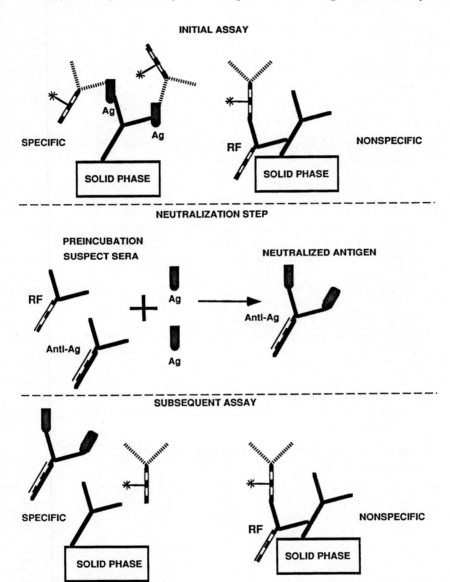

FIGURE 7.7 Illustration of antigen (Ag) neutralization for two-site immunometric assays. After an initial assay, the assay is repeated. Before repeating, exogenous anti-Ag is added to the test sera. The anti-Ag binds the Ag, if it is present, so that the Ag cannot react in the subsequent assay. This causes a decreased level of Ag as compared to the initial assay. If endogenous interfering antibodies such as reumatoid factor (RF) are present, they are not absorbed out and cross-link the capture to the detection antibody in the presence of the neutralizing antibody. Little decrease in apparent concentration from the initial assay occurs. The label is represented by *.

antigen (if present) and prevents its attachment to the solid-phase antibody when the assay is repeated. When viral antigen is present, but the interfering antibody is not, the subsequent assay will show reduced activity while it will not be reduced if only interfering antibody is present (52).

In order to avoid blocking cross-linking antibodies as well as antigen, neutralization antibody must be of human or chimpanzee origin, because reactive human heterophilic antibody does not react with antibody from these species. When viral antigens are being assayed, the neutralization mixture must contain high concentrations of antibodies against all viral subtypes. Sera which contain both the antigen and cross-linking antibody will give an equivocal result.

6.2. Reducing Interference in Two-Site Assays

6.2.1 Immunological Approaches for Reducing Interference with Antigen Assays

Both immunological techniques and chemical treatments have been used to reduce cross-linking interferences. Nonimmune immunoglobulin from the species used to raise the reagent antibodies may block the interfering antibody (41, 52). This technique has been the most common immunological approach used to reduce interference. Yet, the addition of excess nonimmune species-specific immunoglobulin does not always completely eliminate interference (53). In some cases, nonimmune globulin from two or more species may be necessary to eliminate interferences. In most cases, RF would be expected to be absorbed out by this maneuver, but idiotypic Fab–Fab interactions may still cause interference.

Other immunological techniques that have been used to reduce cross-linking interferences include: (i) Using Fab fragments as the capture antibody, rather than whole immunoglobulins. Again, this may not eliminate the effect of Fab–Fab interferences. (ii) Capture and detection antibodies raised in two different species (52). (iii) Combined use of β-galactosidase conjugated F(ab')$_2$ and polyclonal IgG or polymerized monoclonal IgG from the same species used to produce the assay antibodies (54). (iv) The use of chicken antibodies which do not appear to react with human RF (55).

6.2.2. Nonimmunological Approaches for Reducing Interference with Antigen Assays

Nonimmunological techniques usually require a pretreatment step. These include the following: (i) Pretreatment of serum with polyethylene glycol 6000 (130 g/liter) which precipitates all endogenous immunoglobulins, thereby removing all antibodies including idiotypic antibodies (56). (ii) Heating at 90°C has been used to eliminate anomalous activity by denaturing the antibodies (56). (iii) Pretreatment with sulfhydryl agents such as mercaptoethanol or dithiothreitol which will split disulfide bonds inactivating interfering antibodies. (iv) Pretreatment with detergents to inactivate antibodies (46). Evaluation of the utility of any of these pretreatments must carefully control for possible precipitation of or damage to the analyte.

6.2.3. Approaches for Reducing Interference in Specific Antibody Assays

New assays for antibodies include those for anti-endothelial cell and anti-neutrophil cytoplasmic antigens, which appear to be important in identifying and monitoring vasculitis, and the ANA Sm, SS-A/Ro, SS-B/La, RNP, and DNA (41). It must be expected that populations of polyspecific antibodies with various binding capacities will complicate the clinical correlations between the test results and the disease. The interference caused by polyspecific antibodies can be reduced by using highly purified capture antigens to reduce nonspecific binding sites. These are now available due to the emergence of recombinant DNA technologies allowing for the production of recombinant antigens.

6.3. Reducing Interference in Nephelometric and CB Assays

Techniques for reducing interferences with nephelometric and CB assays are similar to those described for two-site assays. Nonimmune immunoglobulin from the species used to raise the assay antibody, Fab fragments, and chicken antibodies may be used to reduce interferences (46, 57). Pretreatment of sera with PEG, sulfhydryl reagents, and detergents have also been used (46).

Since CB assays appear to be affected to a lesser degree than two-site immunometric assays, and nephelometric assays appear mainly to be affected by IgM-RF, less vigorous treatments may be sufficient (i.e., it may not be necessary to use two treatments such as nonimmune globulin combined with Fab fragments). Furthermore, it appears that for conventional nephelometric assays pretreatment with 40 g/liter of PEG, which reduces the IgM concentration about 80%, is sufficient to eliminate interference (46).

7. INTERFERENCES DUE TO MASKING OF ANTIGENS

Interferences may occur as a result of antigenic groups being hidden or altered by associated substances. A good example of this type of interference is illustrated by assays designed to measure endogenous apolipoprotein A-I (apo A-I) in lipoproteins. It has been demonstrated that immunological activity in endogenous apo A-I is increased as much as 60% by treatment with detergents, presumably by releasing lipids which mask epitopes on the protein (58). Since each lipoprotein may be peculiar in its lipid composition and different from an exogenous pure calibration material, it is difficult to obtain accurate analytical results. This type of interference is also seen when attempting to measure antigens in CIC. For example, during early stages of infection by HIV, serum antigen may be bound to anti-HIV antibody, causing it to be unavailable for binding to the assay capture antibody. Early detection of HIV infection in neonates by identifying anti-HIV is complicated by the presence of antibody from the mother in the neonate. Separation of the antigen from antibody improves the antigen detection rate (59).

Solving the problem of hidden antigens may be simple or extremely difficult. In some cases, such as with apolipoproteins, the hidden antigens may themselves be multiple species. For example, lipoprotein (a) consists of multiple isoforms, some of which may be hidden by lipids. Detergents, reducing agents, mild acids, or other chemical treatments may be useful in reducing the interference associated with measuring hidden epitopes (58). These may solubilize and thereby release lipids or other substances masking the epitope, denature the analyte, thereby releasing bound substances, or break bonds between the analyte and the substance hiding it.

It may also be necessary to treat the calibrator in the same way to assure similar behavior of the analyte. For example, treatment of both the sample and the calibrator with iron eliminates interference with transferrin assays (60). Stronger treatments with detergents such as Tween 20, Triton X-100, and sodium cholate have been used to strip lipids from lipoproteins (58). Extremely vigorous treatments, such as guanidine HCl and urea which split hydrogen bonds in proteins, have also been used to remove lipids for measuring lipoproteins (58). After such treatment, it is important to test for parallelism between the analyte and the calibrator to determine whether or not antigenic heterogeneity has been introduced.

8. INTERFERENCE WITH THE INDICATOR MECHANISM

All immunoassays require some indicator mechanism to detect the antigen–antibody complex (e.g., radioactive tracer, enzyme reaction). Some samples may contain compounds that artifactually augment or diminish the magnitude of the indicator response without affecting antigen–antibody binding. For example, diagnostic or therapeutic administration of radioisotopes to a patient often results in detectable radioactivity in samples for RIA. The amount of radioactivity is rarely enough to interfere significantly with the result, but for many of the new nonisotopic assays, analogous interferences have been reported and are more difficult to detect.

For enzyme immunoassays (for reviews see Refs. 61, 62), elevated activity of the detection enzyme in the sample may cause false increases in the measured result. It is also possible for enzyme immunoassays to be affected by the presence of inhibitors or activators of the detection enzyme in the sample. An aspirin metabolite has been reported to shift the ultraviolet absorption spectrum of NADH causing a falsely low absorbances in EMIT drug screens (63, 64). For assays in which the final measured response is fluorescence, as in fluorometric enzyme immunoassays or fluorescence polarization immunoassays, fluorescent compounds or quenchers of fluorescence in the sample may alter the detected signal. Components of serum and urine samples have been reported to interfere with photon emission in chemiluminescence immunoassays (65). As new modes of nonisotopic detection in immunoassays continue to be developed we can expect to encounter additional examples of this type of interference in the future.

9. MATRIX EFFECTS

The matrix of a sample (patient, control, or standard) includes everything present in the sample except the analyte. A matrix effect is an interference caused by a difference in the reactivity of an analyte due to differences in its environment in the sample. Antigen–antibody binding reactions are often quite sensitive to variations in protein concentration, lipid concentration, pH, and ionic strength. Difference in the matrix may also alter the efficiency of separation of bound and unbound fractions and the extent of nonspecific binding of the tracer. The difficulty in matching the artificial matrix of standards, controls, and proficiency samples and the matrix of patient samples often causes marked biases between different assays. Differences in matrix components between patient samples is usually less marked, but occasionally can cause significant inaccuracies.

There are several situations in which matrix effects can be particularly important. When the analyte must be extracted either to remove cross-reactive compounds or to increase sensitivity, it is likely that the extracted sample may have a different matrix than the calibrators unless the calibrators are also extracted. When a result is greater than the analytical range of the assay and must be diluted, use of an appropriate diluent matrix is critical for obtaining accurate results. Matrix interference is common when an assay is performed on body fluids other than the fluid, usually serum, for which the assay was designed.

10. INTERFERENCE PROBLEMS IN THE FUTURE

As mentioned in the introduction to this chapter, there have been many methodological advances in immunoassays in recent years. These advances have allowed great improvements in sensitivity, convenience in terms of automation and rapid turn-around times, and development of immunoassays for many new analytes. These improvements have been accompanied by some new types of interference. In the future, we can expect further developments in detection methods, such as fluorescent, luminescent tags, and increasingly sensitive light scatter assays using latex particles or other techniques, and therefore, we may expect problems of interference to increase. As the assay sensitivity increases and ever lower concentrations of analytes are measured, smaller amounts of endogenous interferents will affect the assays. There is growing interest in assaying low concentrations of antibodies for monitoring the activity of autoimmune diseases and for identifying infectious diseases. Since all sera contain some small amount of heteroantibodies, we may expect that problems related to these will grow. Also, the increasing use of immunotherapeutics is going to complicate testing by increasing the number of sera containing anti-animal antibodies.

As new analytes such as cancer markers, markers for autoimmune disease, and new infectious agents are identified, many of these will have heterogeneous molecular species and hidden epitopes. Thus, we expect that techniques and mechanisms for identifying and reducing interferences will continue to grow in importance.

References

1. Feldman H, Rodbard D, Levine D. Mathematical theory of cross-reactive radioimmunoassay and ligand-binding systems at equilibrium. Anal Biochem 1972; 45:530–56.
2. Pratt JJ, Woldring MG, Boonman R, Kittikool J. Specificity of immunoassays. II. Heterogeneity of specificity of antibodies in antisera used for steroid immunoassay and the selective blocking of less specific antibodies, including a new method for the measurement of immunoassay specificity. Eur J Nucl Med 1979; 4:159–70.
3. Pratt JJ, Woldring MG, Boonman R, Bosman W. Specificity of immunoassays. III. Use of two antisera of differing specificities to improve the specificity of steroid immunoassay. Eur J Nucl Med 1979; 4:171–7.
4. Miller JJ, Valdes R Jr. Approaches to minimizing interference by cross-reacting molecules in immunoassays. Clin Chem 1991; 37:144–53.
5. Vaitukaitis JL, Braunstein GD, Ross GT. A radioimmunoassay which specifically measures human chorionic gonadotropin in the presence of human luteinizing hormone. Am J Obstet Gynecol 1972; 113:751–8.
6. Ozturk M, Bellet D, Manil L, Hennen G, Frydman R, Wands J. Physiological studies of human chorionic gonadotropin (hCG), αhCG, and βhCG as measured by specific monoclonal immunoradiometric assays. Endocrinology 1987; 120:549–58.

7. Mizuochi T, Nishimura R, Taniguchi T, Utsunomiya T, Mochizuki M, Derappe C, Kobata A. Comparison of carbohydrate structures between human chorionic gonadotropin present in urine of patients with trophoblastic disease and healthy individuals. Jpn J Cancer Res 1985; 76:752–9.

8. Puisieux A, Bellet D, Troalen F, Razafindratsita A, Lhomme C, Bohuon C, Bidart J-M. Occurrence of fragmentation of free and combined forms of the β subunit of human chorionic gonadotropin. Endocrinology 1990; 126:687–94.

9. Kardana A, Cole LA. Polypeptide nicks cause erroneous results in assays of human chorionic gonadotropin free β-subunit. Clin Chem 1992; 38:26–33.

10. Temple RC, Clark PMS, Nagi KD, Schnider AE, Yudkin JS, Hales CN. Radioimmunoassay may overestimate insulin in non-insulin-dependent diabetics. Clin Endocrinol (Oxf) 1990; 32:689–93.

11. Pettersson KSI, Söderholm JR-M. Individual differences in lutropin immunoreactivity revealed by monoclonal antibodies. Clin Chem 1991; 37:333–40.

12. Finco B, Bizzaro N, Scomparin D. Pitfalls in measuring lutropin by two-site immunoassay with monoclonal antibodies against the intact molecule. Clin Chem 1992; 38:2159–60.

13. Levinson SS. Studies of Bence Jones proteins by immunonephelometry. Ann Clin Lab Sci 1992; 22:100–9.

14. Yatscoff RW, Copeland KR, Faraci CJ. Abbott TDx monoclonal antibody assay evaluated for measuring cyclosporine in whole blood. Clin Chem 1990; 36:1969–73.

15. Earl R, Sobeski L, Timko D, Markin R. Pentobarbital quantification in the presence of phenobarbital by fluorescence polarization immunoassay. Clin Chem 1991; 37:1774–7.

16. DiPiro JT, Cote JR, DiPiro CR, Bustrack JA. Spironolactone interference with digoxin radioimmunoassay in cirrhotic patients. Am J Hosp Pharm 1980; 37:1518–21.

17. Olsen KM, Gulliksen M, Christophersen AS. Metabolites of chlorpromazine and brompheniramine may cause false-positive urine amphetamine results with monoclonal EMIT d.a.u. immunoassay. Clin Chem 1992; 38:611–2.

18. Martz W, Schütz HW. Synthetic sweetener cyclamate as a potential source of false-positive amphetamine results in the TDx system. Clin Chem 1991; 37:2016–7.

19. Compton R, Lichti D, Ladenson JH. Influence of uremia on four assays for theophylline: improved results with a monoclonal antibody in the TDx procedure. Clin Chem 1985; 31:152–4.

20. Breiner R, McComb R, Lewis S. Positive interference with immunoassay of theophylline in serum of uremics. Clin Chem 1985; 31:1575–6.

21. Roberts WL, Rainey PM. Interference in immunoassay measurements of total and free phenytoin in uremic patients: a reappraisal. Clin Chem 1993; 39:1872–7.

22. Valdes R, Jr. Endogenous digoxin-like immunoreactive factors: false-positive digoxin measurements in clinical groups and potential physiologic implications. Clin Chem 1985; 31:1525–32.

23. Dilena BA, White GH. Interference with measurement of intact parathyrin in serum from renal dialysis patients. Clin Chem 1989; 35:1543–4.

24. Byrn RA, Medrek P, Thomas P, Jeanloz RW, Zamcheck N. Effect of heterogeneity of carcinoembryonic antigen on liver cell membrane binding and its kinetics of removal from circulation. Cancer Res 1985; 45:3137–42.

25. Stibler H, Borg S, Allgulander C. Significance of abnormal heterogeneity of transferrin in relation to alcohol consumption. Acta Med Scand 1979; 206:275–81.

26. Chan DW, Gao Y-M. Variants of prostate-specific antigen separated by concanavalin A. Clin Chem 1991; 37:1133–4.

27. Winkler M, Schumann G, Petersen D, Oellerich M, Wonigeit K. Monoclonal fluorescence polarization immunoassay evaluated for monitoring cyclosporine in whole blood after kidney, heart, and liver transplantation. Clin Chem 1992; 38:123–6.

28. Miller JJ, Straub RW Jr, Valdes R Jr. Digoxin immunoassay with cross-reactivity of digoxin metabolites proportional to their biological activity. Clin Chem 1994; 40:1898–1903.

29. Turnbull JD, Meshriy R, Gere JA, Kochalka G. Caffeine measured in serum from infants with the theophylline channel of the Abbott TDx. Clin Chem 1984; 30:1721.

30. Yatscoff RW, Jeffery JR. Quantification of cyclosporin G (NVa^2 cyclosporin) by radioimmunoassay. Clin Chem 1986; 32:700–1.

31. Chattoraj SC, Turner AK, Pinkus JL, Charles D. The significance of urinary free cortisone and progesterone in normal and anencephalic pregnancy. Am J Obstet Gynecol 1976; 124:848–54.

32. Gault MH, Longerich L, Dawe M, Vasdev SC. Combined liquid chromatography/radioimmunoassay with improved specificity for serum digoxin. Clin Chem 1985; 31:1272–7.

33. Grover S, Griffin J, Odell WD. Ultrasensitive, specific, two-antibody immunoradiometric assay that detects free alpha subunits of glycoprotein hormones in blood of nonpregnant humans. Clin Chem 1991; 37:2069–75.

34. Graves SW, Sharma K, Chandler AB. Methods for eliminating interferences in digoxin immunoassays caused by digoxin-like factors. Clin Chem 1986; 32:1506–9.

35. Etherington L. Testosterone/dihydrotestosterone kit method for diagnostic use. Clin Chem 1985; 31:167.

36. Vining RF, Compton P, McGinley R. Steroid radioimmunoassay—effect of shortened incubation time on specificity. Clin Chem 1981; 27:910–3.

37. Pratt JJ. Steroid immunoassay in clinical chemistry. Clin Chem 1978; 24:1869–90.

38. Parvaz P, Mathian B, Patricot MC, Garcia PI, Revol A, Mappus E, Grenot C, Cuilleron CY. Production of monoclonal antibodies to dehydroepiandrosterone-sulphate after immunization of mouse with dehydroepiandrosterone-bovine serum albumin conjugate. J Steroid Biochem 1989; 32:553–8.

39. Ghosh SK. Production of monoclonal antibodies to estriol and their application in the development of a sensitive nonisotopic immunoassay. Steroids 1988; 52:1–14.

40. Nahm MN, Hoffmann JW. Heteroantibody: phantom of the immunoassay. Clin Chem 1990; 36:829.

41. Levinson SS. Antibody multispecificity in immunoassay interference. Clin Biochem 1992; 25:77–87.

42. Jerne NK. The generative grammar of the immune system. Science 1985; 229:1057–9.

43. Nossal GJV. The basic components of the immune system. N Engl J Med 1987; 316:1320–5.

44. Hunter WM and Budd PS. Circulating antibodies to ovine and bovine immunoglobulin in healthy subjects: a hazard of immunoassays. Lancet 1980; ii:1136–7.

45. Kannisto H, Lalla M, Lukkari E. Characterization and elimination of a factor in serum that interferes with turbidimetry and nephelometry of lipase. Clin Chem 1983; 29:96–9.

46. Müller W, Mierau R, Wohltmann D. Interference of IgM rheumatoid factor with nephelometric C-reactive protein determinations. J Immunol Methods 1985; 80:77–90.

47. Levinson SS, Goldman J, Nathan LE. Erroneous results with routine laboratory testing for immunoglobulins due to interference from circulating immune complexes in a case of hyperviscosity syndrome of autoimmune disease. Clin Chem 1988; 34:784–7.

48. Banfi G, Bonini PA. Interference by cryoglobulins in a light-scatter instument. Clin Lab Haematol 1990; 12:112–4.

49. Wilkin TJ. Receptor autoimmunity in endocrine disorders. N Engl J Med 1990; 323:1318–24.

50. HAMA Survey Group. Interlaboratory survey of methods for measuring human anti-mouse antibodies. Clin Chem 1992; 38:172–3.

51. Massuger LFA, Thomas CMG, Segers MFG, Corstens FHM, Verheijen RH, Kenemans P, Poels LG. Specific and nonspecific immunoassays to detect HAMA after administration of indium-111-labeled OV-TL 3 F(ab')$_2$ monoclonal antibody to patients with ovarian cancer. J Nucl Med 1992; 33:1958–63.

52. Prince AM, Brotman B, Jass D, Ikram H. Specificity of the direct solid-phase radioimmunoassay for detection of hepatitis B antigen. Lancet 1973; i:1346–50.

53. Thompson RJ, Jackson AP, Langlois N. Circulating antibodies to mouse monoclonal immunoglobulins in normal subjects—Incidence, species specificity, and effect on a two-site assay for creatine kinase-MB isoenzyme. Clin Chem 1986; 32:476–81.

54. Vaidya HC, Beatty BG. Eliminating interference from heterophilic antibodies in a two-site immunoassay for creatine kinase MB by using F(ab')$_2$ conjugate and polyclonal mouse IgG. Clin Chem 1992; 38:1737–42.

55. Larsson A, Karlsson-Parra A, Sjöquist JTI. Use of chicken antibodies in enzyme immunoassays to avoid interference by rheumatoid factors. Clin Chem 1991; 37:411–4.

56. Primus FJ, Kelley EA, Hansen HJ, Goldenberg DM. "Sandwich"-type immunoassay of carcinoembryonic antigen in patients receiving murine monoclonal antibodies for diagnosis and therapy. Clin Chem 1988; 34:261–4.

57. Larsson A, Sjöquist J. Chicken antibodies: a tool to avoid false positive results by rheumatoid factor in latex fixation tests. J Immunol Methods 1988; 108:205–8.

58. Levinson SS. Problems with measurement of apolipoproteins AI and AII. Ann Clin Lab Sci 1990; 20:307–17.

59. Miles SA, Balden E, Magpantay L, Wei L, Leiblein A, Hofheinz D, Toedter G, Stiehm ER, Bryson Y. Rapid serologic testing with immune-complex- dissociated HIV p24 antigen for early detection of HIV infection in neonates. Southern California Pediatric AIDS Consortium. N Eng J Med 1993; 328:297–302.

60. Gebbink JAGK, Hoeke JOO, Marx JJM. Influence of iron saturation as a possible source of error in the immunoturbidimetric determination of serum transferrin. Clin Chim Acta 1982; 121:117–22.

61. Pesce AJ, Michael JG. Artifacts and limitations of enzyme immunoassay. J Immunol Methods 1992; 150:111–9.
62. Maxey KM, Maddipati KR, Birkmeier J. Interference in enzyme immunoassays. J Clin Immunoassay 1992; 15:116–20.
63. Wagener RE, Linder MW, Valdes R, Jr. Decreased signal in Emit assays of drugs of abuse in urine after ingestion of aspirin: potential for false-negative results. Clin Chem 1994; 40:608–12.
64. Linder MW, Valdes R, Jr. Mechanism and elimination of aspirin-induced interference in Emit II d.a.u. assays. Clin Chem 1994; 40:1512–16.
65. Tommasi A, Pazzagli M, Damiani M, Salerno R, Messeri G, Magini A, Serio M. On-line computer analysis of chemiluminescent reactions, with application to a luminescent immunoassay for free cortisol in urine. Clin Chem 1984; 30:1597–1602.

8 | LABELING OF ANTIBODIES AND ANTIGENS

EIJI ISHIKAWA

Medical College of Miyazaki
Kiyotake, Miyazaki, Japan

1. INTRODUCTION

A great number of immunological assays have been developed for a variety of purposes and have found wide applications to detect and measure biological and nonbiological substances in many fields. These assays can be divided into two categories, those that use labeled reactants and those that do not. The former provides various advantages over the latter, depending upon the labels employed. The use of labels such as radioisotopes and enzymes, for example, enables immunological assays to demonstrate high sensitivity and excellent reproducibility. However, these advantages are only realized when labeled reactants of well-controlled quality are utilized. Thus, labeling of reactants is one of the most critical factors for developing and performing successful immunological assays.

2. REQUIREMENTS FOR QUALITY OF LABELED REACTANTS

The quality of labeled reactants as essential components of immunological assays needs to be well-controlled in order to meet the desired objectives.

2.1. Detectability

The detectability of labels, as one of many factors which limit the sensitivity of immunological assays, should be preserved as fully as possible after conjugation to reactants. The detectability of labels could be compromised significantly unless appropriate sites are chosen for conjugation. The detectability of enzymes is reduced under drastic conditions such as low or high pH.

2.2. Reactivity

The reactivity or binding ability of reactants including antibodies, antigens, haptens, biotin, avidin, and their derivatives constitutes another critical factor which could limit the sensitivity of immunological assays. Binding ability should be preserved as fully as possible after conjugation to labels. Conjugation of the labels to appropriate sites of reactant molecules is required for preservation of conjugate binding activity. Polymerization of reactants should be avoided, since their reactivity is impaired by steric hindrance. The reactivity of some labeled haptens with antibodies depends upon the presence of spacer structures between haptens and labels.

2.3. Nonspecific Binding

In heterogeneous noncompetitive immunoassays, the nonspecific binding of labeled reactants to solid phase, which limits the sensitivity, should be as low as possible. Polymerization, which is usually a cause of high nonspecific binding, should be avoided.

2.4. Stability

Cross-links generated through conjugation should be stable under appropriate conditions, for example, at 20–37°C for days to months and at 4 or −20°C for as long as possible (preferably years).

3. CHEMICAL REACTIONS FOR CONJUGATION

Some chemical reactions, which take place efficiently at room temperature and are frequently used for conjugation, are shown in Fig. 8.1.

3.1. Reaction of Amino Groups with *N*-Succinimidyl-carboxylates (1, 2)

Amino groups, which are among the functional groups most frequently used for conjugation, readily react with *N*-succinimidyl-carboxylates to form stable cross-links. The reaction is efficient at concentrations higher than 2–3 mmol/liter at neutral pH and at lower concentrations at higher pH (optimal pH~9–10). It should be kept in mind that *N*-succinimidyl-carboxylates also readily react with thiol groups.

3.2. Reaction of Amino Groups with Aldehyde Groups (3, 4)

Amino groups readily react with aldehyde groups at neutral pH to form Schiff bases, which are not stable, and therefore are reduced to stable cross-links. However,

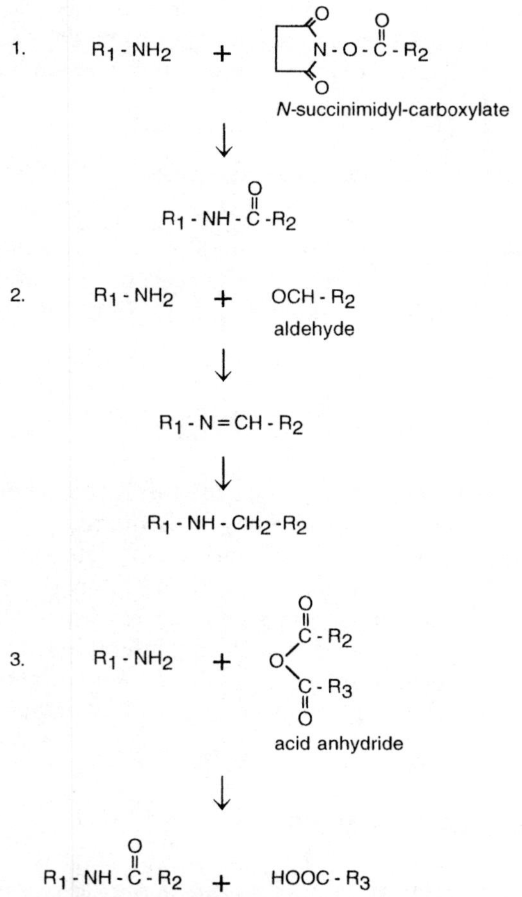

1. $R_1 - NH_2$ + $N - O - C - R_2$

    N-succinimidyl-carboxylate

    ↓

    $R_1 - NH - C - R_2$

2. $R_1 - NH_2$ + $OCH - R_2$
    aldehyde

    ↓

    $R_1 - N = CH - R_2$

    ↓

    $R_1 - NH - CH_2 - R_2$

3. $R_1 - NH_2$ + $C - R_2$ / $C - R_3$

    acid anhydride

    ↓

    $R_1 - NH - C - R_2$ + $HOOC - R_3$

FIGURE 8.1 Chemical reactions frequently used for labeling antibodies and antigens.

the reaction of amino groups with glutaraldehyde forms stable cross-links without reduction. Their exact structures are unknown.

3.3. Reaction of Amino Groups with Acid Anhydrides (1, 2)

Amino groups readily react with acid anhydrides to form stable cross-links.

3.4. Reaction of Amino Groups with p-Benzoquinone (5)

p-Benzoquinone molecules have two sites for reaction with amino groups. After the reaction of one site with an amino group at acidic pH, the other site reacts with another amino group at alkaline pH.

3.5. Reaction of Amino Groups with Isothiocyanate

Amino groups react with isothiocyanates at alkaline pH.

3.6. Reaction of Thiol Groups with Maleimide Groups (1, 2)

Thiol groups readily react with maleimide groups. The reaction is efficient at concentrations higher than $50–100$ μmol/liter and appears not to be dependent on pH. However, maleimide groups are labile at higher pH, and the reaction is usually performed at neutral or lower pH.

3.7. Reaction of Thiol Groups with Pyridyldisulfide Groups (1, 2)

An exchange reaction readily takes place between thiol and pyridyldisulfide groups at concentrations higher than 100 μmol/liter. However, the reaction is less efficient than the reaction between thiol and maleimide groups, since the exchange reaction is reversible.

4. REAGENTS FOR CONJUGATION

A number of reagents reactive with amino groups or/and thiol groups have been tested for conjugation of reactants and labels, and many of them are commercially available. These reagents can be divided into two categories. One category has two identical functional groups and the reagents are called "homobifunctional." The other category has two different functional groups and the reagents are called "heterobifunctional." Homobifunctional reagents such as glutaraldehyde and p-benzoquinone have a disadvantage because they cause self-coupling of antibodies, antigens, and enzymes (homopolymerization). Some commercially available conjugation reagents are shown in Fig. 8.2.

5. CONJUGATION OF ANTIBODY IgG TO ENZYMES

Antibody IgG can be conjugated to enzymes by using one of the various chemical reactions described above.

1. *N*-succinimidyl-6-maleimidohexanoate

2. *N*-succinimidyl-4-(*N*-maleimidomethyl)-
    cyclohexane-1-carboxylate

3. *N,N'-o*-phenylenedimaleimide

4. *N,N'*-oxydimethylenedimaleimide

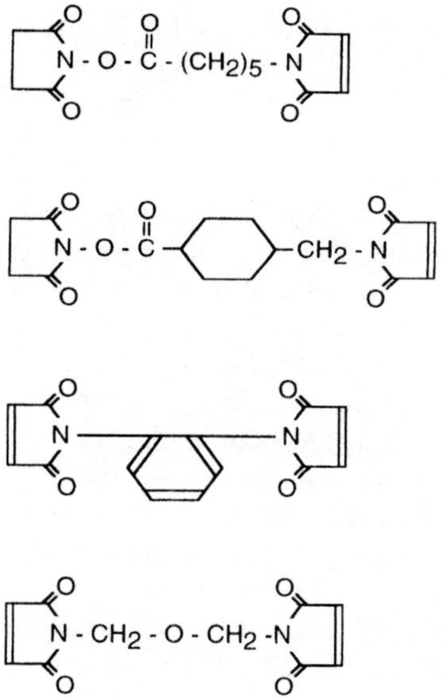

FIGURE 8.2 Reagents for labeling antibodies and antigens.

5.1. Conjugation Using Glutaraldehyde (Glutaraldehyde Method) (3)

IgG and enzymes can be conjugated by addition of glutaraldehyde to a mixture of the two proteins (one-step method). Although this is extremely simple, considerable polymerization leading to formation of homopolymers or/and heteropolymers is inevitable. One exception is the conjugation to horseradish peroxidase, which is treated with glutaraldehyde and, after removing excess of glutaraldehyde, reacted with amino groups of IgG, giving a monomeric IgG–peroxidase conjugate (two-step method). However, the recovery of peroxidase in the conjugate is extremely low (approximately 5%). Polymerization takes place with other enzymes even by the two-step method.

5.2. Conjugation Using Periodate (Periodate Method) (4)

IgG can be conjugated to horseradish peroxidase by using periodate. Aldehyde groups are generated by oxidation of peroxidase, a glycoprotein, with periodate and reacted with the amino groups of IgG. The recovery of peroxidase in the conjugate increases up to 80% with increasing degrees of oxidation. However, this is accompanied by polymerization.

5.3. Conjugation Using *N*-Succinimidyl-maleimidocarboxylates (Maleimide Methods I, II, and III) (1, 2)

IgG can be conjugated to enzymes in two different ways using *N*-succinimidyl-maleimidocarboxylates. In the maleimide Method I, maleimide groups introduced into enzyme molecules using *N*-succinimidyl-maleimidocarboxylates are reacted with thiol groups introduced into IgG molecules using *N*-succinimidyl-*S*-acetylmercaptoacetate or *S*-acetylmercaptosuccinic anhydride. The greater the number of maleimide and thiol groups introduced, the higher the recovery of IgG and enzyme in the conjugate and the greater the extent of polymerization. In the maleimide Method II or maleimide-hinge Method I, maleimide groups introduced into enzyme molecules using *N*-succinimidyl-maleimidocarboxylate are reacted with thiol groups generated in the hinge region of IgG molecules by reduction (for structure of IgG and the hinge region, see Chapter 2). Since thiol groups generated by reduction of IgG are limited in number and localized only in the hinge region of IgG molecules, no polymerization of IgG takes place and the binding ability of IgG is preserved after conjugation. However, the number of IgG molecules conjugated per enzyme molecule varies depending upon the molar ratio of IgG to enzyme used for conjugation. Maleimide groups can be introduced into β-D-galactosidase molecules (the *Escherichia coli* enzyme-containing thiol groups in the native form) with *N,N'-o*-phenylenedimaleimide, and reacted with thiol groups generated in the hinge of IgG molecules by reduction (maleimide Method III or maleimide-hinge Method II).

5.4. Conjugation Using Pyridyldisulfide Compounds (Pyridyldisulfide Method) (1, 2)

Conjugation is possible by replacing the maleimide groups described above with pyridyldisulfide groups.

5.5. Characteristics of IgG–Enzyme Conjugates (1, 2)

Due to the hydrophobicity of the Fc portion of IgG molecules (Fig. 8.3), the nonspecific binding of IgG–enzyme conjugates is higher than that of IgG fragment–enzyme conjugates devoid of their Fc portion. Therefore, the IgG–enzyme conjugates are used only when high sensitivity is not required.

6. CONJUGATION OF ANTIBODY FRAGMENTS TO ENZYMES

Digestion of IgG with pepsin and papain gives rise to IgG fragments called F(ab')$_2$ and Fab, respectively (Fig. 8.3). F(ab')$_2$ is converted to Fab' by reduction, since F(ab')$_2$ consists of two molecules of Fab' bound through disulfide bridge(s) (Fig. 8.3). The nonspecific binding of Fab'– and Fab–enzyme conjugates is lower than that of IgG–enzyme conjugates, providing higher sensitivity of immunological assays. Fab' and Fab can be conjugated to enzymes in different ways as described above for IgG.

6.1. Glutaraldehyde Method (3)

As described for IgG, polymers are formed by the one-step method, and monomeric Fab– and Fab'–horseradish peroxidase conjugates can be prepared by the two-step method, although the recovery of peroxidase in the conjugates is extremely low (approximately 5%) (Fig. 8.4).

6.2. Periodate Method (4)

Fab' and Fab can be conjugated to horseradish peroxidase by the periodate method described for IgG, resulting in the formation of monomeric and polymeric conjugates (Fig. 8.4).

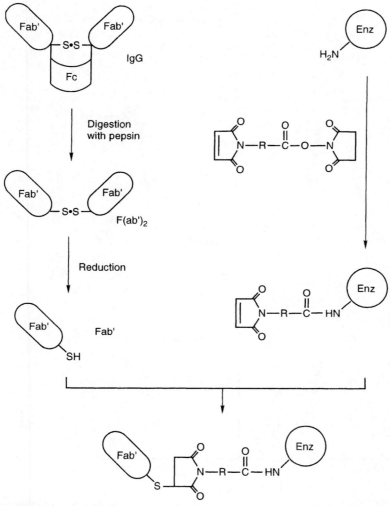

FIGURE 8.3   Conjugation of Fab′ to enzymes by the maleimide-hinge Method I using *N*-succinimidyl-maleimidocarboxylates. Reprinted, with permission, from Masseyeff *et al.,* Methods of Immunological Analysis, Volume 2: Samples and Reagents, 1993 VCH.

6.3.   Maleimide Methods I, II, and III (1, 2)

Fab′ and Fab can be conjugated to enzymes by the maleimide Method I described for IgG. Polymerization depends on the number of thiol and maleimide groups introduced into Fab′, Fab, and enzyme molecules. In contrast, no polymers are formed when thiol groups in the hinge of Fab′ generated by reduction of F(ab′)$_2$ are reacted with maleimide groups introduced into enzyme molecules using *N*-succinimidyl-maleimidocarboxylates (maleimide Method II or maleimide-hinge Method I) (Fig. 8.3). Fab′–horseradish peroxidase conjugate prepared by the maleimide-hinge Method I is exclusively monomeric, since thiol groups are localized in the hinge of Fab′ molecules and are limited in number, and maleimide groups introduced per peroxidase molecule, containing only two or three amino groups, are also limited in number (Fig.

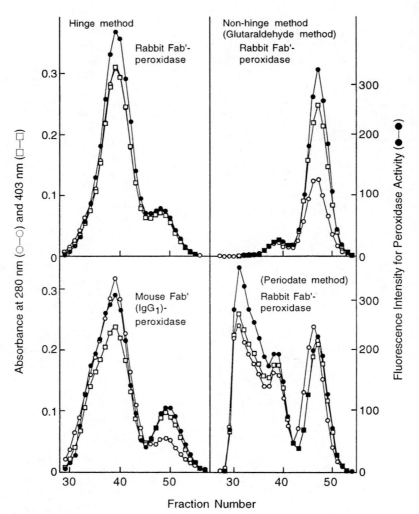

FIGURE 8.4   Elution profiles from a column of Ultrogel AcA 44 of Fab'–horseradish peroxidase conjugates prepared by the maleimide-hinge Method I and the nonhinge methods. Reprinted, with permission, from Masseyeff *et al.*, Methods of Immunological Analysis, Volume 2: Samples and Reagents, 1993 VCH.

8.4). The recovery of Fab' and peroxidase in the conjugate is high (70% or higher) (Fig. 8.4). Maleimide groups can be introduced into β-D-galactosidase molecules from *E. coli* using N,N'-o-phenylenedimaleimide and reacted with thiol groups in the hinge of Fab' (maleimide Method III or maleimide-hinge Method II) (Fig. 8.5).

6.4. Pyridyldisulfide Method (1, 2)

The pyridyldisulfide-nonhinge and hinge methods are possible by replacing maleimide compounds in the maleimide methods with pyridyldisulfide compounds.

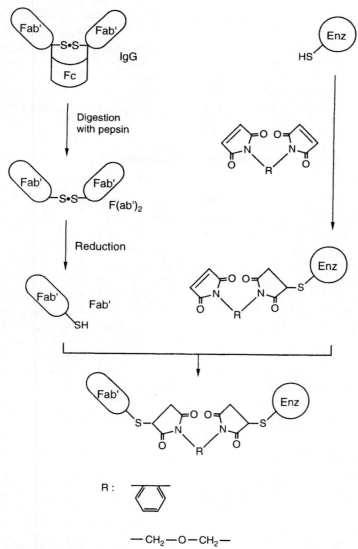

FIGURE 8.5 Conjugation of Fab' to enzymes containing thiol groups by the maleimide-hinge Method II using *N,N'-o*-phenylenedimaleimide. Reprinted, with permission, from Masseyeff *et al.*, Methods of Immunological Analysis, Volume 2: Samples and Reagents, 1993 VCH.

6.5. Characteristics of Fab'– and Fab–Enzyme Conjugates (1, 2)

The nonspecific binding of Fab'–enzyme conjugates prepared by the maleimide- and pyridyldisulfide-hinge methods is lower than that of Fab'– and Fab–enzyme conjugates prepared by the nonhinge methods, including the glutaraldehyde method, the periodate method, and the maleimide Method I. This might be accounted for as follows. Hydrophobic structures in the hinge region exposed by digestion with pepsin are covered by label enzyme molecules in the hinge methods, in which thiol groups of the hinge of Fab' are selectively used for conjugation. However, this is not the case in the nonhinge methods, in which amino groups of Fab' or Fab are randomly used for conjugation. In addition, the specific binding of Fab'–enzyme conjugates prepared by the hinge methods is two- to three-fold higher than that of Fab'– and Fab–enzyme conjugates prepared by the nonhinge methods. Thus, the use of Fab'–enzyme conjugates prepared by the hinge methods makes possible higher sensitivity of immunological assays than that of Fab'– and Fab–enzyme conjugates prepared by the nonhinge methods.

6.6. Protocol for the Conjugation of Fab' to Horseradish Peroxidase (Fig. 8.3) (1, 2)

6.6.1. Pepsin Digestion of IgG to F(ab')₂

(i) Dialyze 3–5 mg IgG in 0.5 ml against sodium acetate buffer, 0.1 mol/liter, pH 4.2–4.9, containing NaCl, 0.1 mol/liter, at 4°C. pH of the buffer is 4.5 for IgG from most animals such as rabbit, goat, sheep, or guinea pig and mouse monoclonals IgG$_{2a}$ and IgG$_3$, and 4.2 for mouse monoclonal IgG$_1$. (ii) Dissolve 0.06–0.2 mg pepsin from porcine gastric mucosa in the dialyzed IgG solution. (iii) Incubate the mixture at 37°C for 6–24 hr. (iv) Adjust the pH of the digested IgG solution to 7 using Tris–HCl buffer, 2 mol/liter, pH 8.0. (v) Apply the digested IgG solution at pH 7.0 to a column (1.5 × 45 cm) of Ultrogel AcA 44 (IBF Biotechnics, Villeneuela-Garenne, France) at a flow rate of 20–30 ml/hr using sodium phosphate buffer, 0.1 mol/liter, pH 7.0. The fraction volume is 1.0 ml. (vi) Concentrate the F(ab')₂ fractions to 0.45 ml in a microconcentrator (Centricon-30, Amicon Corp., Scientific Systems Division, Danvers, MA) by centrifugation at 2000g at 4°C for 30 min. $E_{280} = 1.48$ g^{-1} · liter · cm^{-1} for rabbit F(ab')₂ (1, 2) and 1.4 g^{-1} · liter · cm^{-1} for mouse F(ab')₂ (6). $M_r = 92,000$ for rabbit F(ab')₂ (1, 2) and 95,000–110,000 for mouse F(ab')₂ (6).

6.6.2. Reduction of F(ab')₂ to Fab'

(i) Add, to 0.45 ml F(ab')₂ (2–5 mg), 0.05 ml 2-mercaptoethylamine, 0.1 mol/liter, in sodium phosphate buffer, 0.1 mol/liter, pH 6.0, containing EDTA, 5 mmol/liter. (ii) Incubate the mixture at 37°C for 1.5 hr. (iii) Apply the reaction mixture to a column (1.5 × 45 cm) of Ultrogel AcA 44 at a flow rate of 20–30 ml/hr using sodium phosphate buffer, 0.1 mol/liter, pH 6.0, containing EDTA, 5 mmol/liter. The fraction volume is 1.0 ml. This confirms a complete split of F(ab')₂ to Fab' or separates Fab' from other proteins which are not split by reduction. If this is unnecessary, apply the reaction mixture to a column (1.5 × 45 cm) of Sephadex G-25 (Pharmacia LKB Biotechnology AB, Uppsala, Sweden) at a flow rate of 30–40 ml/hr using the same buffer. (iv) Concentrate the Fab' fractions as described for F(ab')₂. $M_r = 46,000$ for rabbit Fab' (1, 2) and 47,000–58,000 for mouse Fab' (6).

6.6.3. Measurement of Thiol Groups in Fab'

(i) Prepare a sample in a total volume of 0.5 ml sodium phosphate buffer, 0.1 mol/liter, pH 6.0, containing EDTA, 5 mmol/liter, with an absorbance at 280 nm of 0.2–1.0 (0.14–0.71 g/liter, 2.9–14 μmol/liter). (ii) Add 0.02 ml 4,4'-dithiodipyridine (MW 220.3), 5 mmol/liter (1.1 g/liter), to 0.5 ml of the sample solution above. (iii) Incubate the mixture at room temperature for 20 min. (iv) Read the absorbance at 324 nm. (v) Calculate the average number of thiol groups per Fab' molecule using the molar extinction coefficient at 324 nm of pyridine-4-thione, which is 19,800 $mol^{-1} \cdot liter \cdot cm^{-1}$ (1, 2). The average number of thiol groups per Fab' molecule is approximately 1 for rabbit Fab' and 1–3 for Fab' from other animals (1, 2).

6.6.4. 6-Maleimidohexanoyl-peroxidase

(i) Incubate 2 mg (50 nmol) horseradish peroxidase ($E_{403} = 2.275 \, g^{-1} \cdot liter \cdot cm^{-1}$ and $M_r = 40,000$) in 0.3 ml sodium phosphate buffer, 0.1 mol/liter, pH 7.0, with 0.2–0.3 mg (0.6–1.0 μmol) N-succinimidyl-6-maleimidohexanoate (Dojindo Laboratories, Kumamoto, Japan) in 0.03 ml N,N-dimethylformamide at 30°C for 0.5–1.0 hr. (ii) Apply the reaction mixture to a column (1.0 × 45 cm) of Sephadex G-25 at a flow rate of 30–40 ml/hr using sodium phosphate buffer, 0.1 mol/liter, pH 6.0. The fraction volume is 0.5–1.0 ml. (iii) Concentrate pooled fractions as described for F(ab')$_2$. Do not use NaN$_3$ as a preservative, since it inactivates peroxidase and accelerates the decomposition of maleimide groups.

6.6.5. Measurement of Maleimide Groups

(i) Prepare a sample in 0.45 ml sodium phosphate buffer, 0.1 mol/liter, pH 6.0, with an absorbance at 403 nm of 0.7–1.0 (0.31–0.44 g/liter, 7.7–11 μmol/liter). Use 0.45 ml of the same buffer as a control. (ii) Mix 0.01 ml 2-mercaptoethylamine-HCl (MW 113.6), 0.1 mol/liter, freshly prepared and 2 ml EDTA, 50 mmol/liter, pH 6.0. (iii) Add 0.05 ml of the 2-mercaptoethylamine–EDTA mixture to 0.45 ml of the sample. (iv) Incubate the reaction mixture at 30°C for 20 min. (v) Add 0.02 ml 4,4'-dithiodipyridine (MW 220.3), 5 mmol/liter (1.1 g/liter) and incubate the mixture at 30°C for 10 min. (vi) Read the absorbance at 324 nm. Extinction coefficient at 324 nm of pyridine-4-thione = 19,800 $mol^{-1} \cdot liter \cdot cm^{-1}$. The average number of maleimide groups introduced per peroxidase molecule is 1 or 2, and the enzyme activity is fully retained.

6.6.6. Conjugation of Fab' to 6-Maleimidohexanoyl-peroxidase

(i) Incubate 1.8 mg (45 nmol) 6-maleimidohexanoyl-peroxidase with 2.0 mg (43 nmol) Fab' in 1 ml sodium phosphate buffer, 0.1 mol/liter, pH 6.0, containing EDTA, 2.5 mmol/liter, at 4°C for 20 hr or at 30°C for 1 hr. It may be better to block the remaining thiol groups with N-ethylmaleimide. (ii) Apply the reaction mixture to a column (1.5 × 45–100 cm) of Ultrogel AcA 44 at a flow rate of 10–30 ml/hr using sodium phosphate buffer, 0.1 mol/liter, pH 6.5. The fraction volume is 1.0 ml. (iii) Read the absorbance at 280 and 403 nm, and measure peroxidase activity in each fraction (Fig. 8.4). (iv) Store the conjugate at a concentration of higher than 10 mg/liter at 4°C after addition of 1/98 vol of thimerosal, 2–5 g/liter, and 1/98 volume of bovine serum albumin, 100 g/liter, since peroxidase activity in the conjugate tends to decrease with time. Do not use NaN$_3$ as a preservative, since it inactivates peroxidase.

7. CONJUGATION OF ANTIGENS, AVIDIN, AND STREPTAVIDIN TO ENZYMES

Antigens, avidin, and streptavidin can be conjugated to enzymes by the glutaraldehyde method, the periodate method, the maleimide method and the pyridyldisulfide method described above for IgG, Fab', and Fab (2, 7–9).

7.1. Protocol for the Conjugation of HIV-1 Recombinant p24 to Horseradish Peroxidase (7)

7.1.1. Mercaptoacetyl-Recombinant p24 of HIV-1

(i) Incubate recombinant p24 (0.7 mg) in 2.0 ml sodium phosphate buffer, 0.1 mol/liter, pH 7.0, with 0.2 ml N-succinimidyl-S-acetylmercaptoacetate (Boehringer Mannheim GmbH, Mannheim, Germany), 8.25 mmol/liter, in N,N-dimethylformamide at 30°C for 30 min. (ii) Incubate the reaction mixture with 0.1 ml EDTA, 0.1 mol/liter, pH 7.0, 0.2 ml glycine-NaOH, 1 mol/liter, pH 7.0, and 0.28 ml hydroxylamine · HCl, 1 mol/liter, pH 7.0, at 30°C for 15 min. (iii) Apply the reaction mixture to a column (1.0 × 45 cm) of Sephadex G-25 using sodium phosphate buffer, 0.1 mol/liter, pH 6.0, containing EDTA, 5 mmol/liter. (iv) Determine the concentration of recombinant p24 with a commercial protein assay kit using bovine serum albumin as standard. The average number of thiol groups introduced per recombinant p24 molecule is 1.5.

7.1.2. Conjugation of Mercaptoacetyl-Recombinant p24 of HIV-1 to 6-Maleimidohexanoyl-peroxidase

(i) Incubate mercaptoacetyl-recombinant p24 (0.24 mg, 10 nmol) in 55 μl sodium phosphate buffer, 0.1 mol/liter, pH 6.0, containing EDTA, 5 mmol/liter, with 6-maleimidohexanoyl-peroxidase (0.1 mg, 2.5 nmol) in 3.0 μl sodium phosphate buffer, 0.1 mol/liter, pH 6.0, at 4°C for 20 hr. (ii) Incubate the reaction mixture with 10 μl 2-mercaptoethylamine, 10 mmol/liter, in sodium phosphate buffer, 0.1 mol/liter, pH 6.0, containing EDTA, 5 mmol/liter, at 30°C for 15 min and subsequently with 20 μl N-ethylmaleimide, 10 mmol/liter, in sodium phosphate buffer, 0.1 mol/liter, pH 6.0, at 30°C for 15 min. (iii) Apply the reaction mixture to a column (1.5 × 45 cm) of Ultrogel AcA 44 using sodium phosphate buffer, 10 mmol/liter, pH 6.5, containing NaCl, 0.1 mol/liter, and bovine serum albumin, 1 g/liter. The average number of recombinant p24 molecules conjugated per peroxidase molecule is 1.1, which is calculated from the concentration of peroxidase and the total protein concentration determined with a commercial protein assay kit as described above. The amount of recombinant p24–peroxidase conjugate is calculated from peroxidase activity.

8. CONJUGATION OF SMALL MOLECULES TO ANTIBODIES AND ANTIGENS

Small molecules such as biotin, fluorescein, rhodamine, chelating compounds for lanthanides, and any other haptens are conjugated to antibodies and antigens by derivatizing them so as to react with amino groups of antibodies and antigens. Some derivatized substances for this purpose are shown in Fig. 8.2. Small molecules containing amino groups can be readily conjugated to antibodies and antigens, as shown schematically in Fig. 8.6. For example, εN-2,4-dinitrophenyl-L-lysine is treated with N-succinimidyl-6-maleimidohexanoate and reacted with thiol groups introduced into molecules of antibodies and antigens using N-succinimidyl-S-acetylmercaptoacetate (7–9).

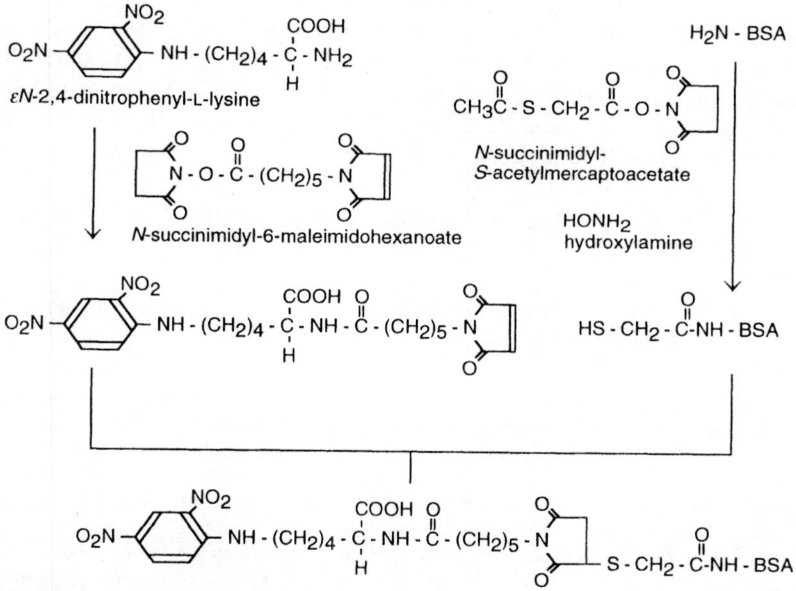

FIGURE 8.6 Conjugation of εN-2,4-dinitrophenyl-L-lysine to bovine serum albumin (BSA).

8.1. Protocol for the Conjugation of εN-2,4-Dinitrophenyl-L-lysine to Bovine Serum Albumin (7–9)

8.1.1. Mercaptoacetyl Bovine Serum Albumin

(i) Incubate bovine serum albumin (10 mg, 150 nmol) in 0.45 ml sodium phosphate buffer, 0.1 mol/liter, pH 7.0, with 50 μl N-succinimidyl-S-acetylmercaptoacetate, 40 mmol/liter, in N,N-dimethylformamide at 30°C for 30 min. (ii) Incubate the reaction mixture with 50 μl Tris–HCl buffer, 1 mol/liter, pH 7.0, 30 μl EDTA, 0.1 mol/liter, pH 7.0, and 60 μl hydroxylamine, 1 mol/liter, pH 7.0, at 30°C for 5 min. (iii) Apply the reaction mixture to a column (1.0 x 30 cm) of Sephadex G-25 using sodium phosphate buffer, 0.1 mol/liter, pH 6.0, containing EDTA, 5 mmol/liter. The amount of bovine serum albumin is calculated from the absorbance at 280 nm by taking the extinction coefficient and the molecular weight to be 0.63 g^{-1} · liter · cm^{-1} and 66,200, respectively. The average number of thiol groups introduced per bovine serum albumin molecule is 5.2.

8.1.2. αN-Maleimidohexanoyl-εN-2,4-dinitrophenyl-L-lysine

(i) Incubate 0.9 ml εN-2,4-dinitrophenyl-L-lysine–HCl (Tokyo Kasei, Tokyo), 11.1 mmol/liter, in sodium phosphate buffer, 0.1 mol/liter, pH 7.0, with 0.1 ml N-succinimidyl-6-maleimidohexanoate, 20 mmol/liter, in N,N-dimethylformamide at 30°C for 30 min.

8.1.3. Conjugation of αN-Maleimidohexanoyl-εN-2,4-dinitrophenyl-L-lysine to Mercaptoacetyl Bovine Serum Albumin

(i) Incubate mercaptoacetyl bovine serum albumin (9 mg, 140 nmol) in 0.9 ml sodium phosphate buffer, 0.1 mol/liter, pH 6.0, containing EDTA, 5 mmol/liter, with 1.1 ml αN-maleimidohexanoyl-εN-2,4-dinitrophenyl-L-lysine solution at 30°C for 30 min. (ii) Apply the reaction mixture to a column (1.0 × 30 cm) of Sephadex G-25 using sodium phosphate buffer, 0.1 mol/liter, pH 7.0. The number of 2,4-dinitrophenyl groups is calculated from the absorbance at 360 nm by taking the molar extinction coefficient to be 17,400 mol^{-1} · liter · cm^{-1}, and the ratio of the extinction coefficient of 2,4-dinitrophenyl groups at 360 nm to that at 280 nm is 1 : 0.32. The average number of 2,4-dinitrophenyl groups introduced per bovine serum albumin molecule is 4.7, as calculated from the absorbance values at 280 and 360 nm.

References

1. Ishikawa E, Imagawa M, Hashida S, et al. Enzyme-labeling of antibodies and their fragments for enzyme immunoassay and immunohistochemical staining. J Immunoassay 1983; 4:209–327.
2. Ishikawa E, Hashida S, Kohno T, et al. Methods for enzyme-labeling of antigens, antibodies and their fragments. In: Ngo TT, Ed. Nonisotopic Immunoassay. New York: Plenum, 1988:27–55.
3. Avrameas S, Ternynck T. Peroxidase labelled antibody and Fab conjugates with enhanced intracellular penetration. Immunochemistry 1971; 8:1175–9.
4. Wilson MB, Nakane PK. Recent developments in the periodate method of conjugating horseradish peroxidase (HRPO) to antibodies. In: Knapp W, Holubar K, Wick G, Eds. Immunofluorescence and Related Staining Techniques. Amsterdam: Elsevier/North-Holland Biomedical Press, 1978:215–24.
5. Chevrier D, Guesdon J-L, Mazié J-C, et al. Enzyme immunoassay for the measurement of histamine. J Immunol Methods 1986; 94:119–25.
6. Ishikawa E, Hashida S, Kohno T, et al. Modification of monoclonal antibodies with enzymes, biotin, and fluorochromes and their applications. In: Schook LB, Ed. Monoclonal Antibody Production Techniques and Applications. New York: Marcel Dekker 1987:113–37.
7. Ishikawa E, Hashida S, Kohno T, et al. Principle and applications of ultrasensitive enzyme immunoassay (immune complex transfer enzyme immunoassay) for antibodies in body fluids. J Clin Lab Anal 1993; 7:376–93.
8. Hashida S, Tanaka K, Yamamoto N, et al. Detection of one attomole of [Arg⁸]-vasopressin by novel noncompetitive enzyme immunoassay (hetero-two-site complex transfer enzyme immunoassay). J Biochem 1991; 110:486–92.
9. Hashida S, Hirota K, Hashinaka K, et al. Detection of antibody IgG to HIV-1 in urine by sensitive enzyme immunoassay (immune complex transfer enzyme immunoassay) using recombinant proteins as antigens for diagnosis of HIV-1 infection. J Clin Lab Anal 1993; 7:353–64.

9 | SOLID PHASES IN IMMUNOASSAY

J. E. BUTLER
Department of Microbiology
The University of Iowa
Iowa City, Iowa 52242

1. INTERFACIAL IMMUNOCHEMISTRY

1.1. General Principles

Interfacial ligand–receptor interactions as exemplified by solid-phase immunoassays (SPI) obey general Mass Law principles, while displaying unique characteristics which differ from ligand–receptor interactions that occur in solution. These differences may complicate data interpretation, can lead to certain misconceptions regarding SPI, and may contribute to less than optimal assay protocols. These characteristics involve: (a) reaction kinetics, (b) reaction volumes, (c) "functional" versus actual reactant concentrations, and (d) the molecular configuration of immobilized versus solution-phase reactants.

1.2. Diffusion Dependence

The time required for static equilibrium to be reached in SPI (except those involving microparticles) is greater than for solution-phase interactions and in-

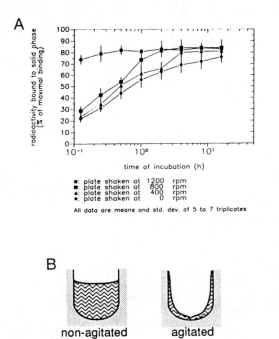

A

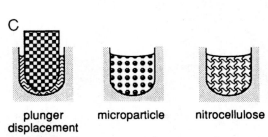

non-agitated   agitated

plunger   microparticle   nitrocellulose
displacement

FIGURE 9.1 The diffusion dependence of solid-phase immunoassay and methods used to reduce its influence. (A) The effect of vortexing (shaking) microtiter wells on establishment of equilibrium (reprinted from Ref. 1). (B) Illustration of the physical effect of vortexing microtiter wells (rotary agitation) on the distribution of the fluid phase relative to the solid phase. The fluid phase is depicted by wavy lines. (C) Alternative methods of confining the reaction volume to within close proximity to the solid phase which displays the immobilized reactant.

creases in proportion to the ratio of the volume occupied by the liquid to that occupied by the interfacial receptor. Interfacial reaction kinetics display a pronounced diffusion dependence when conducted in microtiter wells (Fig. 9.1A). This can be reduced by vortex agitation, which compresses the liquid to a small area in contact with the receptor (reactant)-coated interface (1; Fig. 9.1B). This can also be accomplished by forcing the reactive solution phase into a small volume with an inert plunger, by using a porous matrix with a large surface (such as nitrocellulose), and by using microparticles as the solid phase[1] (Fig. 9.1C). Plastic tubes with internal "fins" to increase surface area have been proposed (2) and microtiter

[1] Microparticles are <1 μm and behave as a colloidal suspension during the assay; "particles" or "beads" are larger and settle out by gravity during nonagitated assays.

"starwells" are now available based on this principle ("Starwells"; NUNC, Roskilde, Denmark). These wells increase surface area and shorten diffusion distances, thus shortening incubation times. The ability to greatly reduce the time required for the establishment of equilibrium using the modification described above supports the view that diffusion dependence is directly correlated with the ratio of the solution-phase volume to the volume of the reactive interface.[2]

1.3. The Reaction Volume of Solid-Phase Immunoassays

The true reaction volume[2] of any SPI, e.g., ELISA, is difficult to determine and may be much less than the total fluid volume of the reaction vessel in which the assay is being performed. One must conceptualize that solid-phase antigen–antibody reactions occur in "microenvironments," i.e., at the fluid–solid phase interface. Interactions probably occur within the attraction distance of the strongest primary bonds, a distance which is <100 Å and probably closer to 10 Å. Diffusion or mass transfer (see above) is needed to move reactants into this true interfacial reaction volume. The reactive surface area of microparticles (Fig. 1C) is much larger than that of microtiter wells and comprises a correspondingly higher proportion of the total volume. The true reactant concentration depends on the true reaction volume which has been estimated but not precisely calculated. The lack of such data complicates the calculation of K_{eq} using common graphic forms of the Mass Law, thus favoring relative and proportional measurements such as "extent of reaction" equations or equations derived by us for evaluating capture antibody (CAb) performance (3). Because of these features of SPIs, mean that values reported for solid-phase antigen–antibody reactions may be incomparable to those obtained for fluid-phase reactions (4).

1.4. Reaction Rates of Interfacial Interactions

Dissociation rates for interfacial reactions, including those on cell surfaces, may be two orders of magnitude lower than those occurring in solution. The similarity between the slow dissociation rates observed for SPI and those occurring on cell surfaces is interesting for a number of reasons. First, many interactions on cell surfaces involve aggregation of the cell surface receptors with a corresponding increase in avidity due to reduced dissociation of multivalent complexes (5). Not surprisingly, we and others have shown that at least passively adsorbed antigens and antibodies also appear to be clustered or aggregated (6, 7), i.e., the active interfacial reactant may be "the cluster." Second, the greater energy needed for dissociation of most antigen–antibody bonds compared to that needed to prevent their association (hysteresis) indicates that secondary bonds have formed after formation of the initial bond. Hysteresis may account for the synergistic behavior of mAbs which bind different epitopes on the same antigen. As more mAbs bind, the avidity of the interaction increases (8). This suggests that in SPI and cell surface reactions, secondary bond formation is important. Third, a very high solid-phase reactant concentration, especially as might occur in clusters, and resulting from

---

[2] The volume of the reactive interface, or reaction volume, does not refer to the total volume in which the SPI is conducted, e.g., the bead volume or the volume of a plastic microtiter well. Rather, it is a theoretical volume at the interface in which the soluble and immobilized reactants interact on the surface of the solid phase.

a confined interfacial reaction volume (see above), could facilitate more rapid reassociation of dissociated analyte than would occur in fluid-phase systems. This might account for the higher K_{eq} of antibodies when tested in SPI versus in solution (9). Fortunately it is this very slow "off-rate" which makes ELISA and SPI technology very forgiving in that the primary receptor–ligand interaction remains associated throughout the repeated washing steps which characterize many of these assays.

1.5. Influence on Apparent Affinity

All immunoassays are affinity dependent, a fact self evident from examination of Mass Law principles governing these interactions. The question arises as to whether SPI and ELISAs are particularly affinity dependent. For example, microtiter SpAbIs, performed using passively adsorbed complex antigens, may display apparent affinity dependence when compared to their solution-phase counterparts (10). This seems paradoxical in light of the stability of solid-phase receptor–ligand interactions until one observes the small proportion of available antibody that is captured by a several log excess of adsorbed antigen (11, 12). This effect could be due to: (a) the small proportion and thus low functional concentration, of antigenic epitopes on adsorbed antigens which survive the passive adsorption process; (b) steric hindrance of epitopes when molecules are crowded into the monolayer or into aggregates; or (c) alteration but not loss of native epitopes, which results in their much lower affinity for their paratopes.

The stable adsorption of 60–80% of most protein antigens as at least a monolayer (13), when passively adsorbed in the range of 1–5 μg/ml, should not result in a deficiency of total antigen. If 500–800 ng of antigen is adsorbed on a microtiter well, a 1/10,000 dilution of serum containing 500 μg antibody/ml should still provide a >10-fold excess of antigen. Considering a reasonable K_{eq} for the interaction, a limitation in total adsorbed antigen does not seem to explain the results. Rather, loss, alteration, or steric unavailability of epitopes seem to be more plausible. Thus, "functional" reactant concentrations in SPIs and ELISA may be much lower than total reactant concentrations. This has been quantitatively demonstrated for adsorbed antibodies (14). The possibility that immobilized reactants may not be conformationally displayed in the same manner as in solution, is supported by a variety of experiments. These are reviewed in Section 3.3.

Steric factors are also operative on solid phases. Antigenic epitopes may become buried during immobilization, either at the solid-phase protein interface or at the protein–protein interface of a tightly packed monolayer. As there is probably some orientational ordering of molecules in the packed monolayer, not all epitopes are likely to be equally affected and not all solid phases behave in the same manner (see below). Steric hindrance may also occur when the specific antibody bound to its epitope cannot be recognized by, e.g., the antibody–enzyme conjugate used in an ELISA (15).

Figure 9.2 shows that the ELISA system is more sensitive than RIA in the range below 10 ng of adsorbed IgG2a, while above 10 ng the RIA plot slopes sharply upward while the ELISA plots tend toward a plateau. In fact, the highest four values in the RIA plot for measuring IgG2a adsorbed on Immulon 2 have a log–log slope of circa 1.0; this is in agreement with the theoretical slope value for the log–log plot of an antigen–antibody interaction. Thus, the ELISA plots in Fig. 9.2 illustrate inhibition at high antigen dose, i.e., the antibody–enzyme conjugate appears hindered from detecting its antigen in this region of the titration plot. In

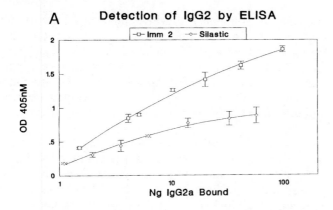

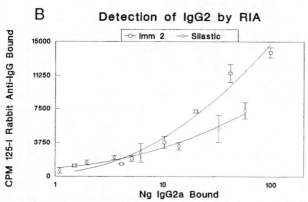

FIGURE 9.2 Detection of IgG2a adsorbed on two different surfaces by ELISA (A) or RIA (B). IgG2a was adsorbed on Immulon 2 (□) or Silastic (◇) at pH 7. ^{125}I-IgG2a was initially employed so that the actual amount of immobilized protein would be known. Detection by indirect ELISA (A) involved the use of a one-step glutaraldehyde antibody–enzyme conjugate. Detection by RIA (B) utilized ^{125}I-anti-IgG. Error bars in both cases reflect standard deviation. For discussion see text.

general, the degree of hindrance seen in ELISA is a function of the molecular size of the conjugate; conjugates composed of only Fab + alkaline phosphatase are the least hindered, whereas "amplified" systems involving a string of antibodies and then the conjugate are most sensitive to steric effects (15).

Detectability may also be more pronounced on certain solid phases than on others. Figure 9.2 also shows that IgG2a adsorbed on silicone is comparatively poorly detected regardless of whether detection is by RIA or ELISA. While this might indicate that greater epitope alteration has occurred on silicone compared to polystyrene, atomic force microscopy studies suggest it may be a steric hindrance problem related to the surface of silicone.

1.6. Blocking and Blocking Reagents

The introduction of a solid phase into reactions involving ligands and their receptors requires that nonspecific interactions (i.e., nonspecific binding, NSB), between the soluble ligand and the solid phase to which the receptor is immobilized, be inhibited or "blocked" so that only the interaction between the receptor and its ligand can occur. Various substances are included in the category of blocking agents, although protein solutions and nonionic detergents are most popular. The choice (or need) for such agents varies with: (a) the solid phase, (b) the empirical experience of the assay designer, and (c) the particular ligand–receptor combination. There are differences of opinion regarding both the need and mechanism of action of blocking agents.

Protein blocking agents, typically solutions of serum albumin, casein, newborn calf serum, or dilute skim milk, are most often added after immobilization of the solid-phase receptor and are believed to "fill in" stretches of the solid phase not occupied by the immobilized receptor. Thus, they reduce NSB by blocking reactive sites on the solid phase. Among the blockers in common use, those based on casein or skim milk appear most effective on both polystyrene and nitrocellulose surfaces. This is believed to be due to the predominance of low-molecular-weight casein and other small proteins or peptides in skim milk, which theoretically would have a greater opportunity to fill in small areas between the larger immobilized receptor molecules. Evidence that this is indeed the mechanism which accounts for their effectiveness is lacking, and would be theoretically difficult to explain if indeed a monolayer of receptor already covers the surface (see 3.2, below). However, the area of reactive, unoccupied surface may vary depending on the configuration of the immunoassay and choice of solid phase. In immunoassays conducted on nitrocellulose, blocking protein solutions (skim milk) are virtually obligatory to reduce NSB and are typically used during every incubation step after receptor immobilization whereas on polystyrene, protein blockers and even nonionic detergents (see below) can be omitted from those reaction steps which come after receptor immobilization and the initial blocking step. The much larger surface area and membranous matrices of solid-phases like nitrocellulose (see 2.2, below) is probably never covered with anything approaching a monolayer of the receptor so that authentic blocking of unoccupied surfaces is more likely to be the mechanism of action for the blocking agents used on such surfaces.

"Leakiness" of blocking agents refers to their failure to suppress nonspecific interactions as the assay proceeds through subsequent reaction steps. It is believed that such failure does not result from the gradual displacement of the blocking agent, but is rather due to the gradual exposure of nonspecific binding sites on the original blocking agent or on the receptor monolayer itself. These observations weaken any concept that the function of protein blocking agents is solely to cover unoccupied reactive sites on the solid phase.

Care must be used in the selection of a blocking agent, if indeed they are at all necessary, for a particular application. For example, commercial blocking agents like Blotto and Superblock (typically concoctions of skim milk protein sometimes containing nonionic detergents and also containing antifoaming agents) either fail to lower NSB on silicone solid phases or actually increase NSB. Thus there is a need for investigators who work with less ubiquitously studied surfaces to empirically test the blocking effectiveness of a particular blocking agent on the solid phase being used, rather than extrapolating experiences encountered with other surfaces.

The second category of blocking agents is detergents. These are low-molecular-weight compounds with distinctive symmetry, i.e., hydrophobic at one end and hydrophilic at the other. The combination of their small size and amphipathic nature means that they can intercalate protein structure, perhaps by bonding hydrophobically to protein and displaying their hydrophilic ends to the solvent. Detergents can be classified as nonionic, ionic, or zwitterionic (Fig. 9.3). Nonionic forms such as Tween, Triton, and Nonident-40 are those most commonly used in immunoassays.

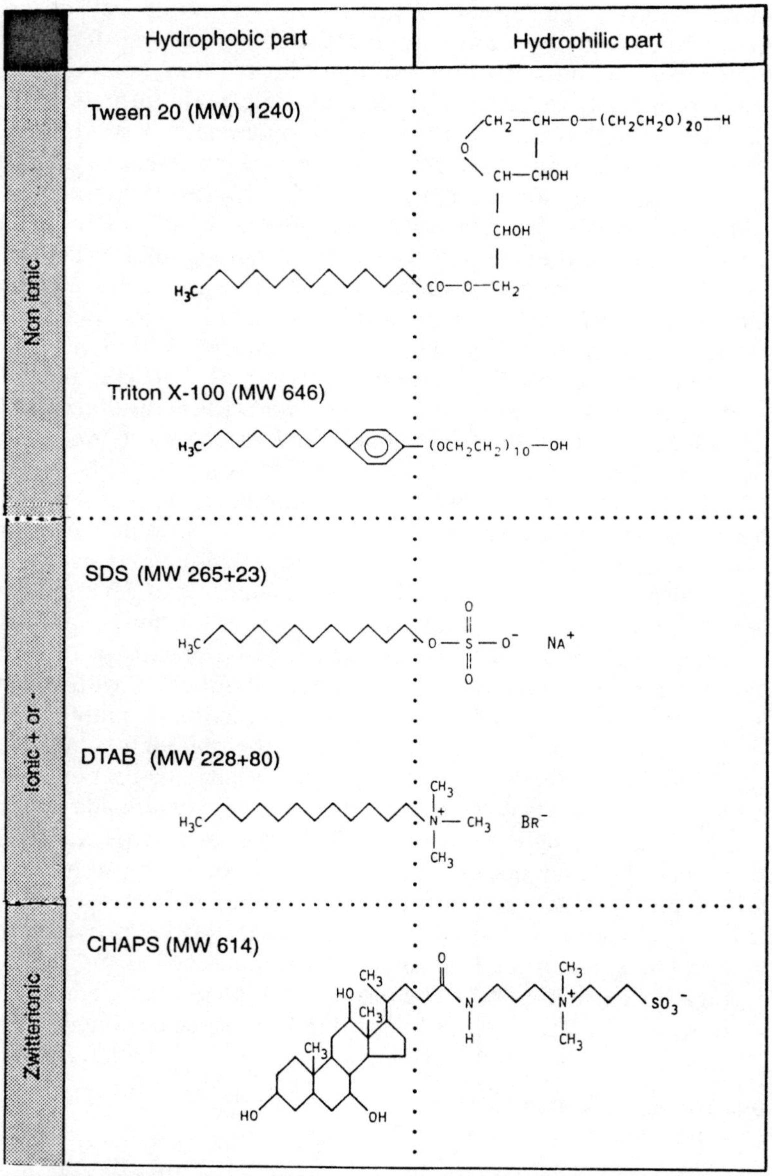

FIGURE 9.3 Chemical differences in the types of detergents used in SPI. Schematic illustration of five detergents commonly used in SPI. Tween 20, ikosaothyethylene sorbitan monolaurate; Triton X-100, octylphenoxy octaethoxy ethanol; SDS, sodium dodecyl sulfate; DTAB, dodecyltrimethyl ammonium bromide; CHAPS, 3-[(cholamidopropyl)dimethylammonio]-1-propane sulfonate. Reprinted with permission from NUNC Bulletin 8, 1990.

Detergents probably act in various ways, but in contrast to protein blockers, their action is generally ascribed to preventing the hydrophobic adsorption of proteins to the solid phase and decreasing the hydrophobic aggregation of macromolecules, rather than filling in unoccupied sites on the solid phase. However, there is little doubt that detergents are capable of dislodging weakly immobilized receptors.

Among the detergents commonly used, Tween-20 appears to be most popular and is unusual in having the capacity of preventing both nonspecific adsorption to polystyrene and nonspecific protein–protein interactions during subsequent steps in an immunoassay conducted on polystyrene. Most other nonionic detergents appear to act principally in preventing nonspecific protein–protein interactions. Therefore, many of the investigators who use polystyrene as a solid phase do not use a separate protein blocking step, but merely conduct all steps of their SPI (e.g., ELISA) after the initial immobilization of the receptor, with only Tween-20 present in the washing and reaction buffers at a concentration of 0.05%. Detergents alone are usually ineffective in preventing NSB on membranous solid phases.

The use of detergents with or without protein blocking agents also has other consequences in the study of receptor–ligand reactions. For example, Qualtiere *et al.* (16) tested the ability of various detergents to interfere with antibody–antigen interactions. Ionic detergents like sodium dodecyl sulfate (SDS; Fig. 9.3) have inhibitory effects on antibody–antigen reactions. The zwitterionic detergent CHAPS (Fig. 9.3) may have the least effect on such interactions but is also less able to block nonspecific interactions, especially adsorption to the solid-phase itself. CHAPS is an example of a detergent that should be used with blocking proteins.

It has been suggested by Avrameas and Terynich (17) that spontaneous autoreactive antibodies, like those seen in nonimmunized individuals, typically: (a) have binding sites which recognize hydrophilic determinants, e.g., CHO; (b) have positively charged residues in their binding sites; and (c) are (often) high avidity IgM antibodies. Immunization appears to shift binding site chemistry to favor more hydrophobic interactions involving IgG (and IgA) antibodies with much higher intrinsic affinity. Hence, unwanted "nonspecific" interactions resulting from hydrophilic interactions might be less inhibitable with nonionic detergents than those interactions involving antibodies resulting from "affinity maturation." While increases in the affinity (avidity) of induced antibodies may overcome any tendency for them to be inhibited by detergent, the inhibition of nonspecific[3] residual or autoreactive antibodies may not occur and may thus contribute to NSB.

The "take home message" on blocking agents is that: (a) the exact mechanism(s) of their actions is unknown; (b) there are two major categories, proteins and detergents; (c) each blocker may behave differently depending on the nature of the ligand–receptor interaction and the chemistry of the solid phase; and (d) blockers may interfere with specific as well as background (nonspecific) interactions.

1.7. A Mass Law for ELISA and Other Solid-Phase Immunoassays

The various immunochemical phenomena observed for SPIs and reviewed above, are the basis for hypothetical Eq. (1).

---

[3] It is important to realize that "specific" and "nonspecific" reactions are operationally defined. In reality, nonspecific reactions may be equally specific, but are simply not the interaction that the assay is designed to measure.

$$Ag_{SOL} + Ab_{SOL} \underset{k_2D}{\overset{k_1D}{\rightleftharpoons}} Ag_{SLD}\text{---}Ab_{SOL}$$

$$\underset{k_2R}{\overset{k_1R}{\rightleftharpoons}} Ag_{SLD} - Ab_{SOL} + Ag_{SOL} - Ab_{SOL} \underset{k_2A}{\overset{k_1A}{\rightleftharpoons}} (Ag_{SLD}Ab_{SOL})_n \qquad (1)$$

Equation (1) describes an interfacial SpAbI using an immobilized antigen (Ag_{SLD}). The equilibrium reaction D governs the diffusion-dependent phase of the reaction, whereas R, governed by rate constants k_1R and k_2R, describes the interaction of Ag_{SLD} and Ab_{SOL} once they have reached the true interfacial reaction volume. Whereas the average forward rate constant (k_1) for solution-phase interaction is $10^7 M^{-1}s^{-1}$, those for reactions on synthetic solid phase and cell surfaces are two to four orders of magnitude slower (18). Equation (1) assumes that this slower k_1 is not the consequence of the kinetics of the interaction within the true interfacial reaction volume, but the result of slower diffusion and lower mass transfer of reactants to the site of interaction. Hence, Eq. (1) distinguishes between D and R and, as described above, k_1D can be greatly increased by a number of means (see Figs. 9.1B, 9.1C).

It is also known that the overall dissociation rate (k_2), from synthetic or cellular interfaces is in the order of 10^{-4} to 10^{-5} s^{-1}, i.e., up to two orders of magnitude slower than for solution-phase systems (19–21). Polyvalent interactions in solution also have higher K_{eq}s which are believed or have been shown to result from lower k_2s (21, 22). This hysteresis effect, combined with the apparent clustering of solid-phase reactants (6, 7), suggests that multivalent interactions involve secondary bonding to other proteins or to the solid phase itself. Extensive cross-linking at the interface may also be associated with surface coagulation or aggregation via translational diffusion (23). This could also increase surface contact and further increase hysteresis and lower k_2. Equation (1) treats this secondary aggregation phase as a third distinct interaction, i.e., interaction A, that is governed by k_1A and k_2A.

Equation (1) is hypothetical, designed both to explain observations made by ourselves and others; moreover, it is a simplistic model for students which simultaneously challenges them with a testable hypothesis.

2. DIVERSITY OF SOLID PHASES

2.1. The Role of the Solid Phase in Immunoassay

Modern immunoassay takes its origin from the historic work of Berson and Yalow (24), who utilized the specificity and sensitivity of the antigen–antibody reaction to quantify biomolecules on the basis of their antigenicity. Their contribution, known as radioimmunoassay (RIA), was based on competitive inhibition and is therefore not dissimilar (albeit considerably more direct) in principle to complement fixation. In spite of its popularity through the 1960s and 1970s, traditional RIA was technically troubled by the difficulty in separating the bound reactant from the free reactant. Hence the observation by, e.g., Catt and Tregear (25) that proteins spontaneously adsorbed to plastic surfaces allowed the simple plastic test tube not only to be a reaction vessel, but also to immobilize the solid-phase reactant and thus provide a convenient means of separating bound reactants from free reactants. For example, once the receptor is adsorbed on the plastic tube, it is allowed to bind its ligand, so that bound ligand and free ligand can be quickly separated by merely inverting the tube. Since the use of pioneer ELISAs and other SPIs in the 1970s, plastic test tubes have given way to microtiter plates, nitrocellulose and nylon membrane, beads of polystyrene and methylmethacrylate, and, somewhat more recently, microparticles. In any case, what constituted the "slowest ship in the RIA convoy (separation of bound and free ligand)" was revolutionarily overcome by the introduction of a solid phase which firmly held the immobilized receptor.

2.2. Characteristics of Common Solid Phases

The popularity of a new principle like SPI often results in its widespread usage on all types of solid phase without regard to the chemical differences among them. It is usually only later that investigations reveal that all solid phases are not created equal, and thus do not behave in the same manner. This has already been illustrated in Fig. 9.2 and mentioned in Section 1.5.

Differences in volume to surface ratios of the various solid-phase surfaces affect both the kinetics and the dynamic range of SPI. Immobilization chemistries also differ among solid phases and specific applications (see Section 3). Table 9.1 summarizes the characteristics of the more commonly used solid phases in terms of parameters which influence their performance in SPI. Solid phases can be grouped into at least three categories with plastic labware, such as tubes and microtiter or tissue culture plates, comprising a rather physically and chemically homogeneous group. Not surprisingly, these materials generally have similar performance, regardless of manufacturer or type.[4] The 96-well microtiter plate is ubiquitous in laboratories where ELISAs, for example, are performed; over a half-dozen companies manufacture plate readers, while a smaller number supply automatic washers and diluters designed for such microtiter plates. Full robotic systems are also available. The most commonly used material for microtiter plates is polystyrene, of which the irradiated versions[4] show somewhat greater capacity to adsorb protein, probably due to covalent bonds made possible by the free radicals produced during the irradiation. Both Costar (Cobind) and NUNC (Covalink) offer functionalized polystyrene and thus covalent attachment. However, the overwhelming influence of the surrounding hydrophobic polystyrene surface in such wells results in the final protein–plastic bonding being essentially hydrophobic, so performance is only slightly different than on nonfunctionalized surfaces. Functionalized plates may differ substantially in performance from nonfunctionized plates when used with small molecules or in special applications.

Polystyrene beads function much like plates, although they provide greater surface area. Their relative inconvenience in use has limited their popularity, whereas microparticle assays have become popular. Microparticles[1] differ from beads in behaving as a colloid, thus greatly increasing surface area and greatly reducing the diffusion dependence of SPI observed on the more traditional solid phases (Fig. 9.1). Magnetic microparticles readily facilitate the separation of the solid phase and its bound reactant from the fluid phase containing the free reactants, after the

---

[4] Subtle differences can affect such things as background, preferential adsorption of certain molecules, and well-to-well variation, but these differences are minor in relationship to differences seen among other categories of solid phases (Table 9.1). On the contrary, irradiated plastics (e.g., NUNC Maxisorp and Immulon 2; Dynatech) have a greater avidity for macromolecules than do untreated polystyrenes.

TABLE 9.1

Solid phase	Bonding force	Relative surface area	Performance characteristics
Plastic labware			
Polystyrene	Hydrophobic	Modest	Low background
Polystyrene-irradiated	Hydrophobic, hydrophilic, and covalent	Modest	Reproducible
Surface-functionalized polystyrene	Hydrophobic and covalent	Modest	Readily adapted to automation
Bead			
Polystyrene (PS) beads	Hydrophobic	Moderate	Yields assays with broad dynamic ranges.
Derivatized PS beads	Covalent, hydrophobic, and hydrophilic	High	Less convenient to use than labware. More difficult to automate.
Beaded agarose and derivatives	Hydrophilic and covalent	High	Minimal protein denaturation. High background and difficult to automate.
Microparticles	Hydrophobic and covalent	Very high	"Solution-phase performance" due to colloidal nature. Wide dynamic range. Magnetized variants make them automatable.
Membranes			
Nitrocellulose (NC)	Hydrophobic and hydrophilic	Very high	Desorption and background problems hinder their use in quantitative assays.
Nylon	Hydrophobic	Very high	Serious background problems reduce signal : noise ratio.
Charge-modified nylon	Hydrophilic, covalent, and hydrophobic	Very high	Problems similar to nylon but perhaps less denaturation and less desorption.
Functionalized nitrocellulose	Hydrophobic, covalent, and hydrophilic	Very high	Similar to NC but less desorption.
PVDF (Immobilon P)	Hydrophobic	Very high	Very high and stable binding. May be best for immunoblotting.

Reprinted from Ref. (11), © 1986, by courtesy of Marcel Dekker.

ligand–receptor interaction has occurred. Magnetic beads are also popular in cell separations, affinity purification of proteins, and preparation of mRNAs.

Beaded materials composed of carbohydrates are unique on the list provided in Table 9.1 in both chemistry and performance. Binding to their hydrophilic surface is usually covalent and proteins immobilized in this manner are only minimally altered (see below). However, hydrophilic beads do not lend themselves to convenient use or to automation and have been largely restricted to affinity chromatography.

The third group of solid phases are membranous and form the basis of ELISA-based immunoblotting. Their adsorptive surface areas are 100–1000 times greater than plastic, presumably due to their immense internal surfaces. Also, the porous nature of membranes allow flowthrough technology to be employed in immunoassay, which is another means of reducing the diffusion-dependent phase of SPI (Eq. (1)). A variety of types exist, including those composed of cellulose nitrate ester (nitrocellulose; NC), nylon, and polyvinylidene difluoride (PVDF). NC and PVDF are preferred for proteins, whereas nylon is popular for nucleic acids. Membranes, especially nylon, have a high propensity toward NSB binding of proteins due in part to their large surface area. Thus, they require "blocking agents" (see Section 1.6) and extensive washing when used in immunoassays. Millipore offers NC in a 96-well format (the well bottoms are NC) and several companies offers assemblies for clamping NC sheets into templates for 96-well systems (e.g., Pierce Chemicals, Rockford, IL). The principal chemical bonds between proteins and nonmodified membranes are hydrophobic, although evidence exists for some hydrophilic bonding. It is possible that a certain amount of the latter represents protein–protein bonds which dissociate under conditions designed to break hydrophilic bonds.

3. IMMOBILIZATION PROCEDURES

3.1. Overview

Solid-phase reactants can be immobilized by four general procedures: (a) passive adsorption, (b) covalent attachment to functionalized solid phases, (c) immuno-chemical immobilization, and (d) other nonadsorbent, noncovalent methods of attachment. The latter includes immobilization via streptavidin–biotin linkages and the use of bacterial Ig-binding proteins, e.g., Protein A. Covalent attachment is most common for hydrophilic beads (agarose) or heavily functionalized polystyrene beads. Passive adsorption is most widely used for ELISAs on microtiter plates and for immunoblotting on NC.

3.2. Immobilization of Proteins by Passive Adsorption

The adsorption of proteins on synthetic surfaces, such as polystyrene latex and glass, was studied as early as 1956 (26) although its popular application to immunoassay dates to Catt and Tregear (25). Figure 9.4 illustrates the characteristics of protein adsorption on nonirradiated polystyrene at alkaline pH. Passive adsorption under these conditions follows typical saturation principles. Compared in percent bound plots, the affinity (avidity)[5] differences among proteins for the plastic is more obvious and avidity appears correlated with molecular weight (Fig. 9.4). Newer formulations of polystyrene, especially irradiated forms, exhibit less difference in their affinity for proteins of different size and conformation than what is shown in Fig. 9.4. Calculations made from saturation analyses indicate that saturation occurs when a monolayer of protein has become adsorbed (6, 13); this is consistent with data showing that fewer large molecules are needed than small molecules (Fig. 9.4). Saturation with IgG antibodies corresponds to the addition of circa 1000 ng/ 200 μl in a microtiter well (13, 27). Most capture antibodies also have their optimal performance when adsorbed at this concentration (3) but not necessarily at alkaline pH.

Nitrocellulose and other membranes show (a) a much higher capacity for adsorption per planar surface area than plastic, and (b) considerable adsorption heterogeneity among membranes and proteins. In contrast, adsorption of IgG on polystyrene microtiter wells from various manufacturers at alkaline pH differs only subtly.

---

[5] The term affinity, as applied to SPI, is probably more correctly avidity, as it reflects a multivalent, aggregation-type interaction. The proportion of added protein which is stably adsorbed is a direct correlate of affinity (avidity; 3).

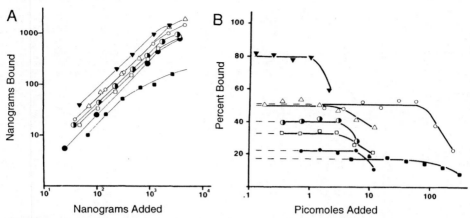

FIGURE 9.4 The characteristics of passive adsorption on polystyrene at alkaline pH. (A) Adsorption behavior of seven different proteins in a log–log saturation plot. (▼) Bovine IgM, 1000 kDa; (△) bovine secretory IgA, 420 kDa; (○) ovalbumin, 44 kDa; (◑) bovine IgG1, 158 kDa; (□) bovine IgG2a, 152 kDa; (●) bovine serum albumin, 69 kDa; (■) bovine α-lactalbumin, 14 kDa. (B) Adsorptive behavior of the same proteins expressed in a molar percentage bound plot. Dashed lines are extrapolations in the region of constant percentage binding for which empirical data were not reported. Same symbols as in (A). Modified from Cantarero *et al.* (13).

The data shown in Fig. 9.4 are based on studies performed at alkaline pH and above the pI of all the proteins studied. Adsorption at alkaline pH was the procedure initially described by Engvall and Perlmann (28) and this procedure has been retained in much of the current ELISA technology. Adsorption at other pHs on polystyrene can give much different patterns. Figure 9.5 illustrates that a linear binding region, i.e., a region in which the proportion of adsorbed IgG (or protein in question) remains constant, is only observed at alkaline pH. At both acid and neutral pH, the proportion which becomes adsorbed is concentration dependent. Because the proportion which is adsorbed is a function of the K_{eq} (avidity) of the interaction (3), the increase in the proportion of IgG adsorbed at acid and neutral pH with increasing amounts of added IgG suggests cooperative binding as may occur during aggregation, i.e., the K_{eq} for adsorption progressively increases with the amount added up to the point at which a monolayer is formed.

Polystyrene is a relatively "pure" hydrophobic surface unless irradiated, so that the pH of the protein has less effect on adsorption than it does, for example, during adsorption on silicone, where polar interactions appear also to be important. At this point, very few studies have been undertaken to determine the macromolecular mechanisms involved in adsorption on surfaces other than polystyrene.

3.3. Stability and Integrity of Adsorbed Proteins

The stability of passively adsorbed macromolecules has been best studied on polystyrene. Studies in our laboratory have shown that for proteins adsorbed to polystyrene within the linear binding region (Fig. 9.4), as much as 15% can desorb during a 16-hr period, provided that both nonionic detergent and blocking proteins are present in the incubation solution. When exchangeable protein is absent from the solution, desorption drops to <10% and when no detergent is used, only 1–2%

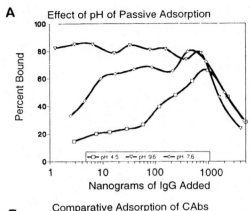

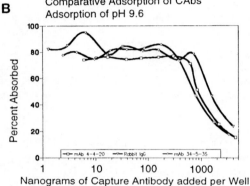

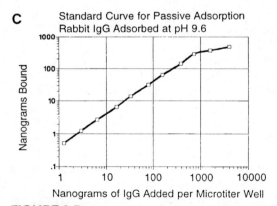

FIGURE 9.5 The effect of pH on the adsorption of IgG on polystyrene. The adsorption characteristics of monoclonal 4-4-20 at pH 4.5, 7.6, and 9.6 are shown. Only at alkaline pH is a region of constant percent adsorption, i.e., an LBR, observed. All IgG studied to date behave similarly. Reprinted from Mol Immunol, 30, Butler et al., The immunochemistry of sandwich ELISAs. VI. 1165–75, © (1993) with kind permission from Elsevier Science Ltd, The Boulevard, Langford Lane, Kidlington OX5 1GB, UK.

of adsorbed protein is released. The ionic detergent SDS can increase desorption, especially from silicone. Protein adsorbed above the linear binding region (which according to calculations is beyond the added concentration that results in a monolayer) generally appears less stable, especially in the presence of SDS. Ionic detergent may cause dissociation of protein–protein interactions that are more likely to form on the surface above saturation. The relatively stable monolayer of protein adsorbed on polystyrene, at least in short-term experiments, is such that a urea/SDS/β-mercaptoethanol cocktail or dilute alkali can be used to remove the immuno-chemically bound reactant after completion of an ELISA without completely dis-lodging the adsorbed layer. This allows the same antigen-coated wells to be reused in subsequent tests. This can result in a major reduction in cost and labware waste, but should not be indiscriminately used until empirically tested in one's own assay system. There is little or no information on the stability of macromolecules adsorbed at other pHs or those immobilized by nonadsorptive methods.

The consequence of passive adsorption of proteins on polystyrene has been studied by various investigators who generally reach the same conclusions. Namely, passive adsorption results in the loss or alteration of antigenic epitopes, the loss of enzymatic activity, the generation of new epitopes, demonstrable physical–chemical changes, and loss of CAb activity–affinity (6, 29; Table 9.2). Losses in antibody activity can exceed 90%, and if the same occurs with antigen, it can explain the discrepancy between total serum antibody measured by quantitative precipitation and that measured by SpAbI (11, 12). At least for polystyrene, there appears to be sufficient evidence that passive adsorption involves conformational changes as proteins unfold to permit internal hydrophobic side chains to form strong hydropho-bic bonds with the solid phase.

The biological consequences of adsorption on various blotting membranes appear to be of less concern to investigators than adsorption on polystyrene. Even if denaturation is on a par with that which occurs on polystyrene, much more protein binds to NC so that a greater amount (not greater proportion) of native protein may survive and denaturation effects are overlooked. Furthermore, evidence that hydrophilic as well as hydrophobic forces are involved in adsorption on immunoblot-ting membranes suggests that conformational alterations on membranes may not be as severe as on polystyrene.

If passive adsorption is so destructive for proteins, why is there continued use of this procedure? The answer is simply that enough molecules survive to make the assay work. For example, if 6% of high-affinity capture antibodies adsorbed on a microtiter well survive in a functional state, it is sufficient to provide a sandwich ELISA with a dynamic range of 2–200 ng/ml; this two log range is adequate for most applications and is typical of assays reported in the literature.

3.4. Immobilization of Other Macromolecules and Peptides

Polysaccharides and heavily glycosylated proteins often have low affinity for polystyrene (reviewed in 29) and often require alternative methods for their immobi-lization. One alternative is covalent immobilization using a suitable cross-linking agent, such as glutaraldehyde, EDAC, or dimethyl suberimidate, to: (a) functional-ized polystyrenes such as aminostyrene that is commercially available as, e.g., "Co-valink" from NUNC (Roskilde); (b) polystyrene first treated with surface modifying agents to produce isocyanate groups or amino groups; or (c) polylysine, phenylala-nine–lysine, octadecylamine, or some irrelevant proteins that have been adsorbed beforehand (reviewed in 29). The same method has been employed for the immobili-zation of proteins which (a) due to their chemistry cannot bind to a hydrophobic surface, (b) are so small that their adsorptive affinity may be very low (Fig. 9.4), or (c) are conformationally altered by adsorption to the extent that they become nonfunctional (30–32). On the other hand, bacterial capsular polysaccharides have been successfully adsorbed on plastic (33) and a surprising number of investigators have merely adsorbed peptides passively to polystyrene or synthesized them directly on polystyrene rods (34). Unfortunately, there are few studies that have addressed the antigenic consequences of passive peptide adsorption. Søndergard-Anderson et al. (32) observed that Angiotensin I and II were 5- to 10-fold more antigenically active when covalently attached than when adsorbed. Lacroix et al. observed that the form of the peptide was important; cyclized peptides appeared more active than their linear counterparts (35).

Another group of biomolecules often studied are those freed from membranes by cell lysis in the presence of detergents. Because detergents are used to block adsorption to hydrophobic surfaces, their presence will inhibit adsorption of the lysate proteins to plastic. Adsorption to NC is possible particularly if detergent concentrations are <0.01%. Triton, Tween, and SDS are the most inhibitory detergents while deoxycholate and octylglucoside have the least effect (36). The fact that detergents are much more inhibitory to adsorption on nylon (Genescreen) than on NC, supports the idea that forces other than hydrophobic ones may be involved in adsorption to NC (Table 9.1).

When detergent levels in cell lysates cannot be diluted to permit adsorption, covalent linkage may be required. Alternatively, materials like SM-2 Bio-Beads can be used to reduce the detergent concentration (37).

3.5. Immunochemical Immobilization

Immunochemical immobilization is an alternative method for immobilizing biomolecules which do not lend themselves to passive adsorption. Investigators have used an adsorbed capture antibody to immobilize the antigen of interest in certain SpAbI (38). The inherent problem with this approach is that only 10–25% of the capture antibody may survive denaturation on polystyrene so that as few as 1 in 10 antibody molecules are available to capture the antigen. This reduces the concentration of antigen much below the total antigen concentration that can be achieved by simple adsorption. Nevertheless, immunochemically immobilized antigen can be 10-fold more active than adsorbed antigen (39) and we have seen total retention of activity for CAb immobilized by this method, whereas only 10% was active when passively adsorbed (14; Fig. 9.6). A major application of immunochemical immobilization is the immobilization of proteins in detergent-containing cell lysates and in samples containing complicating contaminants (see 3.7, below).

3.6. Other Noncovalent, Nonadsorptive Methods

The high affinity of avidin and streptavidin (SA) for biotin provides an alternative, nonadsorptive, noncovalent means of immobilizing both antigens and antibodies. Because of the low affinity of SA for polystyrene, it must be: (a) covalently bound to the surface (40), (b) immobilized by first adsorbing an irrelevant, biotinylated carrier (41), or (c) immobilized by biotin which has been covalently attached to functionalized polystyrene (42). Each of these methods permits the immobilization of antigens and antibodies which (a) bind poorly to plastic or NC, and (b) are denatured beyond use by adsorption.

Lectins and the Ig-binding proteins of bacteria, which are readily adsorbed on plastic or other hydrophobic surfaces, can also be utilized as a bridge between the solid phase and the reactant of interest. Prerequisite is that the adsorption process does not destroy or alter their specificity. Concanavalin A adsorbed to microtiter wells is able to immobilize gp120 of HIV which displays better activity than adsorbed gp120 (43). Both Protein A of *Staphylococcus aureus* and Protein G of *Streptococcus* sp. are capable of stably capturing various IgGs after their adsorption. Background problems connected with the use of Ig-binding proteins in ELISAs are not unexpected, especially in SpAbI in which the Ig binding protein can also bind the specific antibodies that the assay is designed to measure. Assay "short-circuitry" can be a major problem in all immunoassays which involve multiple components such as in ELISA (12).

3.7. Cells, Bacteria, and Viruses as Solid-Phase Reactants

Virus particles can be adsorbed directly on polystyrene in the manner of proteins (see 29). Our experiences reveal two potential problems with this approach. First, the virus must be purified free of tissue culture proteins which can competitively inhibit virus adsorption. Second, virus preparations bound on the solid phase must be free of any antigens (normally of media origin) that may have been present in the vaccine preparation, since the sera of immunized animals or vaccinated humans may also contain antibodies to these proteins. This problem has been overcome by using an adsorbed, virus-specific capture antibody to immobilize the virus (29, 39). Although predictably less virus can be immobilized by this method than by adsorption (39), exposure of internal epitopes due to adsorption-induced denaturation is reduced. Adsorbed CAbs have also been used to detect the presence of virus. NSB is an additional concern with some viruses, e.g., Herpes sp, that express Ig-binding proteins.

Intact cells and bacteria have also been used as solid-phase ELISA antigens. Their heavily glycosylated membranes usually make their stable adsorption difficult, so that simultaneous adsorption and cross-linking to surfaces coated with poly-L-lysine (44), glutaraldehyde (C. Severson and G. A. Bishop, personal communication, 1985, 1990), or the polyaldehyde methyl glyoxal (44) have been used. More serious than in the case of virus, many bacteria have Ig-binding proteins that may increase NSB, thus all but obscuring antibody detection.

3.8. Immobilization Protocols

The considerable diversity of solid phases and the many types of molecules that one may wish to immobilize means that students and scientists should (a) consult the original references cited and (b) empirically optimize their own procedure, i.e., "Vertrauen ist gut aber Kontroll ist besser." However, there are a few general guidelines for adsorption on polystyrene which can provide a starting point for immobilization using this method:

(i) Single-use adsorption solutions used at 5 μg/ml are adequate for most proteins which avidly adsorb to polystyrene and form a monolayer after 4 hr at 37°C or overnight at room temperature (see Fig. 9.4). Some investigators have been known to reuse the same coating solution. When this is done, higher initial concentrations are required.

(ii) There is as yet no proven advantage to adsorbing proteins at a concentration beyond the linear binding region. Higher concentrations encourage desorption and waste reagents. Using less than monolayer-forming concentrations may increase NSB.

(iii) Buffer pH of adsorption can influence adsorption depending on the p*I* of the protein and the nature of the polystyrene used.

4. SPI IN THE FUTURE

4.1. Integrity of the Immobilized Reactant

Table 9.2 summarizes some of the studies that provide evidence that the immobilization of proteins by passive adsorption results in protein alteration. Two observations are particularly noteworthy. First, there was evidence for such alteration nearly 40 years ago (26), and second, the majority of the molecules are affected (14; Fig. 9.6). This historical perspective suggests that the cliché "first time shame on you, second time shame on me" fits well to the field of solid-phase immunoassay. The goal of diagnostic immunoassay development is the construction of systems to accurately measure antibodies or antigens which display the same molecular integrity *in vitro* as they display *in vivo*. If we alter these molecules or block their relevant epitopes or binding site (if antibodies) during the immobilization process, then we are not achieving our objective. Therefore, future designers of SPI will be asked to develop systems which address this issue more carefully than it has casually been addressed in the past.

4.2. Solid-Phase Immunoassays and Molecular Biology

The opportunities afforded by the rapid technical developments in molecular biology and genetics now permit scientific and diagnostic issues to be easily addressed; a decade ago, this seemed technically impossible, or, if possible, could only

TABLE 9.2   Adsorption-Induced Conformational Change

Protein	Phenomenon
Albumin	Conformational change after adsorption on glass
IgG	Concentration-dependent allosteric conformers after adsorption on polystyrene
IgG	Molecule unfolding and changes in antigenicity when adsorbed on polystyrene
IgG	Thermodynamic evidence for conformational change
Monoclonal Ab	Altered specificity after adsorption
Tryptophan synthase	Altered enzymatic and antigenic activity after adsorption
Lactic	Conformational alteration after dehydrogenase adsorption on polystyrene
Monoclonal Ab	Loss of activity after adsorption on polystyrene
IgG, IgA	Loss of antigenicity after adsorption to polystyrene
Ferritin	Cluster formation on silica wafers

Note. The above list is not exhaustive and has been reviewed previously (29, 12).

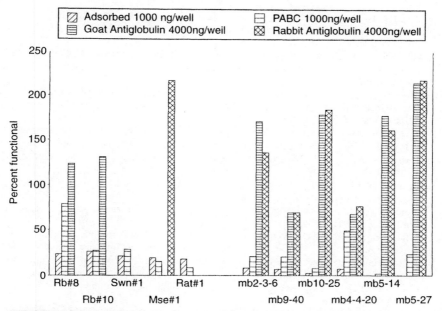

FIGURE 9.6 The proportion of functional capture antibody equivalent (CAbeqv) after immobilization of capture antibodies (CAbs) specific for fluorescein, by different methods. The five CAbs on the left are polyclonals; Rb #8, rabbit 8; Rb #10, rabbit 10; Swn #1, swine 1; Mse #1, mouse 1; Rat #1, rat 1. The six CAbs on the left side are only monoclonal (mb), each with a different number code. CAbeqv is the equivalent of an antibody with two functional sites. Because the standard for this assay was an adsorbed CAb with only one functional site, a value of "200 percent functional" means that 100% of the antibodies are functional with two binding sites. PABC, Protein Avidin Biotin Capture System (41).

provide superficial answers. For example, we can now readily screen patients for defective genes well before the pathological disorder resulting from the defective gene presents itself. Stated otherwise, germline differences can now be detected without waiting for transcription and translation to occur. However, regardless of whether the product of interest is a protein (classically detected by immunoassay) or a gene, most of the ubiquitous technical methods for measuring them involve solid-phase immobilization. For example: (a) hybridizing DNA is detected using a support of nitrocellulose or nylon, (b) phage clones expressing gene products of interest are detected on nitrocellulose plaque lifts using antibodies and ELISA-based technology, and (c) quantitative PCR can be conducted in microtiter wells with one primer immobilized to the solid phase and the amount of product amplified measured by ELISA in a colorimetric plate reader. Hence, the field of immunodiagnostics as we now know it is rapidly changing, and students aspiring to a career in this area will be required to be as much a molecular biologist as a clinical chemist.

References

1. Franz B, Stegemann M. The kinetics of solid-phase microtiter immunoassays. In: Butler JE, Ed. Immunochemistry of Solid-Phase Immunoassay. Boca Raton, FL: CRC Press, 1991:277–84.
2. Park H. A new plastic receptacle for solid-phase immunoassay. J Immunol Methods 1978; 20:349–55.

3. Joshi KS, Hoffmann LG, Butler JE. The immunochemistry of sandwich ELISAs. V. The capture antibody performance of polyclonal antibody-enriched fractions prepared by various methods. Mol Immunol 1992; 29:971–81.

4. Azimzadeh A, van Regenmortel MHV. Antibody affinity measurements. J Mol Recog 1990; 3:108–16.

5. Metzger H. Transmembrane signaling. The Joy of Aggregation. Presidential Address, J Immunol 1992; 1477–87.

6. Butler JE, Ni L, Nessler R, Joshi KS, Suter M, Rosenberg B, Chang J, Brown WR, Cantarero LA. The physical and functional behavior of capture antibodies adsorbed on polystyrene. J Immunol Methods 1992; 150:77–90.

7. Davies J, Dawkes AC, Haymes AG, Roberts CJ, Sunderland RF, Wilkins MJ, Davies MC, Tendler SJB, Jackson DE, Edwards JC. A scanning tunnelling microscopy comparison of passive antibody adsorption and biotinylated linkage to streptavidin on microtiter wells. J Immunol Methods 1994; 167:263–9.

8. Ehrlich PH, Moyle WR, Moustafa ZA. Further characterization of cooperative interactions of monoclonal antibodies. J Immunol Methods 1983; 131:1906.

9. Lehtonen OP. Immunoreactivity of solid phase hapten binding plasmacytoma protein (ABPC 24). Mol Immunol 1981; 18:323–9.

10. Butler JE, Feldbush TL, McGivern PL, Stewart N. The enzyme-linked immunosorbent assay (ELISA): A measurement of antibody concentration or affinity? Immunochemistry 1978; 15:131–6.

11. Dierks S, Butler JE, Richerson HB. Altered recognition of surface-adsorbed compared to antigen bound antibodies in the ELISA. Mol Immunol 1986; 23:403–11.

12. Butler JE. ELISA. In: van Regenmortel MHV, van Oss CJ, Eds. Immunochemistry, Chap. 29. New York: Marcel Dekker, 1994:759–803.

13. Cantarero LA, Butler JE, Osborne JW. The binding characteristics of various proteins to polystyrene and their significance for solid-phase immunoassays. Anal Biochem 1980; 105:375–83.

14. Butler JE, Ni L, Brown WR, Joshi KS, Chang J, Rosenberg B, Voss EW Jr. The immunochemistry of sandwich ELISAs. VI. Greater than 90% of monoclonal and 75% of polyclonal anti-fluorescyl capture antibodies (Cabs) are denatured by passive adsorption. Mol Immunol 1993; 30:1165–75.

15. Koertge TE, Butler JE. The relationship between the binding of primary antibody to solid-phase antigen in microtiter plates and its detection by the ELISA. J Immunol Methods 1985; 83:283–99.

16. Qualtiere LF, Anderson AC, Meyer P. Effects of ionic and non-ionic detergents on antigen-antibody reactions. J Immunol 1977; 119:1645–51.

17. Avrameas S, Terynich T. The natural autoantibody system: between hypotheses and facts. Mol Immunol 1993; 30:1133–42.

18. Nygren H, Werthen M, Czerkinsky C, Stenberg M. Dissociation of antibodies bound to surface-immobilized antigen. J Immunol Methods 1985; 85:87–95.

19. Mason DW, Williams AF. The kinetics of antibody binding to membrane antigens in solution and at the cell surface. Biochem J 1980; 187:1–20.

20. Stenberg M, Nygren H. A receptor ligand reaction studied by a novel analytical tool - the isoscope ellipsometer. Anal Biochem 1982; 127:183–92.

21. Crothers DM, Metzger H. The influence of polyvalency on the binding properties of antibodies. Immunochemistry 1972; 9:341–57.

22. Azimzadeh A, Regenmortel MHV. Measurement of affinity of viral monoclonal antibodies by ELISA titration of free antibody in equilibrium mixtures. J Immunol Methods 1991; 141:199–208.

23. Michaeli I, Absolom DR, van Oss CJ. Diffusion of adsorbed protein within the plane of adsorption. J Colloid Interface Sci 1980; 77:586–7.

24. Berson SA, Yalow RS. Quantitative aspects of the reaction between insulin and insulin binding antibody. J Clin Invest 1959; 38:1996–2016.

25. Catt K, Tregear GW. Solid-phase radioimmunoassay in antibody-coated tubes. Science 1967; 158:1570–2.

26. Bull HB. Adsorption of bovine serum albumin on glass. Biochem Biophys Acta 1956; 19:464–71.

27. Sorensen K, Brodbeck U. Assessment of coating-efficiency in ELISA plates by direct protein determination. J Immunol Methods 1986; 95:291–3.

28. Engvall E, Perlmann P. Enzyme-linked immunosorbent assay (ELISA): quantitative assay of immunoglobulin G. Immunochemistry 1971; 8:871–4.

29. Butler JE. The behavior of antigens and antibodies immobilized on a solid-phase. In: Van Regenmortel MMV, Ed. Structure of Antigens. Boca Raton, FL: CRC Press, 1991:208–58.

30. Shirahama H, Suzawa T. Adsorption of bovine serum albumin onto styrene/acrylic acid copolymer latex. Colloid Polymer Sci 1985; 263:141–6.

31. Lauritzen E, Masson M, Rubin I, Holm A. Dot immunobinding and immunoblotting of picogram and nanogram quantities of small peptides on activated nitrocellulose. J Immunol Methods 1990; 131:257–67.

32. Søndergard-Andersen J, Lauritzen E, Lind K, Holm A. Covalently linked peptides for enzyme-linked immunosorbent assay. J Immunol Methods 1990; 131:99–104.

33. Grantstrom M, Wretlind B, Markman B, Cryz S. Enzyme-linked immunosorbent assay to evaluate the immunogenicity of a polyvalent *Klebsiella* capsular polysaccharide vaccine in humans. J Clin Microbiol 1988; 26:2257–61.

34. Geysen HM, Meloen RH, Barteling SJ. Use of peptide synthesis to probe viral antigens for epitopes to a resolution of a single amino acid. Proc Natl Acad Sci USA 1984; 81:3998–4002.

35. LaCroix M, Dionne G, Zrein M, Dwyer RJ, Chalifour RJ. The use of synthetic peptides as solid-phase antigens. In: Butler JE, Ed. Immunochemistry of Solid-Phase Immunoassay. Boca Raton, FL: CRC Press, 1991:261–8.

36. Palfree RG, Elliott BE. An enzyme linked immunosorbent assay (ELISA) for detergent solubilized Ia glycoproteins using nitrocellulose membrane discs. J Immunol Methods 1982; 52:395–408.

37. Drexler G, Eichinger A, Wolf C, Sieghart W. A rapid and simple method for efficient coating of microtiter plates using low amounts of antigen in the presence of detergent. J Immunol Methods 1986; 95:117–22.

38. Zeiss CR, Pruzansky JJ, Patterson R, Roberts M. A solid phase radioimmunoassay for the quantitation of human reagenic antibody against ragweed antigen. J Immunol 1973; 110:414–21.

39. Herrmann JE, Hendry RM, Collins MF. Factors involved in enzyme-linked immunoassay for viruses and evaluation of the method for identification of enteroviruses. J Clin Microbiol 1979; 10:210–7.

40. Peterman JH, Tarcha PJ, Chu VP, Butler JE. The immunochemistry of sandwich ELISAs. IV. The antigen capture capacity of antibody covalently attached to bromoacetyl polystyrene. J Immunol Methods 1988; 111:271–5.

41. Suter M, Butler JE. The imunochemistry of sandwich ELISAs. II. A novel system prevents denaturation of capture antibodies. Immunol Lett 1986; 13:313–7.

42. Bugari G, Poiesi G, Beretta A, Ghielmi A, Albertini A. Quantitative immunoenzymatic assay of human lutropin, with use of a bi-specific monoclonal antibody. Clin Chem 1990; 36:47–52.

43. Robinson JE, Holton O, Liu J, McMurdo H, Murciano A, Gohd R. A novel enzyme-linked immunosorbent assay (ELISA) for the detection of antibodies to HIV-1 envelope glycoproteins based on immobilization of viral glycoproteins in microtiter wells coated with concanavalin A. J Immunol Methods 1990; 132:63–71.

44. Czerkinsky C, Rees AS, Burgmeier LA, Challacombe SJ. The detection and specificity of class specific antibodies to whole bacterial cells using a solid phase radioimmunoassay. Clin Exp Immunol 1983; 53:192–200.

10 | IMMUNOASSAY CONFIGURATIONS

THEODORE K. CHRISTOPOULOS
Department of Chemistry and Biochemistry
University of Windsor
Windsor, Ontario, Canada N9B 3P4

ELEFTHERIOS P. DIAMANDIS
Department of Pathology
and Laboratory Medicine
Mount Sinai Hospital
Toronto, Ontario, Canada M5G 1X5

1. INTRODUCTION

Most immunoassay configurations can be divided into two large groups, i.e., the "limited reagent" methods (competitive immunoassays) and the "reagent excess" methods (noncompetitive immunoassays). In competitive immunoassays the analyte and the labeled analyte (tracer) are mixed with a limited amount of anti-analyte antibody. After incubation for a certain period, the bound or the free fraction of the tracer is measured and related to the concentration of the analyte in the sample. In noncompetitive immunoassays, an excess of immunoreactant (antibody or antigen) is added, so that all the analyte is practically in the form of an immunocomplex. Then, the immunocomplex is quantified and related to the analyte concentration in the sample.

Noncompetitive assays offer higher sensitivity than competitive ones (1). The ultimate detectability of competitive immunoassays is limited by the affinity constant of the antibody used. In contrast, the ultimate sensitivity of the noncompetitive assays is determined from the nonspecific binding of the labeled immunoreactants. Noncompetitive assays have potential for single molecule detection, by using tracers with extremely high detectability and at the same time a low nonspecific binding (1).

Both competitive and noncompetitive immunoassays require the measurement of immunocomplexes in the presence of free antibodies and/or antigens. In "heterogeneous" immunoassays (competitive or noncompetitive) this is accomplished by first separating the immunocomplex from the free immunoreactants. In "homogeneous" immunoassays, a modulation of the signal occurs as a result of the immunoreaction. Therefore the immunocomplex formation can be monitored directly without prior separation of the bound and free tracer.

Only heterogeneous immunoassays are described in this chapter. Homogeneous assays employ the same general configurations. Detailed description of homogeneous immunoassays is given in the chapters dealing with the various detection systems as applied to immunoassays.

2. COMPETITIVE IMMUNOASSAYS

2.1. Immobilized Antibody Approach

In this type of immunoassays (Figs. 10.1A and 10.1B), an anti-analyte antibody is immobilized on the solid phase (polystyrene microtitration wells, beads, tubes, etc.) either by physical adsorption or covalently. The excess binding sites on the solid phase are then blocked with a protein (e.g., albumin) solution. Analyte, labeled with a radioisotope, an enzyme, or a fluorescent or chemiluminescent label, is used as a tracer. The sample is pipetted onto the solid phase along with the tracer. The analyte competes with the tracer for a limited number of antibody binding sites. After a certain incubation period, the unbound reagents are removed by washing

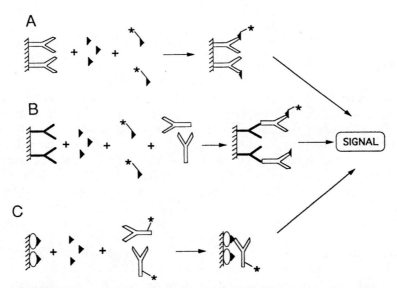

FIGURE 10.1   Configurations for competitive immunoassays. (A) The immobilized antibody approach. Analyte from the sample competes with labeled analyte for a limited number of antibody binding sites. (B) The use of an anti-immunoglobulin-coated solid phase to capture the anti-analyte antibody. (C) The immobilized antigen approach. Here, the analyte from the sample competes with immobilized analyte for binding to labeled antibody molecules. In all cases the signal is inversely related to the analyte concentration.

the solid phase, and the signal from the bound tracer is measured. The signal is inversely related to the analyte concentration.

The anti-analyte antibody used for coating should be affinity purified; otherwise, nonspecific immunoglobulins or other proteins compete for coating. If the antibody can be labeled with biotin or a hapten (e.g., with nitrophenyl groups) without a significant reduction of its binding affinity, then a solid phase coated with (strept)avidin or anti-hapten antibody may be employed. The advantage of this configuration is that a universal solid phase can be used for different assays.

Alternatively, the solid phase can be coated with an affinity-purified antibody which binds to the Fc region of the anti-analyte antibody (see Fig. 10.1B). For instance, a goat anti-rabbit antibody (Fc specific) can be used for coating if the anti-analyte antibody has been raised in a rabbit. This configuration ensures that the anti-analyte antibody is immobilized to the solid phase through its Fc region and therefore has the appropriate orientation to bind analyte more efficiently. As a consequence, significantly less analyte-specific antibody is required for each assay, compared to the direct coating methods.

Delayed addition of the tracer enhances the sensitivity of these assays. In this case, the analyte is first incubated with an antibody-coated solid phase until equilibrium is reached. Then the tracer is added and the immunoreaction is terminated before a new equilibrium is established. The theoretical basis of the increased sensitivity observed is discussed in Chapter 3.

2.2. Immobilization of the Antigen

Protein antigens can be immobilized directly on polystyrene solid phases, by physical adsorption, provided that they are purified. Haptens are first attached to a protein carrier and then incubated with the solid phase. After blocking, the sample and the labeled antibody are added. The analyte from the sample competes with the immobilized analyte for a limited number of antibody binding sites (Fig. 10.1C). The reaction is terminated by washing the solid phase. As the analyte concentration in the sample increases, the concentration of the solid-phase-bound labeled antibody decreases.

If the direct labeling of the anti-analyte antibodies is not feasible, then a crude unlabeled antiserum can be used instead. After the immunoreaction is completed, detection of the solid phase-bound antibody is accomplished by using a labeled anti-immunoglobulin antibody.

3. NONCOMPETITIVE IMMUNOASSAYS

3.1. Two-Site (Sandwich Type) Immunoassays

These assays are applied to the determination of macromolecular antigens, where simultaneous binding of two antibodies to the antigen is allowed without steric hindrance. The sample is pipetted onto a solid phase, which is coated with an excess of affinity-purified anti-analyte antibody (capture antibody) and blocked (Fig. 10.2A). During the subsequent incubation, the capture antibody binds the analyte specifically (immunoextraction). All other sample constituents are washed out and the bound analyte is then quantitated in a second step (two-step assays)

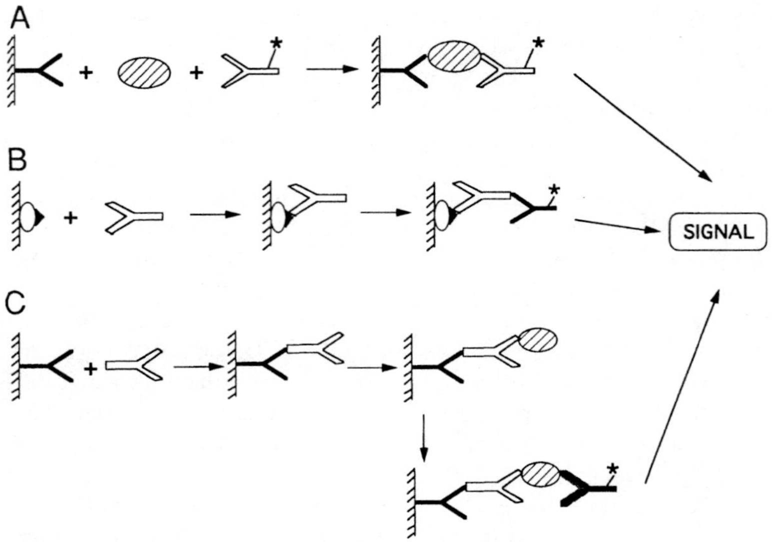

FIGURE 10.2   (A) A two-site (sandwich) immunoassay. The analyte is captured by the immobilized antibody and then is detected by using a labeled antibody. (B) Noncompetitive immunoassay for quantification of antibodies. The sample is incubated with an antigen-coated solid phase. The antibodies bound are then quantified by using a labeled anti-immunoglobulin. (C) An immunoglobulin class capture assay. All the immunoglobulins of the class of interest are first captured on a solid phase which is coated with anti-class antibodies. Then the antigen is added and binds only to specific antibodies of the class. The bound antigen is quantified by using a labeled antibody.

by adding an excess of labeled anti-analyte antibody (detection antibody). After incubation the unbound antibody is washed out and the signal from the solid-phase-bound detection antibody is directly related to the analyte concentration in the sample. Alternatively, the sample is added simultaneously with the detection antibody on the solid phase (one-step assays). Again, after incubation and washing, the signal from the bound detection antibody is measured. This latter method is faster, but problems may arise when the analyte concentration exceeds the binding capacity of the capture and detection antibodies. In this case, the solid-phase antibody becomes saturated and a significant fraction of the analyte remains in solution. The detection antibody is distributed between the two analyte fractions. Immunocomplexes formed in solution are washed away in the next step. As the analyte concentration becomes higher, a smaller fraction of the detection antibody binds to the solid-phase-captured analyte and the signal decreases (high-dose hook effect).

A consequence of the high-dose hook effect is that a sample with very high analyte concentration could give a low signal, thus leading to an erroneous result. This may happen, for example, when measuring tumor markers for monitoring cancer patients. High levels of a tumor marker in the sample may result in a low signal when measured by a one-step noncompetitive immunoassay.

The high-dose hook effect can be detected by repeating the analysis with a diluted sample. The diluted sample gives a higher signal if hook effect is present. Alternatively, the sample is analyzed after the addition of a concentrated standard solution of the analyte. When hook effect is present, the spiked sample gives a lower signal. The hook effect can be eliminated by increasing the concentration of the detection antibody to the point that there is always an excess with respect to the analyte. However, decreased sensitivity may be observed due to the elevated nonspecific binding associated with high detection antibody concentrations. Alternatively, all samples can be diluted several times prior to the assay, if the sensitivity allows for a dilution step.

Two-site noncompetitive immunoassays usually employ two monoclonal antibodies directed against different epitopes of the analyte. Nevertheless, a combination of monoclonal and polyclonal antibodies may be used. Sometimes the same polyclonal antibody serves as the capture and detection antibody.

Because the two-site immunoassays involve two antibodies, they offer better specificity than the competitive assays. Indeed, crossreacting substances that interfere with the competitive assays give no signal in sandwich assays, because usually they do not bind to both the capture and the detection antibodies.

3.2. Immunoassays for Specific Antibodies and Immunoglobulin Class Capture Assays

Noncompetitive immunoassays used in the determination of specific antibodies are included in this group (Figs. 10.2B and 10.2C). The solid phase is coated with the antigen. Protein antigens can be used directly for coating, whereas haptens are first conjugated to protein carriers. The diluted sample is incubated with the solid phase. The antibody bound to the solid phase is then quantified by using a labeled anti-immunoglobulin (Fig. 10.2B). This assay format is particularly useful in screening hybridomas for monoclonal antibody production.

In the immunoglobulin class capture assays (Fig. 10.2C) the solid phase is coated with anti-class antibodies which bind all the antibodies of the same class from the sample. Antibodies of other classes are washed out. Then, the antigen of interest is added and is captured by the specific antibodies on the solid phase. The bound antigen is finally determined by using a labeled antibody against the antigen. Examples of these assays include the determination of IgM in the diagnosis of an acute infection and the determination of IgE against specific allergens.

The immunoglobulin class capture assays are more specific compared to those employing the immobilized antigen approach , especially for antibodies of the minor immunoglobulin classes, since all other antibodies are removed prior to the addition of the antigen.

3.3. Epitope Mapping

In cases where several monoclonal antibodies are available for a single antigen, it may be necessary to determine if they bind to different or overlapping epitopes. A solid phase coated with purified antigen is incubated with a labeled monoclonal antibody in the presence of various concentrations of another unlabeled monoclonal antibody. If the two antibodies bind to identical or overlapping epitopes then, because of competition, the signal will decrease as the concentration of the unlabeled antibody increases. The signal will remain unchanged if the two antibodies bind to two different epitopes.

A slightly modified configuration may be used if a purified antigen preparation is not available for coating. The solid phase is first coated with a monoclonal antibody against the antigen. Then the unpurified antigen solution is added. After incubation and washing out the irrelevant proteins, the solid phase is incubated with two monoclonal antibodies, one labeled and one unlabeled, and the assay is completed as described above.

3.4. Immunoassays of Antigens Immobilized on a Solid Phase

This group involves detection of protein antigens on Western blots (2). Proteins are first separated by polyacrylamide gel electrophoresis and transferred, by electroelution, to a nitrocellulose membrane. The membrane is then incubated with a protein solution (e.g., albumin or nonfat dry milk) to block the remaining binding sites. An antibody specific for the protein of interest is added, and after incubation for a certain period and washing the excess antibody, the immunocomplex formed is detected by using a labeled anti-immunoglobulin directed against the first antibody. This approach offers higher sensitivity than using a directly labeled first antibody. Other strategies employed for detection of the immunocomplexes are described later in this chapter (Section 4).

Monoclonal or polyclonal detection antibodies can be used in immunoblotting. Monoclonal antibodies are more specific but they may fail to recognize epitopes which have been denatured during electrophoresis. On the other hand, a polyclonal antiserum will contain antibodies that will interact with epitopes which remained intact after electrophoresis and transfer. Furthermore, more than one antibody may bind to the same antigen molecule. Thus, polyclonal antibodies give higher sensitivity and are preferred for immunoblotting.

The most widely used labels are enzymes (alkaline phosphatase and horseradish peroxidase). The enzymes convert a soluble substrate to a color or fluorescent precipitate or to a chemiluminescent product. For example, diaminobenzidine is a commonly used hydrogen donor for peroxidase (it yields a brown precipitate) and the mixture of bromochloroindolyl phosphate with nitro blue tetrazolium (which gives a purple precipitate) may be used as substrate for alkaline phosphatase.

3.5. Noncompetitive Immunoassays for Small Molecules

3.5.1. Two-Site Immunoassays for Haptens with Amino Groups

In this configuration (3), all the amino group-containing substances in the sample are first biotinylated by using excess of the N-hydroxysuccinimide ester of biotin. Afterward, the sample is incubated with an anti-hapten antibody-coated solid phase. In this step, the biotinylated hapten is captured from the solid phase, whereas the free biotin along with irrelevant biotinylated molecules are washed away. Subsequently the immunocomplexes are dissociated at pH 1.0 and the solution is reacted with enzyme-labeled anti-hapten antibodies and captured to a streptavidin-coated solid phase. The activity of the enzyme bound to the solid phase is directly related to the concentration of the hapten in the sample.

This configuration is successful only if the biotinylation site is far enough from the epitopic site to allow the simultaneous binding of streptavidin and anti-hapten antibody. Oligopeptides consisting of nine amino acids were determined by this method down to 50 amol. Smaller haptens (such as thyroxin) can be determined by this method only if a spacer is introduced between biotinylation and epitopic sites. These assays are, reportedly, at least 50 times more sensitive than the competitive assays using the same labeled antibodies.

3.5.2. Idiometric Assay

The principle of these assays is as follows (4). The sample is pipetted onto a solid phase which is coated with an anti-hapten antibody (primary antibody). After the immunoreaction is completed, a β-type anti-idiotype antibody is added, which binds to all unoccupied primary antibody binding sites. After washing, a labeled α-type anti-idiotype antibody is added which binds to the hapten/primary antibody complexes. This antibody will not bind to the primary antibody if the β-type is already bound to it. The signal measured is proportional to the hapten concentration in the sample.

3.5.3. Solid-Phase Immobilized Epitope Immunoassay (SPIE-IA)

This is a recently proposed immunoassay configuration (5) for small haptens containing a free amino group which is not a part of the epitope structure. The hapten is first captured on a solid phase coated with an anti-hapten antibody. Then the hapten is covalently linked to the proteins of the solid phase, that is, to the antibody and to blocking proteins as well. This is accomplished by using a homobifunctional crosslinking reagent reactive to primary amino groups, e.g., glutaraldehyde or disuccinimidyl suberate. The reaction is performed under mild conditions which do not disrupt the hapten–antibody complex. A denaturation step follows (addition of methanol or HCl) which serves to dissociate the immunocomplex and expose the immobilized hapten to the detection antibody. The same monoclonal antibody, labeled with acetylcholinesterase, is used as in the detection antibody. Assays of this type are reported to be 70–200 times more sensitive than conventional competitive immunoassays employing the same antibody-coated solid phase and an acetylcholinesterase–hapten conjugate as tracer.

3.5.4. Liquid-Phase Binding Assays (LBA)

The principle of this configuration is as follows (6). The immunoreaction takes place in solution. The analyte reacts with an excess of peroxidase-labeled antibody. After the immunoreaction is completed, the bound and free forms of the antibody are separated by cation-exchange high-performance liquid chromatography. A postcolumn enzyme reaction system is used, where the substrate is mixed with the column effluent in a postcolumn flowthrough coil, followed by fluorometric detection.

In the case of macromolecular antigens (7), the separation of the immunocomplex from the free labeled antibody can be accomplished by gel-filtration high-performance liquid chromatography, since the molecular mass of the immunocomplex is much higher than that of the free labeled antibody.

4. INDIRECT DETECTION OF THE IMMUNOCOMPLEXES

This section describes systems where the signal-carrying or signal-generating molecule(s) (reporter molecule, e.g., radioisotope, enzyme, fluorescent or chemiluminescent label) is not attached directly to one of the immunoreactants but is linked noncovalently and specifically to the immunocomplex after the immunoreaction is completed.

The major advantage of the systems employing indirect detection is that the same reporter molecule-carrying reagent may be used in a variety of immunoassays. Furthermore, the use of indirect detection systems often leads to assays with higher sensitivity, since more reporter molecules are finally bound to the immunocomplex than in assays where the detection antibody is directly conjugated to the reporter molecule.

4.1. Detection of the Immunocomplex with a Labeled Immunoglobulin

In this configuration, the detection antibody is not labeled. After the immunocomplex is formed, a labeled anti-immunoglobulin antibody is added which binds to the constant and variable regions of the detection antibody. This technique is particularly useful when direct labeling of the detection antibody is difficult and results in a significant loss of immunoreactivity. Antibodies against immunoglobulins from various species, labeled with fluorescent or enzyme molecules, are commercially available at a relatively low cost. Moreover this configuration introduces amplification since more than one molecule of labeled anti-immunoglobulin may bind to each detection antibody molecule. In addition, a single labeled anti-immunoglobulin may be used for various detection antibodies from the same species.

A prerequisite for the above configuration is that the capture and detection antibodies should be from different species so that the labeled anti-immunoglobulin does not react with the immobilized capture antibody. Alternatively, Fab or F(ab)$_2$ fragments are employed as capture antibodies along with a labeled anti-immunoglobulin directed against the Fc region of the detection antibody.

4.2. Protein A

Protein A is a 42-kDa protein found in the cell wall of *Staphylococcus aureus*. It binds with high affinity the Fc region of immunoglobulins from various species (8). There are four binding sites for antibodies but only two of them can be used simultaneously. Labeled protein A is useful in the indirect detection of antigens immobilized on a solid support (e.g., microtitration plate or in Western blot). In these assays, an unlabeled detection antibody is added to the solid phase and then the immunocomplex formed is quantified with labeled protein A.

Also, protein A may be used for the indirect detection of imunocomplexes in sandwich type immunoassays, provided that Fab fragments are used instead of whole antibody molecules for coating the solid phase. Alternatively, unlabeled protein A may be used to bridge two antibody molecules, that is, the detection antibody from the immunocomplex and a labeled antibody.

The affinity of protein A for immunoglobulins depends on the immunoglobulin class and the species (8). For example, the affinity is low for mouse IgG$_1$ monoclonal antibodies and high for human and rabbit polyclonal antibodies.

4.3. The Biotin–Streptavidin System (9)

Conjugates of (strept)avidin with enzymes (e.g., alkaline phosphatase, peroxidase) or fluorescent molecules are commercially available. Antibodies can be labeled with several biotins without a significant loss of their affinity to the antigen. As a consequence, more than one molecule of labeled (strept)avidin can bind to each antibody. Therefore, an amplification is introduced which results in enhanced sensitivity. Because streptavidin has four binding sites for biotin, it can act as a bridge between two biotinylated molecules. Biotinylated immunoreactants and labeled (strept)avidin are stable for long periods of time. The biotin–(strept)avidin system can be used in the detection of immunocomplexes as follows (Fig. 10.3):

(a) The detection antibodies or antigens are labeled with biotin. After the immunoreaction is completed and the excess of reagents is washed out, the immunocomplex can be quantified by adding labeled strept(avidin) (Fig. 10.3A). (b) Again, the detection antibodies or antigens are labeled with biotin. After the immunoreaction is completed, the immunocomplex is allowed to react with an excess of unlabeled streptavidin. The unbound streptavidin is washed out and then a biotinylated reporter molecule is added, e.g., biotinylated alkaline phosphatase or peroxidase. Here, streptavidin is used as a bridge between a biotinylated detection antibody and a biotinylated reporter molecule (Fig. 10.3B). (c) (Strept)avidin is first reacted with a biotinylated enzyme and forms macromolecular complexes which involve several enzyme molecules bridged by (strept)avidin (10). The streptavidin to biotinylated enzyme molar ratio can be optimized so that (strept)avidin is not saturated but has at least one site available for binding to biotinylated immunoreactants (Fig. 10.3C).

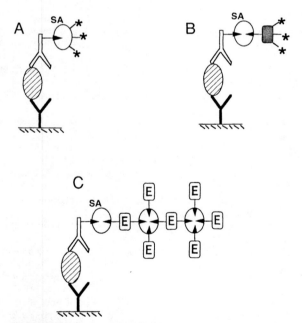

FIGURE 10.3 Indirect detection with the biotin–(strept)avidin system. Biotin is represented by the black arrows. E, enzyme. In all cases the detection antibodies are biotinylated. (A) (Strept)avidin is multiply labeled with a reporter molecule such as an enzyme or a fluorescent or a chemiluminescent molecule. (B) (Strept)avidin is used as a bridge between the biotinylated detection antibody and a biotinylated enzyme. (C) A preformed complex which consists of (strept)avidin and biotinylated enzyme is allowed to react with the detection antibody.

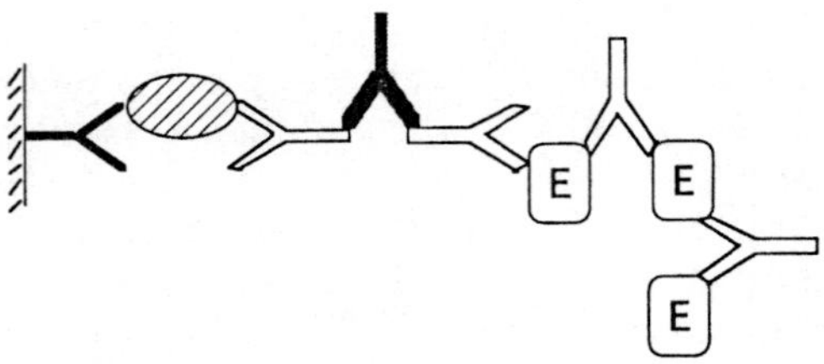

FIGURE 10.4   Indirect detection with enzyme–anti-enzyme complexes. Enzyme–anti-enzyme complexes are first formed by mixing, at the appropriate molar ratio, the enzyme with its specific antibodies. Then, the preformed complexes are linked to the detection antibody by using an anti-immunoglobulin.

4.4. Assays Using Enzyme–Anti-enzyme Complexes (11)

In these assays (Fig. 10.4), the signal-generating molecules are preformed soluble complexes of an enzyme with anti-enzyme antibodies (polyclonal or monoclonal). The anti-enzyme antibodies are from the same species as the detection antibody used in the immunoassay. After the immunoreaction is completed the enzyme–anti-enzyme complexes are bridged to the detection antibody by using an anti-immunoglobulin antibody. Peroxidase anti-peroxidase (PAP) and alkaline phosphatase/antibody complexes are widely used in immunohistochemistry.

References

1. Jackson TM, Ekins RP. Theoretical limitations on immunoassay sensitivity. Current practice and potential advantages of fluorescent Eu^{3+} chelates as non-radioisotopic tracers. J Immunol Methods 1986; 87:13–20.
2. Sambrook J, Fritsch EF, Maniatis T. Molecular Cloning. A Laboratory Manual, 2nd ed. Cold Spring Harbor, NY: Cold Spring Harbor Laboratory Press, 1989.
3. Ishikawa E, Hashida S, Takeyuki K, Hirota K. Ultrasensitive enzyme immunoassay. Clin Chim Acta 1990; 194:51–72.
4. Barnard G, Kohen F. Idiometric assay: A noncompetitive immunoassay for small molecules typified by the measurement of estradiol in serum. Clin Chem 1990; 36:1945–50.
5. Pradelles P, Grassi J, Creminon C, Boutten B, Mamas S. Immunometric assay of low molecular weight haptens containing primary amino groups. Anal Chem 1994; 66:16–22.
6. Taizo H, Nakamura K, Satomura S, Matsuura S. Noncompetitive immunoassay of thyroxine using a liquid-phase binding assay. Anal Chem 1994; 66:351–354.
7. Nakamura K, Satomura S, Matsuura S. Liquid-phase binding assay of human chorionic gonadotropin using high-performance liquid chromatography. Anal Chem 1993; 65:613–6.
8. Harlow E, Lane D. Antibodies. A laboratory manual. Cold Spring Harbor Laboratory Press, Cold Spring Harbor, 1988.
9. Diamandis EP, Christopoulos TK. The biotin-(strept)avidin system: Principles and applications in biotechnology. Clin Chem 1991; 37:625–36.
10. Hsu SM, Raine L, Fanger H. Use of avidin-biotin peroxidase complex (ABC) in immunoperoxidase techniques. J Histochem Cytochem 1981; 29:577–80.
11. Tijsen P. Practice and theory of enzyme immunoassays. In: Burdon RH, Knippenberg PH, Eds. Laboratory Techniques in Biochemistry and Molecular Biology. Amsterdam/New York: Elsevier, 1985.

11 | THE AVIDIN–BIOTIN SYSTEM

EDWARD A. BAYER
MEIR WILCHEK
Department of Biophysics
The Weizmann Institute of Science
Rehovot 76100 Israel

1. INTRODUCTION

The application of the avidin–biotin system in immunoassays does not confer a measure of specificity to the immunoassay system (1, 2). Instead, it serves only to mediate between one of the members of the primary recognition system (namely, the antibody or the antigen) and another component of the immunoassay system (i.e., the solid support or the reporter group). However, in doing so, mediation by the avidin–biotin system frequently improves greatly the performance of the immunoassay system (3). Such improvement is usually manifested either by a substantial amplification of the signal and consequent sensitivity of the assay or simply by convenience. Once a standard immunoassay system has been set up, the primary constituents can easily be substituted by other antibodies or antigens, leading to a versatile and universally applicable immunoassay system for a given laboratory (4).

The use of the avidin–biotin system in immunoassay can be divided into two main categories (2, 5). On the one hand, avidin may be inserted in the immunoassay protocol to mediate between the reporter group or probe and the primary antibody or antigen (see Section 3). On the other, it may be immobilized onto the solid phase in order to improve the characteristics of the capture system (see Section 4).

The nature of the capture system, detection system, or end-point used is really irrelevant. The avidin–biotin system can thus be used in just about any of the immunoassay systems described in the other chapters in this book. In fact, many of the chapters (e.g., see Chapters 10, 14, 19, and 24) include discussion of its use for the particular immunoassay system described. In this chapter, we will thus confine ourselves to a general discussion as to the applicability of the avidin–biotin system in immunoassays and will concentrate on its special properties or consequences of its use. For more details, the reader is referred to Refs. (2, 6, 7).

The use of the avidin–biotin system is a consequence of the exceptionally high affinity constant ($K_a \sim 10^{15}\,M^{-1}$) and specificity shown by the egg-white glycoprotein avidin for the vitamin biotin (1, 4). In addition, avidin occurs in solution mainly as a tetramer, and thus has four biotin-binding sites per molecule. This is particularly useful for immunoassay systems, since the tetrameric structure is one of the major reasons for the observed amplification of the signal. The other reason is the capacity to covalently attach many copies of the biotin moiety to virtually any protein molecule. Multiple copies of biotin on an antibody or protein can then interact noncovalently, but very strongly, with the four binding sites of avidin. This strong noncovalent crosslinking among the components results in an enhancement of the primary interaction.

A very similar biotin-binding protein is also produced by various species of the bacterial genus *Streptomyces,* and "streptavidin" has also been applied very successfully as a substitute for the egg-white glycoprotein in many immunoassay systems. Moreover, other biotin-binding proteins are available; indeed, polyclonal, monoclonal, and single-chain antibodies are currently being used in avidin–biotin-like assay systems. The properties of the various types of avidin-like proteins will be discussed in Section 2.2.

For the purposes of this chaper, and for the avidin–biotin system in general, the rationale in the use of all of the biotin-binding proteins for applicative purposes is essentially the same—i.e., to mediate between an immunochemical component (for immunoassay) and a given probe, reporter group, or solid matrix. This is particularly true for avidin and streptavidin, which exhibit a truly remarkable resemblance in their biotin-binding sites and tetrameric structures. In principle, they are interchangeable. In practice, however, there may be good reasons to employ one or another species of biotin-binding protein for a particular experimental system (as will be discussed later in this chapter). Nevertheless, unless specifically stated otherwise, further reference to any of the biotin-binding proteins—egg-white avidin, bacterial streptavidin, etc.—should be viewed collectively in the broader sense.

There are also many possible permutations of the simple use of avidin and biotin in a given immunoassay system (4). Thus, biotinylated forms of either protein A or secondary antibody can be used either as a universal capture system or detection system (Section 5). In addition, other probes or subsequent treatments can be used to further amplify a signal. Finally, other types of affinity systems (e.g., hapten–antihapten) have become useful replacements or accessories for avidin–biotin mediation (8).

We will end this chapter with some simple protocols which should be instructive for students and researchers in establishing avidin–biotin-based immunoassay systems.

2. COMPONENTS OF THE SYSTEM

2.1. Biotinylation of Immunoassay Components

The first step in the use of the avidin–biotin system is to incorporate the biotin moiety into the experimental system (9). This is usually accomplished by "biotinylating" one of the components of the system, and in the case of immunoassay, this usually means an antibody or an antigen. The biotinylated antibody or antigen is then introduced into the system for interaction with the avidin-containing component.

Biotinylation is a chemical modification which results in a covalent attachment of the biotin moiety to a molecule or to another material (e.g., solid surface). There are many ways to biotinylate a molecule, and today many different chemically reactive, biotin-containing reagents are available commercially for this purpose (10). The procedures for biotinylation are usually very easy, and this is one of the reasons that the use of the avidin–biotin system has become so popular (2, 7, 11, 12).

In the following section, we describe many of the procedures and reagents used for biotinylating a molecule through one of its functional groups. It is desirable that these be located at a distance from the site(s) of biological activity of the molecule (see Section 2.1.3). The molecule can be an antibody, a probe, an antigen, including proteins, glycoconjugates, and even small biologically active molecules such as steroid hormones, haptens, etc. (2, 4).

We begin our descriptions with three very different ways which are particularly suitable for biotinylating an antibody. After this, we present several additional approaches, provisionally for labeling antigens and probes with biotin. However, it should be borne in mind that these procedures are mutually inclusive, and any of the biotinylating approaches described here can be used for antibodies, antigens, and probes. The important criterion for using a given approach is whether the appropriate functional group(s) is available on the target molecule for its effective biotinylation. Equally important is the stipulation that the resultant biotinylated product is biologically active and that its physical properties have been only nominally affected.

2.1.1. Biotinylation of Antibodies

Being a glycoprotein, an antibody can be modified in numerous ways (see overall scheme in Fig. 11.1). Nevertheless, antibodies are usually biotinylated through the resident amino groups (i.e., the lysines and the primary amino group of the N-terminal amino acid). More recently, it has also become popular to biotinylate them through their oligosaccharide moieties. A third method involves the reduction of the disulfide bonds (the cystines) which crosslink the immunoglobulin chains; the sulfhydryls (the cysteines) formed are then biotinylated using a reagent of appropriate specificity.

These three reactions are particularly suitable for the biotinylation of antibodies. In some cases, however, biotinylation using other strategies may be preferred, as detailed in the sections which follow for antigens. Unfortunately, there are no firm guidelines to predetermine a priori the best approach to use. For a given antibody, in particular, and for all proteins, in general, the most suitable method is, ultimately, determined empirically. In most cases (for antibodies, antigens and other probes), biotinylation via lysines is the logical and easiest place to start. If this proves inadequate, then other protocols can be considered.

2.1.1.1. Biotinylation via Lysines   Nearly two decades have elapsed since antibodies were first biotinylated (13). The most popular method of covalently attaching biotin to antibodies is still the original method, which involves interaction of a protein with an N-hydroxysuccinimide ester which contains the biotin moiety. The original biotin derivative used was biotinyl N-hydroxysuccinimide ester (abbreviated BNHS).

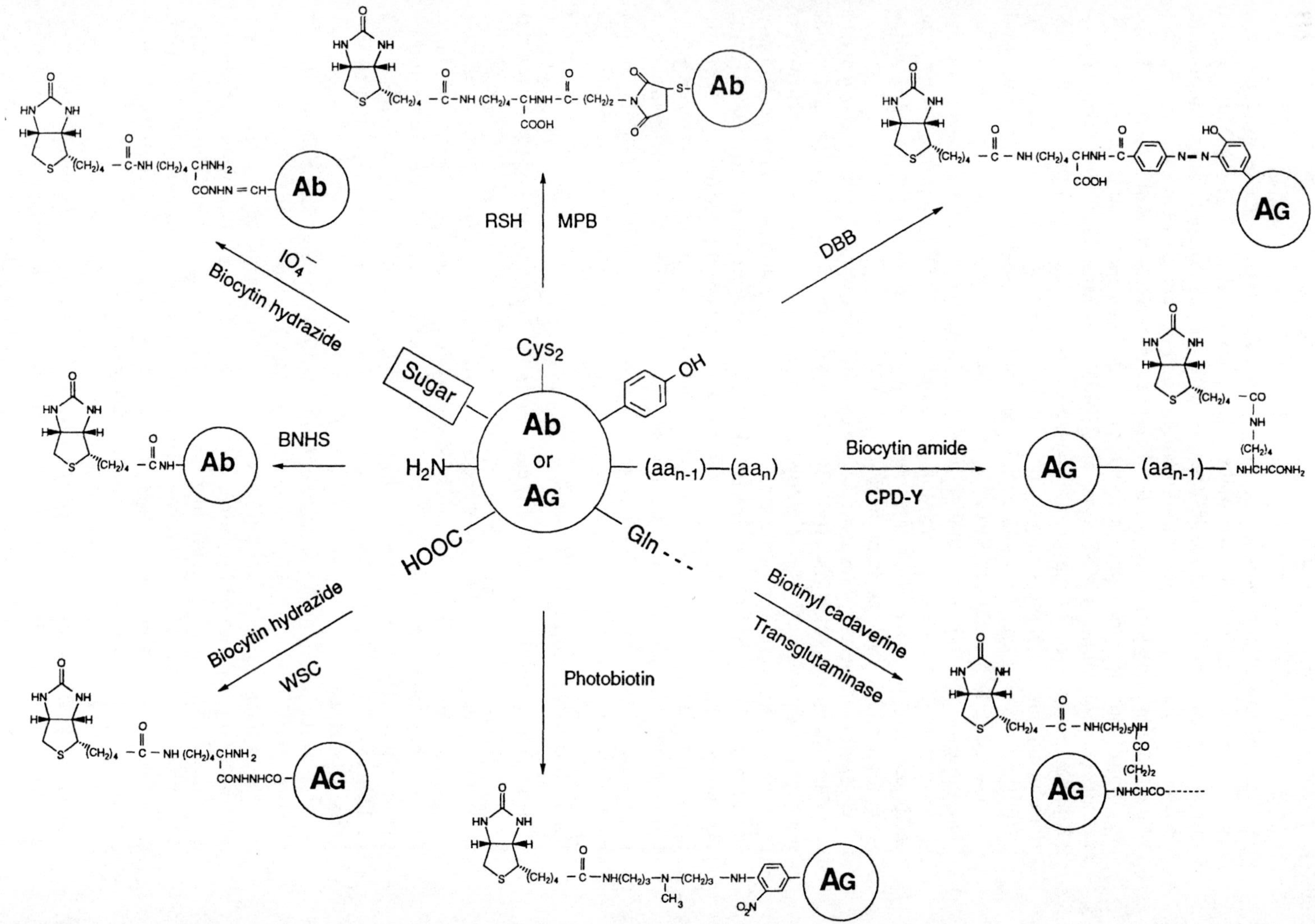

FIGURE 11.1 Biotinylation via various functional groups of antibodies (Ab) or antigens (Ag) using different biotinylating reagents (see text for details).

Students who partake in their first biotinylation reaction using BNHS are invariably astonished at how easy it is to biotinylate a protein. Essentially, one simply weighs a small portion of BNHS, dissolves it in solution, and mixes it with the desired protein solution. After an hour or so, the reaction mixture is dialyzed and ready for use.

More recently, longer-chained derivatives (containing a spacer group which separates and extends the length between the biotin moiety and the chemically reactive group) have been used instead of BNHS. The extra length of the derivative sometimes (but not always) facilitates the interaction of the biotin moiety with the deep biotin-binding pocket of avidin, thus facilitating the overall assay. Otherwise, the chemistry of the reaction and its conditions are identical to those employed for the generic reagent.

The above-described NHS reagents are all fairly insoluble in aqueous solutions. They must therefore be solubilized initially in a water-miscible sovent, usually dimethylformamide or dimethylsulfoxide. Alternatively, water-soluble analogs (the sulfo-NHS derivatives) of BNHS and its relatives are also available. However, they are usually much less efficient than the corresponding NHS analog, since they rapidly undergo autohydrolysis upon contact with water. In any case, the secret in maintaining the efficiency of the NHS derivatives is in their storage. They should not be allowed to become moist. If stored desiccated in the cold, they will retain their full biotinylating capacity indefinitely. On the other hand, if stored on the shelf at room temperature in the absence of desiccant, they hydrolyze rapidly and, after a short time, are no longer reliable.

Since lysines are usually commonly exposed in most proteins and often not directly involved in binding, the BNHS-type reaction has become the predominant starting point when a new antigen is to be biotinylated. Nevertheless, care should be taken not to over-biotinylate a protein using this method (despite the widespread use of very high reagent-to-antibody ratios as reported in many publications). In this context, biotinylation of lysines neutralizes the charge and the antibody molecule thus becomes more acidic and hydrophobic (due to the biotin moieties). Such changes in the physical character of the antibody molecule can have its consequences, vis-à-vis antibody specificity and nonspecific side reactions (see Section 2.1.3). Moreover, some antibody molecules may indeed bear lysine residues which are critical to their combining activity; this is especially crucial if the antibody preparation is monoclonal. It is thus recommended to determine the optimal ratio of reagent to antibody molecule. In our experience, when initially establishing a new biotinylating protocol, a molar ratio of about 20 molecules of reagent to antibody is advised; this value can then be refined empirically, after examining the properties of the biotinylated product.

Another convenience is that biotinylation using BNHS can often be performed successfully on crude antibody preparations—even whole antiserum can be biotinylated. Although all of the proteins in the preparation (mainly albumin) would be biotinylated to varying degrees, it would be expected that during the immunoassay procedure the biotinylated antibody would react with the antigen selectively, and the other unreactive species of biotinylated proteins would be removed during the washings (11).

Finally, antibodies biotinylated using BNHS and related reagents are usually very stable and can be stored for many years in aliquots at −20°C. In some cases, biotinylated antibodies can be maintained indefinitely with no observed alteration in their properties or performance.

2.1.1.2. Biotinylation via Saccharide Residues

Since antibodies are glycoproteins, and the oligosaccharide moieties are not critical to their function, the sugar residues can be biotinylated by a two-step procedure which initially includes mild oxidization with periodate; the aldehydes formed are then available for selective chemical reaction with an appropriate hydrazido derivative of biotin. Originally, biotin hydrazide was used for this type of reaction. Subsequently, longer-chained reagents, such as the aminocaproyl derivative or biocytin hydrazide (ε-biotinyl lysine hydrazide), were substituted for the same reasons that longer-chained NHS derivatives have been used (10).

This reaction has the advantage that the oligosaccharides are in an exposed position at a distance from the antigen-combining site, and the consequences of chemical or steric alterations on the recognition event would be minimized (see Section 2.1.3). In addition, all antibodies are glycoproteins (with the exception of recombinant bacterial preparations), and the geometry of biotinylation would be similar in any native antibody molecule of the same class. On the other hand, the efficiency of the reaction and capacity to incorporate biotin moieties into the antibody molecule are both less than those achieved by NHS-mediated biotinylation.

2.1.1.3. Biotinylation via Cysteines

The four immunoglobulin chains are bound together covalently by disulfide bonds. Their number and relative location in the chains are class specific, but in general, they are positioned in the hinge regions, at a safe distance from the antigen-combining site. They may be converted to cysteines by thiols without disabling the binding capacity of the antibody, and the sulfhydryl groups formed can be biotinylated selectively using an appropriate derivative.

Of the many reagents available for modifying sulfhydryl groups, the maleimides are the most effective. The interaction of maleimido derivatives of biotin is very selective for SH groups, and the covalent bond formed is irreversible. Moreover, unlike the biotinylation of lysines, the reaction does not affect the isoelectric point (pI) of the antibody molecule.

The first reagent described for biotinylation of sulfhydryls was maleimidopropionyl biocytin, or MPB (14). This and other similar analogs are available commercially. Unlike BNHS, MPB is soluble and quite stable in aqueous solutions.

2.1.2. Biotinylation of Antigens and Probes

Proteinaceous antigens, or any other molecule (e.g., hapten) which bears a relevant functional group, are subject to the same procedures for biotinylation as are antibodies. Thus, BNHS-type reagents (Section 2.1.1.1) and maleimido derivatives (Section 2.1.1.3) can be used to biotinylate antigens via amino or sulfhydryl groups, respectively. In many of the cases tested, antigenic activity is maintained even after heavy biotinylation, particularly if the antibody used for its recognition is polyclonal. If, however, a monoclonal antibody is used, it is important to examine whether the biotinylation of the antigen proceeds through a residue which compromises the structure of the given epitope.

For biotinylation of haptens or other small molecules (15), it is frequently recommended to include a long spacer between the biologically active portion of the molecule and the site of the functional group which undergoes biotinylation. This facilitates subsequent interaction with the biotin-binding pocket of avidin.

For biotinylation of the various probes, the character of the probe dictates the strategy to be used. In some cases, the probe is quite rigid and stable, and can be biotinylated profusely. In others, e.g., for certain enzymes, the activity is delicate and even mild biotinylation may be totally destructive to its action. In some enzymes, even if the biotinylation step succeeds and the product is totally active, the enzyme may be completely inactivated upon interaction with avidin.

For antigens or probes which contain oligo- or polysaccharides (with vicinal hydroxyl groups), the procedure described in Section 2.1.1.2 can be used.

In the following sections, we present biotinylation reactions which usually (but not always) involve other types of reagents. The reader is reminded that there are numerous biotin-containing reagents and biotinylation procedures; the descriptions herein serve only as an overview of what is currently available. Some of these approaches have been discussed only sparingly in the literature. Each has its own special properties which may prove ideal for the biotinylation of a given molecule. The last three examples are relatively new approaches for biotinylation which may develop into procedures of choice for many applications.

2.1.2.1. Biotinylation via Tyrosines and Histidines

Diazo derivatives of biotin, e.g., diazobenzoyl biocytin (DBB), selectively modify both tyrosines and histidines in proteins (16). Unfortunately, the diazo group is unstable during storage, but may be activated from its aminobenzoyl precursor upon treatment with $NaNO_2$ and acid. The active reagent must be used immediately. Tyrosines and histidines are not usually abundant in proteins and are generally buried rather than exposed. Moreover, in many proteins, both residues may have important biological or structural contributions. Thus, the extent of biotinylation and its consequences are extremely variable and depend upon the status of these two amino acid residues. Nevertheless, we have found that for certain uses and in certain cases, this approach may indeed be preferred over others.

2.1.2.2. Biotinylation via Carboxyl Groups

Carboxyl groups of proteins (glutamic and aspartic acids and the C-terminus) can be biotinylated using a biotin-containing reagent which bears a terminal amino group (11). The reaction is performed using biocytin hydrazide (the same reagent used to label sugar residues, but a different reaction chemistry). Another type of reagent which is appropriate for this reaction is biotinyl cadaverine (biotin derivatized with a common diamine), also used in Section 2.1.2.5.

The protein is treated with a water-soluble carbodiimide [e.g., 1-ethyl-3-(3-dimethyl aminopropyl) carbodiimide] in the presence of a great excess of the biotin reagent. The carbodiimide reacts temporarily with the carboxyl group, but is displaced by the biotin-containing reagent. One potential problem with this approach is that the biotinylation eliminates the charge of the carboxyl group, and the p*I* of the protein is thereby increased. This problem is thus similar to that of BNHS-type reagents in that the p*I* is altered, but in the opposite direction.

2.1.2.3. Biotinylation Using Photobiotin In some cases, a given antigen or other molecule may be uncommonly resistant to standard biotinylation protocols. This may result from an unusual lack or concealment of functional groups (e.g., $-NH_2$, $-SH$) which are normally available for biotinylation.

In such cases, or in cases where the selective biotinylation of material is not required, photobiotin may be used (17). Upon ultraviolet irradiation, the aromatic azide of photobiotin is activated and the nitrene intermediates formed react in a highly nonspecific manner. Photobiotin can thus be used to biotinylate almost any type of biologically active or inactive organic material. It has particularly been used extensively to label nucleic acids, although it is applicable to proteins, oligosaccharides, and lipids as well.

On the other hand, there are some disadvantages in its use. One intrinsic disadvantage, of course, is that specificity and control over the biotinylation reaction are compromised. Also, the yields obtained are much lower than those observed for most of the other procedures, mainly due to the short half-life of the nitrene intermediates. In addition, exposure to ultraviolet light may have deleterious effects on certain amino acids of some proteins, thereby affecting their structure or activity. Photoactivation can be performed in the high-energy visible range to circumvent this particular problem.

2.1.2.4. Biotinylation via the Carboxy Terminus A fairly recent development in biotinylation protocols is the possibility of attaching a single biotin moiety per polypeptide chain (18). This can be accomplished enzymatically using carboxypeptidase Y and a good biotin-containing nucleophile, such as biocytinamide. The reaction proceeds via transpeptidation of the C-terminal amino acid which is replaced by the biotin reagent. The C-terminus is not usually essential or involved in the biological activity of a protein. Moreover, it is often in an exposed position, and the biotin moiety is thus readily available for interaction with avidin.

The reaction, however, does not usually proceed to completion; yields of about 70% are commonly achieved. Thus, the underivatized protein should be separated from the biotinylated product. Another limitation is that proteins with C-terminal proline residues are not susceptible to the enzymatic modification by carboxypeptidase Y.

2.1.2.5. Biotinylation via Glutamine Residues Another more recent enzymatic method for biotinylation of proteins also involves an acyl transfer reaction—in this case, the incorporation of a primary amino derivative of biotin into glutamine residues of proteins (19). Thus, transglutaminases will replace the amide of an exposed glutamine residue with biotinyl cadaverine, forming a stable covalent bond. The general applicability of this interaction has not been rigorously examined.

2.1.2.6. Biotinylation by Recombinant Gene Technology In nature, the enzyme biotin holoenzyme synthetase functions by covalently attaching a biotin moiety to one of the subunits of the "biotin-requiring" enzymes, i.e., carboxylases, decarboxylases, and transcarboxylases. This natural system can also be used to biotinylate a protein, a process which would be particularly applicable in recombinant host systems. In this context, a 75-residue portion of this subunit has been recognized as the natural subunit for the synthetase (20).

By using peptide libraries, it has been possible to improve the natural substrate and to define a 13-residue substrate (21), which can now be added by recombinant techniques to the N- or C-terminus of either a cloned antigen or a single-chain bacterial monoclonal antibody. In this manner, it should be possible to exploit the natural cellular apparatus to covalently incorporate single biotin moieties in one of the components of an immunoassay during its expression by a host cell system. The recombinant protein would have the biotin moiety bound naturally to the 13-residue extension at one of its termini, which would very likely be spatially displaced from the combining site of an antibody or from important epitopes of an antigen. Short spacers could also be inserted, in order to further separate the biotinylation site from the rest of the molecule.

2.1.3. The Consequences of Biotinylation

In the early days of avidin–biotin technology, when the approach was new and the understanding of its principles and purpose seemingly formidable, we made the initial claim that biotinylation of proteins had only a nominal effect on the target protein (11). When compared to the norm at the time, i.e., the use of protein–protein conjugates prepared by bifunctional crosslinking reagents such as glutaraldehyde, this claim was not unreasonable. In this respect, the consequences of conjugating an enzyme to an antibody were quite dramatic, usually resulting in oligomerization and other severe alterations of the physical and chemical state of both antibody and antigen. The production of functional (both immunochemically and enzymatically) conjugates, amenable to storage and use as shelf reagents, was, and still is, a true art form. Thus, the problems initially encountered upon biotinylation of both antibodies and other proteins were considered by us to be "nominal."

Indeed, when faced with presenting a new "universally applicable" procedure to the scientific community (which was the case two decades ago), to immediately delve into the fine points of its possible shortcomings would have been self-defeating. Today, however, when the virtues of the avidin–biotin system are common knowledge, it would be ludicrous to continue to claim that biotinylation generally has little effect on the biological, chemical, or physical properties of the molecule of interest—for it often does. In fact, in some cases the biological activity of the biotinylated molecule is totally eradicated. In others, the alterations to the chemical or physical properties are so rampant, and the extent of nonspecific (or, more accurately, unwanted) interactions are so prevalent, that the biotinylated molecule (albeit active) is useless.

For the discriminating student of science, when using a given biotinylating reagent or procedure, it is judicious to know *what* and *why* problems might occur, in order to design strategies on *how* to avoid them. The discussion which follows is an introduction to the consequences of biotinylation.

To illustrate the various possibilities (Fig. 11.2), we have drawn an antibody in its interaction with an antigen as a model system for explanatory purposes. Of course, the same principles apply to the biotinylation of antigens, enzymes, other probes, and other biologically active molecules in general. Keep in mind that antibodies constitute a special class of proteins and each type of biologically active molecule may have its own specific set of properties. This should be borne in mind when designing a biotinylation strategy or interpreting its consequences.

The normal, unhindered, immunochemical interaction between an antibody and an antigen is shown schematically at the top of Fig. 11.2. When biotinylating an

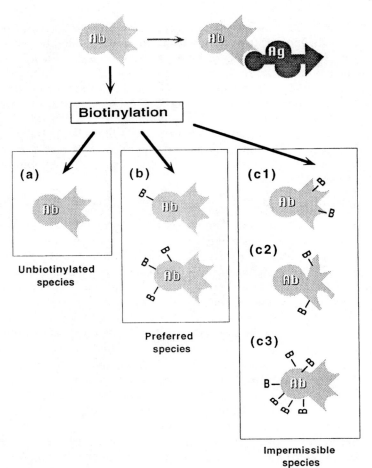

FIGURE 11.2 The consequences of biotinylation. As an example, the biotinylation of an antibody is demonstrated. The normal interaction between an antibody (Ab) and an antigen (Ag) is schematically illustrated at the top of the figure. Biotinylation by one of the procedures described in the text may result in a variety of different types of biotinylated species of antibody, where B—is the biotin moiety. First, as shown in (a), a given percentage of molecules may not have undergone biotinylation at all, due, perhaps, to suboptimal amounts of reagent. In (b), the biotinylation reaction has produced preferred species, in which the biotin residues are both at a distance from the antigen combining site (and hence do not interfere with the primary immunochemical interaction) and in an exposed position (amenable to subsequent interaction with avidin). The species in (c) are all "undesirables." In (c1), the biotin moieties block the combining site, thereby preventing its subsequent interaction with antibody. Likewise, the biotinylation in (c2) has deformed the combining site, which inhibits its interaction or causes spurious interactions with irrelevant components of the system. In (c3), the antibody molecule has been overbiotinylated. The normal physicochemical characteristics of the molecule have been significantly altered, such that it interacts ambiguously with unwanted components of either the experimental system or the immunoassay system.

antibody, it would be desirable to produce a single biotinylated species, in which the biotinylated residue is at a distance from the combining site and in an exposed position favorable for interaction with avidin. Unfortunately, the biotinylation of an antibody usually results in a mixture of different molecular species, both biotinyl-ated and unbiotinylated, as shown at the bottom of the figure.

2.1.3.1. Unbiotinylated Species

The unbiotinylated molecule, shown in Fig. 11.2a, poses a true problem to subsequent steps in the immunoassay. Being underi-vatized, its interaction with the antigen is usually superior to that of the biotinylated species, which often shows some reduction or alteration in affinity or specificity. This is particularly a problem when the biotinylated molecule is part of the detection component of the immunoassay. The unbiotinylated antibody molecule thus success-fully competes with the biotinylated forms in the primary interaction with the antigen. In consequence, they can seriously affect the efficiency of the immunoassay by diminishing both the amplitude of the signal and the overall sensitivity of the assay. The presence of unbiotinylated molecules in the preparation is less of a problem if the molecule is part of the capture system, since they would simply not bind to the avidin in the solid phase and would thus be washed out of the system.

Another similar type of species (not shown in the figure) is a biotinylated antibody molecule in which the biotin moieties are buried or blocked and unavailable for interaction with avidin. Hence, a better definition of this type of species would be molecules which fail to interact with avidin.

2.1.3.2. Preferred Species

As mentioned above, we would like the biotinyla-tion reaction to produce a high proportion of biotinylated species, in which the presence of the biotinylated moiety does not interfere with the antigen–antibody interaction and is positioned favorably for subsequent binding to avidin. Such preferred species are shown schematically in Fig. 11.2b, where the biotin moiety or moieties are all attached to the antibody in a situation isolated from the antigen combining site.

There are two major ways of designing a biotinylation reaction to achieve high ratios of such preferred species. One way is to use a procedure in which the functional group(s) of an antibody is (are) known to be in a desirable position on the molecule. Such is the case for the oligosaccharide moiety and perhaps the disulfide bridges, both of which may be selectively biotinylated (Sections 2.1.1.2 and 2.1.1.3, respec-tively). Another way to impove one's chances of achieving a high proportion of preferred species is to use an indiscriminant biotinylation reagent (e.g., BNHS) to modify an antibody in which the combinding site has been protected. This can be accomplished by immobilizing an antibody on an antigen-containing immunoaffinity column and performing the biotinylation reaction *in situ* on the column. The biotinyl-ated product can be washed (with buffer) to remove excess reagent and subsequently released from the column (e.g., using acidic conditions).

2.1.3.3. Impermissible Species

Impermissible species are also shown sche-matically in Fig. 11.2. In the structure designated c1, residues in or near the combin-ing site have been biotinylated. The covalently attached biotin moiety interferes either sterically or chemically with the immunochemical activity. A second type of species (c2) is one in which the biotinylation has occurred at a site on the antigen molecule which is distant from the combining site per se, but which may be critical to its structure; the covalent attachment of biotin to such residues may cause a deformation of the site. In both cases, the species may simply be inactive but does not necessarily cause nonspecific interactions or interfere with the interaction of other biotinylated species with the antibody. Nevertheless, alteration of the combining site may also affect its specificity and the modified antibody may now recognize extraneous molecules in the experimental system. Another type of impermissible species (not shown in the figure, but which can be grouped with Type c2) is a biotinylated antibody which is active in the free state, but is inhibited or inactivated (or released from its binding with the antigen) upon interaction with avidin.

Another class of impermissible species which may have an adverse effect on the specificity of the immunoassay is shown as Type c3 in Fig. 11.2. In this case, extensive biotinylation of a given type of residue may alter the physicochemical characteristics of the antibody molecule, which may cause nonspecific interactions with other components of the immunoassay system. For example, if lysines or carboxylic acid groups are extensively modified, the pI of the antibody would be significantly altered. Even if the combining site is still active, the dominant interaction of the antibody species may be electrostatic in character. Excessive biotinylation also increases the hydrophobicity of the antibody. In any event, rather than interacting primarily with the antigen, such species may bind nonspecifically to components of the detection or capture system or may even interact directly with the blocking agents or with the solid support. High levels of background would result.

When interpreting the final performance of an avidin–biotin-mediated immunoassay system, it is therefore important to keep in mind the possible consequences that the biotinylation of the given component (antibody, antigen, or probe) may have had on the overall system.

2.2. Avidin and Its Relatives

Initially, the development of the avidin–biotin system was based on the hen egg-white glycoprotein called avidin. Later, other biotin-binding proteins, notably streptavidin, were frequently substituted for the egg-white protein. The purpose of this section is to discuss the characteristics of the different types of avidin which are available today, and to mention some of the possible future developments which may lead to newer and better forms of avidin, streptavidin, or other types of biotin-binding protein.

As mentioned earlier, despite their differences, the character of the interaction of the different types of avidin with biotin is essentially the same, as is the rationale for their use. The original system was worked out with egg-white avidin, and its subsequent substitution by other biotin-binding proteins (e.g., bacterial streptavidin or antibiotin antibodies) simply served to improve the original application (for example, through a lowering of nonspecific binding interactions). By itself, the use of other types of biotin-binding proteins provided no new contribution to the original notion. We therefore consider the term avidin to represent a concept which includes all types of biotin-binding protein, and not necessarily the egg-white protein alone.

Despite the very high affinity constant of egg-white avidin (it is even higher than that of streptavidin, although at such high values, an order of magnitude or two is not particularly significant), it has two intrinsic failings on the molecular level which often restrict its application in many systems. In this context, avidin is a positively charged glycoprotein, and its high pI and presence of oligosaccharide may cause side reactions which lead to high background levels. For this reason, streptavidin has found favor as a replacement for egg-white avidin.

Streptavidin is a neutrally charged unglycosylated bacterial protein. The lack of oligosaccharide and relatively low p*I* has clearly resulted in a better performance in many (but certainly not all) immunoassay systems, thus contributing to its popular usage, despite its high cost, relative to egg-white avidin.

In any case, proteins are complicated molecules which display a multiplicity of attitudes, and one never knows what to expect from a seemingly naive and inert macromolecular component of a system. It should thus not be too surprising that an ambiguous, seemingly nonspecific, biotin-independent interaction of streptavidin was discovered. The source of the interaction turned out to be the inherent presence of an Arg–Tyr–Asp sequence in streptavidin (22). This sequence is similar in structure to the "cell surface recognition motif" (Arg–Gly–Asp) contained in the sequence of various adhesion molecules, such as fibronectin, vitronectin, and fibrinogen. On this basis, streptavidin reacts strongly with the integrins and other related cell surface receptors, and its use should be avoided when assaying cell-derived material.

The problems encountered with streptavidin have aroused a renewed interest in alternatives which include modified versions of both egg-white avidin and the bacterial protein (22). Even in its first use as an immunoassay component, the necessity to reduce the charge on avidin was recognized (3). The native protein has thus been formylated, acetylated, and succinylated in order to reduce its charge. It should be kept in mind that modification of avidin, through the amino groups of lysine, with various reporter groups (e.g., radioactive, fluorescent, chemiluminescent, and chromophoric derivatives) also reduces the charge on the molecule. In fact, this can certainly be an advantage in using avidin over streptavidin, since (due to the additional lysine residues per molecule) higher levels of the desired reporter group can be incorporated into the protein, which leads to higher levels of signal and, consequently, higher levels of sensitivity in the immunoassay system.

Another type of group-specific modification which lowers the overall charge of avidin is via arginine residues. Two different derivatives of this type are commercially available: ExtrAvidin from Sigma Chemical Co. (St. Louis, MO) and NeutraLite Avidin from Belovo Chemicals (Bastogne, Belgium). The latter is also available from a number of other suppliers. In the case of arginine-modified avidins, the lysine groups are still available for subsequent conjugation, i.e., to proteins and other probes.

Regarding the oligosaccharide component of avidin, a procedure to enzymatically deglycosylate the protein has recently been developed (23). This procedure involves a naturally occurring bacterial strain which assimilates the oligosaccharide moiety of avidin, but generally disregards the protein core. This process has been adopted to produce NeutraLite Avidin which is both a deglycosylated and a neutrally charged derivative of the native egg-white protein.

Despite such advances in the alteration of avidin by protein chemical techniques, in the not too distant future we will see a new trend in avidin–biotin technology. In this context, both avidin and streptavidin have now been cloned and expressed (24, 25). It is only a matter of time before a multitude of mutagenized versions of both proteins will become available. These may include neutrally charged (and of course nonglycosylated) versions of avidin, streptavidins which lack the cell-binding motif, and variants of both proteins which are altered in their binding-site residues. The latter alterations may be used to modulate the interaction of avidin or streptavidin with biotin or to augment their binding to another target molecule. In any case, the production of recombinant avidins and streptavidins is currently being considered by many research laboratories both in academia and in industry.

In addition to avidin and streptavidin, other biotin-binding proteins may be appropriate for immunoassay systems. Polyclonal antibiotin antibodies, for example, have been around for nearly 20 years. Monoclonal antibodies of high titre are also available; at least in one case, a monoclonal antibody has been cloned (26) and is currently being expressed as a single-chained polypeptide. In our hands, use of the monoclonal antibiotin antibody results in a superior immunoassay system, when compared with systems which employ either avidin or streptavidin.

Finally, there is a variety of other biotin-binding proteins of relatively high affinity which constitute an untapped resource regarding their potential use in avidin–biotin technology (2). These include the high-affinity biotin-binding protein in egg yolk, biotin receptors from various cells, and the enzymes biotinidase and biotin holocar- boxylase synthetase.

2.3. Avidin Conjugates

The second step in the use of the avidin–biotin system is to prepare an appropriate avidin-containing probe (9). Today, a wide spectrum of different avidin–probe conjugates can be obtained from a variety of companies. These products have usually been analyzed for their designated application, and methods for their long- term storage have been designed for minimal loss of activity (of both components). It is thus recommended that the novice experimentalist purchases the reagents or kits required for setting up a new assay system. On the other hand, one of the major disadvantages of using commercially available reagents and kits is the negative effect it has on one's pocketbook. To synthesize one's own in-house set of biotin- and avidin-containing reagents, when done correctly, is a genuine form of saving your resources.

The same conjugation chemistries used for antibodies, antigens, enzymes, and other probes (see Chapter 8) are applicable to the modification of avidin (or streptav- idin or their relatives) and the production of avidin-containing conjugates. In fact, since both avidin and streptavidin are very stable proteins, their conjugation or derivatization is usually much less detrimental to their activity than that of antibodies or antigens. This, once again, has been a characteristic advantage in using the avidin–biotin system—i.e., the primary components of the system can be used in a more native form, whereas the more damaging chemical modifications can be applied to avidin, which is much less sensitive to such treatments. Representative procedures for producing various avidin derivatives and conjugates can be found in Refs. (2, 7, 9).

Radioactive derivatives of both avidin and streptavidin can easily be prepared. However, since avidin has only one tyrosine residue which is critical to its biotin- binding activity, the chloramine T iodination protocol should not be used with this protein. Instead, the Bolton–Hunter reagent can be used to prepare a highly iodinated derivative of avidin via its amino groups. Similar reagents can be used to tritiate avidin or to incorporate a ^{14}C or ^{3}H label. In contrast to avidin, streptavidin has six tyrosines (only one of which is necessary for biotin binding), and the chlora- mine T procedure has been successfully applied for obtaining highly iodinated prepa- rations.

Fluorescent and chemiluminescent derivatives of avidin are relatively easy to prepare. Since avidin has many lysines, its derivatization often leads to the production of a probe for fluorescent or chemiluminescent immunoassays that is superior to the corresponding streptavidin-based probe. As mentioned in the last section, such derivatizations of avidin also rectify its electrostatic nature, thus circumventing one of the innate problems with this protein. When NeutraLite avidin is derivatized, the product also lacks the oligosaccharide residue, and, to date, is the choice reagent for such purposes.

Many methods are available for conjugation of two protein species. Any method which has been used for conjugating two other proteins together (e.g., an antibody to an enzyme) would also be appropriate for conjugating avidin to another protein. Thus, avidin can be combined with another protein (for example, an enzyme) by the action of homo- or hetero-bifunctional reagents (such as glutaraldehyde, dimethyl adipimidate, or a succinimidyl maleimide derivative) to produce the respective avidin-conjugated enzyme.

Another possibility for preparing avidin-containing conjugates would be to attach extraneous reacting groups to avidin and/or the enzyme. For example, the enzyme β-galactosidase is known to have exposed thiols (cysteines) which are not required for its activity, while avidin does not contain free SH groups. Thus, maleimido groups or bromoacetyl groups can be derivatized onto the avidin molecule which can subsequently be mixed with the β-galactosidase. The same approach is essentially applicable to other enzymes which lack exposed cysteines. In this case, the enzyme can be thiolated (many different reagents are available, e.g., N-acetyl homocysteine thiolactone and 2-iminothiolane), and the product is then subjected to interaction with the appropriate derivatized avidin (e.g., maleimido-avidin).

Still another approach for conjugating avidin exploits the presence of the oligosaccharide residue on the native glycoprotein. In this regard, the sugars of avidin are susceptible to periodate oxidation and the aldehydes formed react with free amino groups. Aldehydes would react with even greater facility with hydrazide groups and these can be derivatized onto proteins (e.g., antibodies or enzymes) using the carbodiimide reaction in the presence of a dihydrazide.

Finally, newer recombinant methods are currently being explored for preparing avidin- or streptavidin-containing conjugates (27, 28). Chimeric constructs, which contain the respective biotin-binding protein together with the desired component of the immunoassay system, can be prepared by genetic means. Thus, either protein can be (and in some cases already have been) fused with recombinant IgG, antigens, or some other immunochemically relevant molecule (e.g., protein A or protein G).

2.4. Avidin Complexes

One of the major advances in using the avidin–biotin system, particularly for immunoassay and immunocytochemistry, has been the introduction of preformed complexes (14, 29). Preformed complexes between avidin (or streptavidin) and biotinylated probes provide a desirable alternative to the use of avidin conjugates by classic covalent crosslinking techniques—particularly for immunoassay. There are several advantages in preparing such complexes rather than preparing conjugates. First of all, the stock solutions of avidin and many of the biotinylated probes (antibodies, enzymes, etc.) are readily stored, sometimes for periods of many years, with little effect on their performance. Their preparation is convenient, reliable, reproducible, and technically very simple. Moreover, the signals achieved using complexes are often superior to those achieved using conjugates.

Complexes are formed by simply mixing predetermined portions of avidin (or a derivative thereof) and a biotinylated molecule. In forming such complexes, it is important to achieve a compromise regarding the amount of biotinylated component which interacts with the avidin. In achieving an optimal ratio, the compromise results in sufficient numbers of free biotin-binding sites on the avidin molecule which allows subsequent interaction with a second biotinylated species in the experimental system. One biotinylated species (the biotinylated probe, e.g., an enzyme) is required to provide a good signal; the other (e.g., a biotinylated antibody or an antigen) is required for the primary interaction. The most effective ratios of the avidin and biotinylated components for complex formation are determined empirically by optimization experiments.

Three different types of complexes are shown in Fig. 11.3. The simplest and most popular type of complex to date is illustrated in Fig. 11.3a. This type of complex consists of avidin (or streptavidin) and a biotinylated enzyme (or other probe). Several enzyme molecules are bound to several molecules of avidin to form the complex. Note that some of the biotin-binding sites are still free for subsequent interaction with a second biotinylated component (e.g., a biotinylated antibody) in the system.

Another possibility would be to prepare a complex which contains both the primary interacting component and the reporter group. One way of accomplishing this is shown in Fig. 11.3b. In this example, a biotinylated antibody is mixed with a conjugate which comprises avidin covalently coupled to an enzyme. In this case, it is not necessary to leave free biotin-binding sites since the complex contains both of the necessary activities for the immunoassay. An alternative would be to prepare an avidin–antibody conjugate which would then be mixed with a biotinylated enzyme. There are, however, few examples of complexes of these types in the literature.

A third type of complex also contains both the primary interacting component and the reporter group (Fig. 11.3c). In this case, and unlike the complex shown in Fig. 11.3b, the preparation of a covalently crosslinked avidin–enzyme or avidin–antibody conjugate is not required. Instead, two biotinylated components (e.g., an antibody and an enzyme) are mixed with avidin. The sequence of mixing, concentrations of the various components, etc., are all determined empirically—there are no rules or guidelines. This approach would also be applicable as a capture system in which the solid phase is biotinylated, as is a capture antibody.

3. AMPLIFIED DETECTION SYSTEMS

The first application of the avidin–biotin system in immunoassay involved the improvement of detection systems (3, 30). By virtue of the four biotin-binding sites of avidin and its stable molecular properties, the system was found to be a convenient and versatile alternative to standard immunoassay technique. Moreover, its mediation frequently resulted in amplified signals and improved sensitivity, sometimes reported at nearly 100-fold that of the conventional immunoassay setup (31).

The avidin–biotin complex has been applied as an improved detection system in the major types of immunoassay (32), i.e., two-site systems and competitive

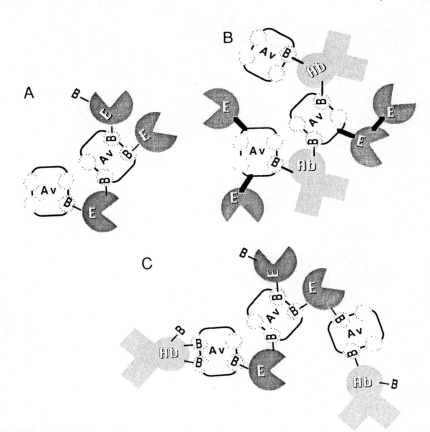

FIGURE 11.3 Some of the possible types of preformed complexes for use in immunoassay. Complex 1 (a) consists of a biotinylated probe (an enzyme) which has been mixed with avidin in an empirically predetermined molar ratio, to form complexes. The complexes should exhibit high levels of both the probe and the free biotin-binding sites for optimal efficiency. Complex 2 (b) consists of a biotinylated antibody incorporated into an avidin–enzyme conjugate. The opposite would be equally feasible, wherein the complex would contain a biotinylated enzyme incorporated into an avidin–antibody conjugate. Complex 3 (c) consists of a biotinylated enzyme and a biotinylated antibody, conjoined via the four biotin-binding sites of avidin. The resultant complex contains multiple copies of all components in an optimal ratio. In Complexes 2 and 3, it is usually not necessary to maintain free biotin-binding sites on avidin once the complexes are formed.

systems (Fig. 11.4). It is appropriate for both heterogeneous and homogeneous systems.

In the two-site format (Fig. 11.4A), the antigen is bound to the solid phase via a capture antibody. Biotinylated primary antibody is then added. Once biotin is present in the system, an avidin-conjugated probe can be used to quantify the amount of antigen. The system is most efficient if a high-affinity monoclonal capture antibody is used for immobilization of the antigen via a distinct epitope. The other epitopes would then be available for interaction with the biotinylated form of either a second monoclonal of alternate specificity or a polyclonal preparation.

Various permutations of this basic format have been examined throughout the years. In place of the interaction with the avidin-conjugated probe, the biotinylated

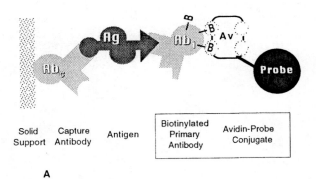

Solid   Capture   Antigen   Biotinylated   Avidin-Probe
Support Antibody   Primary   Conjugate
                               Antibody

A

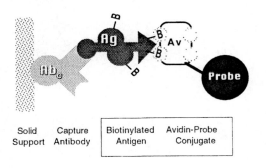

Solid   Capture   Biotinylated   Avidin-Probe
Support Antibody   Antigen   Conjugate

B

FIGURE 11.4   Use of the avidin–biotin complex in the detection system of immunoassays. (A) The two-site immunoassay format, in which an antigen from a complex mixture of molecules is selectively bound to the solid phase via a capture antibody, and detected subsequently via a biotinylated primary antibody and avidin-conjugated probe. (B) The competitive immunoassay format, wherein a biotinylated antigen competes with the native form of the antigen, prior to quantification by the avidin-conjugated probe.

antibody has been detected by sequential addition of an excess of free avidin, followed by a biotinylated probe. In this approach, the avidin molecules are incorporated into the biotin-containing system such that additional free binding sites are available for subsequent interaction with the probe.

Another very efficient alternative to the sequential approach is to apply preformed complexes of avidin instead (see Section 2.3). In this case, the advantage is often twofold over the sequential approach. First, the use of complexes saves one of the steps in the immunoassay, and second, the signal is often higher due to the multiplicity of probe molecules contained in the complex.

The second major type of immunoassy format (Fig. 11.4B) involves the competition between biotinylated and nonbiotinylated antigen molecules for the combining sites of a capture antibody system (33, 34). The nonbiotinylated antigen is of course part of the experimental test system to be assayed, whereas the biotinylated antigen is exogenously added. The amount of biotinylated antigen which successfully competes with the native antigen is then determined by an avidin–probe conjugate or complex. In this case, it is beneficial that the native antigen often gains an advantage in its interaction with the immobilized antibody, by virtue of its higher affinity. Residual free combining sites are then filled by the biotinylated antigen. As described above for the two-site format, sequential treatments with free avidin and biotinylated probe or treatment using the preformed complexes of the two may be substituted for the avidin–probe conjugate.

4. IMPROVEMENT OF CAPTURE SYSTEMS

In the past couple of years, the emphasis on the use of the avidin–biotin complex in immunoassay has shifted from detection systems to the improvement of capture systems. Thus, many of the articles published recently in this field (35–37) have used avidin as a tool for immobilizing a biotinylated antibody or biotinylated DNA (Fig. 11.5).

The use of avidin in this capacity holds several advantages. First of all, one of the weak links of any immunoassay system is that the adsorption of the antibody to the solid phase causes a deformation in its structure which could affect the specificity or overall sensitivity of binding. Avidin, on the other hand, is very stable and the character of its interaction with biotin is normally maintained upon immobilization. Even if one of the sites of the tetramer is inactivated by the adsorption to the solid phase, there are still others available for interaction with a biotinylated antibody. Furthermore, there is more control over the immobilization procedure, since the amount of immunochemically active antibody molecules applied to the solid phase can be more precisely regulated. Moreover, the same solid-phase system may be used for different assays.

5. AUXILIARY ENHANCEMENT SYSTEMS

The use of the avidin–biotin system in immunoassay can be further extended in many ways, either to improve the general applicablility and versatility of a given

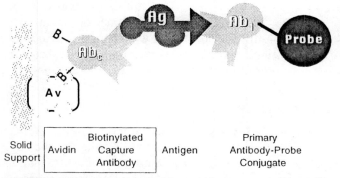

FIGURE 11.5 Use of the avidin–biotin complex as a mediator in capture systems of immunoassays. A biotinylated capture antibody is bound to the solid phase through an avidin bridge. Subsequent sequestering of antigen is quantified by a conjugate consisting of the primary antibody and an appropriate probe.

assay or to increase its sensitivity. Some of the details of the various approaches in this direction will be described in the following sections. In each case, additional components are usually introduced into the system, and although such a strategy is often advantageous in the final analysis, there are also definite disadvantages. In general terms, each new component which is introduced into the immunoassay protocol is a potential source of nonspecific interaction. It should thus be kept in mind, particularly from this point on, that as more components or steps are applied to a system, there is more of a chance for high background levels or false positive signals.

5.1. Secondary Systems

Sometimes, biotinylation of an antibody preparation can cause an alteration in specificity or a loss in its antigen-combining activity. This can be especially problematic when dealing with a monoclonal antibody preparation. One way of evading this particular problem is to incorporate a second recognition molecule into the protocol which would be biotinylated instead of the principal antibody. Recognition molecules of this type include protein A, protein G, and class- or species-specific secondary antibodies (such as anti-IgG$_1$ or goat anti-rabbit antibodies). One of the latter would be biotinylated and used in conjunction with its corresponding underivatized antibody counterpart.

The approach is appropriate for both detection and capture systems (Fig. 11.6). Thus, if an antigen has been immobilized to the solid phase by an appropriate capture antibody and labeled subsequently using a given type of primary antibody (e.g., raised in rabbits), then a biotinylated anti-rabbit Ig can be used for its detection. The same secondary antibody system (together with the avidin–probe) can consequently be used as a general detection system for any primary antibody raised in the same species. Note that in this approach, the primary antibody is used in its native, underivatized form. In fact, the relevant, unprocessed antiserum can be used instead of a purified antibody, since the purification step would take place *in situ* by its application to the solid-phase system.

Likewise, in the application of a general capture system, one of the above-mentioned general recognition molecules can be immobilized to the solid phase via the avidin–biotin complex (Fig. 11.6B). The capture antibody (or antiserum) in the native state can then, in turn, be selectively attached. As an example, we show the immobilization of biotinylated protein A which then binds to the Fc region of an appropriate capture antibody. As stated above, this is a general capture system which can be used when required for analyzing different types of antigen.

5.2. Extended Amplification Systems

Sometimes an immunoassay signal is so low that it is hard to determine whether in fact it constitutes a positive result or not. In some cases, the signal can be further amplified. In order to increase the sensitivity of an immunoassay, several related strategies can be designed which employ the avidin–biotin system. Once avidin and biotin have been introduced into the system with a detectable probe, various methods are available to attenuate a low-level signal by adding additional layers of label. Some of these are shown schematically in Fig. 11.7.

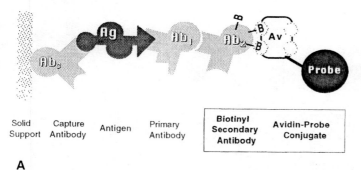

A

| Solid Support | Capture Antibody | Antigen | Primary Antibody | **Biotinyl Secondary Antibody** | **Avidin-Probe Conjugate** |

B

| Solid Support | **Avidin** | **Biotinyl Protein A** | Capture Antibody | Antigen | Primary Antibody-Probe Conjugate |

FIGURE 11.6   Use of biotinylated secondary recognition systems in immunoassay. (A) As an example of a secondary detection system, a biotinylated secondary (e.g., species-specific) antibody is shown which binds to the underivatized primary antibody. (B) As an example of a secondary capture system, biotinyl protein A is bound to an immobilized form of avidin. The resultant matrix can be used to bind immunoglobulins from a variety of different animal species.

The normal approach is shown in Fig. 11.7a. In this case, we show a two-site immunoassay, but the particular format is irrelevant. What is important is that avidin, biotin, and/or the probe are now somewhere in the system, even if the signal itself is very low. One method for further amplification is shown in (b), where an antiavidin antibody (associated with a probe for detection) is used to interact secondarily with the avidin molecules. Alternatively, the avidin molecules can be additionally labeled using another biotinylated protein (c); if desired, the biotinylated protein may be the same probe used for the initial detection in (a). Using this approach, the system now has more biotin moieties than before and can be subjected to further labeling. For example, another layer of avidin–probe conjugates (d) can be applied to the system. Alternatively, avidin and an antiavidin antibody–probe conjugate can be added either sequentially or as preformed complexes (e). Another possibility (f) would be to use antibiotin antibodies, conjugated to the probe, in order to extend the label in (c). The final example shown in the figure, but certainly not the final possibility, is the use of a biotinylated form of an antiprobe antibody (g) to amplify the label in either (a) or (c). The additional biotin moieties thus

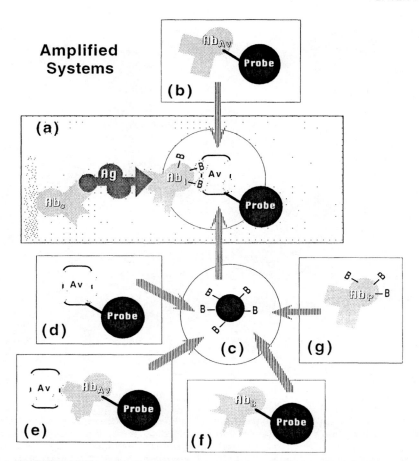

FIGURE 11.7 Amplification of the original signal by supplementary accretion of labels. The original protocol (a), shown here as a two-site assay format, which includes avidin and biotin in the detection system, can be subsequently extended by introduction of additional conjugates. For example, antiavidin antibody (b) or a biotinylated probe or other biotinylated protein (c) can be applied to the system to enhance the original signal. The biotin moieties in (c) can be further enhanced by additional interaction with biotin-binding entities, such as avidin-conjugated probe (d), avidin–antiavidin probe conjugates (e), or antibiotin conjugated to the probe (f). The chain can be lengthened even further by using a biotinylated antiprobe antibody (g), and the additional biotin moieties can be labeled further. The process can theoretically be continued *ad infinitum*, but in practical terms, such extended amplification systems are characterized by high background levels which limit the number of layers one can apply in sequence.

introduced into the system would serve as extra points of accretion for additional layers of avidin-conjugated probes, such as (d), (e), or (f). In any case, strict controls of each layer must be enforced. The increase in detection layers and points of accretion also serve as sources of nonspecific label which strikingly increase the background levels and tendency for false positive signals.

5.3. Dual Labeling Systems

In several of our early reviews on avidin–biotin technology, we expressed the necessity for development of similar high-affinity systems as supplementary tools to assist or extend its application. We suggested (4), for example, the use of high-affinity antihapten antibodies in an approach similar to that used for the avidin–biotin system. Thus, the hapten, like the biotin moiety, could be covalently attached to an antibody or an antigen, and the antihapten antibody could be used for its detection.

It is therefore gratifying that, today, the hapten–antihapten approach (e.g., the anti-DIG system or the antifluorescein system) has indeed come into vogue as an avidin–biotin alternative (8). In fact, the initial use of a hapten–antihapten system (38) actually preceded the flurry of publications which led to the development of avidin–biotin technology (1, 11). By far, however, the most effective use would be to apply both systems together in the same format for a superior and versatile immunoassay system. In this context, the avidin–biotin complex can be used as a capture system and the hapten–antihapten complex can be used in the detection system (Fig. 11.8), or vice versa (39, 40).

The dual labeling approach can also be used in all of the above-described modifications of the original immunoassay protocol, including secondary systems and extended amplification assay systems. A universal assay protocol can conceivably be established using, for example, a biotinylated form of one type of secondary recognition system (see Section 5.1) and a hapten-derivatized form of another. By simply changing the native capture and primary antibodies, the same immunoassay system can be used for different antigens. This approach would be particularly useful for producing universal immunoassay kits.

6. SELECTED PROTOCOLS

In the following sections, we present simple versions of protocols which we have used to establish an avidin–biotin-based immunoassay. The purpose here is not to show how elegant such procedures can be or to introduce the student to the fine details of the approach. Improvements in these procedures and various considerations as to their specificity, applicability, or optimization will become clear to the

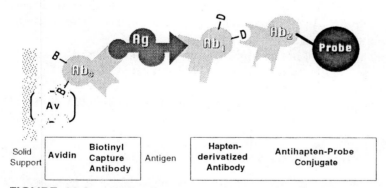

| Solid Support | Avidin | Biotinyl Capture Antibody | Antigen | Hapten-derivatized Antibody | Antihapten-Probe Conjugate |

FIGURE 11.8   Dual labeling system involving the use of the avidin–biotin system and a hapten–antihapten system. In the example shown, the avidin–biotin system mediates the attachment of the capture antibody to the solid phase whereas the hapten–antihapten system mediates the detection of the antigen by the probe. In the example shown, the antigen is recognized by the hapten-derivatized primary antibody. The hapten (—D) is labeled with an antihapten antibody conjugate.

practicing investigator. Instead, we try to be generally instructive. We hope that the protocols we present below will serve as examples or as models for the student to biotinylate an antibody (or antigen) and/or to design his own immunoassay system for a desired antigen. For more information, the interested reader is referred to Refs. (2, 6, 7, 30, 32).

6.1. Biotinylation Procedures

The following two protocols are simple methods for biotinylating either a protein using an NHS derivative of biotin or a glycoprotein using periodate oxidation followed by interaction with a hydrazido derivative of biotin. For other biotinylating approaches, the reader is referred to Refs. (7, 9, 10).

6.1.1. Biotinylation via Amino Groups

Step 1. Dissolve 2 mg of an antibody or antigen into 1 ml of 0.1 M sodium bicarbonate solution (pH 8.5).

Step 2. Dissolve (freshly) 2 mg of biotinyl N-hydroxysuccinimide ester (BNHS) or a similar long-chained analog in 1 ml of dimethylformamide (heat to dissolve, if necessary).

Step 3. Add 25 μl of the BNHS solution into the solution of antibody or antigen. Mix thoroughly. Let the reaction stand at room temperature for 1 hr. This reaction can easily be scaled up or down, depending on how much protein sample is available for biotinylation.

Step 4. Dialyze exhaustively at 4°C against any suitable buffer. Store in aliquots at -20°C.

6.1.2. Biotinylation via Sugar Residues

Step 1. Dissolve 2 mg of an antibody or antigen sample into 1 ml of 0.1 M phospate-buffered saline, pH 7 (PBS).

Step 2. Prepare (freshly) 0.1 M solution of sodium periodate in water.

Step 3. Prepare 10 mg/ml of biotin hydrazide (or, preferably, a longer-chained reagent, e.g., biocytin hydrazide) solution in PBS (heat to dissolve, if necessary).

Step 4. Add 110 μl periodate solution to the sample. Let the reaction stand at room temperature for 30 min.

Step 5. Dialyze for 4 hr at room temperature against 2 liters of PBS.

Step 6. Add 250 μl of the solution containing the hydrazide derivative. Incubate at room temperature for 2 hr.

Step 7. Dialyze exhaustively at 4°C against any suitable buffer. Store in aliquots at -20°C.

6.2. Design of a Typical Avidin-Based Immunoassay

The following procedures provide an approach for establishing a simple two-site immunoassay, mediated by the avidin–biotin system, such as that illustrated schematically in Fig. 11.4A. In this case, we will describe the use of streptavidin–biotinyl enzyme complexes, instead of an avidin or streptavidin conjugate. The particular antigen is not relevant here and we will refer only to "the antigen" or "the antibody" in describing the design and simple optimization of the assay. When setting up a new assay, the optimal amounts or ratios of a given batch of reagents must always be determined anew. Note that in determining the optimal concentration of reagents, we do so from the last step backward. We thus begin by determining the optimal molar ratio of the components required to form active biotin-binding complexes—i.e., a mixture of a biotinyl probe (in this case biotinyl alkaline phosphatase) and avidin (in this case streptavidin).

6.2.1. Preparation of Preformed Complexes: Determination of the Optimal Ratio of Components

In order to determine the optimal ratio of biotinyl alkaline phosphatase and streptavidin required to produce efficient biotin-binding complexes, we need a suitable biotin-containing solid-phase system as a target. For this purpose, a biotinylated form of bovine serum albumin (BSA) or any other biotinylated protein is adsorbed to microtiter plates. By varying the concentrations of the biotinyl enzyme and streptavidin added to the wells, the highest level of signal versus background can be determined.

A similar protocol can be used for examining the ideal ratio for other types of biotinyl probe, solid phase, or other immunoassay designs. For every batch of biotinylated probe, its performance in conjunction with one of the avidins must be determined. Likewise, a preparation which has been stored and unused for long periods of time also should be examined. Reagents should not be used blindly. We have saved countless amounts of time, effort, and heartache by regularly testing the performance of each of our in-house reagents by such assay procedures.

Step 1. Adsorption of biotinyl protein to microtiter plate. To all of the wells of a 96-well microtiter plate, add 100 μl of a solution containing 3 μg/ml of a biotinylated preparation of bovine serum albumin (BSA) in 0.1 M carbonate buffer, pH 9.6. Incubate overnight at 4°C. For a control plate, adsorb an equivalent amount of the unbiotinylated protein to its wells. Block the plates by adding to each well 200 μl of 0.3% BSA solution.

Step 2. Complex formation. In a test tube rack, arrange 24 small test tubes in four rows containing six columns each. To the test tubes in each row, add 0.5 ml of a given concentration of biotinyl enzyme. For example, to each test tube in row 1, add 0.5 ml of 0.3 U/ml biotinyl enzyme; to row 2, 1 U/ml; to row 3, 3 U/ml; to row 4, 10 U/ml. Then, to each column, add various concentrations of avidin (in this example, streptavidin was used). For example, to the first column, add 0.5 ml of water or buffer; to the second, 0.1 μg/ml streptavidin; to column 3, 0.3 μg/ml; to column 4, 1 μg/ml; etc. The result is 24 different solutions, each containing 1 ml of a different ratio and/or concentration of complexes. Let the solutions stand for at least 30 min before continuing with the next step.

Step 3. Application of preformed complexes. Add 100 μl of the 24 types of preformed complexes to quadruplicate wells of the microtiter plate. One possible design of the experimental plate is shown in Fig. 11.9. Incubate for 1 hr at room temperature. Wash the plates with buffer.

Step 4. Assaying the plate. To each well, add 100 μl of substrate solution (for this particular enzyme, an appropriate substrate is 10 mg p-nitrophenyl phosphate in 10 ml of 1 M diethanolamine buffer, pH 9.8, containing 0.5 mM MgCl$_2$). The

Biotinyl enzyme (U/ml)	Well	Streptavidin (µg/ml) 0 (1, 2)	0.1 (3, 4)	0.3 (5, 6)	1.0 (7, 8)	3.0 (9, 10)	10.0 (11, 12)
0.3	A	0.02	0.14	**1.15**	**1.16**	0.43	0.17
	B	0.01	0.01	0.02	0.01	0.00	0.01
1.0	C	0.01	0.07	0.27	**2.53**	**1.39**	0.74
	D	0.05	0.02	0.07	0.06	0.03	0.02
3.0	E	0.00	0.05	0.17	1.42	2.69	1.55
	F	0.00	0.03	0.07	0.23	0.14	0.14
10.0	G	0.03	0.07	0.15	0.76	2.61	2.57
	H	0.01	0.03	0.05	0.25	0.87	0.82

FIGURE 11.9   Determination of the optimal efficiency of preformed avidin-containing complexes for an ELISA-type system. The plate is prepared by coating a biotinylated protein (e.g., BSA) to all of the wells. The complexes are first formed in 24 test tubes, to which were added equal volumes of the indicated concentrations of streptavidin (as the avidin component) and biotinyl alkaline phosphatase (as the biotinyl probe). The final experiment includes samples in quadruplicate. Thus, in the diagram shown, wells A1, A2, B1, and B2 are control samples which contain no streptavidin and 0.15 U/ml of biotinyl enzyme (final concentration); wells A3, A4, B3, and B4 contain 0.05 µg/ml streptavidin and 0.15 U/ml of biotinyl enzyme; and so on. In many cases along the diagonal, the ratio of components is maintained, but their final concentration is increased. For each example, the top value represents the mean of quadruplicate samples for the biotinylated plate; the bottom value shows the data for an unbiotinylated BSA control plate. Bold values show the optimum results. Shaded areas denote the samples which yielded very high background levels in the control plate.

plate can be scanned (at 405 nm, using this particular substrate) at various time intervals in an appropriate ELISA reader.

Comments. The results of a typical experiment are shown in Fig. 11.9. For each combination, the experimental values (for the plates with biotinyl BSA) are given at the top of each box, and the control values (for the unbiotinylated protein) are given at the bottom. For example, the four values for wells A3, A4, B3, and B4 correspond to a mixture of 0.3 U/ml biotinyl enzyme with 0.1 µg/ml streptavidin, giving a mean value of 0.14 for the experimental plate and 0.01 for the control plate. By visually scanning the results in Fig. 11.9, the optimal values (shown in bold type) for complex formation appear to be between 0.3 to 1.0 U/ml biotinyl enzyme and 0.3 to 3.0 µg/ml streptavidin. Within the designated concentration range, the experimental values are highest with very little background. At higher concentrations (shaded boxes), the background values for the control plates are very high, and such complexes should not be applied.

6.2.2. Determination of Optimal Amount of Biotinyl Primary Antibody

Once the optimal ratio for producing efficient biotin-binding complexes is known, the optimal amount of the biotinylated antibody can be determined. This is accomplished much in the same way as shown in the previous section. In this case, various concentrations of the antigen (instead of a biotinyl protein) are used for coating the microtiter plates, in order to provide the abscissa for a titration curve. The biotinyl antibody (at different concentrations) is then added. Finally, the streptavidin-containing complexes (at the predetermined optimal ratio) are applied, and the results are graphed.

Step 1. Adsorption of antigen to microtiter plate. To the wells of each row of a 96-well microtiter plate, add 100 μl of a given amount of antigen in 0.1 M carbonate buffer, pH 9.6. See example in Fig. 11.10 (top plate). Incubate overnight at 4°C. For a control plate, add an irrelevant protein to its wells. Block the plates by adding to each well 200 μl of 0.3% BSA solution.

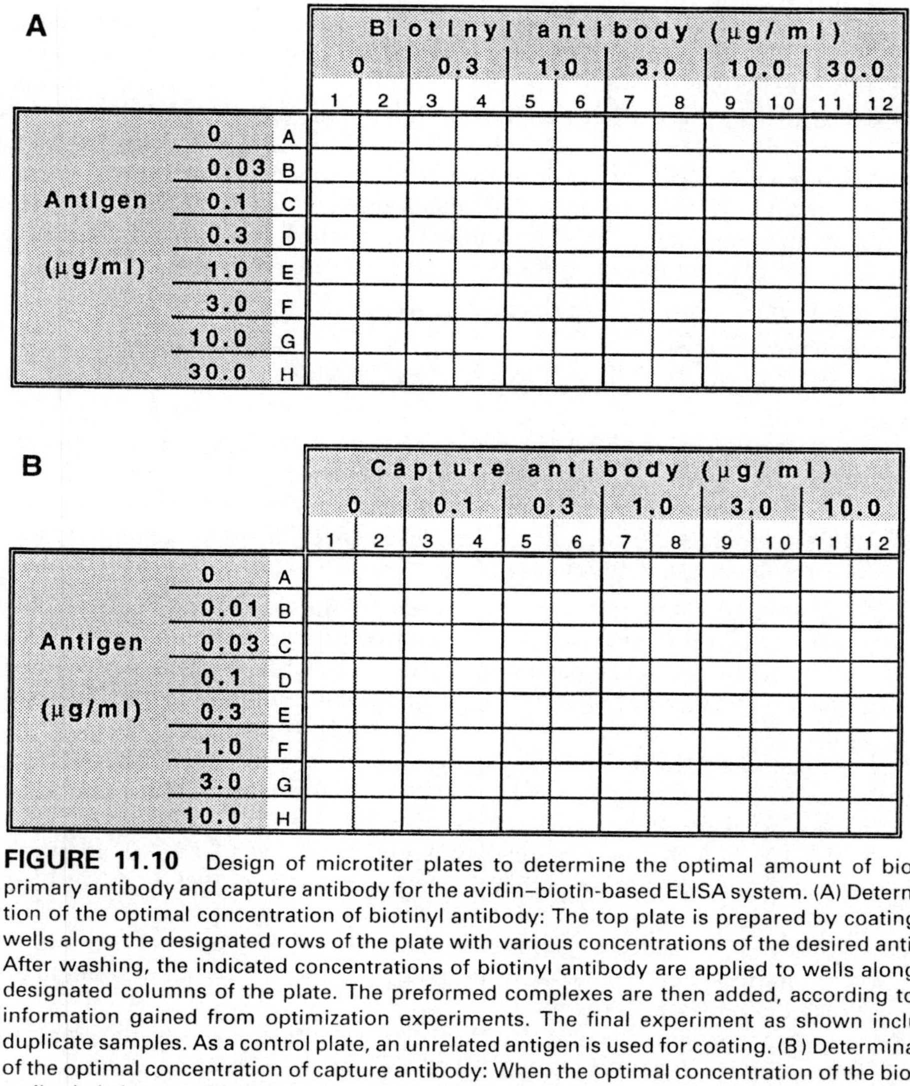

A

			Biotinyl antibody (µg/ml)											
			0		0.3		1.0		3.0		10.0		30.0	
			1	2	3	4	5	6	7	8	9	10	11	12
	0	A												
	0.03	B												
Antigen	0.1	C												
	0.3	D												
(µg/ml)	1.0	E												
	3.0	F												
	10.0	G												
	30.0	H												

B

			Capture antibody (µg/ml)											
			0		0.1		0.3		1.0		3.0		10.0	
			1	2	3	4	5	6	7	8	9	10	11	12
	0	A												
	0.01	B												
Antigen	0.03	C												
	0.1	D												
(µg/ml)	0.3	E												
	1.0	F												
	3.0	G												
	10.0	H												

FIGURE 11.10 Design of microtiter plates to determine the optimal amount of biotinyl primary antibody and capture antibody for the avidin–biotin-based ELISA system. (A) Determination of the optimal concentration of biotinyl antibody: The top plate is prepared by coating the wells along the designated rows of the plate with various concentrations of the desired antigen. After washing, the indicated concentrations of biotinyl antibody are applied to wells along the designated columns of the plate. The preformed complexes are then added, according to the information gained from optimization experiments. The final experiment as shown includes duplicate samples. As a control plate, an unrelated antigen is used for coating. (B) Determination of the optimal concentration of capture antibody: When the optimal concentration of the biotinyl antibody is known, this information is used to determine the optimal concentration of capture antibody. Thus, the wells along the designated columns of the bottom plate are coated with different concentrations of monoclonal antibody. After washing, the indicated concentrations of the antigen are applied to the rows of the plate, followed by the predetermined concentration of the biotinylated antibody and preformed complexes, respectively. As a control, the same plates are used, but an unrelated antigen is substituted for the target antigen.

Step 2. Addition of biotinyl antibody. To the wells of each column, add 100 μl of a designated concentration of biotinyl antibody (see example in Fig. 11.10). Incubate for 3 hr at room temperature. Wash the plates with buffer.

Step 3. Application of complexes. Add 100 μl of the optimal concentration ratio of complexes (determined in Section 6.2.1). Incubate for 1 hr at room temperature. Wash the plates with buffer.

Step 4. Assaying the plate. Add substrate solution and scan the plates at various time intervals in an appropriate ELISA reader.

Comments. For each concentration of biotinyl antibody, the results of the assay are graphed as enzyme activity versus antigen concentration. The results are compared with the control to ensure that the background signal is at a minimum. In this experiment, the antigen is simply adsorbed to the plate and the resultant curve is "artificial" and not necessarily indicative of the actual assay wherein the antigen is concentrated onto the solid phase by virtue of its interaction with the adsorbed capture antibody. Nevertheless, the results of this experiment provide evidence as to the concentration of biotinyl primary antibody which would be appropriate for such an experiment. The final amount of biotinyl antibody can then be adjusted after setting up the next and final stage of the assay system.

6.2.3. Determination of Optimal Amount of Capture Antibody

Now that we know the preferred concentrations of the other components of the immunoassay system, we can determine the best concentration of capture antibody, which is necessary to bind the antigen to the solid phase. For this purpose, various concentrations of the capture antibody are coated onto the microtiter plates. The antigen (at different concentrations) is then added, followed by the biotinyl antibody and the streptavidin-containing complexes (both at the predetermined amounts). The results are then graphed.

Step 1. Adsorption of capture antibody. To the wells of each column of a microtiter plate, add 100 μl of a given amount of capture antibody in 0.1 M carbonate buffer, pH 9.6. See example in Fig. 11.10B. Incubate overnight at 4°C. For a control plate, add equivalent amounts of an irrelevant antibody to the wells. Block the plates by adding to each well 200 μl of 0.3% BSA solution.

Step 2. Addition of antigen. To the wells of each row, add 100 μl of a designated concentration of antigen (see Fig. 11.10B). Incubate for 3 hr at room temperature. Wash the plates with buffer.

Step 3. Application of biotinyl antibody. To each well, add 100 μl of the optimal concentration of biotinyl antibody, as determined in Section 6.2.2. Incubate for 3 hr at room temperature. Wash the plates with buffer.

Step 4. Application of complexes. Add 100 μl of the optimal concentration ratio of complexes (determined in Section 6.2.1). Incubate for 1 hr at room temperature. Wash the plates with buffer.

Step 5. Assaying the plate. Add substrate solution, and scan the plates at various time intervals in an appropriate ELISA reader.

Comments. For each concentration of capture antibody, the results of the assay are graphed as enzyme activity versus antigen concentration. The results are compared with the control to ensure that the background signal is at a minimum.

The composition of the wash buffer and blocking solution can be altered to improve the performance of the immunoassay—particularly to reduce the amount of nonspecific binding of its components. Any change to the system should be examined in a separate model assay protocol.

Using the same basic techniques for determining optimal concentrations of reagents, we can also develop both more sensitive, extended, amplified systems and more universal systems, as described in Section 5.

6.2.4. Final Immunoassay Protocol

In the previous sections, we have determined the optimal concentrations of the reagents. Based on this information, we can now establish a standard immunoassay protocol for these particular reagents and for this particular combination of antibody and antigen.

6.2.4.1. Reagents

Microtiter plates

Preformed complexes: equal volumes of streptavidin (1 μg/ml) and biotinyl alkaline phosphatase (1 U/ml) are diluted in blocking solution and mixed 30 min prior to use

Antigen standard or antigen-containing samples (e.g., serum, cell extract, etc.), diluted in assay buffer

Capture antibody: 1 μg/ml of monoclonal antibody in coating buffer

Biotinyl primary antibody (polyclonal): 3 μg/ml of assay buffer

Coating buffer: 15 mM sodium carbonate-bicarbonate buffer, pH 9.6, brought to 0.01% sodium azide

Wash buffer: 50 mM Tris–HCl buffer, pH 7.8, containing 0.05% Tween 20 and 0.05% sodium azide

Assay buffer: Wash buffer containing 0.5% BSA

Blocking solution: 50 mM Tris–HCl buffer, pH 7.8, containing 0.5% BSA, and 0.05% sodium azide

Substrate solution: 10 mg p-nitrophenyl phosphate dissolved in 10 ml of 1 M diethanolamine buffer, pH 9.8, containing 0.5 mM MgCl$_2$

6.2.4.2. Assay

(i) Coating of wells: Add 100 μl of the monoclonal antibody solution to each well of a microtiter plate. Allow the plate to stand overnight at 4°C. Wash the plate.

(ii) Block with 200 μl of blocking solution. Wash the plate.

(iii) Add 100 μl of the sample or of known concentrations of antigen for a standard curve. Incubate for 3 hr at room temperature. Wash the plate.

(iv) Add 100 μl of the biotinyl antibody solution to each well. Incubate for 3 hr at room temperature. Wash.

(v) Add the preformed complexes. Incubate for 1 hr at room temperature. Wash.

(vi) Add substrate solution. Scan at 405 nm (and at 600 nm for blank).

(vii) Compare experimental signal with standard curve.

References

1. Bayer EA, Wilchek M. The avidin-biotin complex as a tool in molecular biology. Trends Biochem Sci 1978; 3:N237–9.
2. Wilchek M, Bayer EA, Eds. Avidin-Biotin Technology. Methods in Enzymology, Vol. 184. San Diego: Academic Press, 1990:746.

3. Guesdon JL, Ternynck T, Avrameas S. The use of the avidin-biotin interaction in immunoenzymatic techniques. J Histochem Cytochem 1979; 27:1131–9.

4. Wilchek M, Bayer EA. The avidin-biotin complex in bioanalytical applications. Anal Biochem 1988; 171:1–32.

5. Diamandis EP, Christopoulos TK. The biotin-(strept)avidin system: Principles and applications in biotechnology. Clin Chem 1991; 37:625–36.

6. Bayer EA, Wilchek M. Immunochemical applications of avidin-biotin technology. In: Manson MM, Ed. Immunochemical Protocols. Methods in Molecular Biology, Vol. 10. Clifton, NJ: Humana Press, 1992: 149–62.

7. Savage D, Mattson G, Desai S, Nielander G, Morgensen S, Conklin E. Avidin-Biotin Chemistry: A Handbook.Rockford, IL: Pierce Chemical Company, 1992:467.

8. Kessler C, Ed. Nonradioactive Labeling and Detection of Biomolecules. Berlin: Springer-Verlag, 1992:436.

9. Bayer EA, Wilchek M. Avidin-biotin technology. In: Manson MM, Ed. Immunochemical Protocols. Methods in Molecular Biology, Vol. 10. Clifton, NJ: Humana Press, 1992: 137–48.

10. Bayer EA, Wilchek M. Protein biotinylation. Methods Enzymol 1990; 184:138–60.

11. Bayer EA, Wilchek M. The use of the avidin-biotin complex in molecular biology. Methods Biochem Anal 1980; 26:1–45.

12. Wilchek M, Bayer EA. Avidin-biotin immobilisation systems. In: Sleytr UB, Messner P, Pum D, Sara M, Eds. Immobilised Macromolecules: Application Potentials. Springer Series in Applied Biology. London: Springer-Verlag, 1993:51–60.

13. Bayer EA, Wilchek M, Skutelsky E. Affinity cytochemistry: The localization of lectin and antibody receptors on erythrocytes via the avidin-biotin complex. FEBS Lett 1976; 68:240–4.

14. Bayer EA, Zalis MG, Wilchek M. 3-(N-Maleimido-propionyl) biocytin: A versatile thiol-specific biotinylating reagent. Anal Biochem 1985; 149:529–36.

15. Luppa P, Birkmayer C, Hauptmann H. Synthesis of 3-hydroxyestra-1,3,5(10)-trien-17-one and 3,17β-dihydroxyestra-1,3,5(10)-triene 6α-N-(ε-biotinyl)caproamide, tracer substances for developing immunoassays for estrone and estradiol. Bioconjugate Chem 1994; 5:167–71.

16. Wilchek M, Ben-Hur H, Bayer EA. p-Diazobenzoyl biocytin—A new biotinylating reagent for the labeling of tyrosines and histidines in proteins. Biochem Biophys Res Commun 1986; 138:872–9.

17. Forster AC, McInnes JL, Skingle DC, Symons RH. Non-radioactive hybridization probes prepared by the chemical labelling of DNA and RNA with a novel reagent, photobiotin. Nucleic Acids Res 1985; 13:745–61.

18. Schwarz A, Wandrey C, Bayer EA, Wilchek M. Enzymatic biotinylation of the C terminus. Methods Enzymol 1990; 184:160–2.

19. Jeon WM, Lee KN, Birckbichler PJ, Conway E, Patterson MKJ. Colorimetric assay for cellular transglutaminase. Anal Biochem 1989; 182:170–5.

20. Cronan JEJ. Biotinylation of proteins in vivo. A post-translational modification to label, purify, and study proteins. J Biol Chem 1990; 265:10327–33.

21. Schatz PJ. Use of peptide libraries to map the substrate specificity of a peptide-modifying enzyme: A 13 residue consensus peptide specifies biotinylation in Escherichia coli. Bio/Technology 1993; 11:1138–43.

22. Bayer EA, Wilchek M. Modified avidins for application in avidin-biotin technology: an improvement on nature. In: Sim JS, Nakai S, Eds. Egg Uses and Processing Technologies. Wallingford, UK: CAB International, 1994:158–76.

23. Bayer EA, De Meester F, Kulik T, Wilchek M. Deglycosylation of egg-white avidin. Appl Biochem Biotechnol 1995:1–9.

24. Argaraña CE, Kuntz ID, Birken S, Axel R, Cantor CR. Molecular cloning and nucleotide sequence of the streptavidin gene. Nucleic Acids Res 1986; 14:1871–82.

25. Gope ML, Keinanen RA, Kristo PA, Conneely OM, Beattie WG, Zarucki-Schulz, T, O'Malley BW, Kulomaa MS. Molecular cloning of the chicken avidin cDNA. Nucleic Acids Res 1987; 15:3595–606.

26. Bagci H, Kohen F, Kuscuoglu U, Bayer EA, Wilchek M. Monoclonal anti-biotin antibodies simulate avidin in the recognition of biotin. FEBS Lett 1993; 322:47–50.

27. Sano T, Cantor CR. A streptavidin-protein A chimera that allows one-step production of a variety of specific antibody conjugates. Bio/Technology 1991; 9:1378–81.

28. Sano T, Smith CL, Cantor CR. Immuno-PCR: Very sensitive antigen detection by means of specific antibody-DNA conjugates. Science 1992; 258:120–2.

29. Hsu SM, Raine L, Fanger H. Use of avidin-biotin-peroxidase complex (ABC) in immunoperoxidase techniques. J Histochem Cytochem 1981; 29:577–80.

30. Ternynck T, Avrameas S. Avidin-biotin system in enzyme immunoassays. Methods Enzymol 1990; 184:469–81.

31. Barnard G, Bayer EA, Wilchek M, Amir-Zaltsman Y, Kohen F. Amplified bioluminescence assay using avidin-biotin technology. Methods Enzymol 1987; 133:284–8.

32. Kohen F, Amir-Zaltsman Y, Strasburger CJ, Bayer EA, Wilchek M. The avidin-biotin reaction in immunoassay. In: Collins WP, Ed. Complementary Immunoassays. New York: Wiley, 1988:57–69.

33. Rappuoli R, Leoncini P, Tarli P, Neri P. Competitive enzyme immunoassay for human chorionic somatomammotropin using the avidin-biotin system. Anal Biochem 1981; 118:168–72.

34. Wagener C, Fenger U, Clark BR, Shively JE. Use of biotin-labeled monoclonal antibodies and avidin-peroxidase conjugates for the determination of epitope specificities in solid-phase competitive immunoassays. J Immunol Methods 1984; 68:269–74.

35. Kaufman SE, Brown S, Stauber GB. Characterization of ligand binding to immobilized biotinylated extracellular domains of three growth factor receptors. Anal Biochem 1993; 211:261–66.

36. Kalle WHJ, Hazekamp-van Dokkum A-M, Lohman PHM, Natarajan AT, van Zeeland AA, Mullenders LHF. The use of streptavidin-coated magnetic beads and biotinylated antibodies to investigate induction and repair of DNA damage: Analysis of repair patches in specific sequences of uv-irradiated human fibroblasts. Anal Biochem 1993; 208:228–36.

37. Morgan H, Taylor DM. A surface plasmon resonance immunosensor based on the streptavidin-biotin complex. Biosensors Bioelectronics 1992; 7:405–10.

38. Lamm ME, Koo GC, Stackpole CW, Hämmerling U. Hapten-conjugated antibodies and visual markers used to label cell-surface antigens for electron microscopy: An approach to double labeling. Proc Natl Acad Sci USA 1972; 69:3732–6.

39. Jeltsch A, Fritz A, Alves J, Wolfes H, Pingoud A. A fast and accurate enzyme-linked immunosorbent assay for the determination of the DNA cleavage activity of restriction endonucleases. Anal Biochem 1993; 213:234–40.

40. Suzuki K, Craddock BP, Kano T, Steigbigel RT. Chemiluminescent enzyme-linked immunoassay for reverse transcriptase, illustrated by detection of HIV reverse transcriptase. Anal Biochem 1993; 210:277–81.

12 | RADIOIMMUNOASSAY

TIM CHARD

Departments of Reproductive Physiology, Obstetrics, and Gynaecology
St. Bartholomew's and the Royal London School of Medicine and Dentistry
London EC1A 7BE, United Kingdom

With all types of immunoassay it is essential to have a means for determining the distribution between the bound and free fractions. To achieve this, one of the components of the system must be labeled to act as a "tracer." This tracer can be the labeled antigen in a traditional radioimmunoassay (RIA) system or a labeled antibody in immunometric procedures. Any substance which can be measured accurately by simple methods, at levels less than that of direct methods for the measurement of the ligand, can be the label. The most frequently used label was at one time a radioactive isotope, but these are now being replaced by nonisotopic labels (enzymes, fluorescent molecules, etc.). Nevertheless, radioisotopes are still widely used.

1. RADIOACTIVE ISOTOPES

The atomic nucleus contains two main types of particle, protons and neutrons. An element's chemical characteristics are determined by the number of protons, or "atomic number." But with many elements, there is a variable number of neutrons in the nucleus, leading to differences in atomic mass but not in chemical properties. The variable forms are called "isotopes." For example, hydrogen can exist in three isotopic forms. In the simplest there is a single proton in the nucleus. The isotopes in which the mass is increased by the addition of one or two neutrons are "deuterium" (^2H) and "tritium" (^3H).

With some isotopes the nucleus is unstable; these are known as "radioactive isotopes." In this situation the nucleus may undergo spontaneous transformation to a more stable state; it will emit energy in the form of either particles or nonparticulate electromagnetic vibrations. The following processes may be involved:

(i) Expulsion of an α particle (2 protons and 2 neutrons, equivalent to a helium nucleus). This occurs only with heavy elements.

(ii) Conversion of a neutron into a proton, an electron, and a neutrino (a small uncharged particle); the last two are expelled (β emission).

(iii) Conversion of a proton into a neutron, a positron (a positively charged electron), and a neutrino; the last two are expelled (β emission).

(iv) Electron capture, in which a nuclear proton is converted into a neutron by the capture of an orbital electron; the process leads to emission of weak x rays.

(v) Isomeric transition, in which an unstable nucleus changes to a more stable isomer, the excess energy being emitted as γ rays.

(vi) Internal conversion of γ rays leading to emission of an orbital electron.

The rate of disintegration (or "decay") of a particular radioactive isotope is unique to that isotope. It is described by the "half life," the time required for 50% of the radioisotope to decay. The unit of radioactivity was originally defined as the radioactivity of 1 g radium and named the "curie," where:

$$1 \text{ curie (Ci)} = 3.7 \times 10^{10} \text{ disintegrations per second}$$
$$1 \text{ millicurie (mCi)} = 3.7 \times 10^{7} \text{ disintegrations per second}$$
$$1 \text{ microcurie } (\mu\text{Ci}) = 3.7 \times 10^{4} \text{ disintegrations per second.}$$

In the more recent "Systeme Internationale" the unit of radioactivity is the becquerel (Bq) which is one disintegration per second. Typical conversion factors are:

$$1 \text{ curie (Ci)} = 37 \text{ gigabequerels (GBq)}$$
$$1 \text{ millicurie (mCi)} = 37 \text{ megabequerels (MBq)}$$
$$1 \text{ microcurie } (\mu\text{Ci}) = 37 \text{ kilobequerels (KBq).}$$

The radioactivity of a specimen of an isotope thus depends on the amount of isotope present, and the half-life.

2. COUNTING OF RADIOACTIVE ISOTOPES

Quantitation of an isotope in a radioimmunoassay usually depends on a scintillation counter; the essential parts of this system are a scintillator, a photomultiplier tube, and electronic circuits.

A scintillator can be any material which emits light when exposed to ionizing radiation; the intensity of the light varies with the energy of the radiation. Flashes of light from a scintillator are detected by a photomultiplier, which converts them into electrical pulses. The amplitude of these pulses is related to the intensity of the scintillation, and thereby to the energy of the radiation which produced it. The radiation for a given isotope shows a continuous distribution of energies, or spectrum, with a maximum which is characteristic of that isotope. Using pulse-height analysis a scintillation counter can be set to detect pulses within a narrow range of amplitudes, and thus to measure the amount of an isotope with minimum interference from other isotopes or background radiation (Fig. 12.1).

The nature of the scintillator depends on the type of radiation emitted: in practical terms this is either β particles (from isotopes such as ^3H or ^{14}C) or γ rays (from isotopes such ^{125}I).

2.1. Measurement of β Particles

Beta particles have very low penetrating power. Thus they can only be detected when the isotope is in close contact with the scintillator. For this purpose, the isotope is made into a solution together with an aromatic compound which has the property of fluorescing (i.e., emitting light) when excited by ionizing radiation. The most commonly used compound is 2,5-diphenyloxazole (PPO). Because aqueous solutions are relatively insoluble in aromatic solvents such as toluene and xylene, the scintillation "cocktail" includes a nonionic detergent such as Triton X-100. A mixture of this type can accept up to 30% (v/v) of water. The efficiency of a liquid scintillator is greatly reduced by impurities such as proteins. This phenomenon is known as "quenching," and corrections may be necessary if the solutions counted differ widely in composition (e.g., standards prepared in simple buffer while the unknowns are samples of whole serum).

2.2. Measuring γ Rays

Unlike β particles, γ rays have high penetrating power. Close contact between the isotope and the scintillator is not necessary. The scintillator usually consists of

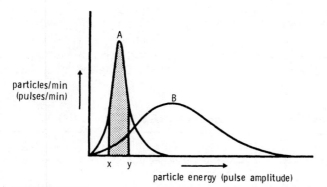

FIGURE 12.1 The energy spectra of two radioactive isotopes, A and B. By setting a "window" on the counter, which sees only energies lying between *x* and *y*, most of the radiation from isotope A, but little of that from isotope B, will be counted. (Modified from Chard, 1990.)

a crystal of sodium iodide coated with thallium, formed as a well. Radiation strikes the molecules making up the crystal lattice causing ionization and thereby results in a light flash which can be detected by the photomultiplier.

Obviously, gamma counting is simpler and cheaper than liquid scintillation counting (Table 12.1). There is no sample preparation, and the specific activities of γ-emitting isotopes are much greater than those of β emitters. Counting times are therefore much shorter. For these reasons, γ emitters are always preferred to β-emitting isotopes for all but a few research assays.

2.3. Choice of Counter

Traditionally, counting was performed using a single-well counter and an automatic sample changer (liquid scintillation counting is still performed in this way). However, for routine γ counting this equipment has now been replaced by manually operated multidetector systems. These are dedicated to isotopes of clinical laboratory interest (^{125}I, ^{57}Co) and have relatively small crystals (2 in. or less). Comparable equipment is now available for β counting (Pharmacia 2450 MicroBeta).

Routine laboratory work does not demand great complexity of counter controls. The only control for which versatility is essential is the count timer, which should be adjustable in steps of 1 sec or less over a range from 1 to 1000 sec. Most counters have a display and an output printer. Sophisticated equipment is invariably connected to an on-line microcomputer.

2.4. Practical Aspects of Isotope Counting

(i) Choice of counting time. The error of a count is roughly proportional to the square root of the total number of counts: for 100 counts the error is 10, or 10%; for 10,000 counts the error is 100 or 1%. All tubes of an assay should be counted for long enough to yield counts with an error less than that introduced by other steps in the assay. This will vary with the dose of analyte (1), but in practice all tubes are counted for the same length of time. As a rule of thumb the minimum number of counts for any tube should be 2000, with an error of approximately 2%. Accumulation of counts greater than 10,000 is usually not required and leads to an unnecessary increase in counting time.

(ii) Background counts and background subtraction. A well-maintained well crystal should not yield more than 50 counts per minute as background. This can usually be ignored, and background subtraction is unnecessary. High background counts (100 cpm or more) may occur for several reasons: (i) mis-setting of controls, (ii) isotope contamination of the crystal, (iii) contamination of a carrier, and

TABLE 12.1   The Characteristics of Commonly Used Isotopes (^{125}I, ^{14}C, and ^{3}H)

	Half-life	Atoms/Ci	Detection efficiency (%)	No. of atoms equivalent to 1 detectable atom of ^{125}I
^{125}I	60 days	1.77×10^{17}	80	1
^{14}C	5730 years	9.65×10^{21}	85	37,010
^{3}H	12.26 years	2.08×10^{19}	55	51.6

(iv) presence of a powerful radioactive source near the crystals. The major problem is contamination of a crystal; this may require repeated washing with detergent and ethanol, and unless carried out with great care the thallium coating can be damaged.

(iii) Precipitates, liquids, paper strips, etc. can be counted in any type of plastic tube which will fit the well of the crystal. If there is a choice between counting the bound fraction and counting the free fraction (e.g., between the precipitate and the supernatant with most separation procedures), the smaller of the two fractions (usually the bound) should be counted.

3. CHARACTERISTICS OF A TRACER

The tracer in an immunoassay system should behave as nearly identically as possible with the unlabeled material (antigen or antibody). By definition, though, it will be slightly different from the unlabeled material. The difference may arise from the sheer presence of the label on the molecule. It may also arise because of alterations in the molecule, or the introduction of impurities in the course of preparation. The general term for variations in the tracer which alter its binding properties is "damage." Any tracer or fraction of the tracer which reacts with a lower affinity than that of the unlabeled ligand or antibody can be described as damaged.

4. PREPARATION OF TRACERS

An isotopic label may be internal or external. With an internal label, an existing atom in the molecule is replaced by a radioactive isotope of that atom (e.g., ^{14}C for ^{12}C, ^3H for ^1H). The tracer should then be virtually identical with the unlabeled ligand. With an external label, an atom of a radioactive isotope (e.g., ^{125}I) is covalently linked to an existing atom on the ligand molecule. This type of tracer is, by definition, not identical with the unlabeled ligand, though in practice its behavior may be virtually identical.

Tracers with an internal label are now used only in research assays for small molecules such as steroid hormones or drugs.

5. IODINATED TRACERS

In RIA the only commonly used isotope is ^{125}I. The use of this will be described in some detail. Less commonly used γ-emitting isotopes include ^{131}iodine, ^{57}cobalt (for vitamin B_{12}; also for thyroxine (2)), ^{75}selenium (in an RIA for cortisol), and ^{32}phosphorus (for labeling of the core antigen of hepatitis B (3)).

6. IODINATION METHODS

Iodine can be substituted onto the aromatic side-chain of tyrosine residues to yield a stable compound which is a highly efficient tracer. Iodine may also substitute onto other amino acids such as histidine and phenylalanine, but the rate of the latter reaction is 30–80 times less than that for tyrosine. The precise nature and location of the substitution onto tyrosine varies with specific activity, the nature of the peptide molecule, and the method for iodination. At low levels of specific activity (one atom of iodine per molecule or less) most substitutions are single (i.e., mono-iodotyrosine); at higher levels of activity diiodotyrosine may be formed. In a given peptide molecule, tyrosine residues may differ widely in their accessibility. Thus, insulin has four tyrosines, in positions 14 and 19 on the A chain, and 16 and 26 on the B chain; most iodine substitution occurs at A14, some at A19, and very few at B16 or B26 (4).

The so-called "direct" methods have in common the conversion of iodide (I^-), which is relatively unreactive, into a more reactive species such as free iodine (I_2), or positively charged iodine radicals (I^+). The basic chemistry of this reaction is poorly understood. The "indirect" methods involve conjugation of ligand to a molecule already labeled with iodine.

6.1. Chloramine T

Chloramine T (5) is an oxidizing agent which can convert iodide to a more reactive form. The procedure requires only mixing of solutions of the protein, sodium iodide (^{125}I), and chloramine T; the reaction is ended by adding a reducing agent, sodium metabisulfite. Practical aspects of the procedure are described below.

6.2. Lactoperoxidase (EC 1.11.1.7)

Enzymatic iodination using lactoperoxidase (6, 7) in the presence of a trace of hydrogen peroxide has the advantage that the peptide is not exposed to large amounts of a chemical oxidizing agent (chloramine T). Thus, use of glucose oxidase (EC 1.1.3.4), which generates hydrogen peroxide from glucose *in situ*, still further reduces the potential for damage. In addition, a reducing agent is not needed since simple dilution will stop the reaction. As an alternative, the lactoperoxidase can be coupled to a solid phase and removed by centrifugation (8).

Tracers prepared by this technique are claimed to suffer less damage than those prepared by the chloramine T method (7, 8), and free iodine is not released into the solution. However, comparison with fully optimized methods using small amounts of chloramine T have shown virtually no difference between the two methods when applied to small peptides (9). Lactoperoxidase has the disadvantage that the preparation of the reagents and the conditions of the reaction itself are more technically demanding than those for chloramine T.

6.3. Iodogen (10)

A sparingly soluble oxidizing agent (1,3,4,6-tetrachlor-3-6-diphenyl-glycouril) is evaporated onto the walls of a reaction vessel from a solution in methylene chloride. The material to be iodinated and ^{125}iodine are added. The reaction ends when the mixture is removed from the vessel and addition of reducing agent is not required.

6.4. Conjugation Labeling

For this procedure a carrier molecule is used: the carrier incorporates a phenol or imidazole group which can be iodinated, and an amine group which can be coupled directly to carboxyl groups on the ligand or its derivatives (11) (Figs. 12.2 and 12.3). There are also carriers for conjugation to amine groups on the ligand (e.g., fluorescein isothiocyanate, N-acetyl-l-histidine). The carrier may be iodinated either before or after attachment to the ligand.

Conjugation labeling has several advantages over direct iodination: it is less damaging to the ligand, it can be applied to peptides without tyrosine residues, the final reaction (mixing of the iodinated ester and the peptide) is very simple, and it can be applied to nonpeptide materials (e.g., steroid hormones) which cannot be iodinated directly. The disadvantages include: (i) the substituted label is considerably larger than the iodine atom and may lead to physicochemical alteration of the tracer; (ii) with haptens such as steroids and drugs, the tracer may bind well to antibody but fail to be displaced by unlabeled material, i.e., a "flat" standard curve; this occurs because the antiserum contains populations of high-affinity antibodies directed toward the bridge between the hapten and the tag (Fig. 12.4). Sometimes this problem can be solved by selection of a particular antiserum (12), by using disequilibrium conditions, or by choosing different bridges or bridge sites for the immunogen and the tracer (13, 14). As a general rule, the steric bulk of the tracer bridge should be greater than that of the immunogen (e.g., in a progesterone assay, an 11-hemisuccinate conjugate should be used for immunisation and an 11-glucuronide conjugate for labeling (15); (iii) iodotyrosine or iodohistamine can itself bind to serum proteins, especially thyroxine-binding globulin, and thus produce artifacts in unextracted samples (16).

6.5. Choice of Iodination Procedure

Many protein molecules are simple to iodinate and yield robust products. For these all methods are equally suitable. Other molecules are more difficult to iodinate and the products may be unstable (ferritin is particularly notorious). The best

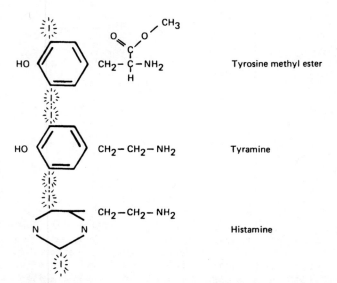

FIGURE 12.2 Compounds which can be used as a "handle" for the indirect attachment of ^{125}I to the ligand. (Modified from Chard, 1990.)

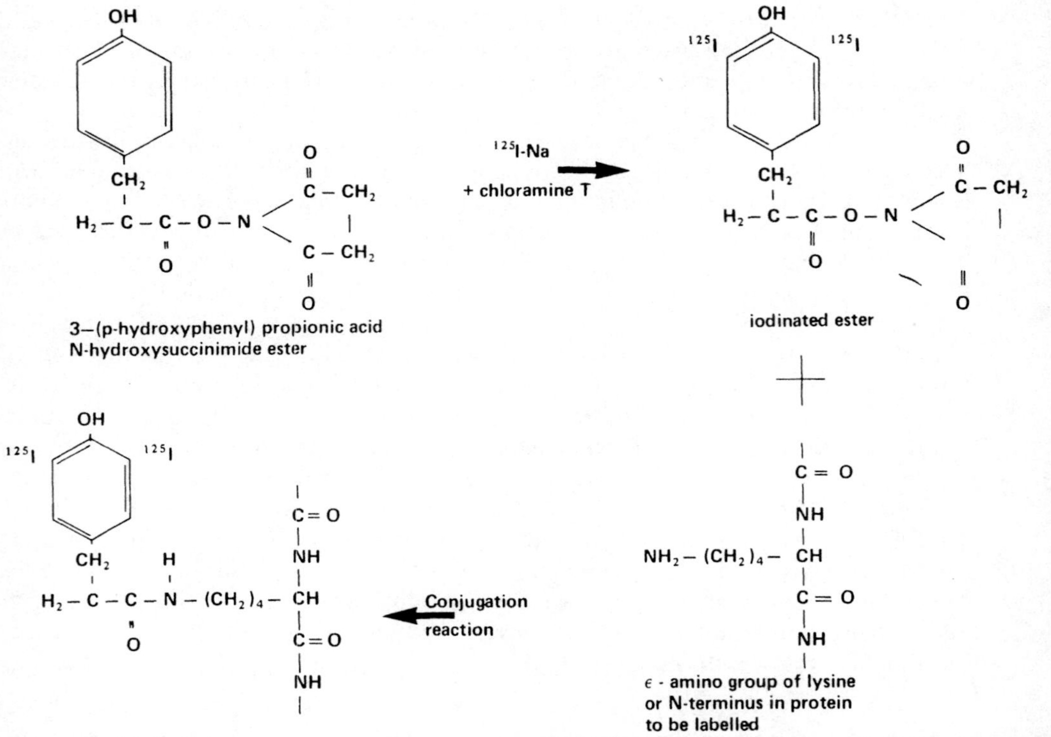

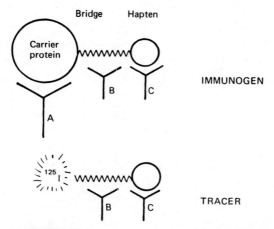

FIGURE 12.3   Schematic of the conjugation labeling technique. (Modified from Chard, 1990.)

FIGURE 12.4   A problem with the conjugation labeling of small molecules (haptens). The antiserum will contain populations of antibodies directed to the carrier protein (A), the hapten (C), and the bridge between the two (B). If the tracer contains the same bridge, then it will be firmly bound by antibodies to the bridge and cannot be displaced by pure hapten (i.e., standard or endogenous material). Greatest sensitivity and slope are achieved when the bridge is dissimilar to that in the immunogen, but unfortunately specificity is often best when the label and immunogen are similar. (Modified from Chard, 1990.)

method has to be found by trial and error, remembering that different preparations of the same molecule may vary in their iodination properties, and that published opinions on the value of different methods are often conflicting.

As a generalization, chloramine T should be tried first. If this does not yield a satisfactory product, then attempts should be made with iodogen or lactoperoxidase. Finally, with the most problematic molecules, conjugation labeling should be considered. With haptens such as steroids the various forms of conjugation labeling are the only possible approach.

6.6. Practical Aspects of Chloramine T Iodination

A procedure for the iodination of a protein using the chloramine T technique is shown in Table 12.2. The exact conditions may vary but should follow certain general principles:

(i) Concentration of reagents: the concentration of all reagents in the reaction mixture should be as high as possible. Usually, this means using the minimum possible volumes.

(ii) Amount of chloramine T: the smallest possible amount should be used. Although originally 50 μg was used, amounts of 10 or even 2 μg are often found to be effective. The minimum required can only be established by trial and error.

(iii) pH of reagents: the pH optimum for the iodination of tyrosine residues is 7.5; above pH 8 there is a tendency for other groups to be substituted and above pH 9 the reaction becomes highly inefficient. Iodine isotopes are usually supplied

TABLE 12.2 Preparation of an Iodinated Protein by Chloramine T (Iodinated hPL)

Diluent buffer: 0.05 M, phosphate, pH 7.4, with no added protein

1. Dissolve purified hPL (50 μg) in 0.02 ml buffer in a small conical vial. It is convenient to prepare aliquots of this type for iodination by freeze-drying the appropriate volume of a solution of hPL in a series of such vials.
2. Add 2 mCi carrier-free sodium ^{125}I (volume approx. 0.02 ml) (obtained from Amersham International, code IMS 30, or similar supplier).
3. Add chloramine T (10 μg) in 0.02 ml buffer. The solution should be freshly prepared immediately before the iodination.
4. Mix thoroughly but briefly (10–15 sec) by flicking with a finger; avoid splashing.
5. Immediately add sodium metabisulfite (20 μg) in 0.02 ml buffer. Mix.
6. Add 0.5 ml diluent buffer containing 2 mg/ml bovine serum albumin.
7. Transfer carefully to a 1 × 15-cm (approx) column of Sephadex G-75, previously washed with diluent buffer containing 2 mg/ml bovine serum albumin.
8. Elute with same diluent buffer. Collect fractions of approximately 0.5 ml.
9. Assess tracer.
10. Store tracer as deep-frozen aliquots.

Note. The procedure outlined has a wide range of possible variations, particularly in the relative amounts of label and protein. However, certain general points should be stated: (i) The volumes of addition should be as small as possible in order to maintain high concentrations. (ii) The amount of chloramine T should be kept to a minimum. (iii) For this type of iodination, which yields one main protein peak and an iodide peak on gel filtration, the column can be relatively small. Total running time is around 30 min and the fractions can be collected manually. In cases where the protein fraction is very heterogeneous a larger column and longer running time are necessary.

as a solution in 0.1 *N* NaOH, and the composition of the other reactants must be such as to buffer this to pH 7.5.

(iv) Mixing of reagents: a common fault leading to poor yield is inadequate mixing, especially when small volumes are used. A small drop on the wall of the tube, if not shaken down into the reaction mixture, may sequestrate 50% or more of one of the reactants.

(v) Speed of mixing: the iodination reaction is virtually instantaneous. Mixing should only proceed long enough to ensure that mixing has occurred, and the whole process should not take more than 20–30 sec.

(vi) Temperature of reaction: some believe that iodination reagents should be cooled in ice.

(vii) Type of reducing agent: milder reducing agents have been suggested as an alternative to sodium metabisulfite, such as 50 μg cysteine or cysteamine (17).

(viii) Quality of isotope: when an iodination has failed it is common to attribute this to poor quality of the isotope. However, this is very unusual.

(ix) Scale of iodination: large-scale iodinations are often of better quality (yield and stability) than small-scale iodinations.

7. IODINATION DAMAGE

Damage is defined as that fraction of the labeled antigen or antibody which will not react with other components of the system. There are several possible causes:

(i) Alteration of the molecule by the presence of an iodine atom: obviously the addition of iodine can affect the reactivity of a smaller molecule more than that of a larger molecule. For example, estrogens, iodinated through their phenolic A ring, may not react with specific antisera. Sometimes the label may alter only part of the molecule and thereby affect the specificity of the system. This is illustrated diagramatically in Fig. 12.5.

(ii) Chemical damage: even mild oxidation can partly split FSH into its α and β subunits, and thus alter the specificity of the resulting assay (18).

(iii) Internal radiation: disintegration of a radioactive iodine atom can disrupt the molecule to which it is attached. In addition, the emitted radiation may generate

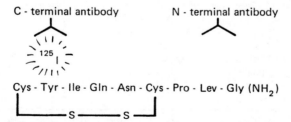

FIGURE 12.5   How iodine substitution could affect the specificity of an assay, in this case that for the nonapeptide oxytocin. If the antiserum contains two populations of antibodies, directed to the C- and N-termini of the molecule, respectively, and if the iodine completely alters the antigenicity of the N-terminus, then only the C-terminal antibodies will be effective in the assay. The assay would measure the intact molecule and C-terminal fragments of the molecule, but not N-terminal fragments. (Modified from Chard, 1990.)

free radicals during passage through the aqueous solution and thus damage other molecules. Internal radiation is not an important cause of damage in the dilute solutions in which tracers are usually stored and can be almost eliminated by including a free radical scavenger such as ethanol. However, it may be important during the actual iodination process when all reagents are at high concentration.

(iv) Decay catastrophe: This term describes the process in which the decay of an attached iodine atom disrupts a molecule bearing another and as yet undecayed iodine atom. The latter is then attached to a fragment which may no longer react with the antibodies because this is still labeled and will appear as damaged tracer in the assay. By definition this type of damage can only occur with molecules which have at least two isotopic iodine atoms. It is therefore characteristic of high specific activity tracers; both decay catastrophe and internal radiation are responsible for the fact that high-activity tracers have the shortest shelf-life in terms of damage. In most assays adequate specific activity is obtained with a substitution level of one atom of iodine per molecule or less, and higher levels should therefore be avoided.

(v) Incubation damage: tracer may be progressively damaged during the assay itself because of the presence of damaging agents in the incubation mixture.

(vi) Impurity damage: the so-called "pure" antigen or antibody used for iodination are often contaminated with irrelevant materials which, since they may take up label but may not react in the system, can be described as damage.

(vii) Iodine release: Deiodination can occur on storage, notably with preparations containing substituents other than monoiodo-tyrosine (19). Free iodide is often the principal component of the damaged tracer (20).

8. COMPARISON OF LABELED AND UNLABELED LIGAND

Several methods are available to compare labeled and unlabeled ligand:

(i) Comparison of iodinated material with material carrying an internal label such as ^{3}H.

(ii) Comparison with unlabeled ligand (21): tubes are prepared which contain a fixed amount of antibody and tracer; to one set, serial dilutions of unlabeled ligand are added; to the other, identical serial concentrations of tracer are added. If the tracer is undamaged, the tubes will contain identical amounts of total ligand and the curves will be superimposable.

(iii) Comparison of the physicochemical properties of the tracer and the unlabeled ligand.

(iv) Comparison of the biological properties of tracer and unlabeled ligand. For example, growth hormone retains full biological activity even with iodine substitution of 2.7 atoms/molecule (22).

9. PURIFICATION OF IODINATED TRACER

The reaction mixture following iodination contains: unlabeled ligand (damaged and undamaged), labeled ligand (damaged and undamaged), free iodide, and salts including the oxidizing and reducing agent. Most standard physicochemical separation procedures can be applied to purification, and should be efficient, simple, and rapid. Several procedures will be described here, though the only commonly used technique for proteins is gel-filtration chromatography.

(i) Dilution: the iodination mixture is usually diluted with albumin-containing buffer once the primary reaction is complete. This reduces the possibility of damage due to internal radiation or high concentrations of chemical agents.

(ii) Adsorption: batchwise addition of ion-exchange resin can remove free iodide and salts from the diluted reaction mixture.

(iii) Ion-exchange chromatography: with the use of appropriate gradients this can readily separate minor variants of a peptide, including damaged and undamaged material, and uniodinated and iodinated material (9). However, it is used relatively little in practice because it can be time-consuming and laborious.

(iv) Group-specific adsorbent chromatography: absorption to concanavalin A–Sepharose, followed by elution with α-methyl-D-glucoside, may considerably improve the immunoreactivity of glycoproteins such as iodinated TSH.

(v) Gel-filtration chromatography: this is the most commonly used technique for purifying iodinated tracers. Column size and material will vary according to the ligand. If it is intended to separate reasonably homogeneous labeled material from free iodide then a small column (e.g., 10 × 0.5 cm) of a low porosity gel (Sephadex G-25 or G-50) will suffice. However, if the tracer is likely to be heterogeneous then a larger column should be used (e.g., G-75, G-100, or G-200). Larger columns are almost always desirable with iodinated proteins because these will very commonly show some degree of heterogeneity (Fig. 12.6).

(vi) Thin-layer chromatography: this is used in the purification of low-molecular-weight tracer ligands, such as steroids and drugs.

(vii) Electrophoresis: separation and purification of ^{131}I-insulin on the basis of the level of iodine substitution was originally demonstrated using starch gel electrophoresis (23). Similar separations have been achieved with isoelectric focusing (24), but the procedure is laborious.

(viii) Immunopurification: a tracer can be separated from irrelevant materials by exposure to solid-phase antibody followed by washing and elution. Relatively low-affinity antibodies can be used and may be desirable since they avoid the damage associated with extreme conditions of elution. A similar approach has been used in the immunoradiometric assay (25) in which purified antibody can be iodinated while actually in combination with solid-phase antigen.

Because of the possibility of progressive damage to the labeled antigen, some workers repurify each stored aliquot by chromatography, after it is thawed for use. This is effective, but very time consuming for a routine assay.

10. CHEMICAL EVALUATION OF TRACER

Chemical evaluation is designed to ascertain the yield, the specific activity, and the absolute concentrations of the tracer. "Yield" is defined as the percentage incorporation of the isotope into the labeled material. Specific activity of the tracer is the radioactivity per unit mass or mole of ligand (e.g., mCi/μg). Concentration of the tracer is simply mass per unit volume. Though this parameter is highly important in assay design, the calculation is often ignored and the tracer distributed as "counts" rather than concentration. If a high proportion of tracer is damaged,

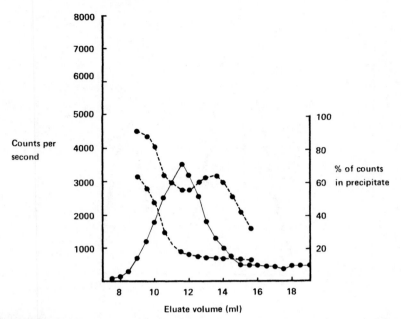

FIGURE 12.6 Chromatography of iodinated pregnancy specific β 1-glycoprotein (MW 80,000) on a 40 × 1-cm column of Sephadex G-200 eluted with phosphate buffer containing 1 mg/ml bovine serum albumin. There is a single but rather broad peak of radioactive protein (—) (the free iodide peak appeared in later fractions and is not shown here). A small aliquot from each fraction was incubated with and without an excess of antibody, and the bound fraction was precipitated with 20% polyethylene glycol. The dashed lines (---) show the percentage of counts precipitated in the presence (upper line) and absence (lower line) of antibody. The earliest fractions give very high blank values, probably due to the presence of aggregates, and would not be suitable for use in an assay. The best fractions are those on the trailing edge of the protein peak which gives the highest antibody bound levels in the presence of a relatively low blank (data kindly supplied by A.T.M. Al-Ani). (Modified from Chard, 1990.)

corrections should be made so that the concentration refers only to undamaged material.

These three parameters can be assessed from the results of the physicochemical purification procedure (Fig. 12.7), with certain provisos. Substantial losses may occur due to absorption onto surfaces such as those of the pipettes, the reaction vessel, and the chromatography matrix. A further problem arises with procedures which separate damaged and undamaged tracer: calculation of specific activity and concentration of the undamaged form is based on the assumption that the level of iodine substitution is equivalent for both. But this may not be true: a small peak of radioactivity could represent a very large amount of protein with a low level of iodination.

It can also be of great value in the setting-up of an assay to estimate the number of iodine atoms per molecule of ligand. This can be worked out from the specific activity expressed in molar terms (the specific activity of ^{125}I at 100% isotopic abundance is approximately 1.8 mCi per nanomole). For example, assume that 20 μg of a peptide hormone of molecular weight 20 kDa is iodinated with 1 mCi of ^{125}I, with a yield of 90%. Ninety percent of 2 mCi is 1.8 mCi, equivalent to

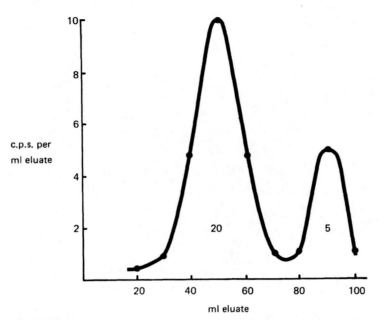

FIGURE 12.7 Theoretical example to illustrate calculation of yield, specific activity, and tracer concentrations after chromatography of an iodinated protein. There are 20 "counts" in the protein peak (first) and 5 in the later iodide peak. Thus the yield is 20/25 or 80%. Assuming that the amount of protein iodinated was 10 μg and the amount of ^{125}I used was 1 mCi the specific activity is 80 μCi/μg. The protein peak has a volume of 40 ml and the concentration of the pooled tracer is 0.25 μg/ml. (Modified from Chard, 1990.)

1 nmol of iodine. Twenty micrograms of the hormone is also equivalent to 1 nmol. The level of substitution is therefore one atom of iodine per molecule of hormone. All other things being equal, substitution of one atom per molecule can be regarded as the optimum; higher levels can alter the immunoreactivity of a molecule, and increase the likelihood of di-substitution with consequent decay catastrophe. Lower levels are not necessary because the tracer will simply be diluted by unlabeled ligand molecules.

11. IMMUNOLOGICAL EVALUATION OF TRACER

This is the most important evaluation of a newly prepared tracer. An aliquot of the pooled tracer is tested for binding in the presence and absence of antibody. The results are compared with previous iodinations to determine performance in terms of assay blank and maximum binding. Sometimes these parameters are not an adequate guide to performance in the assay, and a standard curve and quality controls may have to be included as part of the assessment procedure. When an assay is being developed it is useful to test each individual fraction from a chromatography: frequently this will reveal heterogeneity within the protein peak itself, suggesting that only selected fractions should be used in the assay (see Figs. 12.6 and 12.7).

12. VARIATIONS ON THE USE OF RADIOLABELED TRACERS

12.1. Universal Tracers

Protein A from staphylococci can bind specifically to the Fc region of immuno-globulin molecules and has been used in the separation of bound and free ligand. Protein A has also been used as a "universal tracer" (26). Antibody and ligand are incubated; solid-phase ligand is added and absorbs "free" antibody; the amount of antibody on the solid phase is then measured by addition of ^{125}I-labeled protein A.

A further ingenious suggestion for a universal tracer is the use of purified ^{125}I-labeled antibodies to 2,4-dinitrophenyl (DNP). The primary antibody is labeled with DNP; the anti-DNP is then used as a tracer for bound antibody in a two-site immunometric system.

12.2. Autoradiographic Radioimmunoassay

The assay is set out in a multiwell test plate. After separation of bound and free ligand the plate is exposed to x-ray film; the size and density of the resulting spots reflects the amount of radioactivity (27). The procedure is probably less precise than conventional techniques but might be suitable for assays in which a semiquantitative result is required.

12.3. Internal Sample Attenuators

Incorporation of bismuth oxide into a solid phase effectively blocks radioactive emission from this phase; the liquid phase can then be counted without separation (28, 29).

12.4. Liposome Immunoassay

Antigens are inserted into iodine or fluorescein-labeled lipid vesicles which can be precipitated by antiserum (30).

12.5. Biosynthesized Tracers

Beta-lipotropin (β-LPH) incorporating ^{35}S-methionine, synthesized by pituitary tumor cells, has been used as a recovery marker in assays for this peptide (31).

12.6. Scintillation Proximity Radioimmunoassay

Antibody is linked to microbeads containing a fluorophore. ^{125}I-Antigen binds to the beads: short-range electrons from the ^{125}I excite the fluorophore, and the emitted light can be measured in a scintillation counter (32, 33). This avoids the need for separation of the bound and free fractions. The same approach can also be used for counting β-emitting isotopes (e.g., ^{3}H) without liquid scintillant.

12.7. Double Tracers

Simultaneous determination of LH and FSH has been described using ^{57}Co-FSH and ^{125}I-LH (34).

References

1. Klee GG, Post G. Effect of counting errors on immunoassay precision. Clin Chem 1989; 35:1362–6.
2. Al-Awadi S, Hassan M, Adham K, *et al.* The preparation of a new 57-cobalt-labelled thyroxine for use in single/dual radioimmunoassay techniques. J Immunol Methods 1988; 108:27–32.
3. Wolff W, Gerlich WH. Direct radioimmunoassay of antibody against hepatitis B core antigen using 32-P-labelled core particles. Eur J Clin Microbiol 1984; 3:25–9.
4. Freedlender A, Cathou RE. Iodination. In: Kirkham KE, Hunter WM, Eds. Radioimmunoassay Methods: European Workshop. Edinburgh: Churchill Livingstone, 1971:94–6.
5. Greenwood FC, Hunter WM. The preparation of 131-I-labelled human growth hormone of high specific radioactivity. Biochem J 1963; 89:114–23.
6. Marchalonis JJ. An enzymic method for the trace iodination of immunoglobulins and other proteins. Biochem J 1969; 113:299–305.
7. Thorell JI, Johansson BG. Enzymatic iodination of polypeptides with 125-I to high specific activity. Biochim Biophys Acta 1971; 251:363–369.
8. Karonen S-L, Morsky P, Siren M, *et al.* An enzymatic solid-phase method for trace iodination of proteins and peptides with 125-iodine. Anal Biochem 1975; 67:1–10.
9. Heber D, Odell WD, Schedewie H, *et al.* Improved iodination of peptides for radioimmunoassay and membrane radioreceptor assay. Clin Chem 1978; 24:769–99.
10. Fraker PJ, Speck JC. Protein and cell membrane iodinations with a sparingly soluble chloramide, 1,3,4,6-tetrachloro-3a,6a-diphenylglycoluril. Biochem Biophys Res Commun 1978; 80:849–857.
11. Bolton AE, Hunter WM. The labelling of proteins to high specific radioactivities by conjugation to a 125-I-containing acylating agent. Biochem J 1973; 133:529–39.
12. Jeffcoate SL. Progress towards the wider use of better steroid immunoassays. J Steroid Biochem 1979; 11:1051–5.
13. England BG, Niswender GD, Rees Midgley A. Radioimmunoassay of estradiol-17 beta without chromatography. J Clin Endocrinol Metab 1974; 3842:42–50.
14. Nordbloom GD, Webb R, Counsell RE, *et al.* A chemical approach to solving bridging phenomena in steroid radioimmunoassays. Steroids 1981; 38:161–4.
15. Corrie JET, Ratcliffe WA, Macpherson JS. The provision of 125-I-labelled tracers for radioimmunoassay of haptens: a general approach. J Immunol Methods 1982; 51:159–66.
16. Painter K, Vader CR. Interference of iodine-125 ligands in radioimmunoassay: evidence implicating thyroxine-binding globulin. Clin Chem 1979; 25:797–9.
17. Brown NS, Abbott SR, Corrie JET. Some observations on the preparation, purification and storage of radioiodinated protein hormones. In: Hunter WM, Corrie JET, Eds. Immunoassays for Clinical Chemistry, 2nd ed. Edinburgh: Churchill Livingstone, 1983:267–76.
18. Marana R, Suginami H, Robertson DM, *et al.* Influence of the purity of the iodinated tracer on the specificity of the radioimmunoassay of human follicle-stimulating hormone. Acta Endocrinol 1979; 92:585–98.
19. Krohn KA, Knight LC, Harwig JF, *et al.* Differences in the sites of iodination of proteins following four methods of radioiodination. Biochim Biophys Acta 1977; 490:497–503.
20. Bauman G, Amburn K. The autodecomposition of radiolabeled human growth hormone. J Immunoassay 1986; 7:139–149.
21. Hunter WM. The preparation and assessment of iodinated antigens. In: Kirkham KE, Hunrwe QM, Eds. Radioimmunoassay Methods: European Workshop. Edinburgh: Churchill Livingstone, 1971:3–23.
22. Bartolini P, Ribela MTCP. Influence of chloramine T iodination on the biological and immunological activity of the molecular radius of the human growth hormone molecule. J Immunoassay 1986; 7:129–38.
23. Berson SA, Yalow RS. Iodoinsulin used to determine specific activity of iodine-131. Science 1966; 152:205–6.
24. Dermody WC, Levy AG, Davis PE, *et al.* Heterogeneity of chloramine T- and lactoperoxidase-radioiodinated human calcitonin. Clin Chem 1979; 25:989–95.
25. Miles LEM, Hales CN. The preparation and properties of purified 125-I-labelled antibodies to insulin. Biochem J 1968; 108:611–8.
26. Langone KJ. 125-I protein A: a tracer for general use in immunoassay. J Immunol Methods 1978; 24:269–85.
27. Weiler EW, Zenk MH. Autoradiographic immunoassay (ARIA): a rapid technique for the semiquantitative mass screening of haptens. Anal Biochem 1979; 92:147–55.

28. Thorell JI. Internal sample attenuator counting (ISAC). A new technique for separating and measuring bound and free activity in radioimmunoassays. Clin Chem 1981; 27:1969–73.
29. Erikson H, Mattiasson B, Thorell JI. Combination of solid-phase second antibody and internal sample attenuator counting techniques. Radioimmunoassay of thyroid-stimulating hormone. J Immunol Methods 1984; 71:117–25.
30. Axelsson B, Eriksson H, Borrebaeck C, Mattiasson B, Sjogren HO. Liposome immune assay (LIA). Use of membrane antigens inserted into labeled lipid vesicles as targets in immune assays. J Immunol Methods 1981; 41:351–63.
31. Rosendale BE, Jarrett DB. Biosynthesized [35-S] methionine-labelled pro-opiomelanocortin peptides as novel recovery markers in radioimmunoassay of peptide hormones. Clin Chem 1985; 31:1965–8.
32. Udenfriend S, Gerber L, Nelson N. Scintillation proximity assay: a sensitive and continuous isotopic method for monitoring ligand/receptor and antigen/antibody interactions. Anal Biochem 1987; 161:494–500.
33. Pallesen T, Vangsted A, Drivsholm L, Clausen H, Zeuthen J, Wallin H. Serum immunoassay of a small cell lung cancer associated ganglioside: development of a sensitive scintillation proximity assay. Glycoconjugate J 1992; 9:331–5.
34. Wians FH, Dev J, Powell MM, Heald JI. Evaluation of simultaneous measurement of lutropin and follitropin with Simul-TROPIN (TM) radioimmunoassay kit. Clin Chem 1986; 32:887–90.

13 | ENZYME IMMUNOASSAY

JAMES P. GOSLING
Department of Biochemistry and National Diagnostic Centre
University College
Galway, Ireland

1. INTRODUCTION

Enzymes are the most versatile and popular class of labeling substances used for immunoassays and they have an assured future. The invention of immunoenzymatic staining in the mid-1960s can be said to have been the beginning of enzyme immunoassay (EIA), and this enabled the preparation of permanent photomicroscopic slides with visualization of specific antigens (1, 2). In 1971 enzymes were introduced as alternatives to radioisotopes in immunoassays (3–5). EIA has been the primary subject of a number of books (6–15) and reviews (16–22), and an important concern of other recent books and reviews (23–28).

1.1. Representing Assay Complexes in Text

The complexes formed in assay systems can readily be represented by one-line formulae. For emphasis, the analyte is shown in bold print (e.g., "**Ag,**" "**Ha,**" or "**Ab**" for the general analytes antigen, hapten, and antibody, respectively), a hyphen

("-") represents associations established before commencement of the assay (e.g., conjugations or the coating of antibody onto a solid phase), and the en dash ("–") represents associations formed during the course of the assay procedure. Unusual components are accomodated by spelling out their names. For example, the final complex of a solid-phase (sp) immunoenzymometric assay (IEMA) for an antigen in which biotin is used as primary label is described as: sp-Ab–**Ag**–Ab-biotin–avidin-enzyme. Standard abbreviations are used when the type of antibody (monoclonal, mAb) or antibody fragment (Fab', F[ab']$_2$) or its origin (mouse, M; rabbit, R) is relevant.

2. ENZYMES AS LABELING SUBSTANCES

2.1. Advantages

The general suitability of a labeling substance depends on it having a combination of advantagous physiochemical properties. Enzymes score very well under the criteria for a good labeling substance, except that they are invariably of high molecular weight. Large enzyme-containing conjugates diffuse slowly and may have a greater tendency to bind nonspecifically to reaction vessels, etc., than some other labels. In addition, although properly stored enzyme conjugates usually have shelf lives measured in years, enzymes are more susceptible to inactivation by environmental factors than fluorescent or chemiluminescent compounds. Of the nonisotopic labeling substances, enzymes are measurable by the greatest variety of methods and, with secondary amplification, are measurable in the smallest molecular quantities (see below).

2.2. Variety

Enzymes are perhaps the most varied class of labeling substances and Table 13.1 lists a selection of 10 from the large number of enzymes that have been tested as immunoassay labels. About 1990, the most common enzyme label in new immunoassays was horseradish peroxidase, with alkaline phosphatase in second place (26). A perusal of current issues of relevant journals confirms that this is still true and

TABLE 13.1 Some Enzymes Used as Immunoassay Labels

Enzyme	Source	Enzyme Commission (EC) No.	References
Acetylcholinesterase	*Electrophorus electricus*	3.1.1.7	19, 29
Alkaline phosphatase	Calf intestine	3.1.3.1	20, 30–35
Catalase	Liver	1.11.1.6	19
β-D-Galactosidase	*Escherichia coli*	3.2.1.23	20, 36–38
Glucose oxidase	*Aspergillus niger*	1.1.3.4	19
Glucose-6-phosphate dehydrogenase	*Leuconostoc Mesenteroides*	1.1.1.49	39
β-Lactamase	Bacillus species	3.5.2.6	26, 40
Peroxidase	Horseradish	1.11.1.7	20, 41–44
Pyrophosphatase	*Escherichia coli*	3.6.1.1	45
Urease	Jack bean	3.5.1.5	46

no other enzyme seems likely to challenge their positions in the near future. The popularity of horseradish peroxidase is largely due to its high turnover number, the sensitivity of its colorimetric and luminometric assay systems, its suitability for diverse conjugation procedures [because it is a glycoprotein the "periodate method" may be used (see 11)] and small molecular size (40,000 compared to 100,000 and 500,000 Da for alkaline phosphatase and β-galactosidase, respectively). Alkaline phosphatase is favored for both high-performance and easy-to-use immunoassays because of its simple reaction kinetics, the variety of assay systems available (see below), and the relatively low toxicity of its common substrates. β-D-Galactosidase is sometimes favored when a low detection limit is required and when equipment for fluorimetric determination of the endpoint is available (37, 38). Acetylcholinesterase and β-lactamase are other enzymes characterized by very high turnover numbers and good long-term stability, and they have had many applications (e.g., 29, 40). Glucose-6-phosphate dehydrogenase is common in labels for Enzyme-Multiplied Immunoassay Technique (EMIT) assays (39).

With the growing popularity of biotin and other ligands as primary labeling molecules (26) enzymes are increasingly being used as secondary labels.

2.3. Enzymes as Secondary Labels

Quite often the label determined at the end of an immunoassay procedure is not the primary label; some primary–secondary label combinations used in enzyme immunoassays are listed in Table 13.2. This trend started with the employment of a labeled "second" antibody in solid-phase immunoassays for antigen. For example, if the analyte binds to immobilized sheep antibody (SAb) and unlabeled rabbit antibody (RAb) is used to complete the sandwich (sp-SAb–**Ag**–RAb), the concentration of the bound rabbit antibody may be determined with a labeled goat antibody (GAb) raised against whole rabbit IgG or its Fc fragment (sp-SAb–**Ag**–RAb–GAb-HRP). Here the constant region of the rabbit IgG can logically be said to be the primary labeling substance. Alternatively, protein A–enzyme conjugate can be used as a general purpose reagent for the quantification of immobilized Fc (54). The use of biotin conjugated to antibody (or antigen/hapten) as primary label, with labeled avidin or streptavidin as a secondary label, is a logical, universally applicable extension of the above approach (see Chapter 11). The concentration of biotinylated antibody can be determined by means of avidin conjugated to an enzyme. The use of the avidin–biotin combination is usually justified by citing the high affinity of steptavidin or avidin for biotin ($K_a = 10^{15} M^{-1}$), but a recent study indicated that the affinities of avidin and an anti-biotin monoclonal antibody for biotinylated

TABLE 13.2 Some Enzyme Immunoassays with Secondary Labels

Secondary label	Primary label	References
Anti-FITC–enzyme	Anti-analyte–FITC	47
Anti-species IgG–enzyme	Same-species anti-analyte (IgG)	48–50
Avidin–enzyme	Anti-analyte–biotin	51–53
Biotin–enzyme + avidin	Anti-analyte–biotin	51
Protein A (or G)–enzyme	Anti-analyte (IgG)	54, 55

proteins are similar and much lower than for free biotin (56). Fluorescein isothiocyanate (FITC) is also used to prepare primary labels (rather than to prepare fluorimetric labels), and the concentration of FITC–antigen or FITC–antibody is then determined by means of enzyme-labeled monoclonal antibody to FITC (47).

2.4. Multienzyme Complexes

A recurring approach to maximizing the final signal obtained in immunoassays is to attempt to attach multiple molecules of the final labeling substance to each immune complex to be detected (51, 57). This may be achieved by manipulation of the biotin–avidin system (51; see Chapter 11), or, in enzyme immunoassays, by the use of antibodies to the labeling enzyme. For example, in an assay for lymphocytic antigens (**Ag**) (57) three reagents were used: mouse antibody to antigen (Mab1), complexes of enzyme and mouse anti-enzyme antibodies [(MAb2-β-D-galactosidase)$_n$], and rabbit anti-mouse IgG as bridging molecule (RAb). These were employed with the intention of bringing about the association of multiple copies of the enzyme with each analyte molecule to be detected (sp-lymphocyte-**Ag**–MAb1–RAb–[MAb2-β-D-galactosidase]$_n$). In general, attempts to amplify the signal by assembling large label-containing complexes are inherently limited by steric effects and by high nonspecific binding of label. Therefore, although such tactics may be advantageous in certain circumstances, they are not usually considered relevant to the development of immunoassays with very low detection limits.

Alternatively, the use of liposomes, loaded with many enzyme molecules, as primary labeling substances (58) may lead to amplification when the lysis of each vesicle releases many copies of the trapped enzyme. Such assays are usually "separation-free" (see below).

2.5. Enzymes as Ancillary Reagents

The term enzyme-mediated immunoassay (10) encompasses, as well as all assays with enzymes as labeling substance, assays (usually separation-free) with labels containing enzyme substrates, enzyme inhibitors, coenzymes, or enzyme cofactors. The operation of such assays depends on the use of one or more enzymes as ancillary reagents. Enzymes are also exploited in many other ways for the benefit of immunoassays (Table 13.3).

3. CONJUGATION PROCEDURES

To prepare conjugates with enzyme, the method of conjugation used should be particularly mild so as to retain both immuno- and enzymatic activities. It should also give conjugates which are stable.

3.1. Enzyme–Protein Conjugates

3.1.1. Glutaraldehyde Methods

Glutaraldehyde, a homobifunctional reagent, is very simple to use for linking together proteins via lysine ε-amino and N-terminal groups. In two-step procedures

TABLE 13.3   Examples of Enzymes as Reagents in Immunoassays

Enzyme (EC number)[a]	Use	Reference
Acetylcholinesterase	Enzyme inhibitor immunoassay	59
Alcohol dehydrogenase (1.1.1.1)	Amplified assay of alkaline phosphorylase	35
Diaphorase (1.8.1.4)	Amplified assay of alkaline phosphorylase	35
	Enzyme cofactor immunoassay	59
β-D-Galacatosidase	Substrate-labeled fluorescence immunoassay	59
Glucose oxidase	Enzyme cofactor immunoassay	59
	Generation of H_2O_2 in immunochromatography	60
Lactate dehydrogenase (1.1.1.28)	Enzyme cofactor immunoassay	59
Microperoxidase (a fragment of cytochrome c)	Activation of isoluminol	61
Glucose oxidase	Generation of H_2O_2 in immunochromatography	60
Lactoperoxidase (1.11.1.7)	Radioioiodination	62
Pepsin (3.4.23.1)	Preparation of (Fab')$_2$	24
Range of enzymes for PCR	Immuno-PCR	63

[a] For EC numbers of some enzymes see Table 13.1.

one of the proteins (the enzyme for example) is first allowed to react with glutaraldehyde, the excess reagent is removed, and only then is the second protein (IgG, for example) added and the conjugate allowed to form (64). The coupling efficiency is greater, and higher activty is retained, than with one-step methods, although the recovery of enzyme activity may be very low (<10%).

3.1.2. Periodate Oxidation of Glycoproteins

The oxidation of glycoproteins with sodium periodate (e.g., horseradish peroxidase) cleaves vicinal glycols of the carbohydrate residues to generate dialdehydes capable of reacting with free amino groups on other protein molecules to form Schiff base linkages. The method has been optimized by Tijssen and Kurstak (65) who reported 90% coupling efficiency and 90% retention of peroxidase activity.

3.1.3. Heterobifunctional Reagent Methods

Such methods employ reagents which can react with two different functional groups, one on each of the two proteins to be conjugated. The functional groups most often used are α- or ε-amino (lysine), sulfydryl (cysteine), imidazole (histidine), and phenolic (tyrosine) groups (Table 13.4). While the great majority of proteins and most peptides have free amino groups, free sulfydryl groups are relatively rare in intact proteins and peptides. Important exceptions are Fab' and β-D-galactosidase from *Escherichia coli*. The reaction sequence for the conjugation of an Fab' to an enzyme with free amino groups by means of a heterobifunctional coupling reagent is shown in Fig. 13.1. Fab'–enzyme conjugates normally retain full immunological activity because of the favorable geometry of the linkage and can retain full enzymatic activity because of the mildness of the reaction conditions (42). The absence of the Fc from such conjugates greatly reduces nonspecific binding to sample components. High specific activity, low nonspecific binding conjugates prepared in this way have enabled the development of assays for antigens and specific antibodies with detection limits down to 0.02 amol per tube (20, 21). The use of single-domain Fv fragments in immunoassays may further reduce nonspecific binding and

TABLE 13.4   Reagents for Protein–Protein Coupling, and for Inserting Sulfydryl Groups into Proteins[a]

Acronym	Name	Group 1 reacts with	Group 2 reacts with
ABDP	N-(4-aminobenzoyl)-N'-(pyridyldithiopropionyl)-hydrazine	-SH	-OH (tyrosine)
DPEM	N-[β-(4-diazophenyl)ethyl]maleimide (Ref. 66)	Phenol and imidazole	-SH
—	Glutaraldehyde	-NH$_2$	-NH$_2$
HSAB	N-hydroxysuccinimidyl-4-azidobenzoate	-NH$_2$	Unspecific
MBS	m-Maleimidobenzoyl-N-hydroxysuccinimide ester	-NH$_2$	-SH
SMCC	Succinimidyl-4-(N-maleimidomethyl) cyclohexane-1-carboxylate	-NH$_2$	-SH
SATA	N-hydroxysuccinimide S-acetylthioacetic acid (inserts protected -SH)	-NH$_2$	—
SPDP	N-succinimidyl 3-(2-pyridyldithio) propionate (inserts protected -SH)	-NH$_2$	—
—	2-Iminothiolane (Traut's reagent) (inserts -SH)	-NH$_2$	—

[a] These are available from various suppliers including Pierce (Rockford, IL), Boehringer Mannheim (Mannheim, Germany), and Pharmacia (Uppsala, Sweden).

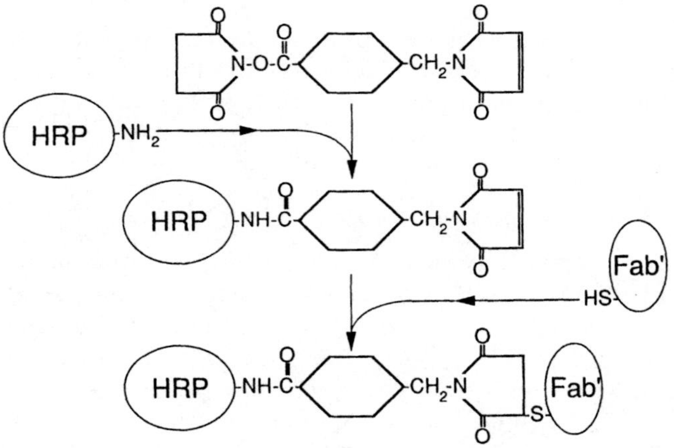

FIGURE 13.1   The conjugation of Fab' to horseradish peroxidase with N-succinimidyl 4-(N-maleimidomethyl) cyclohexane-1-carboxylate (SMCC). The cyclohexane bridge is claimed to give stability to the maleimide group. A sulfonated derivative of SMCC with improved water solubility is also available (Pierce, Rockford, IL). m-Maleimidobenzoyl-N-hydroxysuccinimide ester (MBS) has the same reactive groups but a benzoyl bridge. In the first step SMCC is reacted with a protein containing available free amino groups, and no free sulfydryl group, in this case horseradish peroxidase (HRP). The consequent maleimide-substituted HRP is then reacted with the sulfydryl-containing protein, in this case Fab'. Both reactions proceed efficiently under mild conditions which facilitate retention of enzyme and antigen-binding activities. Abdul-Ahad WG, Gosling JP. Reagent preparation. In: Gosling JP, Basso LV, Eds. Immunoassay: Laboratory and Clinical Applications. Boston, MA; Butterworth-Heinemann, 1994: 31–49.

interference from rheumatoid factors and complement and heterophilic antibodies (see also Chapter 6).

Free sulfydryl groups may be generated by reductive cleavage of native cystine residues with reagents such as dithiotreitol or mercaptoethylamine, or may be introduced chemically. One of a number of available reagents (Table 13.4) may be used, sometimes with a second step to remove a protective group and expose the sulfydryl.

3.2. Enzyme-Labeled Haptens

The most popular procedures for the preparation of enzyme–hapten conjugates link haptens to free amino or sulfydryl groups, but other groups including phenolic, imidazole, or carboxyl (glutamic or aspartic acid) can be the linkage site on the enzyme. On the hapten, a carboxyl or an amino group is most commonly used and, if necessary, one may be added by derivatization. In addition, a spacer group, four to six carbon or oxygen atoms long, between the hapten and the enzyme is usually necessary to allow adequate immunological recognition. A wide variety of common steroids (Steraloids, Wilton, NH; Sigma Chemical Company, St Louis, MO) and other haptens derivatized by the addition of potential bridging groups are available commercially. A range of haptens, including estriol, estradiol-17β, digoxin, theophylline, triiodothyronine, and thyroxine, with both bridging groups and active functions already attached are available from Boehringer Mannheim, Germany (Immunologicals for the Diagnostic Industry Catalog).

In an EIA for hapten, the type of spacer group and its site of attachment to the hapten molecule may be the same in the enzyme–hapten conjugate as in the hapten–protein immunogen used to raise the antibody (homology) or they may be different (heterology). Heterology may concern the bridging group and/or the site of attachment. Site or bridge heterology decreases the affinity of the antibody for the enzyme–hapten conjugate and it used to be widely claimed that heterology is a necessary precondition for an EIA with a low detection limit. But most hapten EIA are homologous and some of these have very low detection limits (26). The length of the spacer arm may be crucial to the operation of a separation-free assay (see below).

The optimum hapten:enzyme ratio in conjugate for an EIA should be investigated each time by preparing a range of test conjugates starting with different ratios of reactant molarities. Often, an incoropration ratio of 1:1 is suitable and a higher ratio results in a decrease in sensitivity (30). Determination of the ratio for hapten–horseradish peroxidase conjugates can be achieved by spectral differences if such exist (as they do for steroids such as progesterone), but radioactive hapten may be used as a quantifiable tracer, or an immunoassay may be used to estimate the accessible haptens. The recovery of enzyme activity should be near 100%, and there should be negligible nonspecific binding; conjugates not meeting these criteria should normally be rejected for use in high-performance assays. The most usual coupling procedures for haptens and enzymes are the mixed anhydride and active-ester procedures.

3.2.1. Mixed Anhydride Procedure

Here the carboxyl group of the hapten is first converted to an acid anhydride that is then allowed to react with a protein amino group. In our own laboratory we have often successfully used the procedure described by Munro and Stabenfeldt (67), by which the hapten reacts with isobutyl chloroformate in the presence of *N*-ethylmorpholine for 2 min at $-20°C$, and is then transferred to react with the protein at the desired molar ratio of hapten:enzyme. It is important to maintain the pH of the protein near its isoelectric point; for example, with horseradish peroxidase a pH of 8.0 should be maintained for efficient incorporation of hapten.

3.2.2. Active Ester Procedure

Here, carbodiimide is used to enable the formation of an active *N*-succinimidyl ester from the carboxyl-containing hapten and *N*-hydroxysuccinimide (30) (Fig. 13.2). The active ester can then be used directly or, more effectively, isolated in solid form. A range of such acivated derivatives of steroid and thyroid hormones is available commercially from Boehringer Mannheim.

4. DETERMINING ENZYME ACTIVITY

The versatility of enzymes as labeling substances has much to do with the range of ways, each with certain advantages, by which enzyme activity may be measured. A wide variety of assay methods have been developed for each of the longer established and most widely used labeling enzymes (Table 13.5). The simplest and least expensive of these will be considered first.

4.1. Visual Assessment

Qualitative and semiquantitative assay procedures that are not dependent on instrumentation are enabled by labeling substances that generate a change in color density, shade, area, or location (or any other visible physical or optical characteristic). Such assays are sold over-the-counter for home use as pregnancy tests, etc., or are used in doctors' offices, operating rooms, or beside the hospitalized patient, and, if inexpensive, are of great value in all situations where laboratory facilities are poor or unavailable. If the color change is permanent the assay device may be retained as a record of the result. Used in conjuction with a simple instrument, such as a reflectance-colorimeter (74), quantitative results may be calculated with reference to a standard, and an easily interpreted, printed result prepared. Although the principle of latex agglutination and the use of labeling substances such as highly colored latex beads or colloidal-gold particles are also used to give immunoassays with visible endpoints, the most widespread and sensitive of such immunoassays use enzyme-containing labels (60, 70, 74).

Most visible endpoint enzymeimmunoassays such as AccuLevel, competitive immunochromatograpy assays for drugs (60), or two-site ICON immunoconcentration assays for antigens (74) are carried out on a paper strip or a membrane. To ensure stable color development the enzyme-substrates used must be converted to a highly colored insoluble product, which precipitates onto, and remains associated with, the paper or membrane. Figure 13.3 shows the Cambridge Biotech dual-analyte, immunoconcentration assay for antibodies to HIV-I and HIV-II.

4.2. Colorimetry

Colorimetric determination is the most common of all the methods used to measure the endpoint of enzyme immunoassays because it is simple, well under-

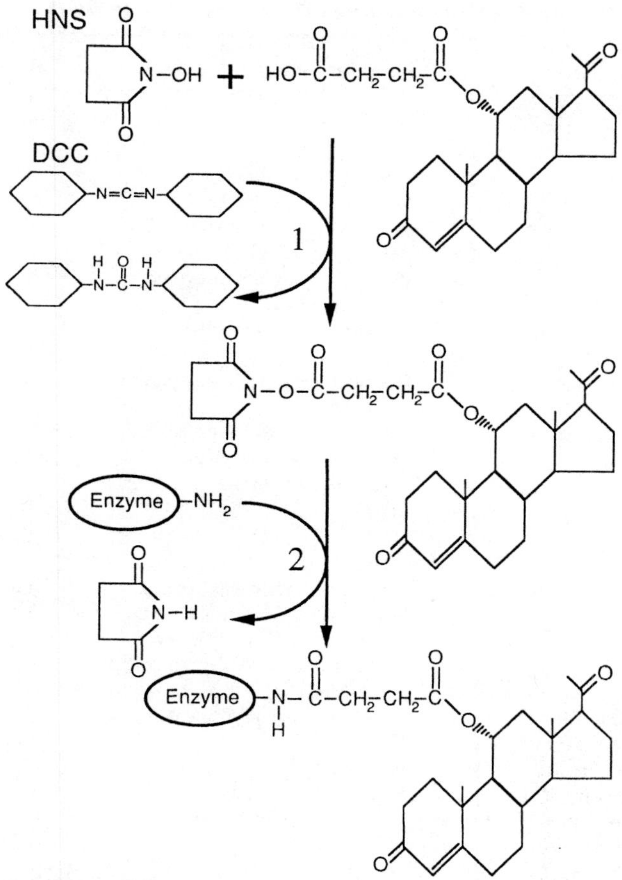

FIGURE 13.2 Active ester procedure for the conjugation of steroid hapten to an enzyme or other protein. This procedure is carried out in two steps (1 and 2), the first to generate the active ester derivative of the carboxyl-containing hapten, which can then be used directly or stored until needed, and the second for the reaction of the activated hapten with the protein. (Step 1) 11α-Hydroxyprogesterone hemisuccinate, the steroid to be conjugated, is reacted with N-hydroxy succinimide (NHS) in the presence of dicyclohexylcarbodiimide (DCC) in dioxane at room temperature (14–20°C) for at least 2 hr, with stirring. As the carbodiimide is transformed to N,N'-dicyclohexyl urea, the NHS active-ester of the 11α-hydroxyprogesterone hemisuccinate is formed. The NHS ester is then isolated after dilution with water and extraction with ethyl acetate, and can be stored until needed. This procedure also removes residual carbodiimide, which could deactivate the protein during step 2, and facilitates the adjustment of the molar ratio of hapten to enzyme for step 2. (Step 2) Here the active ester and enzyme (or carrier protein if an immunogen is being synthesized) are mixed together in 10 mmol/liter phosphate buffer, pH 7.0, and allowed to react at 4°C overnight, before the conjugate is separated from the reactants by means of dialysis (with removal of precipitate by centrifugation) and chromatography on Sephadex G 25. This procedure is similar to that described by Tijssen (11), who reviewed many of the alternative approaches.

stood, and more than adequate for most applications. Efficient, and sometimes highly sophisticated, microtiter plate readers are often already available in the user's laboratory. In my laboratory we have developed colorimetric horseradish

TABLE 13.5   Assay Methods for the Principal Enzymes Used in Immunoassays

Enzyme	Assay method	Substrate etc.	References
Alkaline phosphatase	Amplified (colorimetric, electrometric, fluorimetric)	NADP⁺, etc.	35, 68
	Colorimetric	4-Nitrophenyl-phosphate	20
	Electrochemical	1-Naphthyl phosphate	69
		p-Amino-phenyl phosphate	33
	Luminometric	Adamantyl 1,2-dioxyethane	31
		Phenylphosphate-substituted dioxetane	32
	Time-resolved (TR) fluorimetric	5-Fluorosalicyl phosphate	34
	Visual assessment	Bromochloroindoyl phosphate (BCIP)	70
β-D-Galactosidase	Colorimetric	2-Nitrophenyl-β-D-galactoside	20
	Fluorimetric	4-Methylumbelliferyl-β-D-galactoside (MUG)	71
	Photodensitometry	MUG	71
Horseradish peroxidase	Colorimetric	H_2O_2 and o-phenylene-diamine (OPD)	42, 48, 49, 53
		H_2O_2 and tetramethyl-benzidine	43
		H_2O_2, 3-methyl-2-benzothiazolinone, hydrozone (MBTH), and 3-(dimethylamino) benzoic acid (DMAB)	72
	Fluorimetric	3-p-Hydroxyphenyl-propionic acid	73
	Luminometric (enhanced)	Luminol	41
	Photodensitometry	H_2O_2 and OPD	71
	Visual assessment	H_2O_2 and 4-chloro-1-naphthol	60

peroxidase immunoassays with low detection limits for many steroids (75, 76) and proteins (42, 48).

The limitations of a colorimetric endpoint are directly related to the fundamental limitations of colorimetry itself. By colorimetry, the intensity of the monochromatic light not absorbed by the sample is measured. In order to estimate low concentrations of chromogen small differences in intensity must be measured at high light intensity, limiting the lower detection limit. Also, the relationship between optical absorbance and the intensity of transmitted light is logarithmic. Therefore, at high chromogen concentrations relatively large differences in optical absorbance correspond to very small differences in the intensity of unabsorbed light, limiting the precision and range of measurements. Consequently, it is usually advisable to design enzyme immunoassays so that only optical absorbance readings in the range ~0.1 to ~1.5 are used. This would give a dynamic range of about 15, which is particularly constraining for reagent excess immunoassays.

However, extension of this dynamic range is made possible by simultaneous monitoring of absorbance at two or more wavelengths (77–79). If wavelengths are chosen which correspond to the peak of the chromogen absorption peak and to a point low down on its side, simple computation allows the effective range of the assay to be greatly increased. For example (77), p-nitrophenol (formed by alkaline phosphatase from p-nitrophenol phosphate) absorbs maximally at 405 nm, but at 450 nm the molar extinction coefficient is about 20% of that at 405, so that

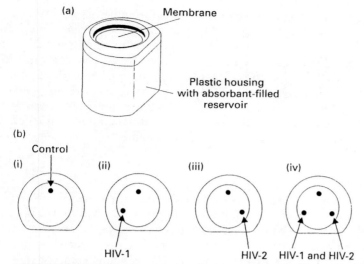

FIGURE 13.3   The recombigen HIV-1/HIV-2 test device of Cambridge Biotech corporation can be used to simultanously detect antibodies to both human immunodeficiency viruses. Basically, the test is an antibody-capture enzyme-linked immunsorbent assay. (a) The test device consists of a small asymmetrical plastic chamber (maximum diameter 30 mm) containing a multilayered absorbant cylinder, fused to the top of which is a glass fiber membrane. During manufacture three discrete, circular areas of the membrane are coated with plastic microspheres previously loaded with antigen or human IgG. None of the three coated spots are visible before use. (b) Operation consists of putting seven drops of patient serum onto the center of the device and adding four drops of conjugate solution, followed by 0.8 ml of wash and four drops of substrate solution. After 3 min, 0.4 ml of stop solution is added and the result is evident. (i) A negative result is indicated by apearance of the control spot only. This spot is coated with human IgG and failure of this spot to appear indicates a procedural or reagent malfunction. (ii) A positive HIV-1 result is indicated by two spots as shown. The extra spot was coated with antigen specific for HIV-1. (iii) A positive HIV-2 result is indicated by two spots as shown. The extra spot was coated with antigen specific for HIV-2. (iv) Coinfected or cross-reactive samples give three spots as shown. This is the most common positive result as there is approximately 30–70% cross-reactivity between HIV-1 and HIV-2 antibodies with the recombinant antigen proteins used. Reproduced by permission of Portland Press Ltd. (27).

dual measurements at these wavelengths can extend the range of enzyme activity readings by about a factor of five. With horseradish peroxidase and 3,3′,5,5′-tetramethylbenzidine (TMB) as cosubstrate, reading at the same two wavelengths allows extension of the measuring range of an IEMA by a factor of about three (78). Alternatively, the dynamic range of the colorimetric determination of enzyme activity may be extended by means of kinetic recording techniques as opposed to fixed time measurements. However, the ranges achieved in these ways may still be limited compared to the dynamic range possible with other enzyme assay methods such as time-resolved fluorimetry (34).

4.3. Fluorimetry

Fluorimetric measurements of very small concentrations of a pure fluorescent compound are precise because they are measured relative to an absence of light and very sensitive light detection systems can be used. Time-resolved fluorimetric measurements reduce interference from contaminating fluorescent compounds, thus enabling much of the theoretical potential of fluorimetry to be exploited (34). However, the potential of fluorimetric measurements of enzyme activities in enzyme immunoassays has long been realized. Ishikawa (20) tabulated the smallest detectable amounts of some enzymes used for immunoassays as determined with different assay systems. With 10-min incubations and a volume of 150 μl, 25, 1000, and 10,000 amol of horseradish peroxidase, β-D-galactosidase, and alkaline phosphatase, respectively, could be determind colorimetrically. Fluorimetrically these limits decreased to 5, 0.2, and 10 amol, respectively. Time-resolved flourimetric determination of alkaline phosphatase is also discussed in Chapter 14.

4.4. Luminometry

Although luminometric assay methods have been developed for alkaline phosphatase (31, 32), luminometric determination of horseradish peroxidase (41) is more common. "Enhanced" luminescence determination implies the addition of certain compounds to the assay buffer that enhance and prolong light emission from a luminescent reaction catalyzed by the enzyme. For example some phenol derivatives, including 4-iodophenol and p-phenylphenol, increase by >1000-fold light emission from the peroxidase-catalyzed oxidation of luminol and prolong light emission over several minutes. This obviates the need for initiation of the light emitting reaction in the counting chamber of the luminometer and enables photographic determination of the endpoint (41). This subject is also discussed in Chapter 15.

4.5. Electrometry

The electrometric determination of enzyme activity has a number of inherent properties that could be highly advantageous for some immunoassay applications. Variably cloudy or colored and even opaque solutions and containers can be monitored electrometrically, and the detection element can, potentially, be a tiny, remotely located probe. Electrometric immunoassays have been recently and comprehensively reviewed (80) and those with the greatest promise for widespread application are enzyme immunoassays with amperometric detection of enzyme activity. Amperometric detection is preferable beacuse there is a linear relationship between the concentration of the detectable substance and the current generated, whereas in potentiometric systems the relationship is logarithmic. Substrates yielding an electrochemically detectable product are used and the continuous operation of the enzyme leads to a large amplification of the measured signal as compared to the use of electrochemically detectable substances themselves in the label. Some electrometric enzyme immunoassays incorporate an extra amplification step (68) (see below).

4.6. Multistage Assay Systems

The elegant amplification method developed by Colin Self depends on alkaline phosphatase (the labeling enzyme) dephosphorylating $NADP^+$ to NAD^+. The NAD^+ then enters a specific redox cycle that cannot utilize $NADP^+$, where it is reduced to NADH by alcohol dehydrogenase, and then reconverted to NAD^+ by diaphorase with the concomitant reduction of p-iodonitrotetrazolium violet reagent

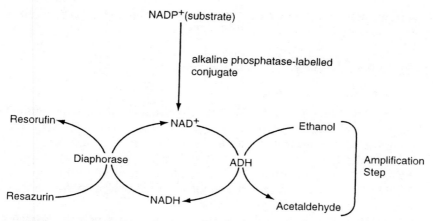

FIGURE 13.4   A fluorimetric amplification assay for alkaline phosphatase. The coenzyme nicotinamide adenine dinucleotide phosphate (NADP$^+$) acts as substrate for the phosphatase and is dephosphorylated to NAD$^+$. Also present in excess are two other enzymes, alcohol dehydrogenase and diaphorase (a lipoyl dehydrogenase which also catalyzes the NAD$^+$-dependent reduction of the nonfluorescent compound resazurin), ethanol, and resazurin. What happens next depends on the fact that the alcohol dehydrogenase used is highly specific for NAD$^+$. As NAD$^+$ is formed a cycle begins, leading to the accumulation of acetaldehyde and resorufin, the highly fluorescent reduced form of resazurin. Therefore, the greater the activity of the phosphatase, the faster the cycle turns and the more resorufin is formed, with many molecules of resorufin formed for each NAD$^+$. Reprinted from Cook DB, Self CH. Determination of one thousandth of an attomole (1 zeptomole) of alkaline phosphatase: Application in an immunoassay of proinsulin. Clin Chem, 1993, courtesy of the American Association for Clinical Chemistry, Inc.

to an intensely purple formazan dye. The NAD$^+$ is thus continuously cycled with the formation of more formazan with every turn of the cycle. Since it was first patented in 1982 this system has been widely applied in research and commercial enzyme immunoassays for antigens and antibodies. Two variations that have since been introduced concern the determination of the endpoint. Stanley *et al.* (68) used amperometric determination of ferricyanide reduced by the diaphorase and reoxidized at the electrode, and Cook and Self (35) used fluorimetric determination of resorufin, formed from nonfluorescent resazurin in the NADH-dependent diaphorase-catalyzed reaction (Fig. 13.4). The flourescent system greatly extended the range of measurements and enabled the measurement of less than 0.001 amol (1 zeptomole) of alkaline phosphatase per microtiter plate well, and, consequently, allowed the measurement of down to 17 amol/liter of proinsulin by IEMA.

5. THE VARIETY OF ENZYME IMMUNOASSAYS

According to the "antibody occupancy principle" of Roger Ekins (81), when an immunoassay relies on the observation of binding sites unoccupied by analyte, the total number of sites available must be small to minimize error in the (indirect) estimation of occupied sites (reagent limited assays); but when an immunoassay depends on the observation of sites occupied by analyte, errors may be minimized by the use of relatively large numbers of sites (reagent excess assays). Essentially all current commercial and research enzyme immunoassays can be classified as reagent-excess or reagent-limited (Table 13.6).

5.1. Reagent-Excess Assays

5.1.1. Assays for Antibodies

Most routine immunoassays for the quantitation of specific antibodies are reagent-excess and the majority of these use enzyme-containing labels (82). Most often, diluted test serum is added to excess antigen immobilized on a solid phase, (sp-Ag) and the amount of specific antibody which binds (or is "captured," sp-Ag–**Ab**) may then be quantified by the employment of labeled antibodies which specifically bind to to the constant region of the immunoglubulin class or classes of interest (e.g., sp-Ag–**IgG₁**–Ab-enzyme).

Alternatively, and much less frequently, an antigen capture approach may be employed. In such assays immobilized anti-immunoglobulin class antibodies (sp-Ab) first adsorb relevant immunoglobulins from the sample (sp-Ab–**IgA₁**), added antigen is then specifically captured only by the antibodies of interest (sp-Ab–**IgA₁**–Ag), and the amount of antigen bound is finally determined, by, for example, the use labeled antibody to antigen (sp-Ab–**IgA₁**–Ag–Ab-enzyme). In one such assay (83) F(ab')₂ fragments of antibody against human IgG₁ were immobilized and excess antigen with enzyme labeled antibody was used (sp-F[ab']₂–**IgG₁**–Ag–Ab-peroxidase). Antigen capture assays may be preferable for specific antibodies of the minor immunoglobulin classes, as less antigen is needed and antibodies of other classes do not interfere because they are discarded after the first step.

The affinity of the Ig synthesized in response to an infection increases as the infection develops and is conquered or controlled. Therefore, both IgM and early IgG antibodies have, in general, lower affinity for pathogen antigens than the IgG antibodies which represent past immunity. This situation is exploited by the use of "protein-denaturing immunoassays" or "avidity ELISA" which are designed to detect only high-affinity antibodies (84–86). For example, diluted patient sera are placed in contact with solid phase coated with pathogen antigen and, instead of the usual washing step, a protein denaturant solution such as 6 M urea is used to

TABLE 13.6   Classification of Enzyme Immunoassays

Class	Analyte type	Subclass	References
Reagent excess	Antibodies	Labeled antibody, two-site	82–88
	Antigens	Labeled antibody, two-site	35, 37, 42–45, 48, 50, 52, 53
	Haptens	Labeled antibody	36
		Selective antibody	89, Chapter 19
Reagent limited	Antibodies	Labeled antibody	82
	Antigens or haptens	Labeled antibody	38, 90
		Labeled antigen or hapten	40, 67, 75, 76, 91
	Haptens	Labeled hapten, separation-free	39, 59, 59
	Haptens, free	Labeled analog	Chapter 20
		Labeled antibody	Chapter 20

elute both nonspecifically adsorbed proteins and lower affinity specific antibodies, before thorough washing and the determination of the remaining bound antibody with labeled anti-Ig or anti-IgG antibody [sp-Ag–**Ab**–Ab-enzyme, where **Ab** represents only high-affinity antibody (85)]. However, the validity of such methods has been questioned (87) and more careful development and validation procedures may be needed (88).

5.1.2. Assays for Antigens

Such assays are almost always two-site sandwich assays equivalent to IRMA, IFMA, and ICLMA and are best referred to as IEMA. The accronym ELISA is used very loosely and, outside certain limited contexts (e.g., reagent excess assays for specific antibodies), often conveys little about the mechanism of the assay so described.

Normally, labeled antibody against the analyte (e.g., Ab-enzyme) is the principal reagent. To separate bound label (e.g., **Ag**–Ab-enzyme) from free, any of a range of adsorption or precipitation reagents can be employed, but usually the antigen–label complex is removed by means of excess immobilized antibody which binds to a separate antigenic site on the analyte. This results in the now classical two-site assay complex in which antigen is sandwiched between two antibodies (e.g., sp-Ab–**Ag**–Ab-enzyme), and plotting the the concentration of labeled antibody bound against the concentration of analyte (**Ag**) gives a direct, linear or nonlinear standard curve. Therefore, specificity is determined by the combined selectivity of two antibodies and such assays are observed to be inherently more specific than single-site assays. However, precautions must be taken that the employment of excess reagents does not lead to high nonspecific binding of label, or degradation of assay specificity (92). It follows that all candidate analytes for such assays must have two antigenic determinants that can be recognized simultaneously, which usually excludes simple steroids, small peptides with less than 15–20 amino acid residues, and most drugs. The most sensitive of such assays in routine use are capable of detecting <1 amol of analyte (20, 26, 35).

A very large number of variations on the basic two-site sandwich assay for antigen have been described. These include indirect labeling and the use of enzyme conjugates with antibody fragments to decrease nonspecific binding (20, 21). In addition, assay schemes and formulations have been developed which are suitable for a wide variety of applications, from highly sensitive TSH assays to home pregnancy detection kits.

There is an increasing interest in multianalyte immunoassays (Chapter 18), which can be very useful in specific clinical screening procedures. While simultaneous enzyme immunoassays with different enzyme activities associated with each analyte are probably less promising for such applications than multiple rare-earth metal-chelates (Chapters 14 and 18), dual enzyme immunoassays may also have a significant future.

Immunoblotting, which often employs enzymes as labeling substances, and has many similarities in principle and in the different strategies and tactics used, with excess reagent immunoassays is reviewed in Chapter 23.

5.1.3. Assays for Haptens

Because the two-site assays described above are unsuitable for analytes with a molecular weight <1000 and because of the inherent limited sensitivity of competitive assays (81), much effort has been put into the invention of reagent excess assays for haptens. In one such system (36), analyte was incubated with a calculated excess of labeled antibody (usually Fab' or F[ab']$_2$) and unoccupied labeled antibody was removed by means of excess immobilized analyte before the label associated with analyte was determined. Note that while the reagents employed here and for labeled-antibody competitive assays may be exactly equivalent, the use of excess label and the determination of the analyte–label complex (**Ha**–Ab-peroxidase, and not immobilized label, sp-Ha–Ab-peroxidase) alters completely the character of the assay. Self (89) and Barnard and Kohen (Chapter 19) have taken another approach to designing reagent excess immunoassays for small molecules.

5.2. Reagent-Limited Assays

5.2.1. Assays for Antibodies

While most assays for specific antibodies are reagent-excess (see above), limited-reagent assays can offer certain advantages for same applications (82). For example, if only antibodies which bind to a specific region of an antigen (a specific epitope) are to be determined, a monoclonal antibody which binds to the same region is selected and labeled. In the assay, the specific antibodies in the sample (**Ab**) are allowed to compete with a limited concentration of the labeled antibody (Ab-enzyme) for the antigen immobilized on a solid phase (sp-Ag). The two possible final complexes are sp-Ag–Ab-enzyme and sp-Ag–**Ab.** Plotting the concentration of labeled antibody bound to the immobilized antigen against the concentration of analyte (**Ab**) gives an inverse standard curve.

5.2.2. Assays for Antigens or Haptens

Enzyme-labeled-antibody reagent-limited assays for antigen or hapten have the advantage that labeled antigens or haptens with undesirable properties, (e.g., low solubility in aqueous media) may be avoided. However, immobilized analyte must also be present in a constant, limited amount in each assay vessel. This approach works well with highly purified monoclonal or affinity-purified polyclonal antibodies, as only then is the nonspecific binding of label not enhanced by contamination with irrelevant antibodies.

Enzyme-labeled-antigen or labeled-hapten assays for antigens or haptens, respectively, are equivalent to classical RIA. The labeled analyte is formed by tagging a derivative of the analyte with an enzyme. After incubation of a limited concentration of label with a limited concentration of analyte-specific antibody and analyte, antibody-bound label and free label are separated to allow the bound enzyme to be determined. Plotting the concentration of label bound to antibody (sp-Ab–Ag-enzyme) against the concentration of analyte (**Ag**) gives inverse, nonlinear standard curves. The detection limits of reagent-limited immunoassays may be improved by the use of high-specific-activity label, but the smallest amount of analyte detectable is ultimately limited by the affinity of the antibody employed (81). The most sensitive of these assays employ enzyme-containing labels and can detect <1 fmol of analyte (26).

5.2.3. Assays for Haptens, Separation-Free

An ideal separation-free (homogeneous) assay requires 100% modulation by the binding reaction of the activity of the enzyme in the label. In practice this is very difficult to achieve and separation-free assays generally have inferior lower-detection limits than immunoassays with separation steps. However, they are characterized by simplicity and speed and are widely employed in monitoring blood and urine levels of therapeutic drugs and of drugs of abuse when low detection limits ($<10^{-9}$ mol/liter) are not required (93).

The activity of the enzyme label may be either decreased or increased by the binding reaction. There are two kinds of EMIT procedures; in some the enzyme activity of the label is decreased when the label is bound by the antibody, and in others the activity is increased on binding (Fig. 13.5). Apart from enzymes, enzyme-mediated separation-free assays may employ as a labeling substance: enzyme prosthetic group, enzyme inhibitor, enzyme fragment, or fluorescent-labeled enzyme substrate (59, 93).

Immunochromatography assays (60) are remarkable separation-free EIA systems in which the concentration of analyte is related to the distance along a chromatographic strip that color develops rather than to the intensity of color develop-

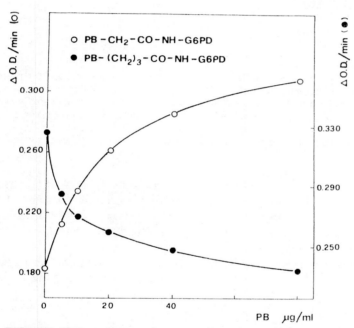

FIGURE 13.5 Whether the enzyme activity in an EMIT is activated or inhibited by increasing concentrations of analyte may be determined by the length of the bridging molecule linking the hapten to the enzyme. Here are examples of dose–response curves for two model EMIT systems for the hapten analyte phenobarbital (PB), reprinted with permission of Kluwer Academic Publishers (7). For the first assay (○) phenobarbital–acetic acid was conjugated to glucose-6-phosphate dehydrogenase. The intrinsic enzyme activity of the label was not significantly reduced by this procedure, but when anti-PB antibody was added the activity was inhibited; as is clear from the dose–response curve, this inhibition was progressively cancelled by increasing concentrations of PB. For the second assay (●) phenobarbital–butanoic acid was conjugated to the enzyme, and the longer bridge gave a conjugate with reduced intrinsic enzyme activity due to steric inhibition by the attached PB. When anti-PB antibody was added the activity was restored and, as is clear from the dose–response curve, this restored activity was progressively cancelled by increasing concentrations of PB. Abdul-Ahad WG, Gosling JP. Reagent preparation. In: Gosling JP, Basso LV, Eds. Immunoassay: Laboratory and Clinical Applications. Boston, MA; Butterworth-Heinemann, 1994: 31–49.

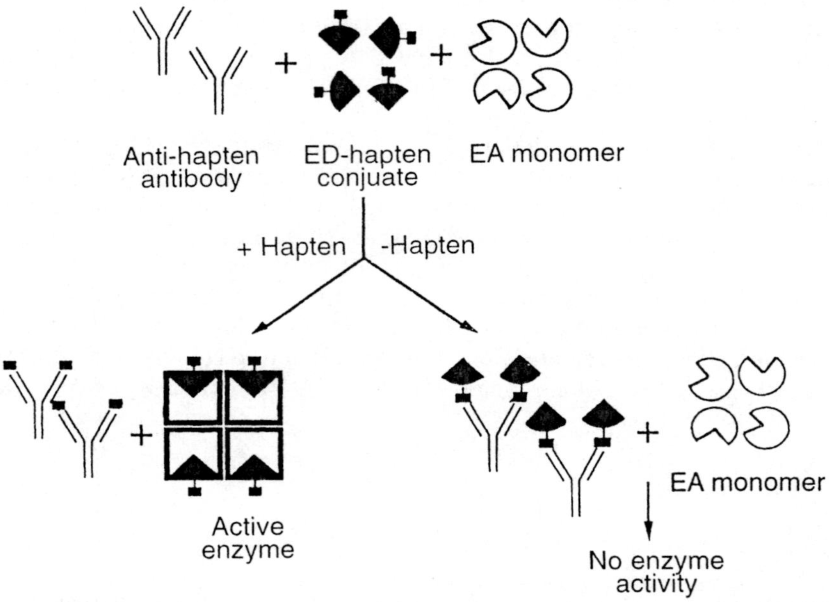

FIGURE 13.6 The principle of CEDIA. The large (inactive) enzyme acceptor protein (EA, 113,000 Da) and the small enzyme donor polypeptide (ED, about 90 amino acid residues) can spontanously associate to form active β-D-galactosidase. The ability to reactivate EA is retained by ED–hapten conjugate, but binding of ED–hapten by anti-hapten antibody prevents reassociation. In this figure the effect of anti-hapten antibody in preventing reassociation is reversed by the presence of free hapten. Reprinted with permission of Macmillan Press Ltd. (59).

ment. To devise combined enzyme donor immunoassay (CEDIA) (94) (Fig. 13.6), recombinant DNA technology was exploited to produce new strains of *E. coli* synthesizing large inactive fragments of β-D-galactosidase (enzyme acceptors) and small inactive fragments of the same enzyme (enzyme donors) which spontaneously associate to give fully active enzyme.

Immunoassays to measure free hormones, which are reviewed in Chapter 20, sometimes employ "analog of analyte"–enzyme or antibody–enzyme conjugates.

6. PROSPECTS

The historical development of immunoassay technology has been partly a process of replacing assays with radioisotopic labels by assays with one or other of the main alternative nonisotopic labels. In addition, instruments for determining endpoints, such as scintillation counters and time-resolved fluorimeters, represent large investments. Therefore, rivalries between manufacturers and users tend to be related to the labeling substance used and the endpoint determination method, and each contender tends to claim all the virtues and all the future for his or her own labeling substance or method. However, as a quick review of the history of video cassette recorder technology reveals, the success of rival technologies can be determined more by broader commercial considerations than by basic specifications. For example, the popularity of enzymes as labeling substances in "in-house" immunoassays has as much to do with their suitability for use in microtiter plates, and on the ready availability of conjugation reagents, etc., as with their versatility and their other intrinsic virtues. The choice of enzymes has also been supported by the non- (or only recent) availability of reagents for the simple preparation of high-quality chemiluminescent or time-resolved flourescent labels. In the commercial domain the choice of a labeling substance and endpoint method is largely determined by research and development resources, the availability and cost of licences, and marketing considerations.

The comparison of immunoassay technologies is regularly the subject of experimental evaluations (e.g., 95) and even of the occasional editorial. While such reviews and comparisons can be very useful they usually have highly sigificant limitations. Certain relevant technologies or technological variants may be absent, or, more importantly, fundamental aspects relevant to their application are ignored. For example, enzyme immunoassays may be found wanting with respect to lower detection limit and range (95) but these limitations may be reduced or transformed by an alternative method of endpoint determination (34, 35). If enzymes have important practical limitations these are more likely to be related to their relative fragility and large size, and on the costs of the measures needed to overcome these. [Perhaps special measures to promote rapid diffusion, such as a short exposure to microwaves, may be of particular benefit to enzyme immunoassays (96).] Therefore, the informed user should keep abreast not just with such published comparisons and individual method evaluations, but, more particularly, with the reports of well established and competent external quality assessment schemes (EQAS). Although these also have limitations, they give important information on the comparability and validity of the results obtained with commercially available assay methods, and it is clear from their collective findings that good comparability and precision are not the prerequisites of any one methodology.

References

1. Nakane PK, Pierce GB. Enzyme-labelled antibodies: preparation and application to the localization of antigens. J Histochem Cytochem 1966; 14:929–31.
2. Avrameas S, Uriel J. Méthode de marquage d'antigénes at d'anticorps avec enzymes et son application en immunodiffusion. Comptes Rendus Hebdomedaires des Seances de l'Academie des Sciences: D: Sciences naturelles (Paris) 1966; 262:2543–5.
3. Engvall E, Perlmann P. Enzyme-linked immunosorbent assay (ELISA): quantitative assay of immunoglobulin G. Immunochemistry 1971; 8:871–4.
4. VanWeeman BK, Schuurs AHWM. Immunoassay using antigen-enzyme conjugates. FEBS Lett 1971; 15:232–6.
5. Avrameas MS, Guilbert B. Dosage enzymo-immunologique de protéines à l'aide d'immunoadsorbents et d'antigènes marqués aux enzymes. CR Acad Sci Paris Série D 1971; 273, 2705–7.
6. Maggio ET, Ed. Enzyme-Immunoassay. Boca Raton: CRC Press, 1980.
7. Malvano R, Ed. Immunoenzymatic Assay Techniques. The Hague: Martinus Nijhoff, 1980.
8. Ishikawa E, Kawai T, Miyai K, Eds. Enzyme Immunoassay. Tokyo: Igaku-Shoin, 1981.
9. Avrameas SP, Dreut P, Masseyeff R, Feldman G, Eds. Immunoenzymatic Techniques. Amsterdam: Elsevier, 1983.
10. Ngo TT, Lenhoff HM, Eds. Enzyme-Mediated Immunoassay. New York: Plenum, 1985.
11. Tijssen P. Practice and Theory of Enzyme Immunoassays. Amsterdam: Elsevier, 1985.
12. Kemeny DM, Challcombe SJ, Eds. ELISA and Other Solid Phase Immunoassays. Theoretical and Practical Aspects. Chichester: Wiley, 1988.
13. Ternynck T, Avrameas S. Techniques Immunoenzymatiques. Paris: Editions INSERM, 1988.
14. Wreghitt TG, Morgan-Capner P, Eds. ELISA in the Clinical Microbiology Laboratory. London: Public Health Laboratory Service, 1990.

15. Avrameas S, Nakane PK, Paramichail M, Pesce AJ, Eds. Enzyme immunoasay techniques. J Immunol Methods 1992; 150:parts 3–4.

16. Wisdom GB. Enzyme-immunoassay. Clin Chem 1976; 22:1243–55.

17. Voller A, Bartlett A, Bidwell DE. Enzyme immunoassays with special reference to ELISA techniques. J Clin Pathol 1978; 31:507–20.

18. Wisdom GB. Recent progress in the development of enzyme immunoassays. Ligand Rev 1981; 3:44–9.

19. Oellerich M. Enzyme-immunoassay: a Review. J Clin Chem Clin Biochem 1984; 22:895–904.

20. Ishikawa E. Development and clinical application of sensitive enzyme immunoassay for macromolecular antigens—a review. Clin Biochem 1987; 20:375–85.

21. Ishikawa E, Hashida S, Tanaka K, Kohno T. Methodological advances in enzymology. Development and applications of ultrasensitive enzyme immunoassays for antigens and antibodies. Clin Chim Acta 1989; 185:223–30.

22. Ngo TT. Enzyme systems and enzyme conjugates for solid-phase ELISA. In: Butler JE, Ed. Immunochemistry of Solid-Phase Immunoassay. Boca Raton, FL: CRC Press, 1991:85–104.

23. Price CP, Newman DJ, Eds. Principles and Practice of Immunoassay. New York: Stockton Press, 1991.

24. Wild D. The Immunoassay Handbook. New York: Stockton Press, 1994.

25. Gosling JP, Basso LV. Immunoassays: Laboratory Analysis and Clinical Applications. Boston: Butterworth-Heienemann, 1994.

26. Gosling JP. A decade of development in immunoassay methodology. Clin Chem 1990; 36:1408–27.

27. Gosling JP. Advanced immunoassays. In: Immunotechnology. London: Portland Press, 1992:91–106.

28. Kricka LJ. Selected strategies for improving sensitivity and reliability of immunoassays. Clin Chem 1994; 40:347–57.

29. Frobert Y, Grassi J. Screening of monoclonal antobodies using antigens labelled with acetylcholinesterase. In: Manson, Ed. Methods in Molecular Biology, Vol. 10. Totowa NJ: Humana Press, 1992:65–78.

30. Hosada H, Takasaki W, Arihara S, Nambara T. Enzyme labelling of steroids by N-succinimidyl ester method. Preparation of alkaline phosphate-labelled antigen for use in enzyme immunoassay. Chem Pharm Bull 1985; 33:5393–8.

31. Bronstein I, Voyta JC, Thorpe GHG, Kricka LJ, Armstrong G. Chemiluminescent assay of alkaline phosphatase applied in an ultrasensitive enzyme immunoassay of thyrotropin. Clin Chem 1989; 35:1441–6.

32. Schaap AP, Akhavan H, Romano LJ. Chemiluminescent substrates for alkaline phosphatase: Application to ultrasensitive enzyme-linked immunoassays and DNA probes. Clin Chem 1989; 35:1863–4.

33. Hadas E, Soussan L, Rosen-Margalit I, Farkash A, Rishpon J. A rapid and sensitive heterogenous immunoelectrochemical assay using disposable electrodes. J Immunoassay 1992; 13:231–52.

34. Christopoulos TK, Diamandis EP. Enzymatically amplified time-resolved fluorescence immunoassay withe Terbium chelates. Anal Chem 1992; 64:342–6.

35. Cook DB, Self CH. Determination of one thousandth of an attomole (1 zeptomole) of alkaline phosphatase: Application in an immunoassay of proinsulin. Clin Chem 1993; 39:965–71.

36. Freytag JW, Lau HP, Wadsley JJ. Affinity-column-mediated immunoenzymometric assay: Influence of affinity-column ligand and valency of antibody-enzyme conjugates. Clin Chem 1984; 30:1494–8.

37. Ruan K-H, Kulmacz RJ, Wilson A, Wu KK. Highly sensitive fluorimetric enzyme immunoassay for prostaglandin H synthase solubilized from cultured cells. J Immunol Methods 1993; 162:23–30.

38. Pauillac S, Halmos T, Labrousse H, Antonakis K, Avrameas S. Production of highly specific monoclonal antibodies to monensin and development of a microELISA to detect this antibiotic. J Immunol Methods 1993; 164:165–73.

39. Beresini MH, Davalian D, Alexander S, Tonton-Quinn R, Barnett B, Cerelli MJ, Berger DE, Blohm WP, Jaklitsch A. Evaluation of EMIT cyclosporine assay for use with whole blood. Clin Chem 1993; 39:2235–41.

40. Prabhasankar P, Ragupathi G, Sundaravadivel B, Annapoorani KS, Damodaran C. Enzyme-linked immunosorbent assay for the phytotoxin thevetin. J Immunoassay 1993; 14:279–96.

41. Thorpe GHG, Kricka LJ, Mosely SB, Whitehead TP. Phenols as enhancers of the chemiluminescent horseradish peroxidase-luminol-hydrogen peroxide reaction: Application in luminescence monitored enzyme immunoassays. Clin Chem 1985; 31:1335–41.

42. Abdul-Ahad WG, Gosling JP. An enzyme-linked immunosorbent assay (ELISA) for bovine LH capable of monitoring fluctuations in baseline concentrations. J Reprod Fertil 1987; 80:653–61.

43. Ikemoto M, Ishida A, Tsunekawa S, Ozawa K, Kasai Y, Totani M. Enzyme immunoassay of liver-type arginase and its potential clinical application. Clin Chem 1993; 39:794–9.

44. Larue C, Calzolari C, Bertinchant J-P, Leclercq F, Grolleau R, Pau B. Cardiac-specifoc immunoenzymometric assay of troponin I in the early phase of acute myocardial infarction. Clin Chem 1993; 39:972–9.

45. Peuravuori H, Korpela T. Pyrophosphatase-based enzyme-linked immunosorbent assay of total IgE in serum. Clin Chem 1993; 39:846–51.

46. Lo CY, Notenboom RH, Kajioka R. An assessment of urease-based enzyme-linked immunosorbent assay. J Immunol Methods 1988; 114:127–37.

47. Harmer IJ, Samuel D. The FITC-anti-FITC system is a sensitive alternative to biotin-streptavidin in ELISA. J Immunol Methods 1989; 122:115–21.

48. Monaghan DA, Power MJ, Fottrell PF. Sandwich enzyme immunoassay of osteocalcin in serum with use of an antibody against human osteocalcin. Clin Chem 1993; 39:942–7.

49. Guérin-Marchand C, Batard T, Brodard V, *et al.* DMISA (dissociated membrane immunosorbent assay), a new ELISA technique performed with blotted samples. J Immunol Methods 1994; 167:219–25.

50. Casl M-T, Grubb A. A rapid enzyme-linked immunosorbent assay for serum amyloid A using sequence-specific antibodies. Ann Clin Biochem 1993; 30:278–86.

51. Avrameas S. Amplification systems in immunoenzymatic techniques. J Immunol Methods 1992; 150:23–32.

52. Yang X, HayGlass KT. A simple, sensitive, dual mAb based ELISA for murine gamma interferon determination: comparison with two common bioassays. J Immunol 1993; 14:129–48.

53. Rønne E, Behrendt N, Plough M, Nielsen HJ, Wöllisch E, Weidle U, Damø K, Høyer-Hansen G. Quantitation of the receptor for urokinase plasminogne activator by enzyme-linked immunosorbent assay. J Immunol Methods 1994; 167:91–101.

54. Reis KJ, Von Mering GO, Karis MA, Faulmann EL, Lottenberg R, Boyle MDP. Enzyme-labelled type III bacterial Fc receptors: a versatile tracer for immunoassay. J Immunol Methods 1988; 107:273–80.

55. Sun S, Lew AM. Chimaeric protein A/protein G and protein G/alkaline phosphatase as reporter molecules. J Immunol Methods 1992; 152:43–8.

56. Vincent P, Samuel D. A comparison of the binding of biotin and biotinylated macromolecular ligands to an anti-biotin monoclonal antibody and to streptavidin. J Immunol Methods 1993; 165:177–82.

57. Durbin H, Bodmer WF. A sensitive micro-immunoassay using β-galactosidase/anti-β-galactosidase complexes. J Immunol Methods 1987; 97:19–27.

58. Canova-Davis E, Redemann CT, Vollmer YP, Kung VT. Use of a reversed-phase evaporation vesicle formulation for a homogeneous liposome immunoassay. Clin Chem 1986; 32:1687–91.

59. Khanna P. Homogeneous enzyme immunoassay. *Op. cit.* (Ref. 23):326–64.

60. Houts T. Immunochromatography. *Op. cit.* (Ref. 23):563–83.

61. De Boever J, Kohen F, Vandekerckhove D. Solid-phase chemiluminescence immunoassay for plasma estradiol-17β during gonadotropin therapy compared with two radioimmunoassays. Clin Chem 1983; 29:2068–72.

62. Edwards R. Radiolabelled immunoassay. In: Price CP, Newman DJ, Eds. Principles and Practice of Immunoassay. New York: Stockton Press, 1991:265–94.

63. Sano T, Smith CL, Cantor CR. Immuno-PCR with a commercially available avidin system. Science 1993; 260:698–9.

64. Avrameas S, Ternynck T, Guesdon JL. Coupling of enzymes to antibodies and antigens. Scand J Immunol 1978; 8:(Suppl. 7):7–20.

65. Tijssen P, Kurstak E. Highly efficient and simple methods for the preparation of peroxidase and active peroxidase-antibody conjugates for enzyme immunoassays. Anal Biochem 1984; 136:451–7.

66. Fujiwara K, Saita T, Kitagawa T. The use of *N*-[β-(4-diazophenyl)ethyl]maleimide as a coupling agent in the preparation of enzyme-antibody conjugates. J Immunol Methods 1988; 110:47–53.

67. Munro C, Stabenfeldt G. Development of a microtitre plate enzyme immunoassay for the determination of progesterone. J Endocrinol 1984; 101:41–9.

68. Stanley CJ, Cox RB, Cardosi MF, Turner APF. Amperometric enzyme-amplified immunoassays. J Immunol Methods 1988; 112:153–61.

69. Athey D, Ball M, McNeill CJ. Avidin-biotin based electrochemical immunoassay for thyrotropin. Ann Clin Biochem 1993; 30:570–7.

70. May K. In-home testing. In: Collins WP, Ed. Complementary Immunoassays. Chicester: Wiley, 1988:451–65.

71. Labrousse H, Avrameas S. A method for the quantification of a colored or fluorescent signal in enzyme immunoassays by photodensitometry. J Immunol Methods 1987; 103:9–14.

72. Geoghegan WD. The Ngo-Lenhoff (MBTH-DMAB) peroxidase assay. *Op. cit.* (Ref. 10):451–65.
73. Tuuminen T, Palomäki P, Rakkolainen A, Welin M-G, Weber T, Käpyaho K. 3-p-hydroxyphenyl-propionic acid—a sensitive fluorogenic substrate for automated fluorimetric enzyme immunoassays. J Immunoassay 1991; 12:29–46.
74. Achord D, Oayne G, Saewert M, Harvey S. Immunoconcentration. *Op. cit.* (Ref. 23):584–609.
75. Howard K, Kane M, Madden A, *et al.* Direct solid-phase enzymoimmunoassay of testosterone in saliva. Clin Chem 1989; 35:2044–7.
76. O'Rorke A, Kane MM, Gosling JP,Tallon DF, Fottrell PF. Development and validation of a mono-clonal antibody enzymeimmunoassay for the measurement of progesterone in saliva. Clin Chem 1994; 40:454–8.
77. Shimizu SY, Kabakoff DS, Sevier ED. Monoclonal antibodies in immunoenzymetric assays. *Op. cit.* (Ref. 10):433–51.
78. Madersbacher S, Berger P. Double wavelength measurement of 3,3',5,5'-tetramethylbenzidine (TMB) provides a three-fold enhancement of the ELISA measuring range. J Immunol Methods 1991; 138:121–4.
79. Madersbacher S, Shu-Chen T, Schwarz S, Dirnhofer S, Wick G, Berger P. Time-resolved immunoflu-orimetry and other frequently used immunoassay types for follicle-stimulating hormone compared by using identical monoclonal antibodies. Clin Chem 1993; 39:1435–9.
80. Green M, Barrance D, Hilditch P. Electrometric immunoassay. *Op. cit.* (Ref. 23):482–515.
81. Ekins RP, Chu FW. Multianalyte microspot immunoassay-microanalytical "compact disk" of the future. Clin Chem 1991; 37:1955–67.
82. Kemeny DM. Titration of antibodies. J Immunol Methods 1992; 150:57–76.
83. Olivieri V, Beccarini I, Gallucci G, Romano T, Santoro F. Capture assay for specific IgE: an improved quantitiative method. J Immunol Methods 1993; 157:65–72.
84. Thomas HIJ, Morgan-Capner P. The use of antibody avidity measurements for the diagnosis of rubells. Rev Med Virol 1991; 1:41–50.
85. Lappalainen M, Koskela P, Koskiniemi M, Ämmälä P, Hiilesmaa V, Teramo K, Raivio KO, Reming-ton JS, Hedman K. Toxoplasmosis acquired during pregnancy: improved serodiagnosis based on avidity of IgG. J Infect Dis 1993; 167:691–7.
86. Ward KN, Gray JJ, Joslin ME, Sheldon MJ. Avidity of IgG antibodies to human herpesvirus-6 distinguishes primary from recurrent infection in organ transplant recioients and excludes cross-reactivity with other herpesviruses. J Med Virol 1993; 39:44–9.
87. Underwood PA. Problems and pitfalls with measurement of antibody affinity solid phase binding in the ELISA. J Immunol Methods 1993; 164:119–30.
88. Goldblatt D, van Etten L, van Milligen FJ, Aalberse RC, Turner MW. The role of pH in modified ELISA procedures used for the estimation of functional antibody affinity. J Immunol Methods 1993; 166:281–5.
89. Self CH. Hapten determination method, its components, its uses and kits including it. Chem Abs 1990; 112:51813.
90. Yonezawa S, Kambegawa A, Tokudome S. Covalent coupling of a steroid to microwell plates for use in a competitive enzyme-linked immunosorbent assay. J Immunol Methods 1993; 166:55–61.
91. Yie S-M, Johansson E, Brown GM. Competitive solid-phase enzyme immunoassay for melatonin in human and rat serum and rat pineal gland. Clin Chem 1993; 39:2322–5.
92. Boscato LM, Egan GM, Stuart MC. Specificity of two-site immunoassays. J Immunol Methods 1989; 117:221–9.
93. Jenkins SH. Homogeneous enzyme immunoassay. J Immunol Methods 1992; 150:91–7.
94. Engel WD, Khanna PL. CEDIA in vitro diagnostics with a novel homogeneous immunoassay technique: current status and future prospects. J Immunol Methods 1992; 150:99–102.
95. Madersbacher S, Shu-Chen T, Schwarz S, Dirnhofer S, Wick G, Berger P. Time-resolved immunoflu-orimetry and other frequently used immunoassay types for follicle-stimulating hormone compared by using identical monoclonal antibodies. Clin Chem 1993; 39:1435–9.
96. Zhang L-Z, Gong Y-F, Fang Y, Zhang Y-S, Gu F-S. Use of microwaves in immunoenzyme techniques. Clin Chem 1993; 39:2021

14 | FLUORESCENCE IMMUNOASSAYS

THEODORE K. CHRISTOPOULOS
Department of Chemistry and
Biochemistry
University of Windsor
Windsor, Ontarior, Canada N9B 3P4

ELEFTHERIOS P. DIAMANDIS
Department of Pathology and
Laboratory Medicine
Mount Sinai Hospital
Toronto, Ontario, Canada M5A 1X8

1. INTRODUCTION

Fluorometry is superior to spectrophotometry in terms of sensitivity and specificity. In general, the sensitivity of fluorescence is 10–1000-fold higher in comparison to absorbance measurements. Fluorometry was introduced in immunological assays to improve immunoassay sensitivity.

An indication of the potential sensitivity of fluorometry is that the search for single-molecule detection has been based almost exclusively on the use of fluorescent compounds. In addition, fluorometric determination could combine several parameters simultaneously, such as excitation and emission wavelength, lifetime, and polarization, thus being a specific and versatile analytical system. Because the above parameters are affected by changes in the microenvironment of the fluorescent compound, fluorescence spectroscopy frequently allows the direct study of molecular processes, such as antigen–antibody interaction, without prior separation of the bound from the free fraction. This forms the basis for the development of homogeneous fluorescence immunoassays. In this chapter, the principles, applications, and limitations of fluorescence immunoassay are discussed along with some future directions.

2. PRINCIPLES OF FLUORESCENCE SPECTROSCOPY

2.1. Fluorescence Emission

Luminescence is generally defined as the emission of photons from excited electronic states. It is divided into fluorescence and phosphorescence. Fluorescence is defined as a radiative transition from the lowest excited singlet state (S_1) to a singlet ground state (S_0) of a molecule. Phosphorescence is defined as a radiative transition from the lowest triplet state (T_1) to the singlet ground state (S_0). In a singlet state, all electrons are paired, i.e., they have antiparallel spin. In a triplet state, two electrons are unpaired, that is, their spins are parallel. The absorption and emission of light is illustrated in the energy flow diagram of Fig. 14.1.

The ground and first excited electronic states are S_0 and S_1, respectively. At each of these energy levels, the molecule can exist in a number of vibrational energy levels (0,1,2, etc.). Following light absorption, a fluorophore is usually excited to a

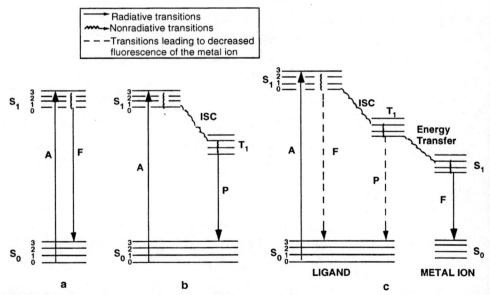

FIGURE 14.1 (a) Energy flow diagram for a fluorescent compound. (b) Energy flow diagram for a phosphorescent compound. (c) Mechanism of fluorescence of a lanthanide chelate. Energy is absorbed by the ligand and through an intramolecular energy transfer process; it flows from the triplet state of the ligand to the metal-ion which subsequently emits ion fluorescence. A, Absorbance; F, Fluorescence, P, Phosphorescence; ISC, intersystem crossing. S and T represent singlet and triplet states, respectively. More details are given in the text.

vibrational level of S_1. It then rapidly (10^{-12} sec) goes to the lowest vibrational level of S_1 by a nonradiative process called "internal conversion." From S_1, the molecule may go to any of the vibrational levels of the ground electronic state, S_0, by emitting fluorescence. Because the emission always takes place from the lowest excited level, the shape of the emission spectrum is independent of the excitation wavelength. The wavelength of fluorescence emission is always longer than the wavelength of excitation because of the nonradiative internal conversion, and also because the molecule can return to any of the excited vibrational levels of the ground electronic state. Both processes are associated with a loss of energy.

Alternatively, the molecule from S_1 can go over to the first triplet state, T_1, by a transition called "intersystem crossing" and subsequently relax to the ground state by emitting phosphorescence (Fig. 14.1b). The S_1 to S_0 radiative transition (fluorescence) is spin-allowed and results in short lifetimes for the excited state, of about 10^{-8} sec, typical for most organic fluorophores (e.g., fluorescein and rhodamine). The T_1 to S_0 transition is spin-forbidden and results in the long lifetimes (10^{-4}–10 sec) characteristic of phosphorescence.

The long-lived fluorescence emitted by chelates of the rare earth metal-ions, Eu^{3+}, Tb^{3+}, Sm^{3+}, and Dy^{3+} (used as labels in time-resolved fluorometric immunoassay), follows a somewhat different mechanism (Fig. 14.1c). Although the fluorescence of simple inorganic salts of these ions is weak, it is dramatically enhanced when the metal-ion forms a chelate with appropriate organic ligands. Radiation is absorbed at a wavelength characteristic of the ligand and is emitted as a line spectrum characteristic of the metal-ion because of an intramolecular energy transfer process from the ligand to the central metal-ion. The organic ligand absorbs energy and is raised from singlet S_0 to S_1 (Fig. 14.1c). Then, intersystem crossing occurs to the triplet state T_1. Afterward, through intramolecular energy transfer, the energy flows from the triplet excited state of the ligand to an appropriate energy level of the central metal-ion which, in turn, moves up to its own excited singlet state and subsequently emits ion fluorescence. For this series of events to take place, the following requirements should be fulfilled: The energy of the ion-resonance level should be just below that of T_1 of the ligand; the deactivating ligand transitions S_1 to S_0 or T_1 to S_0 (radiative or not) should be minimal. The principal emission lines for the four lanthanide ions arise from the transitions: $^5D_0$ to $^7F_2$ (613 nm) for Eu^{3+}; $^5D_4$ to $^7F_5$ (546 nm) for Tb^{3+}; $^4G_{5/2}$ to $^6H_{9/2}$ (643 nm) for Sm^{3+}; and $^4F_{9/2}$ to $^6H_{15/2}$ (483 nm) for Dy^{3+}.

2.2. Fluorescence Lifetime

After instantaneous pulse-excitation of a fluorescent molecule, the fluorescence decay curve follows first-order kinetics described by Eq. (1),

$$F_t = F_o e^{-kt}, \tag{1}$$

where F_o and F_t are the fluorescence intensities at Time 0 and t, respectively, and k is a rate constant. The fluorescence lifetime, τ, is defined as the time required for the fluorescence emission to decay to $1/e$ of its initial intensity following excitation. Substitution of F_t in Eq. (1) by F_o/e (fluorescence intensity after time τ) yields

$$\tau = k^{-1}, \tag{2}$$

indicating that the fluorescence lifetime is equal to the reciprocal of the rate constant. Combining Eqs. (1) and (2) yields:

$$F_t = F_o e^{-t/\tau} \tag{3}$$

$$\ln F_t = \ln F_o - t/\tau. \tag{4}$$

The plot of $\ln F_t$ vs t is a straight line with a slope of $-1/\tau$. If there is only one emitting species, the fluorescence lifetime can be calculated from the linear plot, assuming that the duration of the exciting pulse is substantially shorter than the fluorescence lifetime.

For nanosecond and subnanosecond lifetime measurements, phase-resolved fluorescence, in which the sample is excited by a continuous sinusoidally modulated radiation source, is the method of choice. The emitted fluorescence as a function of time is then phase-shifted and partially demodulated to an extent dependent on the lifetime of the fluorescing species. The fluorescence lifetimes of some common probes are shown in Table 14.1.

2.3. Quantitative Fluorometry

The fluorescence quantum yield (ϕ) is the ratio of the number of photons emitted to the number absorbed. The fluorescence intensity (F) is proportional to the amount of light absorbed,

$$F = \phi(I_o - I) \tag{5}$$

where I_o is the intensity of the incident light and I is the intensity transmitted. Because $I/I_o = 10^{-\varepsilon l c}$ (Beer–Lambert law), the amount of light absorbed is:

$$I_o - I = I_o(1 - 10^{-\varepsilon l c}). \tag{6}$$

By combining Eqs. (5) and (6) we have

$$F = \phi I_o(1 - 10^{-\varepsilon l c}). \tag{7}$$

where ε is the molar extinction coefficient, l is the optical path length, and c is the concentration. When the concentration of the fluorescent compound is low, the fluorescence intensity is given by the equation:

$$F = 2.3\phi I_o \varepsilon l c. \tag{8}$$

TABLE 14.1 Lifetimes of Some Common Fluorescent Probes

Fluorescent probe	Fluorescence lifetime (nsec)
Fluorescein	4.5
Rhodamines	1–3
Dansyl chloride	14
Anilinonaphthalenesulfonic acid	16
Fluorescamine	7
N-(3-Pyrene)-maleimide	100
Europium chelates	$3 \times 10^5 - 10^6$

The linear relationship between fluorescence intensity and concentration holds only for dilute solutions where absorbance is lower than 0.02. From Eq. (8) it can be seen that the fluorescence intensity is proportional to the intensity of the light source. This is the reason for the use of laser light sources to achieve improved sensitivity in fluorometry.

2.4. Limitations of Fluorescence Measurements

Limitations of fluorescence measurements include the following:

(i) Scattering of excitation light from solvent molecules (Rayleigh scattering) or from small particles (Tyndall scattering). Rayleigh or Tyndall scattering have the same spectrum as the excitation light and do not have a lifetime ($\tau = 0$). Furthermore, some excitation light is absorbed by solvent molecules and the resulting scattering occurs at longer wavelengths (Raman scattering). Scattering causes more problems with fluorescent probes having relatively small Stokes shifts (the difference between excitation and emission maxima) because, in this case, the excitation light cannot be effectively filtered out.

(ii) Endogenous fluorescence. Biological fluids used as samples may contain a variety of fluorescent components giving rise to background. Serum proteins (excitation 280 nm) cause high background at 320–350 nm. Bilirubin and NAD(P)H (excitation 330–360 nm) fluoresce at 430–470 nm. Urine may also contain endogenous compounds or fluorescent drugs that can cause high background. The excitation and emission of the fluorescent probes used in fluorescence immunoassays (FIA) should preferably be at longer wavelengths than that of the background emitting species. Endogenous fluorescence is a problem only for homogeneous FIA where the measurement of fluorescence is carried out in the presence of sample constituents. Therefore, sample pretreatment is frequently needed in cases where high sensitivity is required (e.g., serum digoxin assay).

(iii) Quenching. Light-absorbing molecules in serum such as bilirubin and hemoglobin, can absorb either the excitation or the emission energy, causing quenching. Binding of fluorophore-labeled antigens to serum proteins may quench the fluorescence. Binding can also be a source of error for homogeneous FIA because of the disturbance of the equilibrium between antibody-bound and free labeled analyte. Concentration quenching (also known as "inner-filter effect") has been observed during labeling of antibodies with more than one fluorescent probe having a small Stokes shift, e.g., fluorescein. Concentration quenching is likely due to overlapping absorption and emission spectra of the fluorophore. This type of quenching can be seen as a decrease of the quantum yield with increasing load of fluorophore per protein molecule. It is thought that fluorescence emitted by one fluorophore is absorbed by adjacent fluorophores in the same labeled reagent or in solution. Inner filter quenching is not a problem when the fluorophore has a large Stokes shift and there is no overlap between excitation and emission spectra (e.g., the lanthanide chelates).

(iv) Photodestruction. This is the photochemical reaction causing fluorescence to decrease upon continuous excitation. It is strongly dependent on the excitation wavelength. Photodestruction becomes a serious problem when high-intensity excitation and several repeated measurements are used during short intervals.

3. FLUORESCENCE IMMUNOASSAY INSTRUMENTATION

All fluorometers used in fluorescence immunoassay have a light source, excitation and emission filters or monochromators, an optical system which is based either on lenses and mirrors or fiber optics, and a detection system based on photomultiplier tubes with analog or photon-counting signal processing. More dedicated instruments have additional components which may include pipettors, washers, moving carousels, and data reduction units. For time-resolved fluorometric applications the instrument must have electronic circuitry for time-gated measurements. With dedicated instrumentation, all measurement parameters are usually fixed and optimized for the particular chemical system used.

For excitation, the mercury gas discharge lamp which produces high output at 366, 415, and 435 nm is frequently used, e.g., in the Abbott's IMx immunoassay analyzer and in the Dynatech's MicroFluor microplate reader. Xenon lamps are usually employed in spectrofluorometers but are also used in the ARCUS and DELFIA time-resolved fluorometers (Pharmacia-LKB). Halogen lamps, although producing weaker UV light than mercury and xenon lamps, have been used in various FIA systems, e.g., the Ames TD_A, the IDT FIAX, and the Syva Advance fluorometer. Lasers can also be used as high-intensity monochromatic sources of excitation light. A nitrogen laser is used in a time-resolved fluorometer, the CyberFluor 615 Immunoanalyzer.

The optical arrangement used for measurement of the emitted light primarily depends on the requirements of the assay, i.e., emission from solution or solid phase and the type of the solid phase. Microplate fluorometers are usually based on front-surface measurements. They use semireflective dichroic mirrors which reflect excitation light but allow emission light to reach the detector. Many of the fully automated immunoassay analyzers also employ front-surface fluorometers measuring fluorescence emitted directly from the solid phase (filter paper, thin film, microparticles, etc.) or its surrounding liquid.

4. FLUORESCENT LABELS

Table 14.2 summarizes the properties of some fluorescent labels commonly used in FIA (1).

4.1. Fluoresceins

Fluorescein is the most frequently used fluorescent label in FIA because of its high absorptivity and quantum yield. The quantum yield is 0.85 when the molecule is free in an alkaline aqueous solution but it decreases to 0.3–0.5 when fluorescein is conjugated to antibodies. Fluorescein isothiocyanate (FITC, Fig. 14.2), which reacts with aminogroups, is the reagent most commonly used for labeling. The small Stokes shift of fluorescein makes multiple labeling impractical because of the inner filter effect. The optimum labeling for Fab' fragments or IgG is 2 or 4 FITC/antibody molecule, respectively. The overlapping fluorescence emission wavelengths of fluorescein and albumin-bound bilirubin results in a high background interference in homogeneous assays. Also, its affinity for serum proteins may cause errors in FIA.

TABLE 14.2 **Properties of Some Fluorescent Labels Used in Immunoassays (1)**

Label	Ex$_{max}$ (nm)	Em$_{max}$ (nm)	ε LM^{-1} cm^{-1}	ϕ
Fluorescein (FITC, DTAF)	492	516–525	72,000 66,000	0.3–0.85
Carboxy fluorescein (CF)	492	514–518	73,000	0.87
2'-Methoxy-CF	500	534		0.78
TRITC G	535–545	570–580	107,000	
RBITC	545–560	585	103,000	
Texas Red	595	615–620	85,000	0.3
Umbelliferone (U)	325	465		
4-Methyl-U	325	450	16,000	
4-Methyl-U-3-acetate	365	455		
B-PE	545	575	2,410,000	0.59–0.98
C-PC	620	650	580,000	0.51

Abbreviations used: Ex$_{max}$ and Em$_{max}$, excitation and emission maxima; ε, molar extinction coefficient; ϕ, fluorescence yield; FITC, fluorescein isothiocyanate; DTAF, dichlorotriazinyl derivative of amino fluorescein; TRITC G, tetramethylrhodamine isothiocyanate, isomer G; RBITC, rhodamine-B isothiocyanate; B-PE, B-phycoerythrin; C-PC, C-phycocyanin.

A variety of fluorescein derivatives are used for labeling. 4'-(aminomethyl)-fluorescein is used in fluorescence polarization immunoassay (FPIA) reagents. The dichlorotriazinyl derivative of aminofluorescein (Fig. 14.2) is used in a number of FPIA. Carboxyfluorescein, as an *N*-hydroxysuccinimide ester, is used in fluorescence excitation transfer immunoassays (FETI) as an energy donor for tetramethylrhodamine-labeled antibodies. 4',5'-Dimethoxycarboxy fluorescein is an optimal energy acceptor for fluorescein in FETI.

4.2. Rhodamines

Rhodamines are derivatives of the same basic structure as fluorescein. Generally, they emit at longer wavelengths than fluorescein but they have lower quantum yields. Tetramethylrhodamine isothiocyanate (TRITC, Fig. 14.2) is one of the most commonly used rhodamine derivatives in FIA. Because it absorbs where fluorescein emits, it can be used as energy acceptor for fluorescein in FETI assays.

4.3. Coumarins

Derivatives of coumarins (Fig. 14.2) such as umbelliferone (7-hydroxycoumarine) have found wide applications as fluorogenic substrates in substrate-labeled fluorescence immunoassays (SLFIA) and enzyme-linked fluorescence immunoassays (ELFIA). A crucial property of umbelliferone is that its fluorescence is entirely dependent on the excitation of the phenolic form only. Derivatization of the 7-hydroxy group results in nonfluorescent molecules. Umbelliferone and 3'-substituted umbelliferones are used in SLFIA. Here a glycoside or an ester bond is formed between the analyte and the 7-hydroxy group. The conjugate is not fluorescent, but it becomes so after enzymatic hydrolysis of the quenching bond. The phosphate ester of 4-methylumbelliferone is a widely used fluorogenic substrate for ELFIA in combination with alkaline phosphatase as the enzyme label.

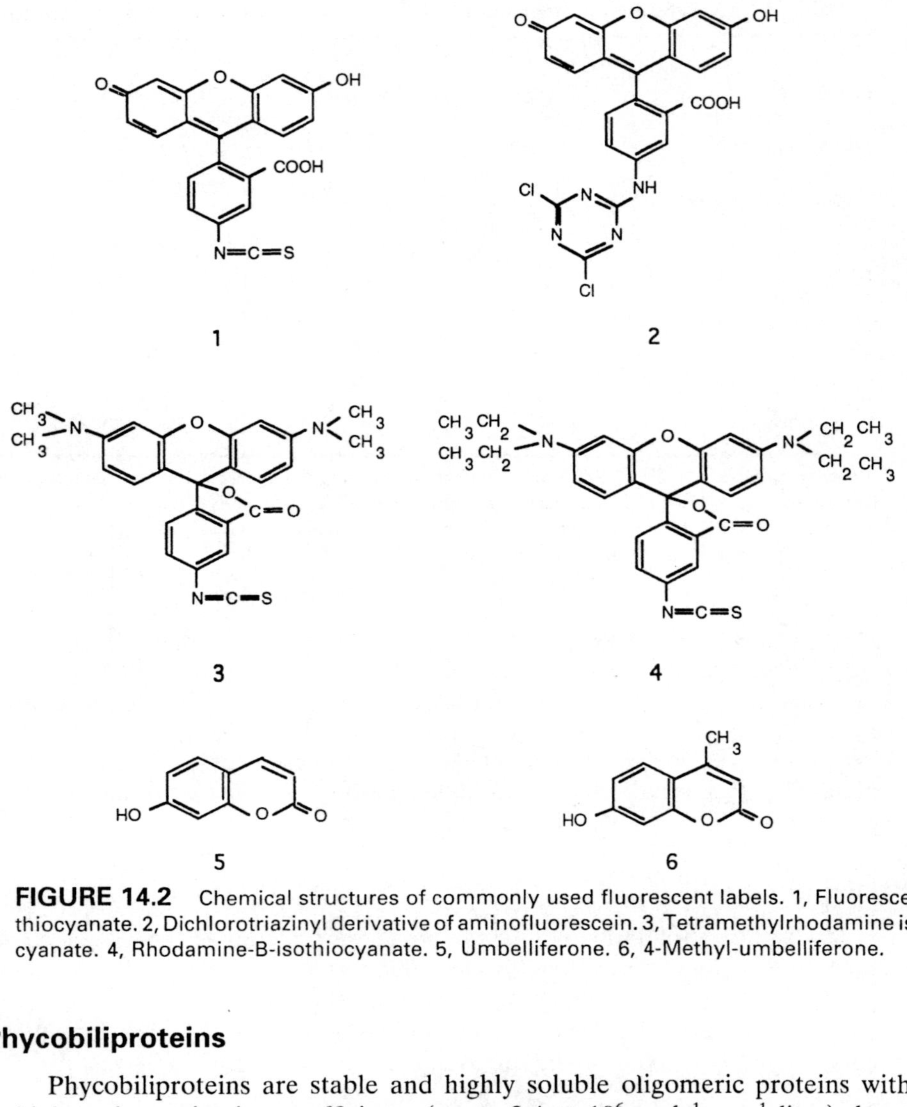

FIGURE 14.2   Chemical structures of commonly used fluorescent labels. 1, Fluorescein iso-thiocyanate. 2, Dichlorotriazinyl derivative of aminofluorescein. 3, Tetramethylrhodamine isothio-cyanate. 4, Rhodamine-B-isothiocyanate. 5, Umbelliferone. 6, 4-Methyl-umbelliferone.

4.4. Phycobiliproteins

Phycobiliproteins are stable and highly soluble oligomeric proteins with very high molar extinction coefficients (up to 2.4×10^6 mol^{-1} cm^{-1} liter) due to the presence of several bilin prosthetic groups. There are three main classes, phycoery-thrin (PE), phycocyanin (PC), and allophycocyanin (APC). They have quantum yields as high as 0.98. In "particle concentration fluorescence immunoassay," PE is commonly used as a fluorescent probe.

5. HOMOGENEOUS FLUORESCENCE IMMUNOASSAYS

5.1. Fluorescence Polarization Immunoassay (FPIA)

The fluorescence polarization principle was first applied to immunoassay proce-dures by Dandiker *et al.* in 1973 (3), but wider use in clinical routine started during the early 1980s, when Abbott introduced the automated TDx instrument. FPIA is one of the most widely used procedures in clinical chemistry. The method is based on the principle that fluorescence polarization gives a direct measure of the bound/free ratio of the labeled analyte without need for their separation (Fig. 14.3).

Fluorescence polarization (2–7) is measured by first illuminating the sample with a plane (e.g., vertically) polarized light. This is accomplished by placing a polarizer in the excitation light path. The emitted light then passes through another polarizer before reaching the detector. The intensity (I) of fluorescence is first measured with the two polarizers having the same orientation ($I_{parallel}$) and then oriented at 90° to each other ($I_{perpendicular}$). The fluorescence polarization value (p) is then calculated using Eq. (9).

$$p = \frac{I_{parallel} - I_{perpendicular}}{I_{parallel} + I_{perpendicular}} \qquad (9)$$

Hypothetical molecules fixed in space with their absorption dipoles parallel to the electrical vector of the excitation light would emit fluorescence completely polarized with $p = 1$ ($I_{perpendicular} = 0$). For randomly oriented molecules, which is the real situation in solution, the probability of light absorption (and excitation) is proportional to $\cos^2 \theta$, where θ is the angle made by the electric vector of the incident light and the absorption dipole of the molecule. Molecules oriented so that θ is small are preferentially excited while the others have little chance to absorb. This $\cos^2 \theta$ distribution of absorption dipoles leads to a variation in the orientation of emission dipoles so that the light emitted from an assembly of molecules is partially polarized.

Thus, for a system of randomly oriented molecules having the absorption axis parallel to the emission axis, the maximum value of p is 0.5, if no rotational Brownian motion occurs. If the molecules are free to rotate, then a further depolarization takes place because of rotation occurring during the time between excitation and emission (typically 10^{-8} sec).

The connection of polarization with the antigen–antibody complex formation arises from the fact that the Brownian motion, and consequently the magnitude of

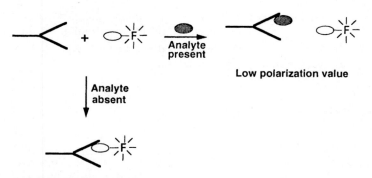

High polarization value

FIGURE 14.3   Fluorescence polarization immunoassay (FPIA). F, fluorescein. Labeled and unlabeled analyte are represented by open and shaded circles, respectively. The polarization value is a direct measure of the bound/free ratio of labeled analyte. The size of the unbound labeled analyte is small and its fast rotation causes depolarization. The bound labeled analyte has a high molecular weight and rotates slowly. In this case, the fluorescence emitted is highly polarized.

depolarization occurring during the excitation lifetime, decreases as molecular size increases. Therefore, the binding of a fluorescein-labeled antigen to its specific antibody causes an increase in the polarization value because of the high molecular weight of the immunocomplex formed. A quantitative description is given by the Perrin equation for steady state (i.e., continuous excitation) measurement of polarization,

$$(1/p - 1/3) = (1/p_o - 1/3) (1 + 3\tau/\rho), \tag{10}$$

where $p_o = 0.5$ (that is, the maximum value of polarization which would be observed in the absence of any Brownian motion), τ is the lifetime of the excited state, and ρ is the rotational relaxation time. For spherical molecules, ρ can be calculated according to Eq. (11).

$$\rho = 3nv/RT \tag{11}$$

Rotational relaxation is directly proportional to the volume (v) of the molecule (size and shape) and viscosity (n) of the medium. R is the gas constant and T is the absolute temperature. From Eq. (10) and (11) it can be seen that polarization increases with molecular size. In a competitive-type immunoassay (Fig. 14.3), the polarization value is maximum when analyte is not present in the sample and all labeled analyte is antibody-bound. With increasing analyte levels in the sample, depolarization occurs because of the fast rotation of the displaced labeled analyte.

For practical purposes, the molecular weight of the antigen (analyte) should be below 20,000; otherwise, the change in molecular size during the immunoreaction is not high enough to cause a significant increase in polarization value.

The technology is employed primarily for therapeutic drug monitoring and screening for illicit drugs, but it is also used for some hormones (e.g., thyroxine, cortisol). Aminomethylfluorescein and FITC are used as labels. Abbott has introduced commercial systems with various stages of automation and even systems which combine the FPIA system for small molecules with a heterogeneous ELFIA system for macromolecules. Other manufacturers such as Roche and CANAM also provide reagents and instruments for FPIA.

Problems in FPIA usually arise either from the nonspecific increase in polarization due to binding of the labeled-analyte to serum albumin or from the high background of the samples. Also, the dynamic range is usually narrow. The sensitivity is limited in the micromolar to nanomolar range.

5.2. Fluorescence Excitation (Energy) Transfer Immunoassay (FETI)

The assay uses two labels, one of which is fluorescent (donor) and the other is an energy-accepting or -quenching molecule (acceptor) (8). The donor is attached to the analyte, whereas the acceptor is attached to the analyte-specific antibody. When the labeled analyte and labeled antibody come to close proximity as a result of the immunoreaction, energy is transferred from the excited electronic state of the donor to the acceptor molecule. This energy transfer occurs without the release of a photon; it is primarily due to dipole–dipole interaction between donor and acceptor and results in quenching of the fluorescence of the donor in the immunocomplex. The free donor-labeled analyte remains fluorescent (Fig. 14.4).

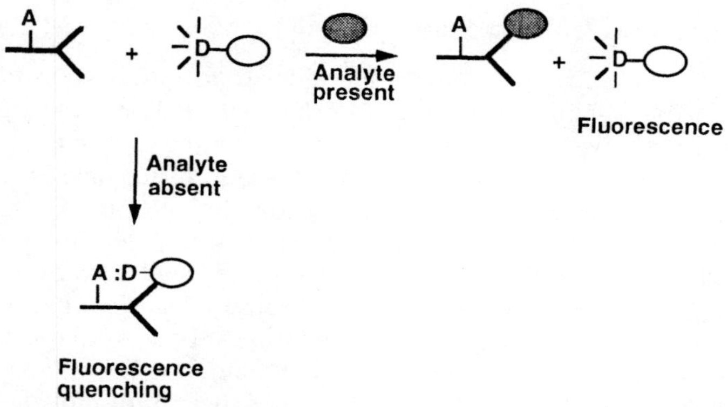

FIGURE 14.4   The principle of fluorescence excitation transfer immunoassay (FETI). Analyte labeled with a fluorescent molecule (energy donor, D) competes with unlabeled analyte for binding to antibodies labeled with an energy accepting molecule (A). The binding of labeled analyte to antibody results in fluorescence quenching because of energy transfer from D to A.

In a typical FETI protocol, the analyte in the sample competes with donor-labeled analyte for a limited amount of acceptor-labeled antibody. Increased analyte concentration causes an increase in the concentration of free labeled analyte and consequently an increase in the intensity of the fluorescence measured.

The energy transfer efficiency is related to the distance, r, between donor and acceptor in the immunocomplex

$$E = (\phi_o - \phi_q)/\phi_o = r^{-6}/(r^{-6} + R_o^{-6}), \tag{12}$$

where ϕ_q and ϕ_o are the fluorescence quantum yields of the donor in the presence and absence of the acceptor, respectively (8). R_o is the distance at which transfer is 50% efficient and has a maximum value of about 8 nm. Most points on the surface of the Y-shaped IgG antibody fall within this distance. Therefore, acceptors conjugated anywhere on the antibody molecule are within potential energy transfer distance of a donor-labeled bound antigen. Strong spectral overlap between the emission of the donor and the absorption of the acceptor molecule is required for an efficient energy transfer.

Automated FETI assays can be performed with the Syva Advance fluorometer. This method has found many applications in the assay of drugs, hormones, and proteins in biological fluids (9). Considerable efforts have been made to find suitable energy donor–acceptor pairs. Fluorescein was chosen as the donor in many applications. Rhodamine was one of the first acceptor molecules tested. Subsequently, many fluorescein derivatives have been tested as donors and dimethoxyfluorescein as acceptor. The 4′,5′-dimethoxyfluorescein has shown good characteristics as an energy acceptor, i.e., good spectral overlapping with fluorescein and practically no fluorescence of its own. Therefore, in this case, the background arising from direct excitation of the acceptor is negligible.

In a noncompetitive assay format for FETI, a portion of the antibody population is labeled with a fluorescent donor and the rest with a nonfluorescent acceptor. When these antibodies bind to a polyhaptenic analyte they come into sufficiently close proximity, which results in energy transfer and fluorescence quenching (8).

5.3. Fluorescence Quenching Immunoassay (FQIA)

In this assay (10), the fluorescence of bound labeled analyte is measured after selective quenching of the fluorescence of free labeled analyte. Analyte in the sample competes with fluorescein-labeled analyte for binding to a limited amount of analyte-specific antibody. The labeled analyte binding to its specific antibody does not affect the fluorescence of the label. After completion of the immunoreaction, anti-fluorescein antibodies are added which bind to the free fraction of the fluorescein-labeled analyte. Anti-fluorescein antibodies are not able to react with the antibody-bound fluorescein-labeled analyte because of steric hindrance. The fluorescence of fluorescein is significantly quenched (up to about 90%) upon binding to anti-fluorescein antibody. Therefore, only the bound fraction of the labeled analyte fluoresces. The fluorescence decreases as the concentration of the analyte in the sample increases, because more of the labeled analyte is available for binding to anti-fluorescein antibodies.

Regardless of the efficiency of quenching, in practical applications the intrinsic fluorescence of samples contributes significantly to the total signal, to a degree that background monitoring and correction is needed. FQIA have been developed for several analytes including albumin, IgG (11), and T4 (12).

5.4. Release Fluoroimmunoassays

The most successful variation of this technique is termed "substrate labeled fluoroimmunoassay" (SLFIA). It is a competitive-type immunoassay (13) where the analyte is labeled with a fluorogenic substrate, i.e., a molecule which is not fluorescent by itself but becomes so after enzymatic hydrolysis. Galactosyl umbelliferone is a suitable fluorogenic substrate.

The nonfluorescent analyte-galactosyl umbelliferone conjugate (shown in Fig. 14.5a) can be hydrolyzed by β-D-galactosidase to galactose and analyte-umbellifer-

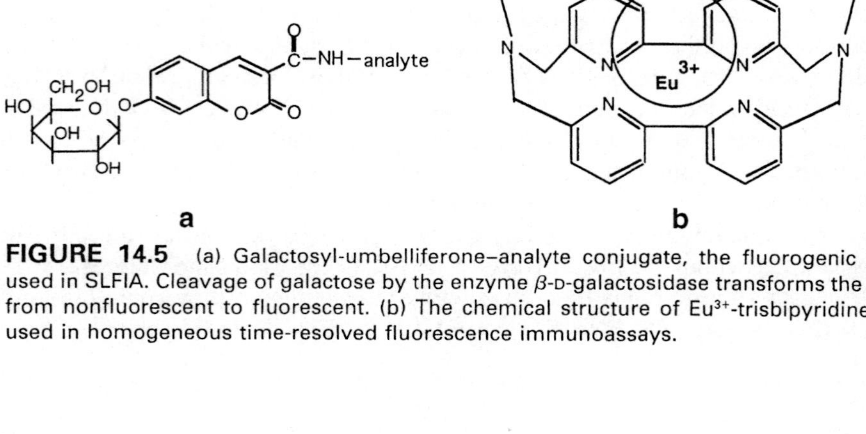

FIGURE 14.5 (a) Galactosyl-umbelliferone–analyte conjugate, the fluorogenic substrate used in SLFIA. Cleavage of galactose by the enzyme β-D-galactosidase transforms the molecule from nonfluorescent to fluorescent. (b) The chemical structure of Eu^{3+}-trisbipyridine cryptate used in homogeneous time-resolved fluorescence immunoassays.

one which fluoresces. The key characteristic of these assays is that the binding of labeled analyte to its specific antibody renders the fluorogenic substrate inaccessible to the enzyme because of steric hindrance. Therefore, only the free (unbound) labeled analyte conjugate can be hydrolyzed by the enzyme and release the fluorescent moiety (umbelliferone).

In a typical assay, the analyte competes with labeled analyte for a limited number of antibody-binding sites. After adding the enzyme β-D-galactosidase, the fluorescence produced is directly related to the level of analyte in the sample.

Ames Division, Miles Laboratories, has commercialized the SLFIA technique primarily for therapeutic drug monitoring (14). Fluorostat is a specially designed fluorometer for SLFIA. As a simple homogeneous assay, SLFIA has also been automated with existing chemistry analyzers, e.g., the Cobas Bio and MULTISTAT II centrifugal analyzers (15).

5.5. Homogeneous Time-Resolved Fluorescence Immunoassay

Homogeneous competitive time-resolved fluorometric immunoassays for thyroxine (16) and estrone-3-glucuronide have been reported. The analytes in this case are labeled with a proprietary, stable, fluorescent europium chelate. Albumin and detergents in the assay buffer enhance the fluorescence of the free labeled analyte but not of the antibody-bound labeled analyte. Therefore, in a competitive assay, the fluorescence measured increases with the concentration of analyte in the sample.

Recently, a novel homogeneous two-site immunometric assay for prolactin was described (17), which combines the principles of fluorescence excitation energy transfer immunoassays (FETI, see above) and time-resolved fluorometry. The assay employs two monoclonal anti-prolactin antibodies, one labeled with the energy donor (a fluorophore with a long fluorescence lifetime) and the other with the energy acceptor (a fluorophore with a short fluorescence lifetime). A Eu^{3+} trisbipyridine cryptate (Eu^{3+}–TBP; see Fig. 14.5b) is the energy donor and allophycocyanin (APC) serves as the energy acceptor. In the Eu^{3+}–TBP complex the bipyridine groups absorb the excitation light. Then, through intramolecular energy transfer, the energy flows to the metal ion which subsequently fluoresces. After excitation at 337 nm (from a nitrogen laser) the Eu^{3+}–TBP complex emits at 580, 620, 650, and 700 nm, the highest peak being at 580 nm. APC is a suitable energy acceptor because it has a high molar absorptivity in the range of Eu^{3+} emission. APC emits fluorescence at 660 nm.

After the immunoreaction is completed, the reaction mixture contains the immunocomplex (sandwich) formed between prolactin and the two labeled antibodies. Free labeled antibodies are also present. The distance between the two labels in the immunocomplex is short enough to allow for an efficient energy transfer from Eu^{3+}–TBP to APC. Because the fluorescence lifetime of the donor is long, the acceptor will also emit long-lived fluorescence (18). Thus, the APC fluorescence at 660 nm due to energy transfer can be distinguished from the short-lived background emission at 660 nm which originates from the direct excitation of free APC-labeled antibodies at 337 nm. Interference from free Eu^{3+}–TBP-labeled antibodies is insignificant because of the different emission wavelengths. Furthermore, serum matrix effects can be avoided by taking the ratio of two time-resolved fluorescence measurements, one at a wavelength characteristic of the donor (e.g., 620 nm) and the other at 660 nm, characteristic of the acceptor.

5.6. Liposome-Based Fluorescence Immunoassay (Homogeneous)

In liposome-based fluorescence immunoassays (19), the tracers are antigens or antibodies conjugated to liposomes. The liposomes are synthetic, closed, and stable vesicles consisting of a glycerophospholipid bilayer membrane that encloses an aqueous solution containing a high concentration of a fluorescent compound.

Liposomes are prepared by injecting an alcoholic solution of phospholipids (e.g., dipalmitoylphosphatidylcholine, dipalmitoylphosphatidylglycerol, dipalmitoylphosphatidylethanolamine) and cholesterol into an aqueous solution of a fluorescent compound (e.g., carboxyfluorescein), or by vigorously mixing a thin phospholipid–cholesterol film with the solution of the fluorescent compound. Once formed, the liposomes are quite stable and may be separated from the solution by centrifugation, dialysis, or size-exclusion chromatography. Antigens or antibodies can be attached to liposomes through the primary amino group of phosphatidylethanolamine.

In a homogeneous, liposome-based, two-site immunosassay for ferritin (19) the sample is first incubated with anti-ferritin antibody (Fab fragments) attached to liposomes. Then, a second anti-ferritin antibody is added along with the complement. The formation of an immunocomplex (sandwich) results in the activation of the complement which causes liposome lysis and subsequent release of the fluorescent compound. The lysis of a single liposome gives thousands of fluorescent molecules in the solution. The fluorescence increases with ferritin concentration. Analyte-independent lysis of the liposomes is the major source of error in these assays.

6. HETEROGENEOUS FLUORESCENCE IMMUNOASSAYS

6.1. Particle Concentration Fluorescence Immunoassay (PCFIA)

In PCFIA (20) commercialized by Pandex, reactions occur on 0.8-mm-diameter latex beads in specially designed, filter-bottom microtiter plates. The large surface area and the Brownian motion of the particles permit fast reaction kinetics. The capture antibody is immobilized on the solid phase either directly (covalently, through surface carboxylic acids) or via a secondary antibody. Labeled analyte or labeled detection antibody are used for competitive or noncompetitive assays, respectively. The fluorescent label for competitive assays is β-phycoerythrin (21), whereas sandwich assays are performed with fluorescein-labeled antibodies. The particles are washed in the wells after the immunoreaction is completed and the fluorescence is measured by a front-surface fluorometer. The system can also use human or microbial cells as solid phases which are useful for screening for antibodies against cell surface antigens. The Pandex Screen Machine is a front-surface fluorometer and pipetting device specially designed for PCFIA applications.

6.2. Time-Resolved Fluorescence Immunoassay (TRFIA)

The introduction of time-resolved fluorometry in immunoassays originated from the realization that the sensitivity of the conventional fluorescence measurement is restricted by the high background signal inevitably present in any routine analysis. Indeed, fluorometric detection under routine conditions is limited to nanomolar concentrations. The rationale behind time-resolved fluorometry is the elimination of background in fluorescence measurements, for the purpose of improving the signal to noise ratio. This is achieved by using fluorescent labels having much longer fluoresence lifetimes than Tyndal, Rayleigh, or Raman scattering ($\tau = 0$), inherent fluorescence of the sample, and background luminescence from cuvettes, filters, and lenses (τ in the order of nanoseconds to a few microseconds). The long fluorescence lifetime of the fluorescent lanthanide chelates ($\tau \approx 10$–$1000~\mu s$) makes them especially suitable for microsecond time-resolved fluorometry.

The principle of the time-resolved fluorescence measurement is illustrated in Fig. 14.6. The sample is excited with a short pulse of light from a laser or flash lamp. The excited molecules emit either short- or long-lived fluorescence. Both types of fluorescence follow an exponential decay curve, but the short-lived one dissipates to zero in less than $100~\mu s$. If no measurements are taken during the first 100–$200~\mu s$ after excitation, short-lived fluorescence and scattered excitation are completely eliminated, allowing for the long-lived fluorescence signals to be measured with high sensitivity. In practice, the only background measured when using lanthanide-chelate labels is the signal produced by the nonspecific binding of the labeled reagents to the solid phases employed in immunoassays.

The classification of time-resolved fluorescence immunoassays is based on the moiety measured after the completion of the immunoreaction. The DELFIA system (Dissociation Enhanced Lanthanide Fluorescence Immunoassay), commercially available from Pharmacia-LKB, is based on the quantitation of Eu^{3+} bound to immunoreactants, after extraction with an enhancement solution. The FIAgen system, commercially available from CyberFluor Inc., uses excess of Eu^{3+} to quantitate the chelator bound to immunoreactants.

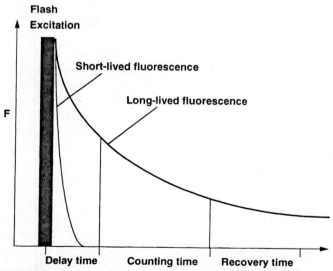

FIGURE 14.6 Principle of time-resolved fluorescence measurement. F, Fluorescence intensity. The solid bar indicates the excitation light and its duration. Measurements are taken only when the short-lived fluorescence dissipates to zero. The cycle is repeated many times during the measurement time which is usually 1 sec/cuvette.

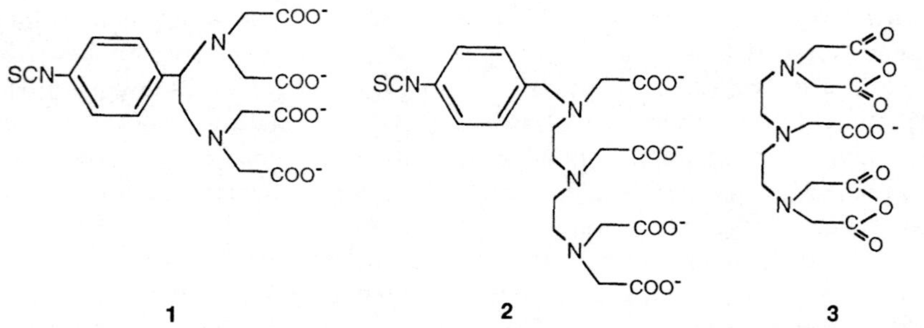

FIGURE 14.7 Chelating agents used for labeling of immunoreactants with lanthanide-ions. 1, Isothiocyanatophenyl EDTA. 2, N_1-p (Isothiocyanatobenzyl) diethylenetriaminetetraacetic acid. 3, Cyclic anhydride of diethyletriaminepentaacetic acid.

6.2.1. Immunoassays Based on Quantitation of Eu^{3+} Bound to Immunoreactants

6.2.1.1. Labeling of Proteins and Other Molecules with Metal-Ions   The most successful strategy for attaching metal-ions like Eu^{3+} to proteins or other molecules involves the use of strong metal chelators (formation constants $>10^{12}$ mol^{-1} liter) of the aminopolycarboxylic acid type (Fig. 14.7).

N-p(Isothiocyanatobenzyl) diethylenetriaminetetraacetic acid is the labeling reagent in all DELFIA products. The anhydride of diethylenetriaminepentaacetic acid (DTPA) can also be used for "in-house" labeling purposes because it is commercially available (e.g., from Pierce Chemical Co., Rockford, IL) and cheap.

These compounds are first reacted with, e.g., an antibody under conditions that favor multiple chelator incorporation with minimal deleterious effects to protein affinity, specificity, solubility, or stability. The metal-ion is then added in excess to saturate all available binding sites (usually 5–15 per antibody molecule) and excess metal-ion is removed by dialysis or gel filtration. Labeled reagents are stable for more than a year.

6.2.1.2. Fluorescence Enhancement   The complexes of Eu^{3+} and other lanthanides with aminopolycarboxylic acids fluoresce very weakly. Thus, in assays employing Eu^{3+}-labeled antibodies or antigens, after the immunoreaction is completed, an enhancement solution is added which (a) has a pH of 3.2 and causes dissociation of Eu^{3+} from the complex, and (b) contains 2-naphthoyltrifluoroacetone (NTA, Fig. 14.8), a β-diketone which is an excellent energy donor and forms highly fluorescent complexes with Eu^{3+} (22).

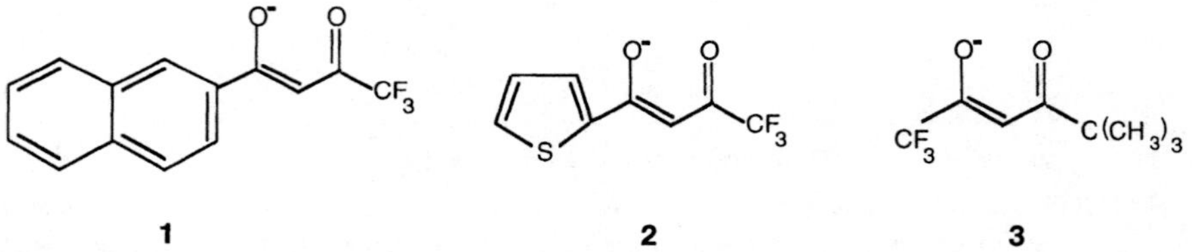

FIGURE 14.8 Chemical structures of: 1, 2-naphthoyltrifluoroacetone; 2, thenoyltrifluoroacetone; and 3, pivaloyltrifluoroacetone.

Thenoyltrifluoroacetone (Fig. 14.8) has also been used as an alternative β-diketone for in-house assay development (23) since NTA was not, until recently, commercially available. A synergistic agent, trioctylphosphine oxide (TOPO, a Lewis base), is also added in the enhancement solution because it insulates the lanthanide–β-diketone complex from quenching by water molecules. The insulation from the aqueous environment is further optimized by adding the detergent Triton X-100. The fluorescent complex consisting of Eu^{3+}, NTA, and TOPO is solubilized in the detergent micelles and gives higher fluorescence. When the optimized solution is used, Eu^{3+} can be quantified by time-resolved fluorometry over a concentration range from 5×10^{-14} to 10^{-7} mol/liter (22).

6.2.1.3. Immunoassay Designs   The noncompetitive, "sandwich" type immunoassay (Fig. 14.9) utilizes capture antibodies, coated on polystyrene microtitration strip wells or other suitable solid phases and Eu^{3+}-labeled detection antibodies. After the immunoreaction is completed, the excess of detection antibody is washed out. Eu^{3+} is then dissociated from the immunocomplex, by adding enhancement solution, and measured by time-resolved fluorometry.

A plethora of assays for peptide hormones, tumor markers, growth factors, and other high-molecular-weight analytes have been developed using the noncompetitive principle (24). In serological assays, the same configuration is applied but instead of capture antibodies, immobilized antigens are used to bind specific antibodies from human serum sample. Eu^{3+}-labeled anti-human antibodies are then utilized as the detection antibodies.

An interesting noncompetitive assay for small molecules, called "idiometric assay," has been proposed recently (25). The protocol is as follows. The sample is

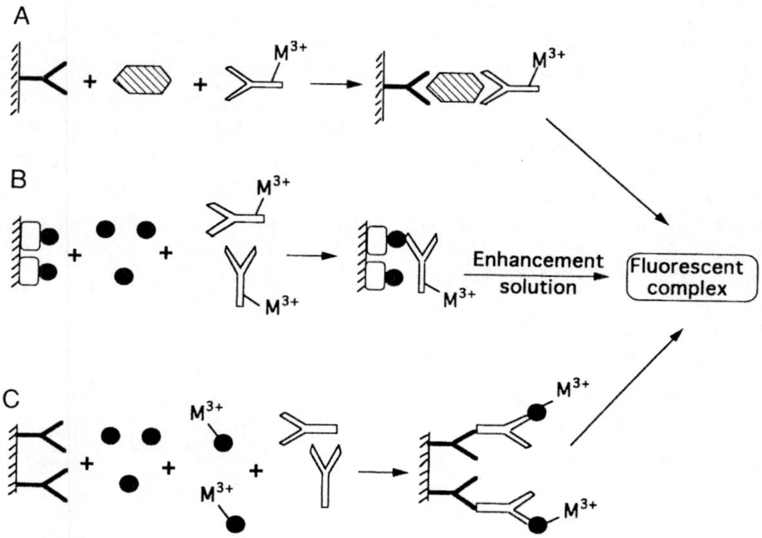

FIGURE 14.9   Immunoassays using Eu^{3+}-labeled reagents. (A) Noncompetitive assay with a solid-phase capture antibody and a Eu^{3+}-labeled detection antibody. (B) Competitive assay using the immobilized antigen approach. (C) Competitive assay using the immobilized second antibody approach. In all assays, Eu^{3+} (M^{3+}) is released and recomplexed in enhancement solution.

pipetted into microtitration wells coated with analyte-specific antibody (primary antibody). After the analyte binding, a β-type anti-idiotype antibody is added, which binds to all unoccupied primary antibody binding sites. After washing, a Eu^{3+}-labeled α-type anti-idiotype antibody is added which binds to the analyte/primary antibody complexes. This antibody will not bind to the primary antibody if the β type is already bound to it. The fluorescence measured is directly proportional to the analyte concentration.

Competitive-type immunoassays are performed either using the immobilized analyte approach and Eu^{3+}-labeled antibodies or by using Eu^{3+}-labeled analyte. Both methods are illustrated in Fig. 14.9. The analyte is immobilized via a protein carrier (e.g., ovalbumin) to polystyrene microtitration wells. The analyte in the sample competes with the solid-phase analyte for binding to a limited amount of Eu^{3+}-labeled antibodies. After washing excess reagents, the amount of bound Eu^{3+} is inversely related to the concentration of analyte in the sample. These assays sometimes suffer from leakage of immobilized analyte from the solid phase, which results in decreased labeled antibody binding.

Applications using Eu^{3+}-labeled analytes are currently more popular. In this case, the solid phase is coated with an excess of secondary antibody (e.g., anti-mouse IgG when the primary antibody is a mouse monoclonal). The competition of the analyte with Eu^{3+}-labeled analyte for binding to primary antibody takes place, at least in part, in solution. The immunocomplex formed is captured by the secondary antibodies. The fluorescence intensity is also inversely related to the analyte concentration (Fig. 14.9).

Competitive assays based on the above principles have been proposed for thyroid and steroid hormones, drugs, aflatoxins, etc. (24).

6.2.2. Immunoassays Based on Quantitation of the Chelator (Ligand) Bound to Immunoreactants

The FIAgen assays (CyberFluor Inc.) use the Eu^{3+}-chelator 4,7-bis(chlorosulfo-phenyl)-1,10-phenanthroline-2,9-dicarboxylic acid (BCPDA) as label (26). The structure of BCPDA is shown in Fig. 14.10. The molecule can be attached to proteins through its sulfonylchloride groups. When excited in the range of 280–340 nm, the Eu^{3+}–BCPDA complex emits strong fluorescence at 615 nm (characteristic of Eu^{3+}) with a lifetime in the range of 0.44–0.76 msec. The detection limit of BCPDA measurement with excess of Eu^{3+} in solution is about 10^{-11} mol/liter. The detection

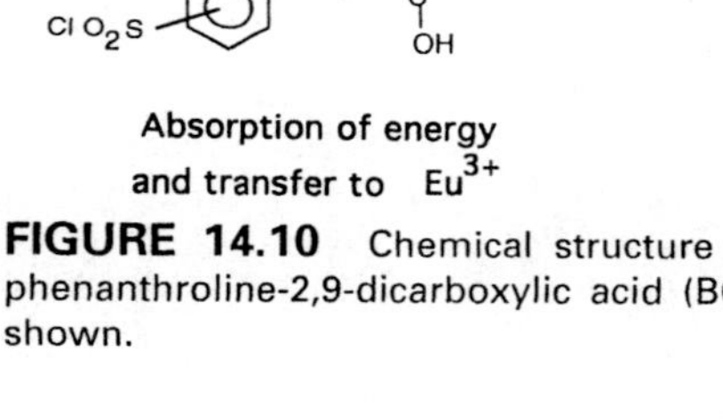

FIGURE 14.10 Chemical structure of the Eu^{3+}-chelator 4,7-bis (chlorosulfophenyl)-1,10-phenanthroline-2,9-dicarboxylic acid (BCPDA). The three major regions of the molecule are shown.

reagent for FIAgen assays (27) is a streptavidin-based macromolecular complex (SBMC) represented by the formula $SA[TG_3(BCPDA)_{480}]$ where SA is streptavidin and TG is thyroglobulin (Fig. 14.11). In this molecule, TG is used as a high-molecular-weight protein carrier labeled with about 160 BCPDA moieties. By incubating $SA[TG(BCPDA)_{160}]$ conjugate with an excess of $TG(BCPDA)_{160}$, in the presence of a suitable amount of Eu^{3+}, a macromolecular complex (SBMC) is formed containing 480 ligands per molecule. In this complex, Eu^{3+} binds two BCPDA molecules, thus acting as a bridge between $TG(BCPDA)_{160}$ and $SA[TG(BCPDA)_{160}]$.

The large Stokes shift (about 290 nm) along with a very narrow emission spectrum (about 10 nm at 50% emission bandwidth) of the Eu^{3+}–BCPDA complex allow for a high degree of protein labeling with no fluorescence quenching effects in the $SA[TG_3(BCPDA)_{480}]$ reagent. This is an important feature of Eu^{3+}-chelates since the fluorescence remains proportional to the number of labels attached to the immunoreactant. When fluorescein is used for multiple labeling of proteins, the emitted fluorescence is much less than expected by the fluorophore load (inner filter effect).

For noncompetitive-type assays, the capture antibody is immobilized on white opaque polystyrene microtitration wells. The sample is added along with biotinyl-ated detection antibodies. The immunocomplex formed is quantitated by adding SBMC and measuring the fluorescence with a front-surface time-resolved fluorome-ter (the 615 Immunoanalyzer). Assays of this type have been developed for thyrotro-pin, choriogonadotropin, ferritin, CK-MB, carcinoembryonic antigen, antibodies to rubella virus, and many other analytes (28, 29).

In the competitive-type assays, analyte immobilized on polystyrene wells via a carrier protein competes with the analyte in the sample for binding to biotinylated specific antibody. After the reaction is completed, SBMC is added to generate the fluorescence signal. The fluorescence measured is inversely related to the analyte concentration in the sample. Alternatively, the solid phase is coated with an analyte-specific antibody and an analyte–biotin conjugate is used as the tracer. After the immunoreaction is completed, the solid-phase-bound biotinylated-analyte is de-

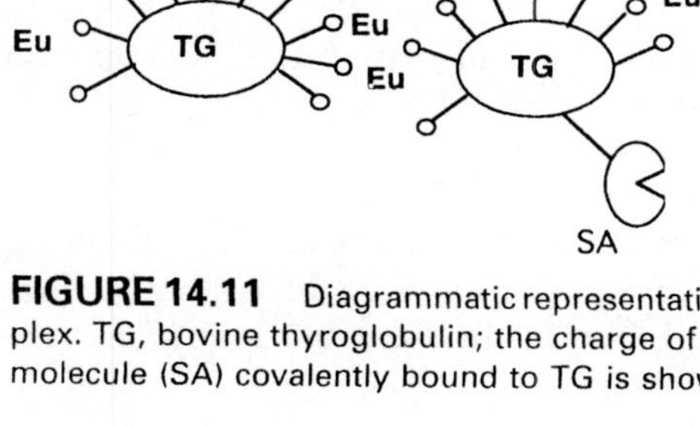

FIGURE 14.11   Diagrammatic representation of the streptavidin-based macromolecular com-plex. TG, bovine thyroglobulin; the charge of Eu^{3+} was omitted for simplicity. One streptavidin molecule (SA) covalently bound to TG is shown. For more details, see text.

tected by adding SBMC. Cortisol, digoxin, thyroxin, and progesterone are examples of competitive immunoassays using the above configurations (28, 29).

6.2.3. Multianalyte Fluorescence Immunoassay

Dual-label immunoassays involving time-resolved fluorometry and either Eu^{3+}– Tb^{3+} or Eu^{3+}–Sm^{3+} (30) as labels have been proposed for the determination of lutropin and follitropin or myoglobin and carbonic anhydrase III, respectively. Also, a quadruple-label immunoassay of thyrotropin, 17α-hydroxyprogesterone, immunoreactive trypsin, and creatine kinase MM based on immunoreactants labeled with Eu^{3+}, Tb^{3+}, Sm^{3+}, and Dy^{3+} was described (31). These label combinations take advantage of the narrow fluorescence emission bands of the lanthanide chelates and the lack of overlap between their emission spectra. In a dual-label assay for LH and FSH, the antibody against the α-subunit was used as a common capture antibody. The anti-β-FSH was labeled with Tb^{3+} and the anti-β-LH with Eu^{3+}. After completion of the immunoreaction, the lanthanides are extracted in a common enhancement solution containing pivaloyltrifluoroacetone (Fig. 14.8), TOPO, and Triton X-100. In the quadruple-label immunoassay, a cofluorescence-based enhancement solution (32) is used which allows the simultaneous measurement of four lanthanides. The solution consists of pivaloyltrifluoroacetone, Y^{3+}, Triton X-100, and phenanthroline.

Multianalyte time-resolved fluorescence immunoassays based on a single label with spatial distribution of the fluorescent areas were also described (33) and applied to the simultaneous assay of LH, FSH, HCG, and PRL in serum. In this system, four small plastic disks are coated with analyte-specific antibodies and attached to a stick, two disks on each side. The stick is immersed in the sample and the analytes bind to their specific antibodies. A cocktail of biotinylated detection antibodies is then added and the sandwich formed is quantified by adding $SA[TG_3(BCPDA)_{480}]$ and measuring the fluorescence of the solid phase, by time-resolved fluorometry, in two sequential measurements (side 1, then side 2 of the stick). The assays developed are highly sensitive, precise, and accurate.

6.3. Enzyme-Linked Fluorescence Immunoassays (ELFIA)

ELFIA is based on enzyme-labeled immunoreactants in combination with fluorogenic substrates. The reason for using enzymes as labels in immunoassays is the high turnover number of substrate molecules in the enzyme-catalyzed reaction which produces an amplification effect. On average, one enzyme is able to generate up to 1000 molecules of colored, fluorescent, or luminescent products per second. The introduction of fluorogenic substrates in enzyme immunoassays offers a dual advantage. First, the sensitivity of enzyme detection is significantly improved in comparison to chromogenic substrates and ELFIA is one of the most sensitive nonisotopic techniques currently in use. Second, fluorometric detection affords a wider assay dynamic range than spectrophotometric detection.

6.3.1. Enzyme Labels and Fluorogenic Substrates

Alkaline phosphatase (ALP), horseradish peroxidase (HRP), and β-D-galactosidase (β-DG) are the most frequently used enzymes in ELFIA. 4-Methylumbelliferyl phosphate (4MUP) is a widely used fluorogenic substrate for ALP. The enzyme-catalyzed hydrolysis of 4MUP is shown in Fig. 14.12.

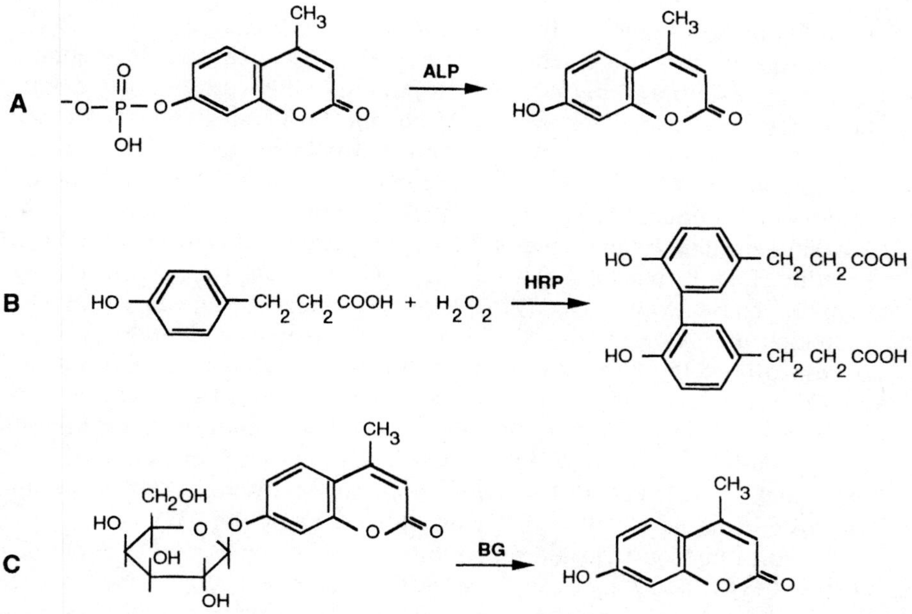

FIGURE 14.12 (A) 4-Methylumbelliferylphosphate (4-MUP) as a fluorogenic substrate for alkaline phosphatase (ALP). (B), p-Hydroxyphenylpropionic acid (HPPA) as a fluorogenic reagent for horseradish peroxidase (HRP). (C) 4-Methylumbelliferylgalactoside as a fluorogenic substrate for β-galactosidase (BG).

Recently, the phosphate ester of 5-fluorosalicylic acid was proposed as a substrate for the determination of alkaline phosphatase activity by time-resolved fluorometry (34,35). The product of the enzymatic hydrolysis, 5-fluorosalicylate, forms a highly fluorescent complex with Tb^{3+}–EDTA in alkaline solution (Fig. 14.13). The ter-

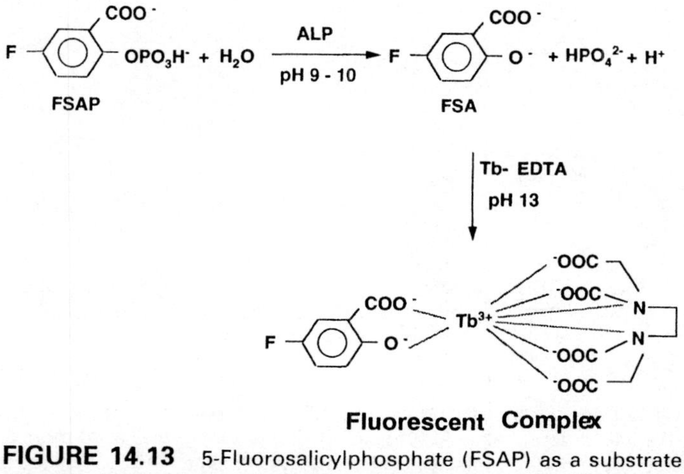

FIGURE 14.13 5-Fluorosalicylphosphate (FSAP) as a substrate for the time-resolved fluorometric determination of alkaline phosphatase activity. The released FSA forms a fluorescent ternary complex with Tb-EDTA, of a long fluorescence lifetime.

nary fluorescent complex absorbs at a wavelength characteristic of the chelator (337 nm) and emits fluorescence characteristic of Tb^{3+}. Ultrasensitive immunoassays for human α-fetoprotein (35), thyrotropin (36), and prostate-specific antigen have been described using this system. Here, the high detectability of time-resolved fluorometry is combined with the amplification introduced by an enzyme label.

The principle of enzyme cycling, in combination with fluorogenic substrates, also offers an exceptional sensitivity (37). This immunoassay system (Fig. 14.14) uses alkaline phosphatase as a label. ALP dephosphorylates $NADP^+$ (nicotinamideadeninedinucleotide phosphate) to NAD^+, which is used as a cofactor by alcohol dehydrogenase (ADH). ADH converts ethanol to acetaldehyde, with a concomitant reduction of NAD^+ to NADH. Subsequently, diaphorase catalyzes the reduction of resazurin to the fluorescent compound resorufin. This reaction regenerates the NAD^+. Therefore, each ALP molecule produces many NAD^+ molecules which are not consumed in the system but are recycled continuously, generating one fluorescent molecule per cycle (Fig. 14.14). The detection limit reported is about 350 molecules of ALP per well. A two-site immunometric assay for proinsulin, based on this system, gave a detection limit of 0.017 pmol/liter (37).

Sensitive fluorometric determination systems for HRP are based on the reaction between H_2O_2 and p-hydroxyphenylcarboxy acids, e.g., acetic, methoxyacetic, and propionic acid. The reaction with hydroxyphenylpropionic acid (Fig. 14.12) gives the highest sensitivity.

4-Methylumbelliferyl-β-D-galactopyranoside(4MUG) is the fluorogenic substrate of choice for assays using β-D-galactosidase as the label.

6.3.2. Applications of ELFIA

An overview of the newly developed automated ELFIA systems for clinical chemistry laboratories reveals that alkaline phosphatase is used almost exclusively as the label and 4MUP is the fluorogenic substrate of choice. HRP and β-DG are used mostly in research applications of ELFIA. Also, most ELFIA applications involve heterogeneous immunoassays.

6.3.2.1. Automated Batch-Analyzing ELFIA Systems
The Abbott IMx System (38), based on the principle of microparticle capture enzyme immunoassay

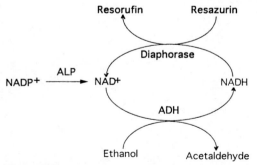

FIGURE 14.14 The principle of enzyme cycling. $NADP^+$, Nicotinamideadeninedinucleotide phosphate; ALP: alkaline phosphatase; ADH, alcohol dehydrogenease. Immunoreactants are labeled with ALP which dephosphorylates the substrate $NADP^+$. The NAD^+ produced is recycled many times by the combination of ADH and diaphorase. Each cycle produces a fluorescent molecule (resorufin).

(MEIA), uses very small (0.47-μm) latex particles as the solid phase to increase the surface area available for the immunoreaction. The particles are coated with analyte-specific antibody. The separation of bound from free labeled fraction is accomplished by capture of the microparticles in a glass–fiber matrix, a process based on the affinity of glass fibers for protein-coated microparticles. The micropar-ticles adhere to the fibers of the glass irreversibly, whereas nonbound material is removed by washing. ALP-labeled detection antibodies and ALP-labeled analytes are used for the noncompetitive and competitive-type assays, respectively. 4MUP is the substrate in both cases. The rate of fluorescence development is measured with a front-surface fluorometer which can detect about 100 nmol/liter of 4MU.

The Stratus II Immunoassay System (from Baxter Diagnostics Inc.) (39, 40) employs filter paper solid-phase cartridges for immobilizing the capture antibodies. The immunoreaction takes place on the filter with either ALP-labeled detection antibodies (noncompetitive assays) or ALP-labeled antigens (competitive assays). When the substrate solution (4MUP) is added, it functions simultaneously as the wash solution, and the unbound conjugate is washed from the central reaction zone of the filter through radial partition (39). The fluorescence of 4MU is measured kinetically from the center of the filter with a front-surface fluorometer. A second ring of fluorescence, due to removed excess of labeled reagent, is also present but is excluded from the analytical measurement.

The FAST System (3M Diagnostics) for allergy testing employs microtitration plates as the solid phase for allergen immobilization. After the immunoreaction is completed, allergen-bound IgE from the sample is detected with ALP-labeled anti-human IgE along with 4MUP as the substrate. In the Pharmacia CAP allergy analyzing system, the allergen is immobilized on a flexible hydrophilic polymer; β-DG is used as the label of anti-human IgE antibodies and 4MUG as the substrate.

6.3.2.2. Automated Random-Access ELFIA Systems

The AIA-1200 immu-noassay system, manufactured by Tosoh Medics Inc. employs chromium dioxide magnetic particles coated with capture antibodies as the solid phase, and ALP-labeled detection antibodies (noncompetitive assays) or ALP-labeled antigens (competitive assays) (41). The substrate is 4MUP and the rate of fluorescence increase is the measured parameter.

The Vista immunoassay system uses streptavidin-coated chromium dioxide mag-netic particles. The capture antibodies are biotinylated. ALP-labeled detection antibodies or ALP-labeled antigens are used for noncompetitive or competitive assays, respectively, and 4MUP is the substrate. The instrument is manufactured by Hitachi and the reagents are available from Syva (42).

The Eclipse ICA system is a centrifugal chemistry and immunoassay analyzer. In a typical noncompetitive-type assay, the sample is mixed with capture antibody and ALP-labeled detection antibody, in solution. The reaction mixture is transferred to the solid-phase chamber by centrifugation. The solid phase contains bromostyr-ene particles coated with a second antibody specific for the capture antibody. After incubation, the excess of labeled antibody is removed by centrifugation through a wash solution and a silicon–oil layer. Because of their specific gravity, only the bromostyrene particles can pass through the oil layer and reach the substrate solution underneath. Unbound low-density material stays at the oil/wash solution interface. The substrate layer contains 4MUP and the rate of fluorescence develop-ment is followed (43).

The OPUS immunoassay system (44, 45) of PB Diagnostics employs two measuring systems. The first is a heterogeneous competitive FIA (Sep-FIA), which takes place on a three-layer agarose film coated on a clear plastic support. The bottom layer (immunoreaction layer) contains immobilized antibody preincubated with rhodamine-labeled analyte. The middle layer is a thin optical barrier where iron oxide particles hide the top layer from excitation light. The top layer contains surfactants, buffer species, or blocking agents. The sample is applied on the top layer. After the immunoreaction is completed, the displaced tracer migrates through the middle thin layer to the upper layer and is shielded from the excitation. The fluorescence is read from below.

The second measuring principle is based on ELFIA. The assay is performed on a glass–fiber filter which contains immobilized capture antibodies. The detection antibodies are labeled with ALP while 4MUP is the substrate. The unbound labeled reagent is washed from the optical window area by radial elution and the rate of fluorescence increase is measured.

The VIDAS immunoassay system (BioMerieux) uses a pipette-tip-like disposable receptacle which serves as the solid phase for the assay as well as a pipetting device. It is coated with capture antibody. Detection antibodies (or antigens) are labeled with ALP and 4MUP serves as the substrate (46).

In the AN2000 immunoassay system (47) from Anagen, monoclonal or polyclonal antibodies are linked directly to spherical (2-μm diameter), ceramic, magnetizable particles. About 12 million particles (a surface of about 2 cm^2) are used per reaction cuvette. ALP-labeled antibodies or antigens are used in the noncompetitive or competitive immunoassays, respectively. 4MUP is the substrate and the fluorescence is measured after a fixed incubation time.

The Abbott AxSYM random and continuous access immunoassay system (48) incorporates three immunoassay technologies, namely, the fluorescence polarization immunoassay (described earlier in this chapter), the microparticle capture enzyme immunoassay (see IMx under automated batch-analyzing ELFIA systems), and the ion-capture immunoassay (ICIA). In ICIA technology the capture antibodies are labeled with a polyanion such as polyglutamate. ALP-labeled detection antibodies or antigens are used in the noncompetitive or competitive assays, respectively. After the immunoreaction is completed, the reaction mixture is transferred on to a glass–fiber matrix which is coated with a cationic (quaternary ammonium) polymer. Because of ionic interactions, the immunocomplex is captured by the solid phase and, after washing out the excess of reagents, it is detected by using 4MUP as the substrate.

6.4. Liposome-Based Fluorescence Immunoassay (Heterogeneous)

A method for serum theophylline which combines flow injection analysis with liposome-based immunoassay has been described recently (49). The method uses immunoreactor columns containing a monoclonal anti-theophylline antibody immobilized on silica particles. The tracer is a theophylline-liposome conjugate. Dimyristoylphosphatidylcholine, cholesterol, dicetyl phosphate, and theophylline-phosphatidylethanolamine are used for the preparation of liposomes. The liposomes contain an aqueous solution of carboxyfluorescein. The sample and the tracer are injected in the column, where they compete for the antibody-binding sites. Subsequently a detergent solution passes through the column, which causes lysis of the bound liposomes and release of carboxyfluorescein. The fluorescence measured is inversely related to the analyte concentration in the sample. Theophylline bound to the column is then dissociated with an excess of buffer. Thus, the column is regenerated (without considerable loss in antibody-binding affinity) and available for the next sample. A 0.25-μl sample is sufficient for the anlysis due to the high sensitivity achieved.

6.5. Other Heterogeneous Fluorescence Immunoassay Systems

One widely used solid-phase FIA system, the IDT FIAX StiQ system (International Diagnostic Technology), is based on a special paddle-shaped dipstick sampler containing an activated cellulose acetate nitrate disk.

For assays of circulating antibodies and for competitive assays, the antigen is immobilized on the activated membrane. For noncompetitive assays, the capture antibodies are immobilized on the membrane. The other side of the disk is used for monitoring nonspecific binding of the label. A typical assay protocol involves incubation of the stick with the sample, washing, incubating with the labeled reagent, washing, and measuring the fluorescence with a front-surface fluorometer (IDT FIAX-100 fluorometer). FITC is used to label immunorectants. The technique is applied primarily to assays of circulating antibodies (50).

References

1. Hemmila IA. Applications of fluorescence in immunoassays. In: Winefordner JD, Ed. Chemistry Analysis, Vol. 117. New York: Wiley, 1991.
2. Dandiker WB, Hsu ML, Levin J, Rao BR. Equilibrium and kinetic inhibition assays based upon fluorescence polarization. Methods Enzymol 1981; 74:3–28.
3. Dandiker WB, Kelly RJ, Dandiker J, Farcuhar J, Levin J. Fluorescence polarization immunoassay. Theory and experimental methods. Immunochemistry 1973; 10:219–27.
4. Dandiker WB, De Saussure VA. Fluorescence polarization in immuno-chemistry. Immunochemistry 1970; 7:799–828.
5. Jolley ME, Stroupe SD, Wang CHT, Panas HN, Keegan CL, Schmidt RL, Schwenzer KS. Fluorescence polarization immunoassay. I. Monitoring aminoglycoside antibiotics in serum and plasma. Clin Chem 1981; 27:1190–7.
6. Popelka SR, Miller DM, Holen JT, Kelso DM. Fluorescence polarization immunoassay. II. Analyzer for rapid precise measurement of fluorescence polarization with use of disposable cuvettes. Clin Chem 1981; 27:1198–201.
7. Jolley ME, Stroupe SD, Schwenzer KS, Wang CJ, Lu-Steffes M, Hill HD, Popelka SR, Holen JT, Kelso DM. Fluorescence polarization immunoassay. III. An automated system for therapeutic drug determination. Clin Chem 1981; 27:1575–9.
8. Ullman EF, Khana PL. Fluorescence excitation transfer immunoassay (FETI). Methods Enzymol 1981; 74:60–79.
9. Calvin J, Burling K, Blow C, Barnes I, Price CP. Evaluation of fluorescence excitation transfer immunoassay for measurement of specific proteins. J Immunol Methods 1986; 86:249–56.
10. Nargessi RD, Landon J. Indirect quenching fluoroimmunoassay. Methods Enzymol 1981; 74:60–79.
11. Zuk RF. Fluorescence protection immunoassay to the measurement of serum proteins. Clin Biochem Anal 1981; 10:83–95.
12. Hassan M, Landon J, Smith DS. A novel non-separation fluoroimmunoassay for thyroxine. J Immunoassay 1982; 3:1–15.
13. Burd JF. The homogeneous substrate-labeled fluorescent immunoassay. Methods Enzymol 1981; 74:79–87.

14. Toseland PA, Wicks JF, Newall RG. Application of substrate-labeled fluorescent immunoassay to the measurement of anticonvulsant and antiasthmatic drug levels in plasma and serum. Ther Drug Monitor 1983; 5:501–9.

15. Tosoni S, Signorini C, Albertini A. Drug monitoring by fluoroimmunoassay with use of a centrifugal analyzer. Clin Chem 1983; 29:991–6.

16. Barnard G, Kohen F, Mikola H, Lovgren T. Measurement of estrone-3-glucuronide in urine by rapid, homogeneous time-resolved fluoroimmunoassay. Clin Chem 1989; 35:555–9.

17. Mathis G. Rare earth cryptates and homogeneous fluoroimmuno-assays with human sera. Clin Chem 1993; 39:1953–9.

18. Morrison LE. Time-resolved detection of energy transfer: theory and application to immunoassays. Anal Biochem 1988; 174:101–20.

19. Ishimori Y, Rokugawa K. Stable liposomes for assays of human sera. Clin Chem 1993; 39:1439–43.

20. Jolley ME, Wang CJ, Ekenberg SJ, Zuelke MS, Kelso DM. Particle concentration fluorescence immunoassay PCFIA: a new rapid immunoassay technique with high sensitivity. J Immunol Methods 1984; 67:21–35.

21. Taber LK, O'Brien P, Bowsher RR, Sportsman JR. Competitive particle concentration fluorescence immunoassay for measuring 5,10-dideaza-5,6,7,8-tetrahydrofolic acid (lometrexol) in serum. Clin Chem 1991; 37:254–60.

22. Hemmila I, Dakubu S, Mukkala V-M, Siitari H, Lovgren T. Europium as a label in time-resolved immunofluorometric assays. Anal Biochem 1984; 137:335–43.

23. Keelan JA, France JT, Barling PM. An alternative fluorescence enhancement solution for use in lanthanide-based time-resolved fluoroimmunoassays. Clin Chem 1987; 33:2292–5.

24. Hemmila I. Lanthanides as probes for time-resolved fluorometric immunoassays. Scand J Clin Lab Invest 1988; 48:389–400.

25. Barnard G, Kohen F. Idiometric assay: noncompetitive immunoassay for small molecules typified by the measurement of estradiol in serum. Clin Chem 1990; 36:1945–50.

26. Evangelista RA, Pollak A, Allore B, Templeton EF, Morton RC, Diamandis EP. A new europium chelate for protein labeling and time-resolved fluorometric applications. Clin Biochem 1988; 21:173–8.

27. Morton RC, Diamandis. Streptavidin-based macromolecular complex labeled with a europium chelator suitable for time-resolved fluorescence immunoassay applications. Anal Chem 1990; 62:1841–5.

28. Diamandis EP, Christopoulos TK. Immunological assays based on time-resolved fluorometry with lanthanide chelates as labels. In: Service Training and Continuing Education (AACC), 1992; 10:9–26.

29. Diamandis EP, Christopoulos TK. Europium chelate labels in time-resolved fluorescence immunoassay and DNA hybridization assays. Anal Chem 1990; 62:1149A–57A.

30. Vuori J, Rasi S, Takala T, Vaananen K. Dual-label time-resolved fluoroimmunoassay for simultaneous detection of myoglobin and carbonic anhydrase III in serum. Clin Chem 1991; 37:2087–92.

31. Xu Y-Y, Pettersson K, Blomberg K, Hemmila I, Mikola H, Lovgren T. Simultaneous quadruple-label fluorometric immunoassay of thyroid-stimulating hormone, 17a-hydroxyprogesterone, immunoreactive trypsin, and creatine kinase MM isoenzyme in dried blood spots. Clin Chem 1992; 38:2038–43.

32. Xu Y-Y. Co-fluorescence enhancement system based on pivaloyltrifluoroacetone and ytrrium for the simultaneous detection of europium, terbium, samarium and dysprosium. Anal Chim Acta 1992; 256:9–16.

33. Kakabakos SE, Christopoulos TK, Diamandis EP. Multianalyte immunoassay based on the spatial distribution of fluorescent areas quantified by laser-excited solid-phase time-resolved fluorometry. Clin Chem 1992; 38:338–42.

34. Evangelista RA, Pollak A, Gudgin-Templeton EF. Enzyme-amplified lanthanide luminescence for enzyme detection in bioanalytical assays. Anal Biochem 1991; 197:213–24.

35. Christopoulos TK, Diamandis EP. Enzymatically amplified time-resolved fluorescence immunoassay with terbium chelates. Anal Chem 1992; 64:342–6.

36. Papanastasiou-Diamandi A, Christopoulos TK, Diamandis EP. Ultrasensitive thyrotropin immunoassay based on enzymatically amplified time-resolved fluorescence with terbium chelates. Clin Chem 1992; 38:545–8.

37. Cook DB, Self CH. Determination of one thousandth of an attomole (1 zeptomole) of alkaline phosphatase: application in an immunoassay of proinsulin. Clin Chem 1993; 39:965–71.

38. Fiore M, Mitcell J, Doan T, Nelson R, Winter G, Grandone C, Zeng K, Haraden R, Smith J, Harris K, Leszczynski J, Berry D, Safford S, Barnes G, Scholnick A, Ludington K. The Abbott IMx automated benchtop immunochemistry analyzer system. Clin Chem 1988; 34:1726–32.

39. Giegel JL, Brotherton MM, Cronin P, D'Aquino M, Evans S, Heller ZH, Knight WS, Krishnan K, Sheiman M. Radial partition immunoassay. Clin Chem 1982; 28:1894–8.

40. Plant DS, McLellan WN. The Baxter Diagnostics, Inc., Dade Stratus II automated fluorometric immunoassay system. J Clin Immunoassay 1991; 14:120–5.

41. Loebel JE. TOSOH AIA-1200/AIA-600 automated immunoassay analyzers. J Clin Immunoassay 1991; 14:94–102.

42. Chen R, Nguyen T, Li TM. Development of a thyroxine (T4) assay on the random-access VISTA immunoassay system. Clin Chem 1992; 38:1087.

43. Mahoney WC, Opheim KE, Fleck TM, Schueler PA, Enfield DL, Kingsley JT, Eclipse ICA: An immunoassay and clinical chemistry system. In: Chan DW, Ed. Immunoassay Automation. A Practical Guide. San Diego: Academic Press, 1992.

44. Grenner G, Inbar S, Meneghini EW, Long EW, Yamartino EJ, Bowen MS, Blackwood JJ, Padilla AJ, Maretsky D, Staedrez M. Multilayer fluorescent immunoassay technique. Clin Chem 1989; 35:1865–8.

45. Olive C. PB Diagnostics' OPUS Immunoassay system. J Clin Immunoassay 1991; 14:126–32.

46. Picelli G, Chakamian J, Mercier I, Fleury B, Aubry C. Performance of the HCG assay on BioMerieux VIDAS. Clin Chem 1992; 38:1085.

47. Clements JA, Forrest GC, Jay RF, Jeffery M, Kemp PM, Kjeldsen NJ, Rattle SJ, Smith A. The anagen system for automated fluorometric immunoassay. Clin Chem 1992; 38:1671–7.

48. Smith J, Osikowicz G and others. Abbott AxSYM random and continuous access immunoassay system for improved workflow in the clinical laboratory. Clin Chem 1993; 39:2063–9.

49. Locascio-Brown L, Plant AL, Chesler R, Kroll M, Ruddel M, Durst RA. Liposome-based flow-injection immunoassay for determining theophylline in serum. Clin Chem 1993; 39:386–91.

50. Fayram SL, Akin S, Aarnaes SL, Peterson EM, DeLa Maza LM. Determination of immune status in patients with low antibody titers for rubella virus. J Clin Microbiol 1987; 25:178–86.

15 | CHEMILUMINESCENCE IMMUNOASSAY

LARRY J. KRICKA

Department of Pathology and Laboratory Medicine
University of Pennsylvania
Philadelphia, Pennsylvania

1. INTRODUCTION

Chemiluminescent labels were initially tested as possible alternatives to radioisotopes in the 1970s (1). This type of label has become very popular and today a wide range of assays and associated analyzers are available commercially. Chemiluminescent reactions have also found use in enzyme immunoassay to quantitate enzyme labels (e.g., alkaline phosphatase, horseradish peroxidase) (2).

Chemiluminescence is the light emission that is produced in certain chemical oxidation reactions (3, 4). The light emission arises from the decay of chemi-excited intermediates or product molecules to the electronic ground state. Molecules with diverse structural features will produce chemiluminescence; some representative examples are collected in Table 15.1. The majority of chemiluminescent reactions are oxidation reactions because the production of visible light requires highly energetic reactions (71.3 kcal/mol for visible light at 400 nm and 38.0 kcal/mol for light at 750 nm) (5). The most extensively studied chemiluminescent reaction is the oxidation of luminol (5-amino-2,3-dihydro-1,4-phthalazinedione) (Fig. 15.1).

337

TABLE 15.1   Chemiluminescent Reactions

Acridinium ester + peroxide + base
Adamantyl 1,2-dioxetane aryl phosphate + alkaline
phosphatase
Benzylamine + benzoyl chloride
Benzylphenylketone + O_2
Cyanomethyl indole + O_2 + base
Cyclopentanone + O_2
Cysteine + O_2 + Cu(II)
Diphenyl peroxide + rubrene
Lophine (2,4,5-triphenylimidazole) + peroxide + base
Lucigenin + peroxide + base
Lithium diphenylphosphide + O_2
Luminol + peroxide + base
Nitric oxide + ozone
Oxalyl chloride + peroxide + anthracene
Phenyl magnesium bromide + O_2
Polystyrene + dicyclohexyl peroxydicarbonate
Pyrogallol + formaldehyde + peroxide
Tetrachloroethylidene carbonate + H_2O_2 + fluorophore
Tetrakisdimethylaminoethylene + oxygen
Tetralin hydroperoxide + zinc tetraphenylporphyrin
bis(2,4,6-Trichlorophenyl)oxalate + peroxide + fluorophore

The precise mechanism of the reaction is not fully elucidated, but luminol reacts with an oxidant (e.g., perborate, peroxide) in the presence of a catalyst (e.g., microperoxidase, horseradish peroxidase, Co(III), Cr(III), $Fe(CN)_6^{3-}$) to form either a hydroperoxide or a cyclic endoperoxide intermediate (Fig. 15.1) (4). This interme-

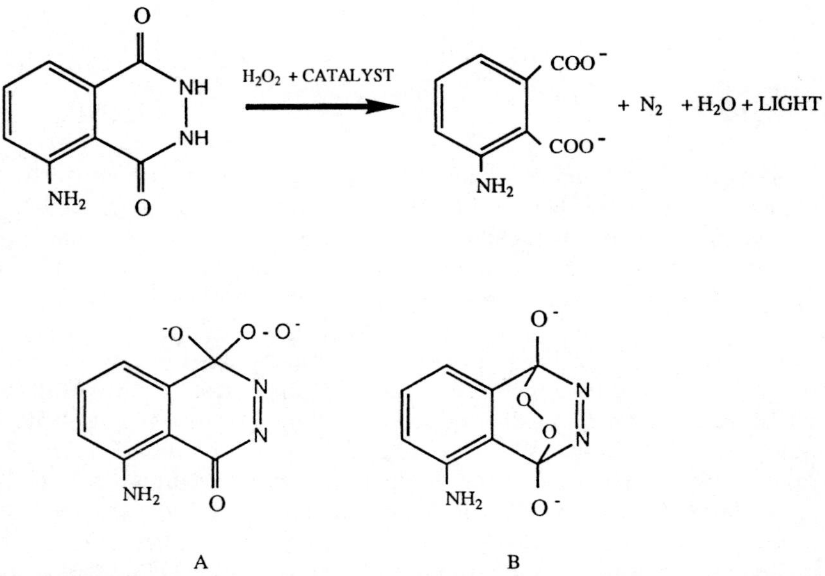

FIGURE 15.1   Chemiluminescent luminol reaction and reaction intermediates A and B.

diate decomposes to produce 3-aminophthalate molecules in an electronically excited state, and these decay to the ground state; some of the energy is released as light as a broad emission (375–550 nm) centered at 425 nm. The luminol reaction is very inefficient, and the quantum yield for chemiluminescence is 1.2% (4). The chemiluminescence quantum yield (ϕ_{CL}) is the product of three components ($\phi_{CL} = \phi_C \times \phi_{EX} \times \phi_F$)—the fraction of molecules entering the chemiluminescent reaction pathway (ϕ_C), the fraction of these molecules that become electronically excited (ϕ_{EX}), and the fluorescence quantum yield of the excited state emitter (ϕ_F). Other reactions have higher quantum yields than the luminol reaction, e.g., the oxidation of bis(2,4,6-trichlorophenyl)oxalate ($\phi_{CL} = 27\%$), and certain naturally occuring reactions, e.g., the bioluminescent firefly luciferase reaction which has a quantum yield of >88% (Table 15.2). Despite the inefficiency of chemiluminescent reactions, they have proved analytically useful and there are many highly sensitive assays based on compounds such as luminol with quantum yields of <10%. The reader is directed to various books, reviews, and literature surveys for additional information on chemiluminescence and its analytical applications (1–8).

2. CHEMILUMINESCENT LABELS AND LABELING

The most popular labels are derivatives of isoluminol and acridinium esters. Other chemiluminescent molecules have been tested as labels but have been abandoned, or perhaps currently there is insufficient data to make a realistic assessment of their potential as labels (e.g., pyridopyridazine derivatives).

2.1. Cyclic Diacyl Hydrazides

Luminol and isoluminol were the first chemiluminescent molecules to be tested in an immunoassay (1). The 5-amino group of luminol provides a convenient site of attachment for antigens and antibodies using a range of chemical conjugation

TABLE 15.2   Bioluminescence (A) and Chemiluminescence (B) Quantum Yields

	Chemiluminescence quantum yield (%)
A	
Firefly luciferase + luciferin	88
Vargula luciferase + luciferin	30
Aequorin	5
Renilla luciferase + luciferin	5
B	
Oxalate ester + fluorophore	5–50
Luminol	1.2
Aminobutylethyl luminol	1
Lucigenin	1
Isoluminol	0.1
4-Chlorophenyl magnesium bromide	10^{-4}–10^{-6}
Benzylamine + benzoyl chloride	10^{-12}

procedures, e.g., diazonium reaction. However, substitution of this group reduces the chemiluminescence efficiency 10-fold. Substitution of the heterocyclic ring abolishes the chemiluminescence of luminol and is thus not a useful site for attachment of other molecules (5). The 6-amino isomer (isoluminol) (Fig. 15.2) has a chemiluminescence efficiency of 0.1% (4). However, when this molecule is reacted via the 6-amino group the chemiluminescence efficiency increases 10-fold, and thus this

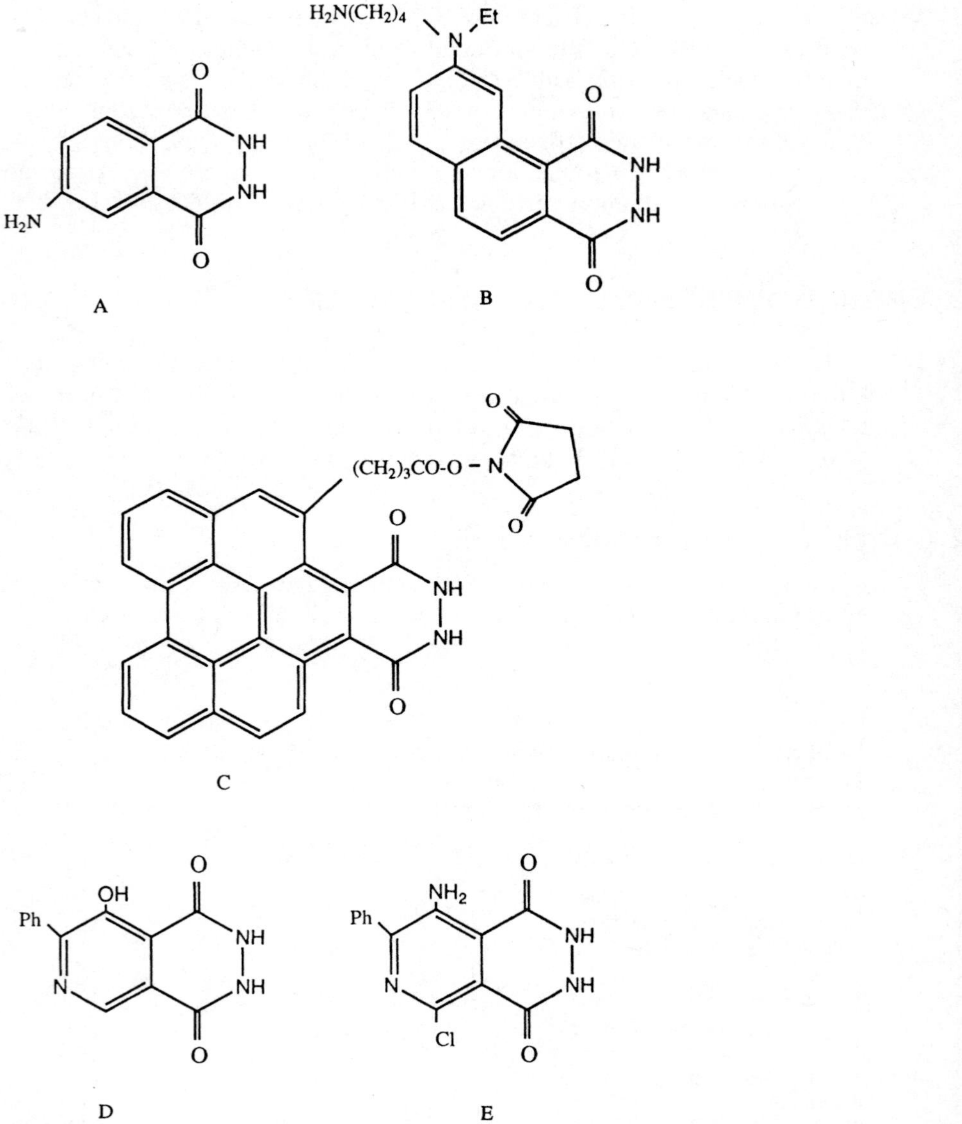

FIGURE 15.2 Isoluminol and related labels. A, isoluminol; B, naphthalene-1,2-dicarboxylic acid hydrazide derivative; C, benzo[ghi]perylene-1,2-dicarboxylic acid hydrazide 4-butanoic acid-N-hydroxysuccinimidyl ester; D, 8-hydroxy-7-phenyl pyridopyridazine; E, 8-amino-5-chloro-7-phenylpyridopyridazine.

molecule and its derivatives have become preferred as labels. A range of isoluminol derivatives have been synthesized and tested (5) (Table 15.3), and the influence of the polymethylene chain length on light emission has been investigated. In this regard some conflicting trends have been observed. For example, the light emission of N-ethylisoluminol–progesterone conjugates separated by a hexamethylene spacer group was higher than that of the corresponding conjugates with ethylene or pentamethylene spacers (6). In contrast, for an N-ethylisoluminol–estrone-3-glucuronide conjugate the detection limit for the conjugate improved as the spacer group was shortened [e.g., $-(CH_2)_4-$, 218 fg; $-(CH_2)_2-$, 126 fg (7)]. Full substitution of the 6-amino group is beneficial; this is illustrated by the improvement in the detection limits for the monosubstituted conjugate cortisol–aminobutylisoluminol, and the fully substituted conjugate cortisol–aminobutyl-N-ethylisoluminol, 1 vs 0.2 fmol, respectively (8). Labeling is achieved using one of several different conjugation reactions, e.g., isothiocyanate, mixed anhydride, aldehyde, or active ester reaction. An HPLC method for the purification and quality control of isoluminol labels has been described based on reverse-phase chromatography on a Hypersil ODS (5-μm) column (9).

Various naphthalene-1,2-dicarboxylic acid hydrazides have been synthesized and tested as labels (10, 11) (Figure 15.2). These analogs of luminol are more efficient than luminol (>twofold) (4), but have found few applications, probably because of limited availability of the labels. A more complex activated benzoperylene analog of luminol has also been synthesized—benzo[ghi]perylene-1,2-dicarboxylic acid hydrazide 4-butanoic acid-N-hydroxysuccinimidyl ester (Fig. 15.2) (12). The detection limit for the label is 0.1 fmol, and although this label has a higher quantum efficiency than luminol it has not found a role as a label in chemiluminescent immunoassays.

2.2. Acridinium Esters and Related Compounds

The synthesis and analytical application of this class of chemiluminescent compound was first described in 1977 (13). Acridinium ester labels were the first to be successfully commercialized. An acridinium ester label is quantitated very simply by reaction with hydrogen peroxide in alkaline solution. The mechanism of chemilu-

TABLE 15.3 Isoluminol Labels

6-Amino substituents (6-NRR¹)		
R	R¹	Abbreviation
H	H	—
Et	$(CH_2)_2 NH_2$	AEEI
Et	$(CH_2)4 NH_2$	ABEI
Et	$(CH_2)5 NH_2$	APEI
Et	$(CH_2)6 NH_2$	AHEI

Note. For isoluminol structure refer to Fig. 15.2. ABEI, N-(4-aminobutyl)-N-ethylisoluminol; AEEI, N-(2-aminoethyl)-N-ethylisoluminol; AHEI, N-(6-aminohexyl)-N-ethylisoluminol; APEI, N-(5-aminopentyl)-N-ethylisoluminol.

minescent decomposition of an acridinium ester involves attack of a peroxide anion at the C-9 ester to form a hydroperoxide, followed by loss of an alcoholate leaving group to produce an unstable dioxetanone. This species decomposes to carbon dioxide and N-methylacridone in an electronically excited state (14) (Fig. 15.3). Decay of this molecule to the ground state is accompanied by light emission at 430 nm. The detection limit for a monoclonal antibody labeled with this type of label is about 0.8 amol (0.8×10^{-18} mol) (antibody:label ratio = 1:2.8) (15).

A complication for an acridinium ester is that above pH 7 a chemiluminescently inactive carbinol is formed by attack of base at the C-9 position. This compound is in equilibrium with the acridinium ester form and thus basic conditions are avoided in order to minimize its formation (5). Studies with a series of acridinium esters has shown that the light emission intensity and kinetics correlate with the pK_a of the conjugate acid of the leaving group, hence methylacridinium esters (MeO^- leaving group) are less efficient than phenylacridinium esters (PhO^- leaving group) (16, 17).

In the course of the detection reaction the excited state emitter product (N-methylacridone) formed by oxidation of the label is released into solution. This minimizes any influence of the microenvironment created by the substance (antigen, antibody) to which the label is attached. It is possible to enhance the chemilumines-cence of an acridinium ester up to threefold using different additives, e.g., Triton X-100, Brij-35, sodium dodecyl sulfate (SDS), cetyltrimethylammonium chloride (CTAC), α-, β-, γ-, and methyl-β-cyclodextrins (18, 19). The mechanism of this

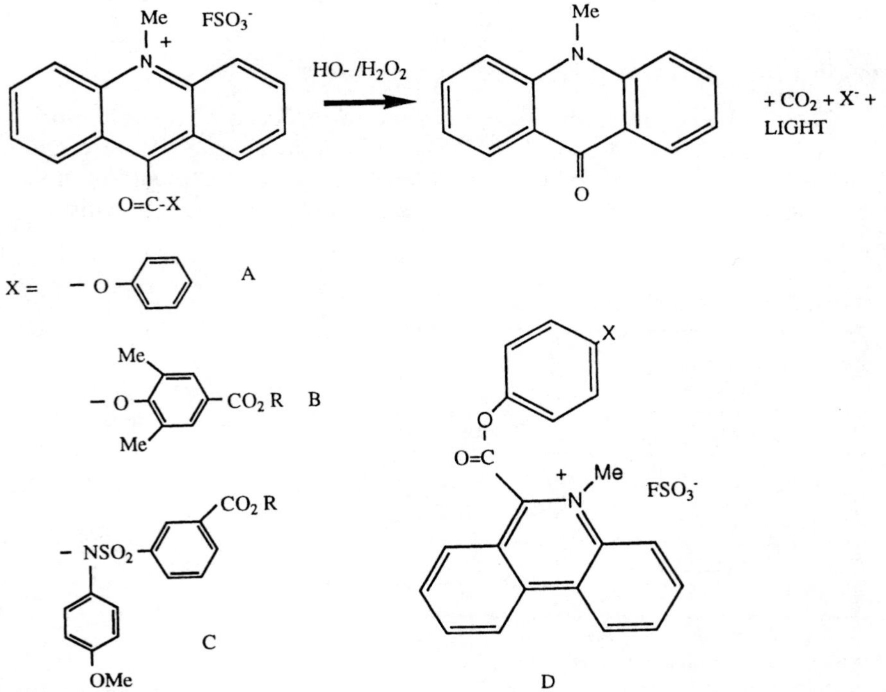

FIGURE 15.3 Acridinium esters and analogs. A, acridinium ester; B, dimethyl substituted acridinium ester; C, acridinium N-sulfonyl carboxamide; D, phenanthridinium ester derivative.

effect probably involves the sequestration of the excited state emitter into a more hydrophobic micellar environment or into the cavity of the torus-shaped cyclodextrins.

A problem with the early acridinium ester derivatives was that the ester bond was labile to hydrolysis, thus limiting long-term storage at pH > 4. This was remedied by synthesizing the dimethyl-substituted compound shown in Fig. 15.3B. The two methyl groups hinder hydrolysis of the ester bond and thus increase stability (20). Several different reactions can be used in acridinium ester labeling, but the N-hydroxysuccinimidyl active ester reaction is now the method of choice (21).

Various analogs of acridinium esters have been synthesized including thioester and sulfonyl carboxamide derivatives, e.g., acridinium-9-(N-sulfonyl)carboxamide and phenanthridinium esters (22) (Figure 15.3). Detailed studies of a series of sulfonylcarboxamides revealed that this class of compound is more stable than the ester analog, and the light emission kinetics can be controlled by appropriate selection of the sulfonamide substituents as illustrated in Table 15.4. Generally, electron withdrawing groups increased the reaction rate and bulky electron donating groups reduced the rate of the chemiluminescent reaction (23).

2.3. Pyridopyridazines

This class of molecules is the latest addition to the armamentarium of chemiluminescent labels, and a range of derivatives have been synthesized (Fig. 15.2). Light is produced by oxidation in the presence of a catalyst (e.g., hydrogen peroxide + microperoxidase). Comparative studies indicate that these new molecules are superior to luminol (Table 15.5), and that the 8-amino-5-chloro-7-phenyl- and 8-hydroxy-7-phenyl derivatives, will be useful as labels and as cosubstrates for detection of peroxidase labels (24, 25).

TABLE 15.4   Substituent Effects on the Chemiluminescence of 10-Methylacridinium-9-(N-sulfonylcarboxamide) Salts

R	R¹	Time for >90% of the light emission to occur (sec)	Time to reach the maximum light output (sec)
Ph	CF$_3$	1	0.22
Ph	2-NO$_2$Ph	2	0.23
Ph	4-BrPh	2	0.24
iPr	CF$_3$	2	0.25
nBu	4-NO$_2$Ph	2	0.25
iPr	2-NO$_2$Ph	2	0.25
Ph	4-CH$_3$Ph	2	0.27
nBu	2-NO$_2$Ph	2	0.29
nBu	2,4-di-NO$_2$Ph	2	0.32
nBu	4-BrPh	3	0.44
iPr	4-BrPh	6	0.44
nBu	4-CH$_3$Ph	6	0.98
iPr	4-CH$_3$Ph	10	0.96
nBu	2,4,6-(i-Pr)$_3$P h	20	4.08
nBu	2,4,6-(CH$_3$)$_3$Ph	50	11.6

Note. iPr, isopropyl; nBu, n-butyl; Ph, phenylmethylacridinium CONRSO$_2$R¹.

TABLE 15.5 Comparison of Chemiluminescent Properties of pyridopyridazines and luminol[a]

Pyridopyridazine	Relative light emission (10 pg microperoxidase)
8-HO, 7-Ph	5541
8-NH$_2$, 7-Ph	124
8-HO, 7-(4-MeOPh)	3740
8-HO, 7-[3-H$_2$N(CH$_2$)$_3$O)Ph]	3533
8-NH$_2$, 5-Cl, 7-Ph	102
8-NH$_2$, 5-MeO, 7-Ph	34
Luminol	100

[a] Refer to Fig. 15.2 for chemical structures. Data derived from Ref. (24).

2.4. 1,2-Dioxetanes

Adamantylidene adamantane 1,2-dioxetane is stable ($t_{1/2} = 1.2 \times 10^4$ years at 25°C) and will chemiluminesce when heated to above ca. 200–250°C. The molecule cleaves symmetrically to form excited-state adamantanone molecules (chemiluminescence quantum yield $= 1 \times 10^{-4}$). Derivatives of adamantylidene adamantane 1,2-dioxetanes have been synthesized with a reactive group at the 4-position on one of the adamantane rings (Fig. 15.4). This type of label was tested in a

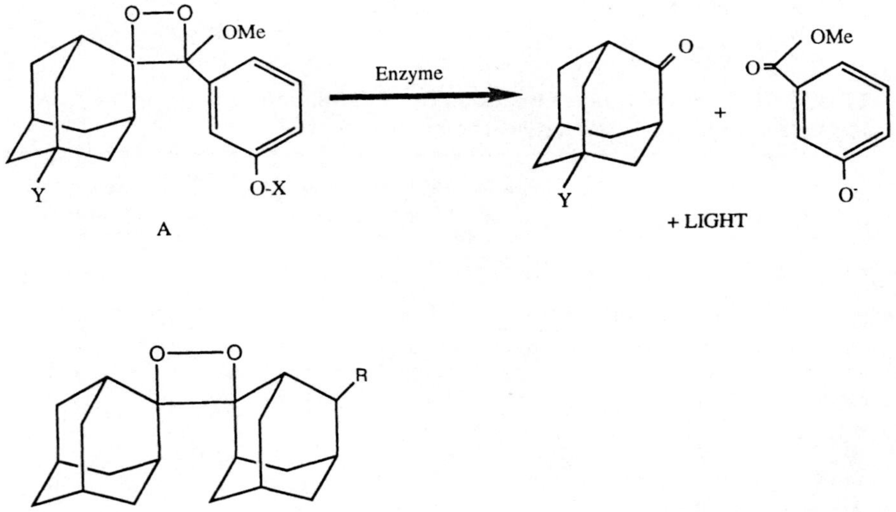

FIGURE 15.4 1,2-Dioxetanes. (A) Adamantyl 1,2-dioxetane aryl derivatives, Y = H or Cl; X = phosphate or galactoside; Y = H, X = 2-methyl-4-hydroxynaphthylphosphate. (B) Adamantylidene adamantane. R = H, and an activated derivative for labeling R is succinic acid monoamide N-hydroxysuccinimide ester.

thermochemiluminescent immunoassay for carcinoembryonic antigen (CEA) (26). In order to withstand the high temperature of the detection step, it was necessary to use a special plastic (Kapton 500H) for the fabrication of the assay reaction vessel. A further problem was that light emission from this label was very weak, but this was in part remedied by an energy transfer strategy using 9,10-diphenylanthracene. This highly efficient fluorescer ($\phi_{CL} = 0.8-1.0$) was activated (2-[-O-(N-succinimidyl)carboxypropyl]-9,10-diphenylanthracene derivative) and used as a second label so that it was in close proximity to the dioxetane label for efficient energy transfer. These two labels were tested in an immunoassay for CEA which was linear in the CEA concentration range of 1–10 ng/ml. The high temperature and need for special equipment and reaction vessels have discouraged further development of this type of immunoassay.

3. DETECTION OF LABELS

The kinetics of the chemiluminescence light emission determines what type of instrumentation (luminometers) can be used to detect a chemiluminescent label. Various parameters can be measured and related to the label concentration; these include peak light intensity, the integral or partial integral of the light emission, and rate of light production. The kinetics of light emission varies considerably, ranging from the rapid flash of light produced when acridinium esters are oxidized (decay half-life 0.9 sec), to the much slower emission from an aminobutyl-N-ethylisoluminol conjugate that can last for longer than 25 sec, and the protracted glow (minutes–hours) from enzyme-label-catalyzed chemiluminescent reactions.

A wide range of luminometers for measuring light emission have been constructed and are the subject of a periodic survey (27). Manual, semiautomatic, and fully automatic luminometers suitable for tubes or microwells, which use photomultiplier tubes in a photon current or the more sensitive photon counting mode, are available. In addition, qualitative and semiquantitative results can be obtained with camera luminometers which use photographic film to record the light emission. A current trend is toward photon imaging systems based on a different type of camera (e.g., charge-coupled device), and these are particularly effective for chemiluminescent immunoassays performed in two-dimensional arrays, such as a 96-well microplate (28).

4. TYPES OF CHEMILUMINESCENT IMMUNOASSAY

Both heterogeneous immunoassays (competitive and sandwich assays) that require a separation of bound and free labeled fractions, and homogeneous (nonseparation) immunoassays, which do not require a separation step, have been described. Proteins in biological samples quench chemiluminescence, and so the separation and washing steps in sandwich-type immunoassays provide a means of eliminating these interferents.

4.1. Heterogeneous

Separation of bound and free fraction can be achieved using adsorption (dextran-coated charcoal) (29), Sephadex chromatography (30), or antibodies immobilized to microparticles (31), beads (32), or the inside surface of tubes (33) or microwells (34).

4.2. Homogeneous (Nonseparation)

The advantage of a nonseparation assay format is that the assay can be performed in one step in a single tube, and is more adaptable to implementation on an automatic analyzer. All of the nonseparation chemiluminescent immunoassays are experimental and none have undergone development to a commercially available product. Exceptions to this generalization are the DNA probe assays based on acridinium ester labels (hybridization protection assay format) (35) and an electrochemiluminescent immunoassay for TSH based on a ruthenium tris(bipyridyl) label (36). Two different types of nonseparation chemiluminescent immunoassays have been described. One is based on the enhancement of light emission when a labeled antigen binds to a specific antibody. The other exploits an energy transfer between chemiluminescently labeled and a fluorophore-labeled assay components, as illustrated in Fig. 15.5.

4.2.1. Enhancement

The observation that the light emission from a biotin–isoluminol conjugate was increased 10-fold when it bound to avidin prompted the development of a nonseparation assay for biotin. Biotin samples were incubated with fixed amounts of a biotin–isoluminol conjugate and avidin. The light emission was inversely proportional to biotin concentration due to competition between biotin and labeled biotin for binding sites on the avidin. The 10-fold difference in light emission between bound and free conjugate was sufficient to produce a 5-min assay for biotin with a working range of $50–400$ nM (37). Similar enhancements occur when steroid–isoluminol conjugates bind to specific anti-steroid antibodies. For example, a 4-fold increase in light emission occurs when a progesterone–aminohexyl-N-ethyl isoluminol conjugate binds to an anti-progesterone antibody (38). Steroid in a sample modulated this enhancement and provided the basis for an assay that required a 50-min incubation and detects 25 pg of progesterone. This type of assay is also applicable to other steroids including estriol (39).

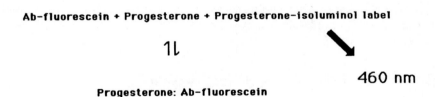

Ab–fluorescein + Progesterone + Progesterone–isoluminol label

$1↓$

460 nm

Progesterone: Ab–fluorescein

+

isoluminol label–Progesterone: Ab–fluorescein

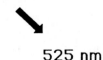

525 nm

FIGURE 15.5 Chemiluminescence energy transfer immunoassay. AB, anti-progesterone antibody. (Emission from unbound conjugate 460 nm; emission from bound conjugate 525 nm due to energy transfer to fluorescein.)

Binding of antibody to a steroid–isoluminol conjugate can also modulate the kinetics of the light emission. The peak light emission from a cortisol–aminopropyl-N-ethylisoluminol conjugate is decreased and the total light emission slightly increased in the presence of an anti-cortisol antibody. The kinetics of the decay of light emission is much slower in the presence of the antibody. Cortisol in a sample modulates these effects as a result of competition with the conjugate for binding sites on the antibody. Thus, by measuring the light intensity at a point on the decay part of the light–time curve it is possible to quantitate cortisol in a sample in the range 20–2000 pg (2-hr assay) (40). This assay, like other nonseparation assays described above, requires that the steroid be extracted from the sample in order to avoid interference by substances present in serum, plasma, and urine. The mechanism for the enhancement effects is unknown but it may be as a result of a more hydrophobic environment created around the label when it is bound in the complex (biotin : avidin or antigen : antibody).

A variant on the enhancement strategy is to use a strong base (2 M NaOH) to selectively enhance light emission from the unbound label (41). This strategy was tested in an immunoassay for estrone-3-glucuronide based on an N-aminoethyl-N-ethylisoluminol label. The detection limit for estrone-3-glucuronide was 8 pg/tube.

4.2.2. Energy Transfer

A chemiluminescent label can act as a source of excitation light for a fluorophore label, and assay formats can be designed that modulate this transfer of energy and hence produce nonseparation immunoassays (Fig. 15.5). Assays for both low- and high-molecular-weight analytes have been developed, and this assay principle is the subject of a patent (42, 43).

5. CHEMILUMINESCENT DETECTION OF ENZYME LABELS

A continuing trend is the development of chemiluminescent endpoints for enzyme labels (Table 15.6). The new endpoints are more sensitive than the colorimetric and fluorometric alternatives, and have been adopted for the detection of alkaline phosphatase, peroxidase, and glucose oxidase labels. The following section provides a brief account of the different chemiluminescent detection reactions for enzymes; the reader is refered to various recent books and reviews for additional information (2, 5, 8, 44).

5.1. Alkaline Phosphatase

There is now a diverse range of chemiluminescent assays for alkaline phosphatase (EC 3.1.3.1) labels. The most sensitive are based on adamantyl 1,2-dioxetane aryl phosphates, such as disodium 3-(4-methoxyspiro[1,2-dioxetane-3,2′-tricyclo[3.3.1.1$^{3.7}$]decan-4-yl]phenylphosphate) (AMPPD) and the 5-chloro-substituted analog (CSPD) (Fig. 15.4). Alkaline phosphatase dephosphorylates these substrates to produce a phenoxide intermediate and this decomposes to produce light emission at 470 nm (45–47). The 5-chloro derivative exhibits more rapid emission kinetics than the unsubstituted parent compound. This is most likely due to a hyperconjugation effect of the remote chloro substituent which modulates the decomposition of the dephosphorylated dioxetane. The detection limit for the

**TABLE 15.6   Chemiluminescent Detection Reactions
for Enzymes**

<hr>

Alkaline phosphatase (AP; EC 3.1.3.1)

1. AMPPD $\xrightarrow{AP}$ light
2. Ascorbic acid 2-O-phosphate $\xrightarrow{AP}$ ascorbic acid
   Ascorbic acid + lucigenin + $O_2 \xrightarrow{OH^-}$ light
3. 4-Nitrophenyl phosphate $\xrightarrow{AP}$ 4-nitrophenol
   Change in pH $\xrightarrow{lucigenin}$ light
4. $NADP^+ \xrightarrow{AP} + NAD^+ + P_i$
   $NAD^+ + CH_3CH_2OH \xrightarrow{alcohol\ dehydrogenase} NADH + CH_3CHO$
   $NADH + 1\text{-}MPMS \longrightarrow 1\text{-}MPMSH_2 + O_2^-$
   $O_2^- + luminol \xrightarrow{microperoxidase}$ light
5. Galactose 1-phosphate $\xrightarrow{AP}$ galactose + P_i
   Galactose + $NAD^+ \xrightarrow{galactose\ dehydrogenase}$ galactonate + NADH
   NADH $\xrightarrow{1\text{-}MPMS,\ luminol,\ microperoxidase}$ light
6. Glucose 1-phosphate $\xrightarrow{AP}$ glucose + P_i
   Glucose + $O_2 \xrightarrow{glucose\ oxidase}$ gluconate + H_2O_2
   $H_2O_2 + isoluminol \xrightarrow{microperoxidase}$ light
7. 4-Iodophenyl phosphate $\xrightarrow{AP}$ 4-iodophenol
   4-Iodophenyl $\xrightarrow{HRP\ +\ luminol\ +\ H_2O_2}$ light
8. 4-Nitrophenyl phosphate $\xrightarrow{AP}$ 4-nitrophenol
   p4-nitrophenol $\xrightarrow{HRP\ +\ luminol\ +\ H_2O_2\ +\ 4\text{-}iodophenol}$ light

β-Galactosidase (GAL; EC 3.2.1.23)

1. AMPGD $\xrightarrow{GAL,\ OH^-}$ light
2. Lactose $\xrightarrow{GAL}$ glucose + galactose
   Glucose $\xrightarrow{glucose\ oxidase,\ isoluminol,\ microperoxidase}$ light
3. Lactose $\xrightarrow{GAL}$ glucose + galactose
   Glucose $\xrightarrow{glucose\ oxidase}$ H_2O_2
   $H_2O_2 \xrightarrow{TCPO\ +\ ANS}$ light

Glucose oxidase (GO; EC 1.1.3.4)

1. Glucose + $O_2 \xrightarrow{GO}$ gluconolactone + H_2O_2
   $H_2O_2 \xrightarrow{isoluminol,\ microperoxidase}$ light

(Horseradish peroxidase (HRP; EC 1.11.7)

1. Luminol + H_2O_2 + 4-iodophenol $\xrightarrow{HRP}$ light

Invertase (EC 3.2.1.26)

1. Sucrose $\xrightarrow{invertase}$ fructose + glucose
   Reducing sugar + lucigenin + $O_2 \xrightarrow{HO^-}$ light

Microperoxidase (EC 1.11.1.7)

1. Luminol + $H_2O_2 \xrightarrow{microperoxidase}$ light

Urease (EC 3.5.1.5)

1. Urea $\xrightarrow{Urease}$ CO_2 + NH_3
   Change in pH $\xrightarrow{lucigenin}$ light

Xanthine oxidase (EC 1.1.3.22)

1. Xanthine + $O_2 \xrightarrow{xanthine\ oxidase}$ hypoxanthine + H_2O_2
   $H_2O_2 + luminol + Fe\text{-}EDTA \longrightarrow$ light

<hr>

Note. Adapted from Ref. (2). Abbreviations: AMPGD and AMPPD, disodium 3-(4-methoxyspiro[1,2-dioxetane-3,2′-tricyclo-[3.3.1$^{3.7}$]-decan-4-yl]phenyl-galactoside and phosphate; ANS, 8-anilino-1-naphthalenesulfonic acid; 1-MPMS, 1-methoxy-5-methylphenazinium methyl sulfate; 1-MPMSH$_2$, reduced form of 1-MPMS; P$_i$, inorganic phosphate; TCPO, bis(2,4,6-trichlorophenyl)oxalate.

enzyme is 1 zmol (10^{-21} mol) and the light emission is a long-lived glow (>1 hr), thus making this an ideal system for use with membrane-based immunoassays (e.g., Western blotting) (48). Light emission from this reaction can be enhanced by a nylon membrane surface and by certain polymers, e.g., polyvinylbenzyl(benzyldimethylammonium) chloride, and by detergent–fluorescein mixtures (49, 50). For nylon, enhancement is due to sequestering of the dephosphorylated intermediate in hydrophobic domains—these stabilize and minimize nonluminescent decomposition of the intermediate.

The benefits of replacing a colorimetric by a more sensitive chemiluminescent detection reaction for an alkaline phosphatase label has been demonstrated in several studies (51). For example, the dose–response curves (expressed as signal to background vs dose) for identical enzyme immunoassays for α-fetoprotein using a colorimetric and a chemiluminescent detection reaction for the alkaline phosphatase label were compared (51). The detection limit was improved from 2 to 0.03 μg/liter by substituting the chemiluminescent endpoint for the conventional colorimetric endpoint.

A wide selection of immunoassays has now been developed (45) and the dioxetane substrates are being exploited in several commercial automated chemiluminescent enzyme immunoassay analyzers (e.g., Access, Sanofi; Immulite, DPC; Lumipulse, Fujirebio).

A recent patent application discloses the concept of time-resolved heterogeneous chemiluminescence immunoassay in which an acridinium ester and an alkaline phosphatase label are combined in a simultaneous assay for morphine and phencyclidine (52). The labels are detected after an incubation period with the substrate for the alkaline phosphatase. Addition of the signal-generating reagent triggers a rapid burst of light from the acridinium ester label, and after a delay, the longer-lived signal from the alkaline phosphatase label is measured.

5.2. Galactosidase

A β-galactosidase (EC 3.2.1.23) label can be quantitated using the coupled-enzyme assay scheme shown in Table 15.6. NADH formed as a result of the reaction of the β-galactose product with galactose dehydrogenase reduces oxygen in the presence of an electron mediator to form peroxide. Peroxide is quantitated using a mixture of isoluminol and microperoxidase. The detection limit for the enzyme is 0.33 zmol, and the reaction was successfully used in an enzyme immunoassay for 17-α-hydroxyprogesterone (53). Enzyme-catalyzed cleavage of the galactoside group from the 3-position of the aromatic ring of an AMPGD substrate (Fig. 15.4) produces a phenoxide intermediate which then decomposes to produce light. The detection limit for the enzyme using this chemiluminescent assay is 30 zmol, but as yet it has not found significant application in immunoassay.

5.3. Glucose Oxidase

A number of chemiluminescent assays for glucose oxidase (EC 1.1.3.4) are available. Luminol or isoluminol in the presence of a microperoxidase catalyst can be used to assay peroxide produced by the action of a glucose oxidase label on glucose (Table 15.6). (54). Alternatively, the peroxide can be measured using a chemiluminescent fluorophore-sensitized bis(2,4,6-trichlorophenyl) oxalate reaction (55). The isoluminol–microperoxidase detection system is currently used in a commercial enzyme immunoassay system manufactured by Sankyo (54).

5.4. Glucose-6-phosphate Dehydrogenase

A glucose-6-phosphate dehydrogenase (EC 1.1.1.49) label has been quantitated in an immunoassay for 17-α-hydroxyprogesterone using the assay scheme shown in Table 15.6. The detection limit for the label was 1 amol and the assay was linear from 1 amol to 10 fmol (53).

5.5. β-N-Acetylglucosaminidase

A nonluminescent luminol-based substrate (δ-aminophthalylhydrazido-N-acetyl-β-D-glucosaminide) for β-N-acetylglucosaminidase (EC 3.2.1.30) has been synthesized. The substrate is converted to a luminescent product by the enzyme, and its use to detect this particular label in an enzyme immunoassay has been proposed (56).

5.6. Peroxidase

Luminol and related cyclic diacylhydrazides are cosubstrates for peroxidases, and the catalytic effect of these enzymes on the chemiluminescent oxidation is used to quantitate peroxidase labels in immunoassay. The first chemiluminescent enzyme immunoassay used a mixture of luminol and peroxide to measure a horseradish peroxidase label in an assay for cortisol (57). The sensitivity and utility of this assay were improved by the discovery of enhancers for this reaction. These molecules increased light emission and reduced the assay reagent background, hence dramatically improving the signal to background ratio for detection of the label. Various types of molecules act as enhancers of the reaction, including substituted phenols (4-iodophenol, 4-bromophenol, 4-hydroxycinnamic acid), naphthols (1-bromonaphth-2-ol), amines (4-methoxyaniline), and boronates (4-iodophenylboronic acid) (58, 59). Enhanced chemiluminescent detection of peroxidase labels has found a wide range of applications, including immunoassay and Western blotting, and has been commercialized by several companies (e.g., Amersham, Kodak, and DuPont).

5.7. Invertase

The detection limit for an invertase (EC 3.2.1.26) label using the chemiluminescent assay scheme shown in Table 15.6 is 0.74 fmol. This label has been tested in an enzyme immunoassay for 17-α-hydroxyprogesterone (53).

5.8. Xanthine Oxidase

A xanthine oxidase (EC 1.1.3.22) label can be assayed using a mixture of an iron–EDTA complex and luminol (60). The assay is very sensitive (detection limit 3 amol) and a particular advantage is that the light emission from the xanthine oxidase-catalyzed chemiluminescent reaction is very long-lived (>96 hr). Several chemiluminescent enzyme immunoassays have been developed using this combination of label and detection reaction (e.g., TSH, thyroxine, IgE) (60).

TABLE 15.7 **Chemiluminescence Immunoassay Analyzers**

Label	Analyzer
Acridinium ester	ACS:180 (Ciba Corning)
Acridinium sulfonyl carboxamide	BeriLux (Behring)
Alkaline phosphatase	Access (Sanofi)
	Immulite (DPC)
	Lumipulse (Fujirebio)
Glucose oxidase	Luminomaster (Sankyo)
Isoluminol	LIA-mat (Byk-Sangtek)
Horseradish peroxidase	Amerlite (Kodak Clinical Diagnostics)

6. AUTOMATED CHEMILUMINESCENT IMMUNOASSAY SYSTEMS

Table 15.7 lists the current range of automatic and semiautomatic chemiluminescent immunoassay analyzers, and the label used in the immunoassay. Both glow- and flash-type chemiluminescent reactions are in use, and the different analyzers exploit the relative benefits of these contrasting emission kinetics (i.e., rapid signal generation and acquisition with the flash-type reactions, and flexibility in signal generation and measurement with the glow-type chemistries). The reader is referred to the recent book by Chan (61), a survey (62), and to Chapter 21 for a detailed account of automatic immunoassay analyzers.

References

1. Kricka LJ. Ligand-Binder Assays. New York: Dekker, 1985.
2. Kricka LJ. Chemiluminescent and bioluminescent techniques. Clin Chem 1991; 37:1472–81.
3. Campbell AK. Chemiluminescence. Chichester: Horwood, 1988.
4. Gundermann KD, McCapra F. Chemiluminescence in Organic Chemistry. Berlin: Springer, 1987.
5. Pringle MJ. Analytical applications of chemiluminescence. Adv Clin Chem 1993; 30:89–183.
6. DeLuca MA, McElroy WD, Eds. Bioluminescence and chemiluminescence. Methods in Enzymology, Vol. 133. New York: Academic Press, 1986.
7. Nozaki O, Kricka LJ, Stanley PE. Bioluminescence and chemiluminescence literature—immunoassay and blotting assays. J Biolumin Chemilumin 1992; 7:263–98.
8. Szalay A, Kricka LJ, Stanley PE, Eds. Bioluminescence and Chemiluminescence: Status Report. Chichester: Wiley, 1993.
9. Jansen EHJM, van den Berg RH, Zomer G. HPLC method for purification and quality control of isoluminol labels. In: van Dyke K, van Dyke R, Eds. Luminescence Immunoassay and Molecular Applications. Boca Raton: CRC Press, 1990:99–118.
10. Buckler RT, Schroeder HR. Dimethyl 7-[w-N-(phthalimido)alkyl]aminonaphthalene-1,2-dicarboxylates. US Patent 1980: 4,238,395.
11. Buckler RT, Schroeder HR. Chemiluminescent naphthalene-1,2-dicarboxylic acid hydrazide-labeled polypeptides and proteins. US Patent 1980: 4,225,485.
12. Zomer G, van den Berg RH, Jansen EHJM. Synthesis and chemiluminescence of benzo[ghi]perylene-1,2-dicarboxylic acid hydrazide 4-butanoic acid-N-hydroxysuccinimidyl ester. In: Scholmerich J, Andreseen R, Kapp A, Ernst M, Woods WG, Eds. Bioluminescence and Chemiluminescence: New Perspectives. Chichester: Wiley, 1987:443–6.
13. McCapra F, Tutt RE, Topping RM. Assay method utilizing chemiluminescence. UK Patent 1977; 1,461,877.
14. McCapra F, Perring KD. General organic chemiluminescence. Clin Biochem Anal 1986; 16:259–320.

15. Weeks I, Campbell AK, Woodhead JS. Two-site immunochemiluminometric assay of human alpha$_1$-fetoprotein. Clin Chem 1983; 29:1480–3.
16. McCapra F, Whatmore D, Sumun F, Patel A, Beheshti I, Ramakrishnan K, Branson J. Luminescent labels for immunoassay—from concept to practice. J Biolumin Chemilumin 1989; 4:51–8.
17. Zomer G, Stavenuiter JFC. Chemiluminogenic labels old and new. Anal Chim Acta 1989; 227:11–19.
18. Bagazgoitia FJ, Garcia JL, Diequez C, Weeks I, Woodhead JS. Effect of surfactants on the intensity of chemiluminescence emission from acridinium ester labeled proteins. J Biolumin Chemilumin 1988; 2:121–8.
19. Howie CL, Grayeski ML. Effect of micelles and cyclodextrin solutions on acridinium chemiluminescence. In: Scholmerich J, Andreseen R, Kapp A, Ernst M, Woods WG, Eds. Bioluminescence and Chemiluminescence: New Perspectives. Chichester: Wiley, 1987:415–8.
20. Law SJ, Miller T, Piran U, Klukas C, Chang S, Unger J. Novel poly-substituted aryl acridinium esters and their use in immunoassay. J Biolumin Chemilumin 1989; 4:88–98.
21. Weeks I, Beheshti I, McCapra F, Campbell AK, Woodhead JS. Acridinium esters as high-specific-activity labels in immunoassay. Clin Chem 1983; 29:1474–9.
22. Mayer A, Schmidt E, Kinkel T, Molz P, Neuenhofer S, Skrzipczyk H. Hydrophilic acridinium-9-carboxylic acid derivatives used as labels in luminescence immunoassays. In: Stanley PE, Kricka LJ, Eds. Bioluminescence and Chemiluminescence: Current Status. Chichester: Wiley, 1991:99–102.
23. Mattingly P. Chemiluminescent 10-methyl-acridinium-9-(N-sulphonylcarboxamide) salts. Synthesis and kinetics of light emission. J Biolumin Chemilumin 1991; 6:107–14.
24. Masuya H, Kondo K, Aramaki Y, Ichimori Y. Pyridopyridazine compounds and their use. Eur Patent Appl 1992; 491,477.
25. Ii M, Yoshida H, Aramaki Y, et al. Improved enzyme immunoassay for human fibroblast growth factor using a new enhanced chemiluminescence system. Biochem Biophys Res Commun 1993; 193:540–5.
26. Hummelen JC, Luider TM, Wynberg H. Stable 1,2-dioxetanes as labels for thermochemiluminescent immunoassay. Methods Enzymol 1986; 133:531–57.
27. Stanley PE. Commercially available luminometers and imaging devices for low-light measurements and kits and reagents utilizing bioluminescence or chemiluminescence: survey update I. J Biolumin Chemilumin 1993; 8:237–40.
28. Leaback DH, Haggart R. The use of CCD imaging luminometer in the quantitation of luminogenic assays. J Biolumin Chemilumin 1989; 4:512–22.
29. Pazzagli M, Kim JB, Messeri G, Martinazzo G, et al. Luminescent immunoassay (LIA) for progesterone in a heterogeneous system. Clin Chim Acta 1981; 115:287–96.
30. Schroeder HR, Yeager FM, Boguslaski RC, Vogelhut PO. Immunoassay for serum thyroxine monitored by chemiluminescence. J Immunol Methods 1979; 25:275–82.
31. Weerasekera DA, Kim JB, Barnard GJ, Collins WP. Measurement of serum thyroxine by solid-phase chemiluminescent immunoassay. Ann Clin Biochem 1983; 20:100–4.
32. Kohen F, Lindner HR, Gilad S. Development of chemiluminescence monitored immunoassays for steroid hormones. J Steroid Biochem 1983; 19:413–8.
33. Kim JB, Barnard GJ, Collins WP, Kohen F, Linder HR, Eshhar Z. Measurement of plasma estradiol-17β by solid-phase chemiluminescence immunoassay. Clin Chem 1982; 28:1120–4.
34. Schroeder HR, Hines CM, Osborn DD, et al. Immunochemiluminometric assay for hepatitis B surface antigen. Clin Chem 1981; 27:1378–84.
35. Arnold Jr. LJ, Hammond PW, Wiese WA, Nelson NC. Assay formats involving acridinium-ester-labeled DNA probes. Clin Chem 1989; 35:1588–94.
36. Blackburn GF, Shah HP, Kenten JH, et al. Electrochemiluminescence detection for development of immunoassays and DNA probe assays for clinical diagnostics. Clin Chem 1991; 37:1534–9.
37. Schroeder HR, Boguslaski RC, Carrico RJ, Buckler RT. Monitoring specific protein-binding reactions with chemiluminescence. Methods Enzymol 1978; 57:424–45.
38. Zomer G, van den Berg RH, Jansen EHMJ. Fast homogeneous immunoassay for progesterone based on antibody-enhanced chemiluminescence. In: Scholmerich J, Andreseen R, Kapp A, Ernest M, Woods WG, Eds. Bioluminescence and Chemiluminescence: New Perspectives. Chichester: Wiley, 1987:305–8.
39. Kohen F, Kim JB, Lindner HR, Barnard G. An immunoassay for urinary estriol-16-glucuronide based on antibody-enhanced chemiluminescence. In: DeLuca MA, McElroy WD, Eds. Bioluminescence and Chemiluminescence. New York: Academic Press, 1981:351–6.
40. Kohen F, Pazzagli M, Kim JB, Lindner HR. An immunoassay for plasma cortisol based on chemiluminescence. Steroids 1989; 36:421–37.

41. Kim JB, Kwon OJ, Barnard G. A novel homogeneous immunoassay for estrone-3-glucuronide based on antibody protected effects on the enhancement of chemiluminescence by NaOH. In: Stanley PE, Kricka LJ, Eds. Bioluminescence and Chemiluminescence: Current Status. Chichester: Wiley, 1991:111–4.

42. Woodhead JS, Weeks I, Campbell AK. Immunological procedure for detecting or quantifying substances. UK Patent 1986:2,129,553.

43. Patel A, Davies CJ, Campbell AK, McCapra F. Chemiluminescence energy transfer: A new technique applicable to the study of ligand interactions in living systems. Anal Biochem 1983; 29:162–9.

44. Bronstein I, Kricka LJ. Clinical applications of luminescent assays for enzymes and enzyme labels. J Clin Lab Anal 1989; 3:316–22.

45. Bronstein I, Kricka LJ. Chemiluminescence: Properties of 1,2-dioxetane chemiluminescence. In: Kessler C, Ed. Nonradioactive Labeling and Detection of Biomolecules. Berlin: Springer, 1992:168–75.

46. Bronstein I, Juo RR, Voyta JC, Edwards B. Novel chemiluminescent adamantyl 1,2-dioxetane enzyme substrates. In: Stanley PE, Kricka LJ, Eds. Bioluminescence and Chemiluminescence: Current Status. Chichester: Wiley, 1991:73–82.

47. Bronstein I. Chemiluminescent 1,2-dioxetane-based enzyme substrates and their applications. In: van Dyke K, van Dyke R, Eds. Luminescence Immunoassay and Molecular Applications. Boca Raton: CRC Press, 1990:256–74.

48. Bronstein I, Voyta JC, Murphy OJ, Bresnick L, Kricka LJ. Improved chemiluminescent western blotting procedure. BioTechniques 1992; 12:748–53.

49. Voyta JC, Edwards B, Bronstein I, McGrath P. Chemiluminescent enhancement of enzyme-activated decomposition of enzymatically cleavable chemiluminescent 1,2-dioxetanes. US Patent 1992: 5,145,772.

50. Schaap AP, Akhaven J, Romano LJ. Chemiluminescent substrates for alkaline phosphatase: applications to ultrasensitive enzyme-linked immunoassays and DNA probes. Clin Chem 1989; 35:1863–4.

51. Thorpe GHG, Bronstein I, Kricka LJ, Edwards B, Voyta JC. Chemiluminescent enzyme immunoassay for alpha-fetoprotein based on an adamantyl dioxetane phosphate substrate. Clin Chem 1989; 35:2319–21.

52. Khalil OS, Genger KR, Cotter SM, et al. Simultaneous determination of multiple analytes using time-resolved heterogeneous chemiluminescence assay. PCT Intl Appl 1992:12,255.

53. Tsuji A, Maeda M, Arakawa H. Enzyme immunoassays monitored by chemiluminescence reactions of lucigenin and NADH. In: van Dyke K, van Dyke R, Eds. Luminescence Immunoassay and Molecular Applications. Boca Raton: CRC Press, 1990:157–72.

54. Sekiya K, Saito Y, Ikegami T, Yamamoto M, Sato Y, Maeda M, Tsuji A. Fully-automated analyzer for chemiluminescent enzyme immunoassay. In: Stanley PE, Kricka LJ, Eds. Bioluminescence and Chemiluminescence: Current Status. Chichester: Wiley, 1991:123–6.

55. Arakawa H, Maeda M, Tsuji A. Chemiluminescence enzyme immunoassay of 17-alpha-hydroxy-progesterone using glucose oxidase and bis(2,4,6-trichlorophenyl)oxalate-fluorescent dye. Chem Pharm Bull 1982; 30:3036–9.

56. Sasamoto K, Okhura Y. A chemiluminogenic substrate for N-acetyl-beta-D-glucosaminidase, delta-aminophthalylhydrazido-N-acetyl-beta-D-glucosaminide. Chem Pharm Bull 1990; 38:1323–5.

57. Arakawa H, Maeda M, Tsuji A. Chemiluminescence enzyme immunoassay of cortisol using peroxidase as a label. Anal Biochem 1979; 97:248–4.

58. Thorpe GHG, Kricka LJ. Enhanced chemiluminescent reactions catalysed by horseradish peroxidase. Methods Enzymol 1986; 133:331–53.

59. Kricka LJ. Chemiluminescent enhancers comprising organoboron compounds. UK Patent Appl 1993:2,265,459.

60. Baret A, Fert V. T_4 and ultrasensitive TSH immunoassays using luminescent enhanced xanthine oxidase assay. J Biolumin Chemilumin 1990; 4:149–53.

61. Chan, D. Ed. Immunoassay Automation. New York: Academic Press, 1992.

62. Stanley PE. A survey of some commercially available kits and reagents which include bioluminescence or chemiluminescence for their operation: Including immunoassays, hybridization, labels, probes, blots and ATP-based rapid microbiology. Products from more than forty companies. J Biolumin Chemilumin 1993; 8:51–63.

16 | BIOLUMINESCENCE IMMUNOASSAYS

REINHARD ERICH GEIGER
BioAss
D 86911 Diessen
Federal Republic of Germany

DUSICA GABRIJELCIC
BioAss
D 86911 Diessen
Federal Republic of Germany

WERNER MISKA
Hautklinik der Universität Gießen
D 35392 Giessen
Federal Republic of Germany

1. INTRODUCTION

Bioluminescence is a natural phenomenon found in many lower forms of life (1–3). Naturally occurring bioluminescent systems differ with regard to the structure and function of enzymes and cofactors as well as in the mechanism of the light-emitting reactions (4, 5). Because of its high sensitivity (down to 10^{-15} mol/liter of ATP or D-luciferin can be detected) firefly (*Photinus pyralis*) bioluminescence has been used for many years for the sensitive determination of ATP (6) and many different analytes (7–10). Bacterial bioluminescence is also widely used for scientific applications (11–13). Furthermore, luciferase genes, applied in a large number of molecular biological and biochemical systems, have become an established tool for research (14–18).

2. PRINCIPLES OF BIOLUMINESCENT LIGHT EMISSION

Depending on the respective bioluminescent system light is formed in different ways. In Eq. (1), light production by firefly luciferase (bioluminescence of *P. pyralis;* 19) is shown schematically (PP, pyrophosphate). Luciferase catalyzes the oxidation of D-luciferin in the presence of ATP and Mg^{2+} to oxyluciferin, with emission of light at 546 nm.

$$\text{D-Luciferin + ATP + Mg}^{2+} \xrightarrow{\text{luciferase}} \text{Light + Oxyluciferin + AMP + PP} \qquad (1)$$

The mechanism for light emission by bacteria (bacterial bioluminescence) is quite different from the luminescence of firefly bioluminescence (for review see 20). A substrate delivers NAD(H) and the energy of the reaction is transfered to $FMNH_2$. $FMNH_2$ is the necessary cofactor which is used by bacterial luciferase to emit light. During further reaction steps $FMNH_2$ is oxidized, and the oxidized $FMNH_2$ oxidizes aldehydes, e.g., acetaldehyde or other aldehydes, to form carbonic acids under light emission.

Other bioluminescence systems and compounds are reviewed elsewhere (21–23). In renilla bioluminescence (21) the luciferase substrate is a complex heterocyclic organic compound. During the enzymatic reaction with renilla luciferase, renilla luciferin is oxidized followed by carbon dioxide release. A high-energy intermediate is formed which is converted under light emission to oxyluciferin.

Calcium-triggered luminescence of aequorin produces the blue-fluorescent protein (BFP; 22), which contains dissociable coelenteramide. The protein part of BFP regenerates aequorin on aerobic incubation with coelenterazine.

Light emission using bioluminogenic substrates (24–26; Fig. 16.1) is based on the release of D-luciferin from D-luciferin derivatives by the action of hydrolytic

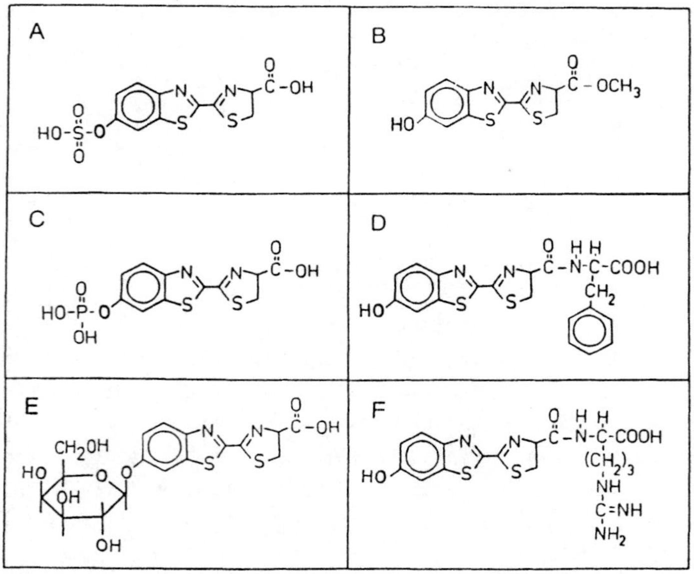

FIGURE 16.1   Structures of some D-luciferin derivatives. (A) D-luciferin-O-sulfate, (B) D-luciferin methyl ester, (C) D-luciferin-O-phosphate, (D) D-luciferyl-L-phenylalanine, (E) D-luciferin-O-β-galactoside, (F) D-luciferyl-L-*N*-arginine.

enzymes (Fig. 16.2). Released D-luciferin can be quantified by a luminometric detection system (see Fig. 16.6). The high sensitivity of these bioluminogenic substrates is obtained, on one hand, by the amplification which occurs in the releasing step (e.g., one molecule of alkaline phosphatase can convert more than 1000 molecules of D-luciferin-O-phosphate to D-luciferin per second), and, on the other hand, by the highly sensitive bioluminescence system (*P. pyralis,* concentrations of 5×10^{-12} mol/liter of D-luciferin can be detected; Fig. 16.3, Eq. (2)).

$$\text{D-Luciferin} + \text{ATP} + \text{Mg}^{2+} \xrightarrow{\text{luciferase}} \text{Light} + \text{Oxyluciferin} + \text{AMP} + \text{PP} \qquad (2)$$

These new substrates can be used for unmodified enzymes and for enzyme conjugates, and are suitable for enzyme immunoassays, for protein blot analysis, and for nucleic acid hybridization tests (27–32).

3. BIOLUMINESCENCE IMMUNOASSAY INSTRUMENTATION

A large variety of commercially available luminometers and imaging devices for bioluminescence measurements are on the market at present. For interested readers we recommend two detailed surveys (33, 34).

4. ENZYME LABELS AND BIOLUMINOGENIC SUBSTRATES

Bioluminescence-enhanced enzyme immunoassays are similar to conventional enzyme immunoassays in the immunological part of the test. They differ only in the detection reaction in which D-luciferin derivatives are cleaved by the respective enzymes and light is produced by oxidation of liberated D-luciferin by luciferase (see Section 2). In Table 16.1 bioluminogenic detection systems and enzyme labels are listed.

5. BIOLUMINESCENCE ENZYME IMMUNOASSAYS

5.1. Immunoassays Based on Alkaline Phosphatase as Label

In these assays (36) the bound alkaline phosphatase–antibody conjugate or analyte–alkaline phosphatase conjugate cleave D-luciferin-O-phosphate liberating D-

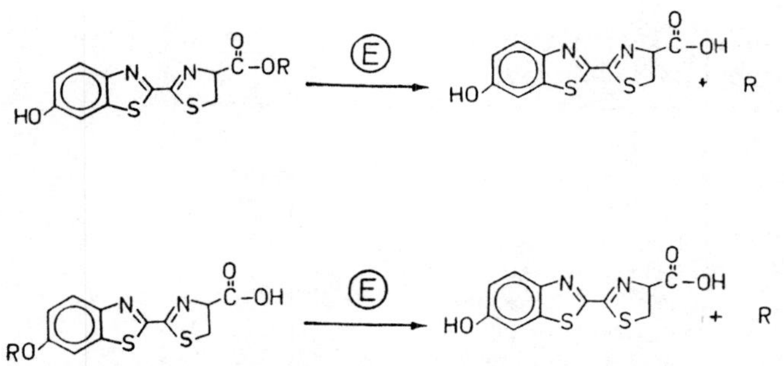

FIGURE 16.2 Scheme of an enzymatically enhanced bioluminescence detection system; E, respective enzyme. The released D-luciferin is quantified using the luciferase-catalyzed reaction in the presence of ATP and Mg^{2+}.

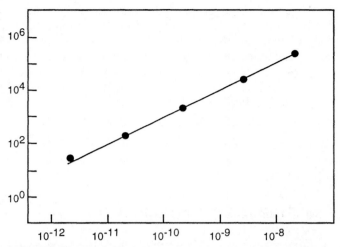

FIGURE 16.3   Determination of D-luciferin in the luminometric assay. The detection limit is around 5 × 10⁻¹² mol/liter.

luciferin. D-Luciferin is oxidized by luciferase with light emission. The principle is illustrated in Fig. 16.2 and Eqs. (3) and (4) for competitive and immunometric enzyme immunoassays.

$$\text{D-Luciferin-O-phosphate} \xrightarrow{\text{alk. phosphatase}} \text{luciferin} + \text{P} \qquad (3)$$

$$\text{Luciferin} + \text{O}_2 + \text{ATP} \xrightarrow[\text{(Mg}^{2+})]{\text{luciferase}} \text{oxyluciferin} + h \cdot v + \text{AMP} + \text{PP} \qquad (4)$$

5.2. Immunoassays Based on β-Galactosidase as Label

In these tests (37) bound β-galactosidase–antibody conjugate or analyte–β-galactosidase conjugate cleave D-luciferin-O-β-galactoside, liberating D-luciferin. D-luciferin is oxidized by luciferase with light emission. The principle is illustrated in Fig. 16.5. The liberated D-luciferin is measured as shown in Figure 16.4.

TABLE 16.1   Enzyme Labels and Substrates for Bioluminogenic Enzyme Immunoassays

Enzyme label	Substrate (D-luciferin derivative)	Reference
β-Galactosidase	D-luciferin-O-β-galctoside	(25)
β-Glucosidase	D-luciferin-O-β-glucoside	(35)
Alkaline phosphatase	D-luciferin-O-phosphate	(24, 26)
Arylsulfatase	D-luciferin-O-sulfate	(24, 26)
Carboxypeptidase B	D-luciferyl-L-Nᵃ-arginine	(24, 26)
Carboxypeptidase N	D-luciferyl-L-Nᵃ-arginine	(24, 26)
Carboxypeptidase A	D-luciferin-L-phenylalanine	(24, 26)
Carboxylic esterase	D-luciferin methyl ester	(24, 26)

a

b

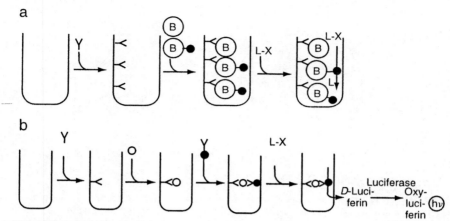

FIGURE 16.4.(a)   Scheme of the competitive bioluminescence enzyme immunoassay for bradykinin. B, bradykinin; L-X, D-luciferin-O-phosphate; L, luciferin; B–●, bradykinin–alkaline phosphatase conjugate; Y, anti-bradykinin antibody; P, phosphate; PP, pyrophosphate. (b) Scheme of the immunometric enzyme immunoassay for human immunoglobulin E. Y, immunoglobulin G directed against IgE; Y-●, immunoglobulin G–alkaline phosphatase conjugate; ○, immunoglobulin E; L-X, D-luciferin-O-phosphate.

5.3.   Immunoassays Based on Other Labels

In these enzymatically enhanced bioluminescence immunoassays (38), bound enzyme–antibody conjugate or analyte–enzyme conjugate cleave D-luciferin derivatives liberating D-luciferin. D-Luciferin is then oxidized by luciferase with light emission. The principle is illustrated in Fig. 16.4.

6.   OTHER BIOLUMINESCENCE IMMUNOASSAY SYSTEMS

A number of other bioluminescent reactions have also been used in immunoassays. For example, enzyme cofactors have been used to label antigens and antibodies (39–41). Examples are given below.

6.1.   Bioluminescent Conjugates

In this type of assay, antigens or antibodies are conjugated to bioluminescent substrates such as D-luciferin (*P. pyralis;* 42).

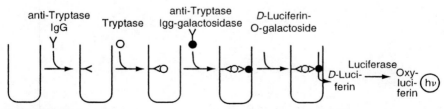

FIGURE 16.5   Scheme for the bioluminescence enzyme immunoassay of tryptase based on a β-galactosidase enzyme label. This scheme has general applicability.

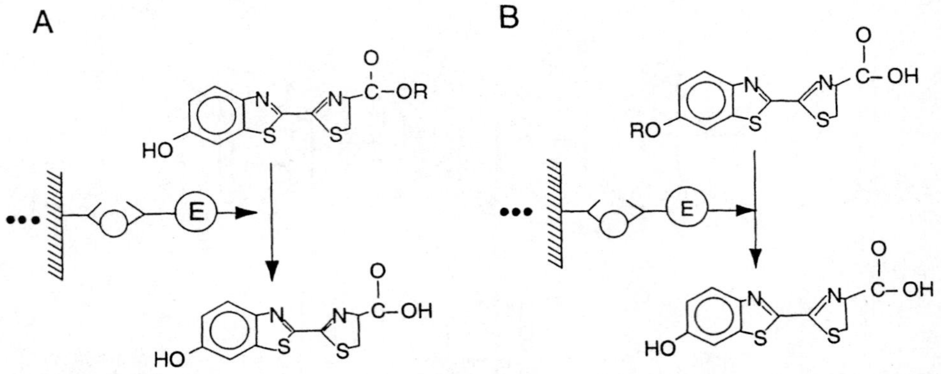

A

B

FIGURE 16.6 General scheme for the bioluminogenic detection of enzyme-labeled antibodies. (A) Liberation of luciferin from luciferin derivatives substituted at the carboxyl group; (B) release of luciferin from luciferin derivatives substituted at the hydroxyl group; Y, antibody; O, antigen; >E, enzyme–antibody conjugate.

6.2. Bioluminescent Cofactors

Cofactors such as ATP and NAD which participate directly in a bioluminescent reaction have been used for labeling antigens and antibodies (39).

6.3. Bioluminescent Enzyme Labels

In this type of assay, bioluminescent labels such as bacterial or firefly luciferase have been used for labeling antigens or antibodies (43).

6.4. Bioluminogenic Precursors

D-Luciferin (*P. pyralis*) derivatives are cleaved, releasing luminometrically active D-luciferin. Luciferin derivatives can be used as very sensitive enzyme substrates in enzyme immunoassays, producing a bioluminescent endpoint signal which can be detected with high sensitivity (24, 44).

7. AVAILABILITY OF BIOLUMINESCENCE IMMUNOASSAYS

BioAss has successfully developed a large number of bioluminescence immunoassays for research. Bioluminescence immunoassays for routine application are not as yet available.

References

1. DeLuca M. Bioluminescence and chemiluminescence. Methods in Enzymology, Vol. 57. New York Academic Press, 1978.
2. DeLuca M, McElroy WD. Bioluminescence and chemiluminescence, Part B. Methods in Enzymology, Vol. 133. New York: Academic Press, 1986.
3. Herring PJ. Systematic distribution of bioluminescence in living organisms. J Biolum Chemilum 1987; 1:146–63.

4. Burr GJ. Chemi- and Bioluminescence. New York: Marcel Dekker, 1985.
5. Schölmerich J, Andreesen R, Kapp A, Ernst M, Woods WG. Bioluminescence and Chemilumines-cence. New Perspectives. Chichester: Wiley, 1987.
6. Lundin A, Richardsson A, Thorpe A. Continous monitoring of ATP-converting reactions by purified firefly luciferase. Anal Biochem 1976; 75:611–20.
7. Kricka LJ, Stanley PE, Thorpe A, Whitehead TP. Analytical applications of bioluminescence and chemiluminescence. New York: Academic Press, 1984.
8. Wood WG. Luminescence immunoassays: Problems and possibilities. J Clin Chem Clin Biochem 1984; 22:905–18.
9. Gould SJ, Subramani S. Review. Firefly luciferase as a tool in molecular and cell biology. Anal Biochem 1988; 175:5–13.
10. Kricka LJ. Review. Clinical and biochemical applications of luciferase and luciferins. Anal Biochem 1988; 175:14–21.
11. Kricka LJ, Wienhausen GK, Hinkley, JE, DeLuca M. Automated bioluminescent assays for NADH, glucose-6-phosphate, primary bile acids and ATP. Anal Biochem 1983; 129:392–7.
12. Hastings JGM. Luminescence in clinical microbiology. In: Schölmerich J, Andreesen R, Kapp A, Ernst M, Woods WG, Eds. Bioluminescence and Chemiluminescence. New Aspects. Chichester: Wiley, 1987:453–61.
13. Wieland E, David A, Kather H, Armstron VW. Bioluminometric determination of aldehydic lipid peroxidation products during the oxidation of low density lipoproteins (LDL). In: Stanly P, Kricka LJ, Eds. Bioluminescence and Chemiluminescence. Current Status. Chichester: Wiley, 1991:455–8.
14. Wood KV, DeLuca M. Photographic detection of luminescence in Escherichia coli containing the gene for firely luciferase. Anal Biochem 1987; 161:501–7.
15. DeWet JR, Wood KV, DeLuca M, Helinski DR, Subramani S. Firefly luciferase gene: Structure and expression in mammalian cells. Mol Cell Biol 1987; 7:725–37.
16. Israel S, Honigman A. A bioluminescence assay for gene expression by continously growing mamma-lian cells: Application for detection of human immunodeficiency virus type I (HIV-1). Gene 1991; 104:139–45.
17. Kajiyama N, Nakano E. Isolation and characterization of mutants of firefly luciferase which produce different colors of light. Prot Eng 1991; 4:691–3.
18. Steiner C. Advantages of firefly luciferase as a reporter gene. Bio Forum Eur 1992; 9:123–7.
19. DeLuca M, McElroy WD. Purification and properties of firefly luciferase. Methods Enzymol 1978; 57:3–15.
20. Hastings JW. Bacterial bioluminescence: an overview. Methods Enzymol 1978; 57:125–35.
21. Cormier MJ. Application of renilla bioluminescence: an introduction. Methods Enzymol 1878; 57:237–44.
22. Johnson FH, Shimomura O. Introduction to the bioluminescence of medusae, with special reference to the photoprotein aequorin. Methods Enzymol 1978; 57:271–91.
23. Johnson FH, Shimomura O. Introduction to the cypridina System. Methods Enzymol 1978; 57:331–64.
24. Miska W, Geiger R,. Synthesis and characterization of luciferin derivatives for use in bioluminescence enhanced enzyme immunoassays. New ultrasensitive detection systems for enzyme immunoassays, I. J Clin Chem Clin Biochem 1987; 25:23–30.
25. Geiger R, Schneider E, Wallenfels K, Miska W. A new, ultrasensitive bioluminogenic enzyme substrate for β-galactosidase. Biol Chem Hoppe Seyler 1992; 373:1187–91.
26. Miska W, Geiger R. A new type of ultrasensitive bioluminogenic enzyme substrates. I. Enzyme substrates with D-luciferin as leaving group. Biol Chem Hoppe Seyler 1988; 369:407–11.
27. Geiger R, Miska W. New ultrasensitive detection systems for bioluminescence-enhanced enzyme immunoassys. In: Modern Methods in Protein Chemistry, Vol. 3, Tschesche H, Ed. Berlin: de Gruyter, 1989.
28. Hauber R, Geiger R. 1987. A new, very sensitive, bioluminescence-enhanced detection system for protein blotting. Ultrasensitive detection systems for protein blotting and nucleic acid hybridization, I. J Clin Chem Clin Biochem 1987; 25:511–4.
29. Hauber R, Miska W, Schleinkofer L, Geiger R. The application of a photon-counting camera in very sensitive, bioluminescence-enhanced detection system for protein blotting. Ultrasensitive detection systems for protein blotting and nucleic acid hybridization, II. J Clin Chem Clin Biochem 1988; 26:147–8.
30. Hauber R, Geiger R. The application of a photon-counting camera in very sensitive, bioluminescence-enhanced detection system for nucleic acid hybridization. Ultrasensitive detection systems for protein blotting and nucleic acid hybridization, III. J Clin Chem Clin Biochem 1989; 27:361–3.

31. Geiger R, Hauber R, Miska W. New, bioluminescence-enhanced detection systems for use in enzyme activity tests, enzyme immunoassays, protein blotting and nucleic acid hybridization. Mol Cell Probes 1989; 3:309–28.

32. Berger J, Hauber J, Hauber R, Geiger R, Cullen BR. 1988. Secreted placental alkaline phosphatase: a powerful new qualitative indicator of gene expression in eukaryotic cells. Gene 1988; 66:1–10.

33. Stanley PE. A survey of more than 90 commercially available luminometers and imaging devices for low-light measurements of chemiluminescence and bioluminescence. Including instruments for manual, automatic and specialized operation, for HPLC, LC, GLC and Microtitre Plates. Part 1:Descriptions. J Biolum Chemilum 1992; 7:77–108.

34. Stanley PE. Commercially available luminometers and imaging devices for low-light measurements and kits and reagents utilizing bioluminescence or chemiluminescence. Survey Update I. J Biolum Chemilum 1993; 8:237–40.

35. Finkenzeller C, Geiger R, Miska W. A new, ultrasensitive bioluminogenic enzyme substrate for β-glucosidase. Biol Chem Hoppe Seyler 1993; in press.

36. Schröter A, Gabrijelcic D, Geiger R, I. Determination of human immunoglobulin E by bioluminescence-enhanced two-site immunometric assay, J Biolum Chemilum 1994; in press.

37. Schneider E, Gabrijelcic D, Geiger R. Determination of human mast cell tryptase by bioluminescence-enhanced two-site immunometric assay. Eur J Clin Chem Clin Biochem 1992; 30:871–3.

38. Schneider E, Geiger R. The use of carboxypeptidas N as a marker enzyme in bioluminescence-enhanced enzyme immunoassay. Eur J Clin Chem Clin Biochem 1994; in press.

39. Wandlund J, Azari J, Levine L, DeLuca M. A bioluminescent immunoassay for methotrexate at the subpicomole level. Biochem Biophys Res Commun 1980; 96:440–8.

40. Kricka JL, Carter TJN. Clinical and Biochemical Luminescence. Kricka JL, Carter TJN, Eds. New York: Dekker, 1982:153.

41. Kohen F, Pazzagli M, Serlo M, deBoevers J, Vandekerckhove D. Chemiluminescence and bioluminescence immunoassays. In: Collins WP, Ed. Alternative Immunoassays. Chichester: Wiley, 1986:103–16.

42. Carrico RJ, Johnson RD, Boguslaski RC. ATP-labelled ligands and fire fly luciferase for monitoring specific protein-binding reactions. Methods Enzymol 1978; 57:113–8.

43. Wienhausen G, DeLuca M. Bioluminescent assays using coimmobilized enzymes. Methods Enzymol 1986; 133:198–208.

44. Geiger R, Miska W. Bioluminescence enhanced enzyme immunoassay. New ultrasensitive detection systems for enzyme immunoassays, II. J Clin Chem Clin Biochem 1987; 25:31–8.

17 | NEPHELOMETRIC AND TURBIDIMETRIC IMMUNOASSAY

DANIEL J. MARMER
Department of Pathology and
Laboratory Medicine
Diagnostic Immunology Laboratory
University of Cincinnati Hospital
Cincinnati, Ohio

PAUL E. HURTUBISE
Department of Pathology and Laboratory
Medicine
Diagnostic Immunology Laboratory
University of Cincinnati Hospital
Cincinnati, Ohio

1. INTRODUCTION

Classical methods for the detection and quantitation of antigens or antibodies using methods such as immunoprecipitation in gels, complement fixation, and numerous particle agglutination assays use only the observation of the late stages (secondary and tertiary) of the antibody–antigen reaction to provide observable and measurable end-products. This late-stage reaction can take hours to days to develop. In addition, these methods are often dependent upon the participation of other moieties than the antibody or antigen to make the observation that a reaction has taken place. These assays, especially gel immunoprecipitation, require up to several days to acquire a stable end-product. The original radial immunodiffusion procedures developed by Mancini *et al.* (1) for the immunoquantitation of proteins required up to 7 to 10 days to reach equilibrium for a stable measurement. Fahey and McKelvery (2) modified this technique and reduced the endpoint measurement time to within 18 to 24 hr. In the contemporary clinical laboratory, waiting for test results can be costly in the total management of patient care.

Other techniques such as equilibrium dialysis, polarization, fluorescence quenching, and radioimmunoassay allow quantitation or detection of an antigen or antibody by observing the primary stages of the antibody reaction. Some of these methods frequently use potentially hazardous materials or are only available in research labs. They are often labor intensive and time consuming.

For many antigen–antibody systems, especially the measurement of specific serum proteins and numerous haptenic groups, the measurement of the primary binding of an antibody to its specific antigen, which occurs rapidly (seconds to minutes) in solution, can be observed and measured by an increase in light scatter at various angles to the incident light. The presence of small immune complexes formed in antibody excess cause the light scatter to occur, and as long as the complexes remain small in relation to the wavelength of the incident light ($<\lambda/10$), the intensity of the light scattered is proportional to the molecular weight and concentration of the complexes formed. These types of measurements are valid when the reactants are in dilute solution. With the current availability of nephelometric and turbidimetric instruments, the specific measurement of serum proteins and other serum analytes can be generated rapidly and with significant cost effectiveness.

2. HISTORICAL PERSPECTIVE

Since the first observation of the precipitation reaction was described in the late 1800s by Kraus (3), the scientific community has been stimulated to develop new techniques and instruments to measure antigen–antibody reactions (see Table 17.1).

TABLE 17.1 Historical Landmarks Leading to Today's Clinical Immunonephelometers and Immunoturbidimeters

Year	Investigator(s)	Historical Contribution
1897	R. Kraus	Precipitin reaction (3)
1929	H. Heidelberger F. Kendall	Quantitative serology (4)
1934	J.R. Marrack	Lattice theory of antigen–antibody complex formation (6)
1938	R.L. Libby	"Photronreflectometer" (8)
1947	A. Boyden	Monitored immunoprecipitation reaction by photoelectric method (11)
1947	B.F. Chow	First quantitated human serum protein; albumin (12)
1964	K. Hellsing	Nonionic polymers in enhanced immunoprecipitin reaction (22)
1967–69	R.F. Ritchie	Described measuring proteins with standard lab spectrophotometers (14) and first automated nephelometer for clinical use (16)
1970	I. Eckman et al.	First reported automated continuous flow analyzer (17)
1970	J. Savory et al.	Kinetic antigen–antibody reactions (19)
1974	G. Buffone et al.	First to use a laser optical system in nephelometry (29)
1975	M. Blom H. Hjorne	First reported use of an automated centrifugal analyzer (18)

The original work of Heidelberger and Kendall was the first to use a quantitative immunoprecipitin reaction for the estimation of small quantities of specific polysaccharides (4), and subsequently Goettsch and Kendall (5) applied the procedure to estimate albumin and globulin in serum. In 1934, Marrack published the lattice theory of the precipitation and agglutination of antigens by antibodies based on the assumption that antibodies are multivalent (6). In subsequent studies these techniques were modified to quantitate proteins in semisolid medium or agar gel by tube diffusion, crossed immunoelectrophoresis (CIE) or two-dimensional immunoelectrophoresis, radial immunodiffusion (RID) (1, 2), and electroimmunodiffusion (EID).

As investigators became experienced with the immunoprecipitin procedures for RID and EID, it was soon apparent that these techniques raised important technical problems that were influenced by diffusion and electrophoretic characteristics of molecular configuration or genetic variants of the proteins studied (7). The immunoprecipitin reactions can be labor intensive, subject to errors associated with the measurement of diffusion diameters or length of the "rocket-technique," and limited to relatively tight ranges of quantitation. Consequently, with these limitations in mind, improved reagent systems and new instrumentation using the principle of molecular light scatter were developed to circumvent many of the obvious problems.

In 1938 two instruments were developed independently, the "photronreflectometer" by Libby (8) and the "photoelectric apparatus" by Pope and Healey (9). These instruments broke ground for a relatively simple, rapid, and accurate quantitative method for measuring turbidity or opalescence produced by the precipitation of antigen–antibody reactions (10). Other reports quickly surfaced in the literature describing the use of the photoelectric method to measure immunoprecipitation. The concept of using turbidimetric measurements to monitor immunoprecipitation reactions was introduced in 1947 by Boyden et al. (11). During the same year, Chow (12) was the first to quantitate a human serum protein (albumin) by nephelometry or light-scattering measurements of antibody–antigen reaction, using rabbit antiserum; in 1951, Gitlin and Edelhoch quantitated albumin using equine antiserum (13). In 1967 the work of Ritchie (14, 15) described a sensitive, simple, manual technique and direct method for measuring antigen–antibody reactions of individual serum proteins in dilute fluids with a standard spectrophotometer available in most laboratories at that time.

It was not until 1969 that automated nephelometers became available for use in the clinical laboratory (16). The earliest reported automated immunoturbidimetric method by a continuous flow and a centrifugal analyzer was in 1970 and 1975, respectively (17, 18). During the 1970s, the work of Savory et al. paved the way for distinct nephelometric systems by examining the kinetics of the antigen–antibody reaction (19). At this time, the automated systems encouraged the development of important refinements to improve the overall accuracy, sensitivity, and precision of these instruments and their reagents. Improvements involved the standardization and development of high avidity antibodies (20), use of polymer (21, 22), microparticle (23, 24) and hapten conjugate (25) enhancements, automated sample handling (26), timed incubation period (27), and new optical systems (28, 29). As illustrated in Fig. 17.1, application of immunonephelometry and immunoturbidimetry has grown rapidly over the past 15 years in the clinical laboratory and has replaced RID as the method of choice for the specific quantitation of individual serum proteins (30, 31).

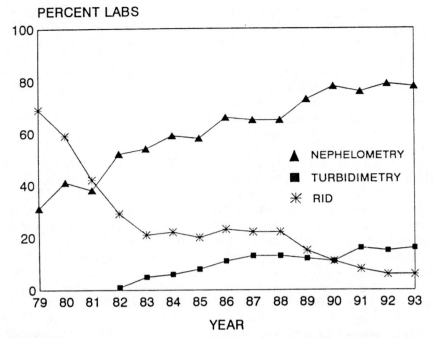

FIGURE 17.1 Laboratory utilization of radial immunodiffusion (RID), nephelometry, and turbidimetry over a 15-year period for quantitation of IgG, IgA, and IgM, based on average CAP proficiency survey participants.

3. CHARACTERISTICS OF THE IMMUNOPRECIPITIN REACTION

When soluble protein antigen combines with antibody in a solution, a visible product may appear. This reaction product is known as "precipitate" and consists of insoluble antibody–antigen complexes that are formed by the process referred to as immunoprecipitation. The amount of precipitate is dependent on the ratio of antibody to antigen concentration. At the molecular level, simple antibody–antigen complexes involve the mixture of individual binding sites on antibody with single ligand sites, or epitopes, on an antigen. Ranging from substantial antibody excess to slight antigen excess, the reaction can be regarded as a series of sequential reactions represented by

$$\text{Ag} + \text{Ab} \underset{k_1'}{\overset{k_1}{\rightleftarrows}} \text{AgAb} \underset{k_2'}{\overset{k_2}{\rightleftarrows}} (\text{AgAb})_x \text{ intermediate complexes} \overset{k_3}{\rightarrow} \text{precipitin}, \qquad (1)$$

where Ag is antigen, Ab is antibody, AgAb is the primarily formed antigen–antibody complex, $(\text{AgAb})_x$ is the soluble AgAb lattice of variable composition, k is forward reaction rate, and k' is reverse reaction rate constant ($k_1 > k_1'$ and $k_1 \gg k_2$ or k_3). In the antigen excess zone the reaction may be reflected as:

$$2\text{Ag} + \text{Ab} \underset{k'}{\overset{k}{\rightleftarrows}} \text{Ag}_2\text{Ab}. \qquad (2)$$

The association is noncovalent and follows the law of mass action as demonstrated in the equations above. The antigen–antibody reaction is a reversible reaction that can be rearranged in conventional form to yield an expression for the association constant, k_a, in terms of the reactant and product concentrations.

$$\frac{[AgAb]}{[Ag][Ab]} = \frac{k}{k'} = k_a \text{ (association constant)} \tag{3}$$

$$\frac{[Ag][Ab]}{[AgAb]} = \frac{k'}{k} = k_d \text{ (dissociation constant)} \tag{4}$$

Large k_a values are consequently ideal for good immunoassays. The interpretation of k_a is that the equilibrium reaction falls far to the right, resulting in minimal dissociation of the antigen–antibody complex once it has formed. If antibodies are able to bind to antigen in both a concentrated and dilute solution, then the antibodies have a strong affinity for the antigen. A small dissociation constant (k_d) is interpreted to mean that the antibody is bound firmly to the specific antigen. That is, the fit between the antigen and the antibody is optimal and the binding forces have been maximized; therefore, the dissociation constant, k', is minimized.

For a given antibody–antigen reaction to proceed to form a precipitate, several chemical and physical conditions must exist (32). Other factors that influence the degree of precipitation formation include antibody avidity, ionic strength, pH, temperature, reaction time, the presence of molecules with hydrophilic or hydrophobic properties, the nature and concentration of anions, and viscosity of the medium (33–35). First, both antigen and antibody molecules must have multiple binding sites specific for one another. Second, the relative concentration of antibody–antigen in the mixture must be optimal for that system, usually corresponding to approximately equal amounts of antibody and antigen.

Heidelberger and Kendall (4) performed the classic quantitative precipitation reactions, as illustrated in Fig. 17.2, confirming the lattice theory of immunoprecipi-

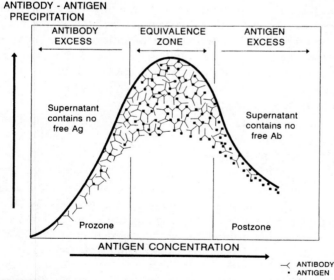

FIGURE 17.2 Heidelberger–Kendall immunoprecipitin curve: amount of antibody precipitated as a function of antigen concentration at fixed antibody concentration with a schematic representation of antibody–antigen complexes present in antibody excess, equivalence, and antigen excess.

tation (6). The lattice theory states that a precipitate is formed as a result of random, reversible reactions, where each antibody binds to more than one antigen and each antigen can bind to more than one antibody, eventually forming a lattice of antibody and antigen that exceeds the critical volume for solubility.

Immunoprecipitation requires the presence of either bivalent or multivalent antibodies, and an antigen with at least two antigenic determinants per molecule. The reaction between antigen and antibody is described in terms of three zones of precipitation reactivity: antibody excess, equivalence, and antigen excess (see Fig. 17.2). Most precipitins of the IgG class are bivalent whereas the precipitating antigens are multivalent. The antigen–antibody reaction occurs in a series of consecutive steps that ultimately lead to large aggregates of immune complexes that can no longer be supported in solution and precipitate. The consecutive steps are summarized as follows: (a) primary interaction of the antibody with the antigen forming simple immune complexes: (b) a secondary interlinking or lattice formation through the reaction of the components of simple complexes with themselves to form larger complexes; and (c) the tertiary formation of large aggregates to produce a visible precipitate through hydrophobic and charge-based interactions (32).

Relating these steps to the immunoprecipitation curve in Fig. 17.2, in the zone of antibody excess (prozone), all available antigen is bound to antibody and only simple complexes form as $Ag(Ab)_m$, where m is the valence of the antigen. Precipitation is minimal at the antibody excess zone because lattice formation of these simple complexes are impeded since there are no available reactant sites on the multivalent antigen. The concentration of antibody is such that individual antigen sites are covered so extensively that no cross-linkage of antigens take place. In this case, the antigen–antibody reaction results in soluble complexes. In the zone of equivalence, the lattice formation occurs from the initially formed simple complexes. At this point the antigen and antibody concentrations have reached optimal proportions and maximum precipitation occurs. If a divalent antibody is used, virtually every antibody is attached to two different antigen molecules. All of the antigen and antibody in the reaction precipitates. In the zone of antigen excess (postzone), the concentration of antigen far exceeds the binding capacity of the concentration of antibody. Soluble complex formation occurs as Ag_2Ab, with excess antigen, but subsequent precipitation is hindered because of a lack of free antibody present to form the lattice necessary for precipitation.

4. PRINCIPLES OF LIGHT SCATTERING

Light scattering is a physical phenomenon caused by the interaction of light with a particle in solution. Nephelometry and turbidimetry are methods used to measure light scatter. When light, a form of electromagnetic radiation, strikes a particle in solution, it causes the electrons around the particle to oscillate in synchronism with the energy of the incident light. Thus, the incident light creates an oscillating dipole in the particle. The strength of this dipole moment is proportional to the energy of the incident light. This oscillating dipole is a source of energy-scattering light in all directions at the same wavelength as the incident light. To understand this light scattering there are several factors to consider. These include particle size, wavelength dependence, the distance of the observation of the light scattering, and the concentration and molecular weight of the particles.

4.1. Particle Size

An important element in the observation of light scattering is the size of the particle interacting with the incident light. When the particle is smaller than the wavelength of the incident light ($<\lambda/10$), the entire particle is subjected to the same energy field strength at the same time. The resultant scattered-light wavelengths are all in phase and reinforce each other. When the particle is larger than the wavelength of the incident light, the wavelengths of the scattered light are no longer all in phase, and reinforcement occurs in some directions and destructive interference in others. The scattering patterns of large particles are a function of the size and shape of the particle.

4.2. Wavelength Dependence of Light Scattering

The wavelength of the incident light and its relationship to the measurement of scattered light is expressed in the following equation, derived by Rayleigh in 1871,

$$\frac{i_s}{I_o} = \frac{16\,\pi^2 a \sin^2 \theta}{\lambda^4 r^2}, \tag{5}$$

where i_s is the intensity of the scattered light, I_o is the intensity of the excitation light, a is the polarizability of the small particle, λ is the wavelength of the incident light, θ is the angle of observation, and r is the distance from the light scattering to the detector. It is evident from this equation that the intensity of the light scattered will increase to the fourth power as the wavelength is decreased, and the measurement of light scatter is influenced by the square of the distance from the light-scattering particle to the detector of the light scattered. These issues are very important in the design of instruments to measure light scatter.

4.3. Other Factors

There is a direct relationship to the concentration and molecular weight of particles and the amount and directional intensity of light scatter. Figure 17.3 shows that light scatter intensity and direction are dependent upon the size of the particle. Figure 17.3A characterizes Rayleigh light-scattering principles when the scattering particle is small (e.g., IgG and albumin) and significantly less than the wavelength of the incident light ($<\lambda/10$). The light is scattered both forward and backward, as well as 90° from the incident light. As the particle size increases ($>\lambda/10$), the light scatter pattern changes to a more forward direction and less in the backward and 90° directions (Fig. 17.3B). This characterization is identified as Rayleigh–Debye scattering, and is observed with large proteins such as IgM, forming immune complexes, and chylomicrons. Very large particles such as blood cells and bacteria display an even more complex pattern of angular dependence with the predominance of scattered light in a more forward direction. This type of pattern in called Mie scattering.

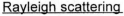
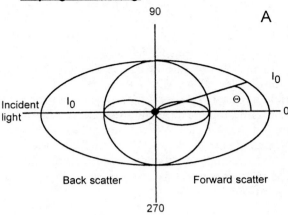

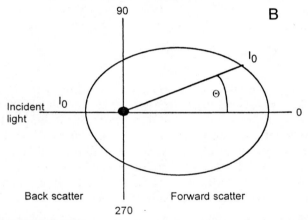

FIGURE 17.3 The influence of particle size on light scatter. (A) Small particles, (B) large particles.

The Rayleigh and Rayleigh–Debye characterizations of light scattering by small and intermediate-size particles are useful and important in developing instrumentation to measure light scatter.

5. DEFINITION AND PRINCIPLES OF NEPHELOMETRY AND TURBIDIMETRY

5.1. Basic Definition

Light is scattered in all directions when it passes through a transparent medium containing particles from a secondary phase manifestation of an antibody–antigen immunoprecipitation reaction. Nephelometry and turbidimetry are general terms used to refer to the measurement of scattered light.

5.2. Nephelometry

More specifically, nephelometry, from the Greek nephele', νεφελη, meaning cloud or mist, refers to the detection of light scattered after exciting a solution at some angle other than that of the incident beam (see Fig. 17.4A). The ideal measurement of light scatter is performed in a dilute sample suspension to minimize reflection and absorption of light. Since scattered light is characteristically of very low intensity in relation to incident light, high-intensity light sources and photodetectors are required. Since particles of the size of immunocomplexes appear to scatter light more in the forward direction, there is an increased signal-to-noise ratio as the photodetector is positioned nearer the transmitted path at 0°. Most light scatter of antibody–antigen complexes in serum is essentially Rayleigh–Debye ($d > \lambda$) and ranges in size from 250 to 1500 nm, which is near to or larger than the wavelengths used in most nephelometers. The blank signal, described best by Rayleigh scatter ($d < \lambda/10$), is not as affected by an altered angle of detection.

Although most early nephelometers detected light scattered at 90° to the incident light beam, newer nephelometers take advantage of enhanced light scattering at

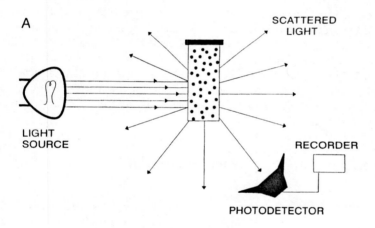

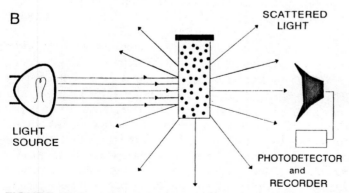

FIGURE 17.4   Basic nephelometric (A) and turbidimetric (B) optical system.

lower detection angles of 31° or less to optimize, and in many cases, to give the highest signal-to-noise ratio for the instrument's optics. Obviously, detection at 0° is not possible because of the high intensity of the transmitted beam, but some laser-equipped fast analyzers using a mask to block the transmitted beam are able to operate at quite low angles. Therefore, nephelometers that measure scattered light in a more forward direction have the advantage of providing greater sensitivity and will be less affected by interferences from endogenous proteins, chylomicrons, lipid molecules, and aggregated immunoglobulins, particularly after freezing and thawing serum (28). Nephelometry may be used to measure either antigen or antibody in suspension. Routine use in the clinical laboratory most often uses antibody reagents to detect antigen in patient specimens.

5.3. Turbidimetry

Turbidimetry measures the cloudiness or turbidity of a solution. As demonstrated in Fig. 17.4B, the photodetector is placed such that it is in direct line with the incident light and the solution, usually referred to as either a 0° or 180° angle. The light source should emit a wavelength in the near ultraviolet range (290–410 nm). The photodetector must be aligned with the incidence source and collect the beam after passage through the solution, therefore measuring a decrease in signal or the reduction in light intensity that occurs as a result of the combination of reflection, absorption, or scatter of incident light. Turbidimetric analysis is influenced by both Rayleigh and Mie light scattering. The current application in the clinical field of immunoturbidimetry is limited because the technique measures a decrease in a large signal of transmitted light and is limited primarily by the photometric accuracy and sensitivity of the instrument.

5.4. Monitoring Antigen–Antibody Reactions by Light Scatter Detection

5.4.1. Theory and Principle

Nephelometric or turbidimetric immunoassay systems must operate in the antibody excess zone where the concentration of antibody is held constant and the amount of antigen–antibody complex formed depends directly on the concentration of antigen in the mixture. This permits the formation of complexes of a constant size, providing a reproducible, stoichiometric relationship between the number of complexes formed at a given antigen concentration (32).

Polymers or hydrophilic agents are added to accelerate the immunoprecipitation in both nephelometry and turbidimetry (22, 36). The most desirable characteristics of the polymer are high molecular weight, a high degree of linearity, and high aqueous solubility. The effect of polymers on immunoprecipitation enhancement is most likely due to steric exclusion of water, which has the effect of: (a) decreasing the solubility of protein molecules, (b) driving the antigen–antibody interaction toward immunoprecipitin formation, (c) increasing the slope of the antibody excess area of the immunoprecipitation curve, and (d) displacing equivalence toward higher antigen concentration (34). The most effective agent to expedite complex formation, that markedly shortens reaction time and increases peak rate as much as tenfold (22), is polyethylene glycol (PEG) with a molecular weight of 8000 Da.

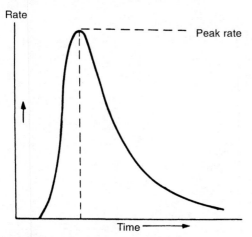

FIGURE 17.5   Rate of change of light scatter signal verses time. Reprinted with permission from the Beckman Array 360 system operating manual, Beckman Instruments, Inc. (43).

5.4.2. Kinetic and Endpoint Methodology

There are two methods commonly used for the quantitation of the immunoprecipitin reaction by light scatter: (i) kinetic and (ii) endpoint (quasi-equilibrium) nephelometry or turbidimetry. Several articles are available for in-depth review of these methodologies (27, 34, 37–42). Kinetic or rate assays measure the peak rate of immunocomplex formation (see Fig. 17.5), whereas endpoint methods, also known as steady state, measure light scatter immediately after addition of the antiserum and then again after a constant time interval (Fig. 17.6). Several instruments are available commercially that perform immunonephelometric and immunoturbidimetric measurements in either a kinetic or endpoint mode or both (Table 17.2). Listed in Table 17.3 are the more commonly requested clinical analytes measured

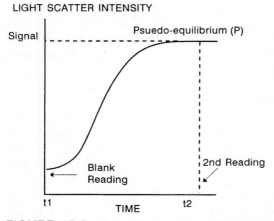

FIGURE 17.6   The endpoint (steady state) measuring the light scattering signal at near equilibrium (P).

**TABLE 17.2   Clinical Instruments
Commonly Used to Quantitate Proteins
by Immunoprecipitation**

Nephelometers	Turbidimeters
Abbott TDx - Turbo	ABA 100
Beckman Nephelometers[a]	Abbott VP
Behring Nephelometers[a]	BNC Cedia
Hyland Nephelometer	Beckman CX 4,5
IL Miltistat III	Behring TurbiTime System[a]
Kallestad QM 300[a]	Boeringher Mannheim/Hatachi[a]
Technicon Nephelometer	Dupont ACA[a]
	Roche Cobas BIO System
	Roche Cobas FARA System[a]
	Roche Cobas MIRA System
	Technicon RA 1000
	Hitachi 911 Analyzer

[a] Instruments listed on CAP Diagnostic Immunology Proficiency survey S1-B summary report with 10 or more participating labs (44).

by immunoassay procedures from biological fluids that include serum, plasma, cerebrospinal fluid (CSF), and urine.

5.4.3. Analyte Standardization

During the last two decades professional organizations and commercial manufacturers have produced large numbers of secondary reference materials used worldwide that are traceable to several different primary standard reference materials distributed by the World Health Organization (WHO) or the National Institutes of Health (NIH). Unfortunately, variations in analyte quantitation have been evident in quality assessment surveys, both in Western Europe and in the United States (45, 46).

Depending on the analyte and the reference material used, values for a particular protein may vary as much as 50–100% (47). The reasons for the variability of analyte quantitation are complex but many can be attributed to (i) the poor understanding of the proper use of the primary reference materials, including nature of the dilution matrix, (ii) value drifting of secondary materials from their primary counterparts, (iii) insufficient quantity of primary materials on a worldwide basis, and (iv) dated primary reference preparations that are not suited for measurement on state-of-the-art optical systems (48). This situation has resurrected the interest of a worldwide effort for restandardization of protein quantitation to permit more consistent clinical results between instrumentations and laboratories (48–50). To accomplish a global restandardization, sufficient quantities of a widely available reference preparation for plasma proteins that could be used worldwide by manufacturers, professional organizations, and laboratories would be required.

In 1989, the International Federation of Clinical Chemistry (IFCC) Committee for Plasma Protein Standardization initiated the process of preparing, characterizing, and calibrating a new international reference preparation for proteins in human serum (RPPHS) for 14 protein analytes (see Table 17.3, analytes marked with [a]). The Committee also intends to assign values for additional proteins to the RPPHS

TABLE 17.3   Analytes Available Clinically for Immunonephelometry and Immunoturbidimetry Quantitation

Serum proteins	Urine proteins
Albumin	Albumin
Alpha$_1$ acid glycoprotein[a]	Alpha$_1$ microglobulin
Alpha$_1$ antichymotrysin[b]	Immunoglobulin G
Alpha$_1$ antitrypsin[a]	Transferrin
Alpha$_2$ macroglobulin[a]	CSF Proteins
Antistreptolysin O	Albumin
Apolipoprotein A$_1$	Alpha$_2$ macroglobulin
Apoliprotein B	Immunoglobulin A
Beta$_2$ macroglobulin	Immunoglobulin G
Ceruloplasmin[a]	Immunoglobulin M
Circulating immune complexes	Total protein in CSF
Complement C3[a]	Therapeutic drugs[d]
Complement C4[a]	Amikacin
C-reactive protein[a]	Carbamazepine
Haptoglobin[a]	Digoxin
Hemopexin[b]	Gentamicin
Immunoglobulin A[a]	Lidocaine
Immunoglobulin G[a]	Phenobarbital
Immunoglobulin G1, 2, 3, 4	Phenytoin
Immunoglobulin M[a]	Primidone
Immunoglobulin E	Procainamide
Light chain - kappa	N-Acetyl-procainamide
Light chain - lambda	Quinidine
Microalbumin	Theophylline
Myoglobin[c]	Tobramycin
Prealbumin (transthyretin)[a]	Valproic acid
Properidin factor B	Vancomycin
Retinol binding protein	Other analytes
Rheumatoid factor	B12
Total protein	Cortisol[c]
Transferrin[a]	Ferritin[c]
Plasma proteins	Folate[c]
Antithrombin III	
Fibrinogen	
Fibronectin	
Plasminogen	
Prothrombin	

   [a] Proteins standardized to the IFCC international preparation for plasma proteins, lot CRM470, certified by BCR and designated Reference Preparation for Proteins in Human Serum (RPPHS), lot 91/0619, by CAP.

   [b] Available except in U.S.A.

   [c] In development.

   [d] Performed by rate-neph. inhibition immunoassay.

as resources become available. The material was accredited as a Certified Reference Material (CRM 470) in 1993 by the Bureau Communitaire de Reference of the European Economic Community (47) and was jointly released by the College of American Pathologists in 1994 to manufacturers of immunochemical analytes.

The IFCC Committee does not intend the RPPHS material to be directly used in laboratory assays but rather as a serum-based reference for transfer of values to tertiary preparations, such as calibration standards and controls. Each diagnostic manufacturer must validate their analytes against the RPPHS reference material. Reassignment of reference ranges is necessary, either through analysis of new reference groups or by the use of conversion factors supplied by manufacturers of commercial protein calibrants. The expected benefit is decreased interlaboratory variation in serum protein assays, resulting in improvement in patient testing and clinical research.

5.5. Kinetic Immunonephelometry and Immunoturbidimetry

The basic principles of kinetic immunonephelometry and immunoturbidimetry are similar. In this section only a general kinetic immunonephelometric assay will be discussed in detail. In kinetic nephelometry, a light beam is directed through a disposable flow cell containing buffer, diluted serum, and dispensed antiserum specific to a particular analyte. The intensity of light as it is scattered by complexes in suspension is measured. A specimen blank is not required since background scatter constitutes a constant background signal and has no effect on the rate measurement. As shown in Fig. 17.5, the rate of light scatter increases until the peak rate of change is reached.

The initial signal response prior to a valid reaction in a nephelometric assay is illustrated in Fig. 17.7. Small but detectable Rayleigh scatter is initially present and then increases slightly as the specimen and subsequent antisera are added to the reaction mixture. A progression of the primary and secondary immunochemical reactions will intensify the light scatter, creating a sigmoidal response. The scatter will eventually reach a maximum (plateau) and then begin to decrease as larger immunocomplexes begin to settle out. As illustrated in Fig. 17.8, at a fixed concentration of antibody, the slope of this curve can be changed by increasing the antigen concentration in the reaction mixture. The slope becomes steeper when the antigen concentration is increased, indicating more immunocomplexes formed per unit of time. The rate signal will become larger until an approximately linear region is achieved, beyond which the rate will progressively decrease as the antigen concen-

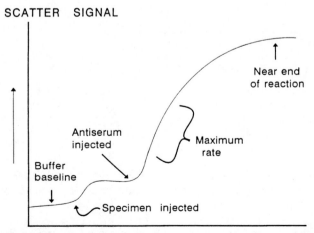

FIGURE 17.7 Scatter signal developed verses time. Reprinted with permission from the Beckman Array 360 system operating manual, Beckman Instruments, Inc. (43).

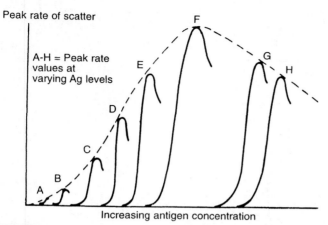

FIGURE 17.8 Kinetic precipitin curves representing various degrees of peak rate of scatter produced by mixing increasing antigen concentrations to a constant antibody concentration. Reprinted with permission from the Beckman Array 360 system operating manual, Beckman Instruments, Inc. (43).

tration moves into the antigen excess zone. The slope becomes more shallow when the antigen concentration is decreased. The maximum rate occurs at the kinetic equivalence point (F), and the regions at lower (A) and higher (H) antigen concentration are described as antibody and antigen excess, respectively.

A valid nephelometric rate measurement must be performed at optimal antigen and antibody proportions with a reaction containing excess antibody. Each lot of antibody released from production by the supplying vendor is adjusted to a concentration compatible with the optimized sample dilution so the initial measuring range of each analyte will cover the majority of expected values. To ensure accuracy of measurement, a diluted test specimen is examined to determine whether the rate scatter signal falls within predefined high and low limits (Fig. 17.9) for each analyte and, if required, it is analyzed again with the next appropriate dilution. Figure 17.9 is a dose–response curve for samples B through F, which contain increasing antigen concentration and produce respective increasing rate scatter signals. When the scatter signals are located on the linear and ascending area of the dose–response curve, only then will the measurement be considered legitimate.

Depending on the peak rate scatter for a specimen, the nephelometer program will perform one of two functions. It will either retest the next specimen dilution or perform an antigen excess inspection. Sample D in Fig. 17.9, containing an intermediate concentration of antigen, demonstrates a valid dose–response peak. Samples containing extremely low (B) or high (F) concentration of antigen generate curves whose peak rates are recognized as being out of the predefined range. In these particular cases, the nephelometer will repeat the analysis at a less or more dilute sample. Samples E and H produce similar scatter signals. The difference is that the scatter signal of sample H is on the descending portion of the dose–response curve, where antigen is in excess and there is insufficient antibody available. Both specimens E and H produce a signal that spontaneously triggers a check to verify the presence or absence of excess antigen. Consequently, rate nephelometers are programmed with a standard antigen excess procedure check to differentiate between a reaction that is in antibody excess and one that is in antigen excess.

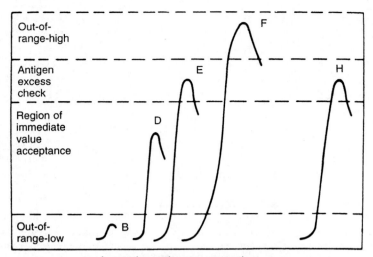

FIGURE 17.9 Kinetic precipitin curves representing peak rate of scatter values of acceptance, out of range, and antigen excess. Reprinted with permission from the Beckman Array 360 system operating manual, Beckman Instruments, Inc. (43).

This checking procedure is performed by dispensing a calibrator containing surplus antigen immediately into the reaction well after the routine analysis is performed. One of two events will occur as the diluted calibrator is injected into the reaction cell as demonstrated in Fig. 17.10. Additional scatter is generated by the formation of antibody complexes if specimen is in antibody excess, as in example E (see Figs. 17.9 and 17.10). The initial peak rate scatter is verified as a valid curve and the result held in memory of the nephelometer. On the other hand, if the

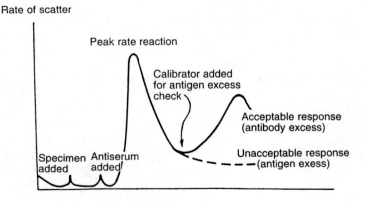

FIGURE 17.10 Sequence of events for monitoring antigen excess. Antigen and antibody reagent are injected into reaction cuvette and a peak rate of light scattering is generated. Additional antigen is added to cuvette and observed for an antibody excess response or an antigen excess response.

specimen contains excess antigen, as in sample H, the addition of calibrator produces no response and therefore no additional light scatter is measured. At this point, the nephelometer automatically takes the next higher specimen dilution and analyzes the peak rate of scattered light. If necessary, performance of the antigen excess check may be repeated to verify a valid rate of scatter.

5.6. Endpoint Immunonephelometry and Immunoturbidimetry

In the endpoint assay, light-scattering measurements are performed when the antigen–antibody reaction has gone to pseudo-equilibrium (near completion) or reached a steady state. For the purpose of this discussion such conditions will be referred to as pseudo-equilibrium because true equilibrium is not reached within a reasonable time for ideal test assays. As shown in Fig. 17.6, the reaction requires an incubation interval (t_2) before a measurement is made. The incubation period may be as long as 2 hr after the initiation of the reaction. A single measurement of the light scatter signal is taken at a time interval when the rate of change is minimal (P). A specimen blank reading is necessary, especially for immunoturbidity, to correct for high background light-scattering signals caused by endogenous proteins and other factors in the specimen. This problem may be minimized by using a high sample dilution by pretreating the sample to remove interfering substances. The measured values are compared with a reference curve and converted to concentration units.

A modification of the endpoint assay is the fixed-time method for measurement of analytes as shown in Fig. 17.11. This method accelerates the analysis time and makes it more appealing in the clinical laboratory. Fixed time makes two sequential scattered measurements, one taken a very short time after initiation of the reaction (t_0) and the second measurement at another time interval (t_2). The difference in scattered light intensity between both readings is converted to concentration units by comparing the value to a reference curve previously stored in the instrument's computer memory. Calibration is performed by either a single-point or a multipoint calibration method.

LIGHT SCATTER INTENSITY

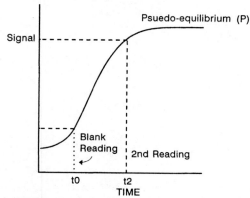

FIGURE 17.11   Fixed time method measuring the light scattering signal at two specific time intervals (t_0, t_2).

5.7. Nephelometric Inhibition Immunoassay

A competitive binding method known as the nephelometric inhibition assay was developed for the indirect measurement of small molecules such as haptens. Haptens typically have a small molecular weight and do not induce an immunologic response alone, but can react with antibodies that are specific to themselves. In 1942, Pauling described the inhibition effect of haptens on the precipitation of antisera (51). Cambiasco *et al.* reported the development of a nephelometric inhibition immunoassay that permitted the indirect measurement of hapten molecules (52). In this type of immunoassay, polyvalent haptens are coupled to a high-molecular-weight carrier protein or a latex particle, historically referred to as the "developer antigen" (34). As demonstrated in Fig. 17.12, the developer antigen competes with free hapten, the analyte being measured, for combining sites on a fixed amount of antibody. The development of maximal light scattering will occur at equivalence, where appropriate ratios of antibody and developer antigen results in cross-linking and antibody–antigen complex formation.

The light-scatter and rate signals during the reaction are similar to a rate nephelometric assay. The haptens on this developer antigen then compete with added free haptens for the hapten-specific recognition sites on the antibody surface. A known antibody concentration is used, and any excess of free hapten inhibits formation of the antibody–developer antigen precipitate. The nephelometric light-scatter signal is inversely related to the concentration of free hapten. Therefore, the higher the concentration of free hapten, the smaller the amount of antibody–developer antigen precipitate. The assay is more sensitive than conventional nephelometric immunoassays and is commonly used to quantitate therapeutic drugs (Table 17.3).

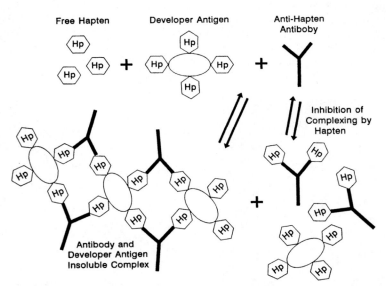

FIGURE 17.12   Nephelometric inhibition immunoassay. Free hapten and anti-hapten antibody compete to bind with developer antigen. The anti-hapten antibody binding to the developer antigen forms insoluble immunoprecipitin complexes. The free hapten inhibits the formation of anti-hapten antibody–developer antigen complex.

5.8. Immunoassay Sensitivity

The sensitivity of nephelometric techniques has been much improved through the years, especially when automation essentially replaced the manual methods. This is due, in part, to the detection of antigen excess, to the incorporation of polymers to increase immunoprecipitation formation, and to discrimination between background scatter and scatter intrinsic to the antigen–antibody complex (by measuring light scatter at a forward direction rather than a 90° angle, and by electronically subtracting background signals, as in kinetic immunonephelometry, or taking a blank reading, as with endpoint immunonephelometry). Endpoint nephelometry can measure protein analytes with concentrations as small as 1–10 ng/liter and requires a minimum of 20 min to 4 hr incubation time, whereas the kinetic nephelometry assays may detect analytes of proteins at concentrations less than 1 ng/liter with an assay time of approximately 1 min.

The choice between immunonephelometry and immunoturbidimetry depends on the particular application and requirements of analysis by the available instrumentation. Until recently, the assertion was often made that nephelometry was the method of choice because fluids with 95% or more transmittance of light in a forward direction characteristically have small changes in absorption due to turbidity and were difficult to measure with good accuracy and precision. However, with the advent of stable, high-resolution, microprocessor-driven photometric systems, turbidimetric measurements have become competitive in sensitivity with nephelometric methods for immunological quantitation of serum proteins. Nephelometry, however, still offers some advantage in sensitivity of serum protein detection at the lower limits of 1–10 ng/ml. Improved sensitivities are obtained in fluids such as CSF and urine because of their lower lipid and protein concentrations that result in a better signal-to-noise ratio.

6. INSTRUMENTATION

6.1. General Considerations

The principle considerations of light-scatter instrumentation are: (a) wavelength, (b) excitation intensity, (c) sample cuvette distance from the detection source, (d) sample slits, and (e) maximum reduction of external stray light. Instrument components generally consist of a (a) light source, (b) collimating optics, (c) sample cell, and (d) collection of optic parts, which includes the light-scattering optics, detector optical filter, and a detector. Some of the commonly used light sources in light-scattering analyzers having wavelengths of 320 to 650 nm are: tungsten–halogen lamps at a wavelength from 400 to 620 nm, mercury arc (357 nm), helium–neon lasers (632 nm), and, more recently, infrared high-performance, light-emitting diode (LED) at 840 nm. Depending on the particular instrument, the collection optics components that measure the light scatter are located at different angles from the incident light beam.

The companies that have the largest market for clinical immunonephelometers or immunoturbidimeters are listed in Table 17.2. Beckman Instruments, Behring Diagnostics, and Sanofi Diagnostic Pasteur have instrumentation solely dedicated to clinical immunonephelometry and offer the largest menu of protein and drug analyte immunoassay tests (see Table 17.3) for clinical use, whereas the remaining companies have limited immunoassay kits available for the nephelometric or turbidimetric analysis. These companies and others represent the successful efforts to automate quantitative measurements of both proteins and drug levels. The easily operated systems are dedicated and provide the user with increased throughput, accuracy, linearity, and precision (53). Representative key instrumentation attributes are listed in Table 17.4.

6.2. Beckman Array 360 CE Nephelometer

The Beckman Array 360 CE is a fully automated, microprocessor-controlled, kinetic nephelometer that quantitates proteins from most body fluids and serum therapeutic drug levels. The instrument houses a tungsten–halogen source lamp and uses bandpass filters and focusing lenses to direct light to a temperature (26.7°C)-controlled flow cell. The immunoprecipitation reaction takes place in one of two sets of optics with light scatter detected at a forward angle of 70° in the 400–650 nm bandwidth range by a silicon photocell. The broad bandwidth is crucial since light-scatter signals from a heterogeneous mixture of various immunoprecipitin sizes are averaged. Depending on the sample concentration and test sequence the nephelometer has a maximum throughput of 40–80 tests per hour.

Antigen excess testing mode using a dilution of the appropriate calibration is optional. When this check mode is activated, results that are out-of-range are

TABLE 17.4 Representative Instrumentation Used for Immunonephelometric and Immunoturbidimetric Assays

Vendor:	Beckman Instruments	Behring Diagnostics	Boehringer Mannheim (BM)	Roche
Model:	Array 360 CE	BNA 100	BM–Hitachi Analyzer Systems (704, 705, 717, 736, 911)	Cobas Centrifugal Analyzer Systems
Principle:	Kinetic nephelometry	Endpoint nephelometry	Kinetic, endpoint (EP), or EP with blanking turbidimetry	Endpoint or kinetic turbidimetry and nephelometry
Light source:	Tungsten–halogen lamp	Helium–neon laser	Tungsten–halogen lamp	Pulsed xenon flashtube
Wavelength (nm)	400–650	632.8	340–800 (12 options)	285–750
Light angle:	70°	13–24°	Incident light	Incident light or 90°
Test/hr:	80	225	180–600	240–400
Temp. control (°C)	26.7	Ambient	variable	variable
Antigen excess check:	Yes	No (analytical range extended)	No	No
Sensitivity limits:	ng/liter	ng/liter	μ-mg/liter	μ-mg/liter
Sample volume:	7–100 μl	5–150 μl	1–20 μl	5–95 μl
Reagent volume:	42 μl	40–80 μl	50–500 μl	1–370 μl
Blanking mode:	No	Yes	Yes	Yes
Calibration:	Single point (stable 14 days)	Single or multiple point (stable 7 days)	One or two point rate	Single or multiple point

automatically retested at the next suitable sample dilution, unless the particular dilution is obstructed by programmatic constraints. The instrument may be programmed for nonstandard dilutions for any analyte and calibration is based on a single-point method with a stability for 2 weeks. Microprocessor cards are supplied with each reagent kit containing important calibration data and reagent lot characteristics necessary to standardize the particular assay run. Assay sensitivity is as low as 1 ng/liter. There are level detectors for the test sample and antisera cups but not for the buffer and diluent containers.

6.3. Behring Nephelometer

The Behring nephelometer utilizes a 6-min fixed time (accelerated equilibrium) measurement of light scatter produced by antigen–antibody immunoprecipitation. The availability of high-titered, high-affinity, and high-avidity antisera permits extremely high concentrations of serum proteins to be quantitated. During the 6-min reaction time two sequential light-scatter measurements are taken. The first measurement is taken at 10 sec after initiation of the reaction. This is a sample turbidity check and a check for rapid-reacting sample. The second reading is made 6 min into the reaction. After the reaction occurs in the cuvette located on a rotating wheel, it indexes every 8 sec to allow for light-scatter detection at a forward angle of 13–24°. The high throughput of 225 tests per hour is assisted with a unique feature that eliminates antigen excess testing by using extended measuring ranges and a warning system that identifies possible antigen excess.

Antisera, mode of measurement, and optimized reagents have the effect of shifting the classic Heidelberger curve to the right, toward the area of higher concentration. As a result of this shifting effect, a measurement that would be taken on the descending portion of the Heidelberger curve is now measured on the ascending portion of the optimized curve. A "theoretical maximum concentration" in sera was determined, that is, the point at which protein is no longer soluble in serum. That point is still on the ascending portion of the optimized curve and within the measuring range of the instrument. If the sample reads beyond the specified limit of an analyte, at that time the instrument will flag the sample result.

Samples of high concentration are automatically remeasured at the next highest dilution and any test sample may be programmed for a nonstandard dilution. Calibration uses either a single-point or a multipoint calibration method, which is stable for 7 days. A status message on the CRT screen and an audible alarm are activated by sensors that detect low levels of samples and all reagents used. The resident computer program offers up to 10 user-defined profiles, stat sample analysis, quality control limits and monitoring, and up to three reference ranges per analyte.

6.4. Turbidimetric Instrumentation

Turbidimetric measurements are easily performed on photometers (continuous flow and centrifugal fast analyzers) or spectrophotometers and require minimal optimization. The most widely employed automated systems for immunoturbidimetric analysis have been adapted to centrifugal analyzers because the parallel nature of the analytical process permits concurrent evaluation of standard and test samples in identical circumstances. Reagents are pipetted into separate chambers, spun into a reaction cell under centrifugal force, and mixed by changes in acceleration within 3–5 sec of contact. The effects of centrifugal force, however, may cause the settling of large immunocomplexed particles formed by concentrated reactants. The sample and control cuvettes are measured simultaneously within 1 sec after reagents are combined. The absorption signal for each mixture is then monitored by a microprocessor system as the cuvette is moved through the light beam. This measurement is often used as a combined blank for sample and reagent.

Many clinical analyzers incubate reactants under no centrifugal force, and a few offer constant mixing as the reaction carousel advances into various positions. In these systems, samples may be assayed undiluted with concentrated antibody. These instruments, however, mix samples and calibrators at different temperatures and must rely on precise timing of equivalent reading. Furthermore, measurements usually cannot be taken within 15 sec of reactant mixing, necessitating separate sample and reagent blanks. Multicuvette systems use flat, highly polished optical windows that reduce internally reflected or stray light. Flowthrough systems, as compared to centrifugal analyzers, have the advantage of using the same cell chamber for all measurements.

The centrifugal fast analyzer provides rapid analysis of specific analytes with an excess of 500 results per hour. Precision is acceptable; however, the application for many of the specific proteins found in low concentration may limit the sensitivity issue. The use of an endpoint methodology and a separate blank run is also required by most applications. The principle concern of turbidimetric measurements is signal-to-noise ratio. Photometric systems with electro-optic noise range not more than ± 0.0002 absorbance units are effective for turbidity measurements. Several commercially available automated instruments in the clinical laboratory are capable of measuring turbidimetric light scatter (Table 17.2).

6.5. Advantages, Disadvantages, and Limitations

Nephelometric immunoprecipitation assays have several distinct advantages for protein quantitation: (a) highly automated, (b) rapid assay time, (c) simple to operate, (d) capabilities of using small sample and reagent volumes (1–10 μl) (e) high sensitivity (less than 1 ng/liter), and (f) superb precision. A limitation of kinetic nephelometry is the restricted measuring ranges and requirement for controls and checks to guard against underestimation caused by antigen excess. Antigen-excess checking may lead to the increased consumption of reagents and higher cost per test. Instruments that rely on endpoint and fixed time methods must be capable of monitoring antigen excess. This was recently addressed by the technique extending the assay ranges by using a two-parameter calibration method while conserving reagent (54).

Another limitation of nephelometry and especially turbidimetry is background scatter from particulate matter or lipoproteins and chylomicrons in a lipemic specimen which interfere with accurate scattered light measurements (28, 41). Results can be affected by other extraneous factors in turbidimetric measurements, such as the presence of dust or dirt particles. Dust and other large interfering particles can be eliminated by centrifugation of the specimen or by filtering all reagents used in the reaction cuvette. A useful technique to reduce background interference is rate measurements in which the immunoprecipitin blank is eliminated.

The major advantage of turbidimetry in the clinical laboratory is that it can be performed with centrifugal analyzers, automated spectrophotometers, and other routine multipurpose instruments. A disadvantage with these types of instrumentation is the limited immunoprecipitation assays commercially available for quantitation of protein analytes. The major disadvantage of turbidimetry is that it requires the presence of a relatively high particle concentration. As a result, optical quality and alignment are extremely important for accurate turbidimetric quantitation to measure relatively small changes in light intensity caused by absorbance. As previously mentioned, although sensitivity has been limited in the past, because of the detection of a small decrease in a large signal, current instruments have improved discrimination and can better quantify small changes in signal, thereby allowing turbidimetric measurements to achieve high sensitivity. Whicher *et al.* (34) report that good spectrophotometers can detect 50–100 ng of target analyte protein per cuvette with little specimen pretreatment.

References

1. Mancini G, Carbonara AO, Hermans JF. Immunochemical quantitation of antigens by single radial immunodiffusion. Int J Immunochem 1965; 2:235–54.
2. Fahey JL, McKelvery EM. Quantitative determination of serum immunoglobulins in antibody-agar plates. J Immunol 1965; 94:84–90.
3. Silverstein AM. In: A History of Immunology. San Diego: Academic Press, 1989:51.
4. Heidelberger M, Kendall FE. A quantitative study of the precipitin reaction between type III pneumococcus polysaccharide and purified homologous antibody. J Exp Med 1929; 50:809–23.
5. Goettsch E, Kendall FE. Analysis of albumin and globulin in biological fluids by the quantitative precipitin method. J Biol Chem 1935; 109:221–31.
6. Marrack JR. The chemistry of antigen and antibodies. Br J Exp Pathol 1934; 32:212.
7. Grubb A. Quantitation of immunoglobulin G by electrophoresis in agarose gel containing antibodies. Scand J Clin Lab Invest 1970; 26:249–55.
8. Libby RL. The photronreflectometer: an instrument for the measurement of turbid systems. J Immunol 1938; 34:71–3.
9. Pope CE, Healey M. A photo-electric study of reactions between diphtheria toxin and antitoxin. Br J Exp Pathol 1938; 19:397–410.
10. Libby RL. A new and rapid quantitative technic for the determination of the potency of types I and II antipneumococcal serum. J Immunol 1938; 34:269–79.
11. Boyden A, Bolton E, Gemeroy D. Precipitin testing with special reference to the photoelectric measurement of turbidity. J Immunol 1947; 57:211–27.
12. Chow BF. The determination of plasma or serum albumin by means of a precipitin reaction. J Biol Chem 1947; 167:757–63.
13. Gitlin D, Edelhoch H. A study of the reaction between human serum albumin and its homologous equine antibody through the medium of light scattering. J Immunol 1951; 66:67–77.
14. Ritchie RF. A simple, direct, and sensitive technique for measurement of specific protein in dilute solution. J Lab Clin Med 1967; 70:512–17.
15. Alper CA, Ritchie RF. Comparison of immunochemical techniques. In: Ritchie RF, Ed. Automated Immunoanalysis, Part I. New York: Dekker, 1968:139.
16. Ritchie RF, Alper CA, Graves JA. Experience with a fully automated system for immunoassay of specific serum proteins. Arthritis Rheum 1969; 12:693.
17. Eckman I, Robbins JB, Van der Hamer CJA, Lentz J, Scheinberg IH. Automation of a quantitative immunochemical microanalysis of human serum transferrin: A model system. Clin Chem 1970;16:558–61.
18. Blom M, Hjorne H. Immunochemical determination of serum albumin with a centrifugal analyzer. Clin Chem 1975;21:195–8.
19. Savory J, Buffone G, Reich R. Kinetics of the IgG anti-IgG reaction as evaluated by conventional and stopped-flow-nephelometry. Clin Chem 1974; 20:1071–5.
20. Schotters SB, McBride JH, Rodgerson DO, Higgins S, Pisa M. Standardization for four protein analytes with the Behring nephelometer. Clin Chem 1988; 34:1870–2.
21. Lizana J, Hellsing K. Polymer enhancement of automated immunological nephelometric analysis, as illustrated by determination of urinary albumin. Clin Chem 1974; 20:415–20.

22. Hellsing K. Enhancing effects of nonionic polymers on immunochemical reactions. In: Price CP, Spencer K, Eds. Centrifugal Analysers in Clinical Chemistry. London: Praeger, 1978:67–112.

23. Cuilliere ML, Montagne P, Bessou T, El Oari R, Riochet D, Varcin P, Laroche P, Prud'homme P, Marchand J, Flecheux O, Pau B, Duheille J. Microparticle-enhanced nephelometric immunoassay (Nephelia^R) for immunoglobulins G, A, and M. Clin Chem 1991; 37:20–5.

24. Cliquet F, Montagne P, Cuilliere ML, Varcin P, Duheille J. Development of a rapid microparticle-enhanced nephelometric immunoassay for serum myoglobin in acute myocardial infarction. J Clin Lab Anal 1992; 6:176–81.

25. Grenier FC, Granados EN, Schick BC, Kolaczkowki L, Pry TA. Enhanced sensitivity immunoassay for TDx analyzer. Clin Chem 1987; 33:1570.

26. Kahan J, Sunobald L. Automated immunochemical determination of beta-lipoproteins. In: Automation in Analytical Chemistry, Vol. II. New York: Mediad, 1967:361.

27. Lizana J, Jansson L, Hellsing K. Electronic timing of a high-speed immunonephelometric continuous-flow systems. Clin Chem 1975; 21:762–4.

28. Kusnetz J, Mansberg HP. Optical considerations: nephelometry. In: Ritchie RF, Ed. Automated Immunoanalysis, Part 1. New York: Dekker, 1978:1–43.

29. Buffone GJ, Cross RE, Savory J, Soodak C. Measurement of laser-induced near front surface light scattering with a parallel fast analyzer. Anal Chem 1974; 46:2047–9.

30. Ritchie RF, Rippy JH. Performance on immunoglobulins IgG, IgA, and IgM tests in CAP survey specimens. Am J Clin Pathol 1982; 78:644–50.

31. College of Americam Pathologists (CAP). Proficiency surveys from 1976 to 1993 for immunology analytes. Northfield, IL.

32. Sternberg JC. Rate nephelometry. In: Rose NR, Friedman H, Fahey JL, Eds. Manual of Clinical Laboratory Immunology, Vol. 6, 3rd ed. Washington DC: American Society of Microbiology 1986:33–37.

33. Ouchterlony O, Nilsson LA. In: Weir DW, Ed. Handbook of Immunology I. Oxford: Blackwel Scientific, 1986.

34. Whicher JT, Price CP, Spencer K. Immunonephelometric and immunoturbidimetric assays for proteins. CRC Crit Rev Clin Lab Sci 1983; 18:213–57.

35. Tedford MC, Stimson WH. Molecular recognition in antibodies and its applications. Experientia 1991; 47:1129–38.

36. Otsuji S, Kamada T, Matsura T, Seki M, Tanaka K, Shibata H, Honda T. A rapid turbidimetric immunoassay for serum antistreptolysin-O. J Clin Lab Anal 1990; 4:241–5.

37. Anderson J, Sternberg JC. A rate nephelometer for immunoprecipitin measurement of specific serum proteins. In: Ritchie RF, Ed. Automated Immunoanalysis, Part 2. New York: Dekker, 1978:409–69

38. Deaton CD, Maxwell KW, Smith RS. Laser nephelometry. In: Ritchie RF, Ed. Automated Immunoanalysis, Part 2. New York: Dekker, 1978:375–408.

39. Normansell DE. Quantitation of serum immunoglobulins. CRC Crit Rev Clin Lab Sci 1982 17:103–69.

40. Whicher JT, Perry DE. Nephelometric methods. In: Butt WR, Ed. Practical Immunoassay: The State of the Art, Vol. 6. New York: Dekker, 1984:117–77.

41. Price CP, Spencer K, Whicher J. Light-scattering immunoassay of specific proteins: a review. Ann Clin Biochem 1983; 20:1–14.

42. Gosling JP. A decade of development in immunoassay methodology. A review. Clin Chem 1990 36:1408–27.

43. Beckman Array 360 System Operations Manual. 015-248545-B. Brea, CA: Beckman Instrument Inc., Diagnostic Systems Group, 1991:3-1, 3-2, 3-5, 3-7, 3-8.

44. Participant summary report, College of American Pathologists survey program, Diagnostic Immunol ogy - series 1, set S1-B, CAP, Northfield, IL: 1995.

45. Bullock DG, Dumont G, Vassault A, Aguzzi F, Chambers RE, Milford-Ward A, Whicher JT Bienvenu J. Immunochemical assays of serum proteins: a European external quality assessmen survey and the effects of calibration procedures on interlaboratory agreement. Clin Chim Acta 1990; 187:21–35.

46. Whicher JT. Calibration is the key to immunoassay but the ideal calibration is unattainable. Scand J Clin Lab Invest 1991; 51(Suppl. 205):21–32.

47. Johnson AM. A new international reference preparation for proteins in human serum. Arch Patho Lab Med 1993; 117:29–31.

48. Whicher JT, Ritchie RF, Johnson AM, Baudner S, Bienvenu J, Blirup-Jensen S, Carlstrom A Dati F, Milford-Ward A, Svendsen PJ. New Internaltional reference preparation for proteins in human serum (RPPHS). Clin Chem 1994; 40:934–8.

49. Marcovina SM, Albers JJ, Henderson LO, Hannon WH. International federation of clinical chemistry standardization project for measurement of apolipoproteins A-1 and B. III. Comparability of apolipoprotein A-1 values by use of international reference material. Clin Chem 1993; 39:773–81.
50. Reimer CB, Smith SJ, Wells TW, Nakamura RM, Keitees PW, Ritchie RF, Williams GW, Hanson DJ, Dorsey DB. Collaborative calibration of the U.S. National and the College of American Pathologists reference preparations for specific serum proteins. Am J Clin Pathol 1982; 77:12–9.
51. Pauling L, Pressman D, Grossberg AL. The serological properties of simple substances. VII. A quantitative theory of the inhibition by haptens of the precipitation of heterogeneous antisera with antigens, and comparison with experimental results for polyhaptenic simple substances and for azoproteins. J Am Chem Soc 1944; 66:784–96.
52. Cambiasco CL, Riccomi Ha, Mason PL, Hermans JF. Automated nephelometric immunoassay. II. Its application to the determination of hapten. J Immunol Methods 1974; 5:293–302.
53. Emancipator K, Elin RJ, Fleisher TA. Comparison of two automated nephelometers. J Clin Lab Anal 1992; 8:399–404.
54. Tillyer C. Calibration in three dimensions: optimizing a two-parameter calibration technique to extend the range of an immunoturbidimetric urinary albumin assay into antigen excess. Clin Chem 1990; 36:307–12.

18 SIMULTANEOUS MULTIANALYTE IMMUNOASSAYS

LARRY J. KRICKA
Department of Pathology and Laboratory Medicine
University of Pennsylvania
Philadelphia, Pennsylvania

1. INTRODUCTION

Immunoassays are usually performed as discrete tests, i.e., a single analyte is measured in each assay tube. An alternative option that is attracting increasing interest is simultaneous multianalyte immunoassays in which two or more analytes are measured simultaneously in the same assay tube (1, 2).

A simultaneous multianalyte immunoassay has a number of potential advantages:

(i) Work simplification—The number of assay tubes required for the assay is reduced, and there is a concomitant reduction in the number of pipetting, washing, and decanting operations.

(ii) Increase in test throughput—The time required for a simultaneous immunoassay is generally the same as that required for each individual immunoassay, hence providing a considerable saving in assay time and increasing test throughput.

(iii) Reduced overall cost per test—The time and labor component of the overall cost per test is reduced for a simulaneous multianalyte immunoassay compared to the same tests performed on an individual basis.

A simultaneous multianalyte immunoassay protocol is most attractive for analytes which are grouped in panels (e.g., allergen tests, thyroid function tests, "triple test" for Down's syndrome) (3, 4) (Table 18.1) and in situations where a single positive test result in a group of tests is significant, e.g., testing of units of blood for antibodies against infectious agents (HIV, HTLV-I, hepatitis, CMV). The latter

TABLE 18.1   Diagnostically Related Groups of Tests Suitable for the Simultaneous Immunoassay Format

Allergen testing
    Allergen-specific IgE and IgG antibodies
Blood banking
    Antibodies to HIV-1, HTLV-I, hepatitis B and C virus, CMV
Cardiac markers
    Myosin light chains, troponin, creatine kinase MB isoenzyme, myoglobin
Dried blood spot analysis
    17-α-Hydroxyprogesterone, thyrotropin, immunoreactive trypsin, creatine kinase MM isoenzyme
Drugs of abuse testing
    Cocaine, amphetamines, opiates
Dual and triple testing (Neural tube defects, Down's syndrome)
    AFP, free-beta hCG
    AFP, estriol, hCG
Fertility testing
    Lutropin, follitropin, hCG, prolactin

Note. Adapted from Kricka (1).

situation is the least technically demanding, because there is no need to distinguish which analyte(s) gave the positive result. Hence the same label can be used as in a recent simultaneous assay for antibodies to HTLV-1 and HIV-1 using alkaline phosphatase as the label (5, 6).

2. LABELS AND IMMUNOASSAY FORMATS

A number of immunoassay formats have been developed in pursuit of the goal of simultaneous multianalyte testing (Figs. 18.1 and 18.2). They can be classified into two main formats—assays based on more than one label (7–21), and assay formats based on spatially separated test zones (22–35) (Tables 18.2 and 18.3).

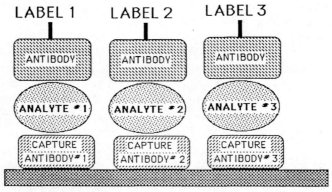

FIGURE 18.1   Multiple label strategy for simultaneous multianalyte immunoassays.

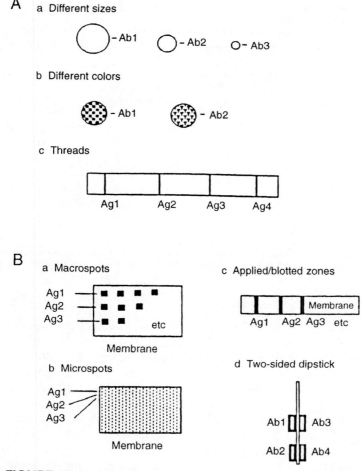

FIGURE 18.2   Solid-phase formats for simultaneous multianalyte immunoassays. (A) Discrete solid phases. (B) Discrete zones on a single solid phase. Reprinted, with permission, from Ref. (1).

3. LABELS

Selecting combinations of labels (one per analyte) has proved difficult and, until recently, had not progressed beyond combinations of two labels (Table 18.2).

3.1. Dual Labels

Two radioisotopic labels, ^{125}I and ^{131}I (7) or ^{125}I and ^{57}Co, have been combined in dual-analyte assays, e.g., SimulTROPIN assay for lutropin (LH) and follitropin (FSH) based on ^{125}I and ^{57}Co (8). Fluorophore labels provide a broad range of fluorescent signals, distinguishable on the basis of both lifetime and wavelength of emission. Europium (III) and terbium (III) labels and europium (III) and samarium (III) labels have been effectively combined for dual-analyte immunoassays (9–13).

**TABLE 18.2 Combinations of Labels Used in Dual-Label
Simultaneous Immunoassays**

Label 1 (detection method)	Label 2 (detection method)	Reference
	Radioisotope labels	
^{125}I (scintillation counting)	^{131}I (scintillation counting)	(7)
^{125}I (scintillation counting)	^{57}Co (scintillation counting)	(8)
	Fluorescent labels	
Eu (III) (TRF)	Sm (III) (TRF)	(9–13)
Eu (III) (TRF)	Tb (III) (TRF)	(14)
	Metal labels	
Co_2 $(CO)_6$ (FT-ir)	Cyclopentadienyl $Mn(CO)_3$ (FT-ir)	(15)
	Enzyme labels	
β-Galactosidase (fluorometry)	Phosphodiesterase (fluorometry)	(16)
β-Galactosidase (photometry)	Alkaline phosphatase (photometry)	(17, 18)
Alkaline phosphatase (photometry)	Peroxidase (photometry)	(19, 20)
	Enzyme/radioisotope label combinations	
Alkaline phosphatase (photometry)	^{125}I (scintillation counting)	(21)

Note. FT-ir, Fourier transform infrared spectroscopy; TRF, time-resolved fluorometry. Adapted from Kricka (1).

These labels have differing emission wavelengths and fluorescence lifetimes (Table 18.4), and by judicious choice of wavelength and time at which the fluorescence measurement is made, the two labels can be easily distinguished (36).

Attempts to combine two or more enzyme labels have had limited success. The enzymes commonly used as labels in immunoassay have markedly different requirements for optimum enzyme activity, e.g., the pH optima for the three most popular labels (37), horseradish peroxidase, alkaline phosphatase, and β-galactosidase, are 5–7,8–10, and 6–8, respectively. A simultaneous assay of two or more enzyme labels inevitably involves a compromise in the final assay conditions, and a further problem is that the absorption spectra of the commonly used enzyme substrates and products are broad and overlapping. The absorption maxima of the colored products produced by the action of peroxidase on 2,2′-azinobis(3-ethylbenzthiazolinesulfonic acid (ABTS), ortho-phenylene diamine (OPD), and

**TABLE 18.3 Discrete Test Zone
Formats for Simultaneous Immunoassay**

Format	Reference
Colored beads	(22)
Two-sided dipstick	(23)
Microspots	(24–26)
Macrospots	(27, 28)
Different diameter microparticles	(29–31)
Threads	(32)
Zones on a membrane	(33, 34)
Radially disposed test chambers	(35)

Note. Adapted from Kricka (1).

TABLE 18.4 Spectral and Lifetime Characteristics of Time-Resolved Fluorescent Lanthanide Pivaloyltrifluoroacetone (PTA) Chelates

Lanthanide PTA chelate	Excitation max (nm)	Emission max (nm)	Fluorescence decay time (μsec)
Eu (III)	295	612	925
Sm (III)	295	643	60
Tb (III)	295	543	96

Note. Adapted from Kricka (1) and Lovgren and Pettersson (36).

3,3′,5,5′-tetramethylbenzidine (TMB), and alkaline phosphatase on 4-nitrophenyl-phosphate (PNPP) all lie between 400 and 500 nm, thus making accurate measurement of individual products difficult. However, a sequential detection protocol eliminates some of these difficulties (19, 20). This dual-analyte immunoassay for α-fetoprotein (AFP) and free-β human chorionic gonadotropin (hCG) is based on a microwell coated with a mixture of anti-AFP and anti free-β hCG. The captured analytes are reacted successively with a mixture of goat anti-AFP and biotinylated anti free-β hCG, and then a mixture of alkaline phosphatase-labeled anti-goat IgG and a horseradish peroxidase–streptavidin conjugate. Bound label is quantitated sequentially. First the alkaline phosphatase is measured using 4-nitrophenyl phosphate as substrate, then the well is washed and the peroxidase quantitated using 3,3′,5,5′-tetramethylbenzidine. This assay was developed as a screening assay for neural tube defects and Down's syndrome (20).

The introduction of fluorescent substrates has also facilitated the use of two enzyme labels in a simultaneous immunoassay. The enzyme labels, β-galactosidase and phosphodiesterase, have been combined in a dual assay for the drugs phenobarbital and phenytoin. The fluorescent products generated from a 4-methylumbelliferyl galactoside and a phosphodiester derivative were measured sequentially, using two different excitation wavelengths (20 min/330 nm and 35 min/410 nm, respectively) (16). Other enzyme–label combinations (e.g., β-galactosidase and alkaline phosphatase) can also be assayed simultaneously using kinetic assays monitored at two wavelengths (17, 18).

New chemiluminescent enzyme substrates based on aryl-substituted adamantyl 1,2-dioxetanes (e.g., AMPPD, CSPD) offer an alternative route to simultaneous immunoassay. There are substrates available that produce characteristic chemiluminescence emissions when triggered by an enzyme—e.g., blue (459 nm) and green (555 nm) chemiluminescence. Hence, it would be possible to design assays in which the concentration of different analytes is determined using a series of enzymes and the appropriate substrates, and monitoring the chemiluminescent emissions at specific wavelengths (38).

3.2. Quadruple Labels

Quadruple labeling using four different fluorescent lanthanide labels has been achieved (39). This was used in a simultaneous immunoassay for TSH, 17-α-hydroxyprogesterone (17OHP), immunoreactive trypsin (IRT), and creatine kinase

MM (CK-MM). The assay was performed in a single microtiter well that had been coated with a mixture of anti-TSH, anti-17OHP, anti-IRT, and anti-CK-MM antibodies. The sample was reacted with a mixture of the four antibodies each labeled with an EDTA complex of a different lanthanide as follows—anti-TSH/Eu(III), anti-17OHP/Tb(III), anti-IRT/Sm(III), anti-CK-MM/Dy(III). After incubation and washing the individual labels were detected in a time-resolved fluorometric assay at different wavelengths (Sm^{3+} 644 nm, Dy^{3+} 573 nm, Tb^{3+} 545 nm, Eu^{3+} 613 nm). One slight complication was that the detection sensitivity of two of the labels (Sm^{3+}, Dy^{3+}) was poor. In order to increase the detection sensitivity a dissociative cofluorescent enhancement procedure was utilized based on pivaloyl phenanthroline, trifluoroacetone, and yttrium(III) ions (40). The detection limits for the four lanthanice labels were: Eu(III), 0.035; Tb(III), 0.34; Sm(III), 7.9; Dy(III), 46 pmol/liter. The detection limits for the four analytes were 0.1 mIU units/liter for thyrotropin, 2 nmol/liter for 17-α-hydroxyprogesterone, 2 μg/liter for immunoreactive trypsin, and 4 U/liter for creatine kinase MM isoenzyme.

A similar quadruple label concept has been proposed for simultaneous analysis of multiple firefly luciferase reporter genes based on different click beetle (*Pyrophorus plagiothalamus*) luciferases (41). A series of four different beetle luciferase genes have been cloned that express luciferases which catalyze the oxidation of firefly luciferin to produce light at 548, 560, 578, and 590 nm.

4. DISCRETE TEST ZONES

The use of discrete test zones on a single device has been the most successful route to multianalyte immunoassays (Fig. 18.2). (See Table 18.3 for representative examples of this type of assay.)

4.1. Beads, Microparticles, and Threads

In this sandwich immunoassay strategy the capture reagents (antigen or antibody) are immobilized on discrete and distinguishable solid phases. The earliest examples of these assays used color-coded beads coated with different antibodies (22). A mixture of red-stained human IgG-coated beads, orange-stained human serum albumin-coated beads, blue-stained horseradish peroxidase-coated beads, and un-stained (white) ovalbumin-coated beads was incubated with the sample containing a mixture of antibodies and a peroxidase–anti-IgG conjugate. Conjugate bound to the individual beads was then detected using diaminobenzidine as substrate. The beads which had reacted with antibody contained in the sample became brown due to deposition of the insoluble product on the surface of the bead, thus obscuring the original color of the bead. Qualitative inspection of the mixture of beads revealed which beads had reacted and hence which antibodies were present in the sample.

Microparticles with different diameters in combination with a flow cytometer form the basis of another format for simultaneous immunoassays (42). In one application, 5-, 7-, and 9.3-μm-diameter polystyrene particles were coated with different *Candida albicans* antigens (a whole cell extract, a cytoplasmic protein extract, and a cell wall polysaccharide). The coated microparticles were then reacted sequentially with a serum sample and a fluorophore–anti-human IgG conjugate. The fluorescence associated with the different sized particles was measured after separation of the particles by electronic volume gating (30). Anti-HIV-1 antibodies specific for p24, p31, gp 41, and gp 120 have been measured using a similar strategy (29). An array of individual cellulose threads is another way of forming discrete reaction zones in a simultaneous immunoassay device. This strategy is used in the MASTpette device for allergy testing (IgE and IgG antibodies). It contains a series of up to 36 threads, each coated with a different allergen, and a positive and negative control thread (32). Specific IgE antibody bound to the threads is detected using a peroxidase conjugate and the chemiluminescent cosubstrate luminol. Light emission from individual threads in the array is recorded on photographic film contained in a special cassette (Fig. 18.3).

4.2. Multiple Test Zones on a Single Solid Phase

An array of individual reaction zones on a single solid phase has become the most popular format for simultaneous immunoassays. The principal advantage of this assay format is that only one immunoassay label is required. A limitation is that this assay format must be used with a detection system capable of serial or simultaneous quantitation of signal associated with the individual test zones.

4.2.1. Membranes

The principal example of a membrane-based simultaneous immunoassay is Western blotting, and the most common clinical laboratory application is in the detection of antibodies to specific HIV-1 virus antigens (33). Western blotting uses a membrane (e.g., nitrocellulose) onto which are blotted HIV-1 virus antigens that have been separated electrophoretically by size on a polyacrylamide gel. The membrane is cut into narrow strips, and a strip of the membrane is incubated sequentially with a serum sample and an enzyme-labeled anti-human IgG conjugate. The strip is then incubated with a substrate which produces an insoluble product at locations where the conjugate has bound to the blotted HIV-1 antigen. Several variants of this technique have been described, one of which is the "multicolor" Western blot. This combines multiple discrete test zones and two labels (alkaline phosphatase and horseradish peroxidase) (34). This assay has been used to detect different types of interferon (α-1, α-2, and γ) blotted on a nitrocellulose membrane. Following sequential incubation with anti-interferon antibodies and alkaline phosphatase- and peroxidase-conjugated anti-species antibodies, the membrane was developed using diaminobenzidine (peroxidase substrate) and 5-bromo-4-chloro-3-indolyl phosphate (alkaline phosphatase substrate). Any bound peroxidase conjugate was visualized as a brownish-green band and any bound alkaline phosphatase appeared as a turquoise-colored band. An alternative to blotting antigens from a gel is to apply the antigens directly to the membrane in parallel lines. This technique ("line immunoassay") has been used to detect antibodies to treponemal antigens (43).

Discrete spatially separated zones can also be produced by simply dotting or chemically immobilizing antigens onto a membrane. For example, a simultaneous multianalyte immunoassay has been developed based on a nitrocellulose strip embossed to form a 5 × 6 array of small (2.5-mm diameter) islands (Abbott MATRIX) (Fig. 18.4). The different capture proteins are immobilized on the embossed areas to form a multianalyte test array comprising recombinant HIV-1 antigens p17, p24, p31, p41, p66, gp120, and HIV-2 antigen p41 (28). This array also includes a proce-

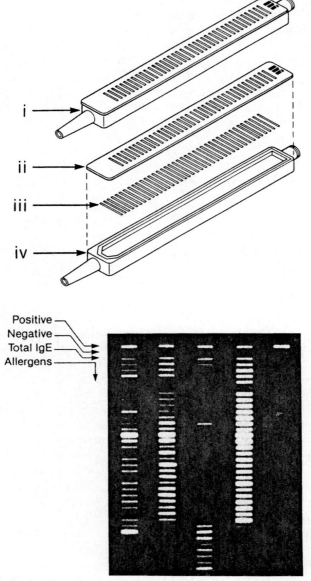

FIGURE 18.3 MASTpette test chamber (top) and photograph of result from four patients with positive responses and one patient with a negative response (bottom). (Reprinted from Ref. (32), courtesy of the American Association for Clinical Chemistry, Inc.)

dural control and a negative control. The embossed membrane is held in a special test cell and the test is processed by an automatic bench-top analyzer.

The most active area of development for multianalyte immunoassays is in testing for drugs of abuse. There are several test devices available, including the Triage Ascend MultiImmunoassay (Biosite Diagnostics, San Diego, CA) and the Mach IV Screen (Drug Screening Systems Inc, Blackwood, NJ), which test urine simultaneously for seven and four different drugs of abuse, respectively. The Biosite device

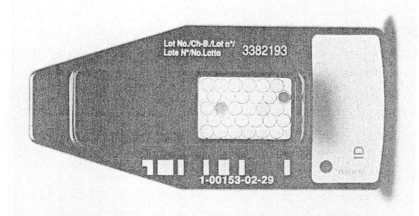

FIGURE 18.4   Matrix (Aero Plus) test device. (Reproduction of "Matrix Aero Plus" has been granted with approval of Abbott Laboratories, all rights reserved by Abbott Laboratories.)

tests urine for the presence of phencyclidine, benzodiazepines, cocaine, amphetamines, tetrahydrocannabinol, opiates, and barbiturates in a 10-min assay (44, 45) (Figure 18.5). A 140-μl sample of urine is mixed with a cocktail of monoclonal anti-drug antibodies and colloidal gold particles coated with the drugs. After a short incubation, the mixture is transferred onto the assay membrane, which is coated with discrete bands of monoclonal drug antibodies. The unbound drug-colloidal gold particles are captured by the respective immobilized antibodies and appear as purple bands. The assay is designed to operate above certain thresholds, e.g., amphetamine, 1000 ng/ml. If the concentration of the drug in the sample exceeds the threshold concentration, it competes with gold-labeled drug for binding sites on the soluble antibody and more of the gold-labeled drug is available to bind to

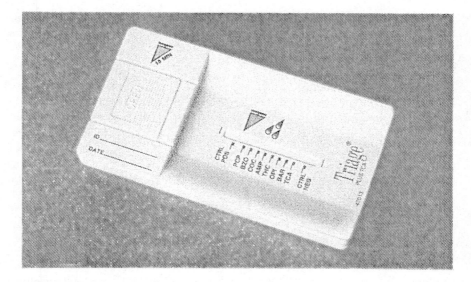

FIGURE 18.5   Triage drugs of abuse test device (photograph courtesy of Biosite Diagnostics).

the immobilized anti-drug antibody. Bound gold-labeled drug appears as a purple band on the membrane, signifying a positive result.

The MACH IV device operates on an immunochromatographic assay principle. A urine sample is applied at one end of a porous membrane. The sample is drawn along the membrane by capillary action and it mobilizes the antibody-coated colored microparticles on the membrane. The resulting mixture of sample and reagent moves along the membrane to a zone containing immobilized drug. If a particular drug is present in the urine sample above the preset threshold concentration then the particles do not bind and no colored band is visible (positive result). However, if the urine sample is free of that drug then the immobilized drug captures the antibody coated microparticles and a colored band forms, denoting a negative result.

The use of microspots of capture antigen or antibody on membranes is a recent development in simultaneous multianalyte immunoassays (24–26). The spotted reagent (e.g., antibody) covers an area of approximately 100 μm^2 and the microspot contains a very small concentration of antibody binding sites (e.g., 10^{-13} mol/liter). The fractional occupancy of the antibody binding sites at this very low antibody concentration depends only on the ambient concentration of analyte in the sample to which the microspot is exposed. In one example of the assay, a Texas Red-labeled monoclonal anti-thyrotropin was spotted onto the surface of a small piece of polystyrene. Immobilized monoclonal antibody in the spot was incubated with a sample containing thyrotropin and then incubated with a fluorescein-labeled monoclonal anti-thyrotropin antibody. The ratio of the bound fluorescein and Texas Red labels in the spot was measured using a dual-channel laser scanning confocal microscope. The assay is extremely sensitive and Ekins has presented a detailed account of the theory underlying this type of fractional occupancy immunoassay (24–26). The potential sensitivity of this assay technique is $<10^{-15}$ mol/liter and as many as 10,000 assays could be performed on a 1×1-cm polystyrene surface. An assay for a single analyte (TSH) illustrates the potential of this technique. The detection limit for TSH was 0.0002 mIU/liter (80,000 molecules/ml) in an overnight incubation assay and 4 μIU/liter in a one-step 30-min assay (46).

4.3. Two-Sided Dipstick

Macrodevices have also been fabricated for simultaneous immunoassays. In one example a two-site (sandwich) time-resolved fluoroimmunoassay for lutropin, follitropin, choriogonadotropin (hCG), and prolactin in serum was developed based on a series of four antibody-coated plastic disks attached to a dipstick (two disks on each side of the dipstick). A europium chelate was chosen as the label in the sandwich assay. Label bound to the disks was detected by time-resolved fluorometry in two sequential measurements (side 1, then side 2 of the stick) (23) (see also Chapter 14).

4.4. Radially Disposed Test Chambers

A recent device for testing drugs of abuse (Advisor) makes use of a series of radially disposed test chambers in order to achieve simultaneous immunoassays

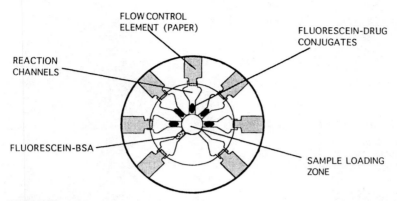

FIGURE 18.6 Advisor-laminated test card. BSA, bovine serum albumin. (Reprinted from Ref. (1), courtesy of the American Association for Clinical Chemistry, Inc.)

(Fig. 18.6) (35). This assay system utilizes red cells stained with Remazol Brilliant Blue R as the label. The cells are coated with antifluorescein antibodies. When the coated cells are mixed with a cocktail of anti-drug antibodies and drug–fluorescein conjugates, an agglutination reaction occurs. In the presence of a specific drug, the agglutination is inhibited (Fig. 18.7). The immunoassays are performed on a laminated card that has seven test chambers, containing drug–fluorescein conjugates, radially disposed around a central application well. Five of the test chambers are used for drug assays (amphetamines, cannabinoids, cocaine metabolites, opiates, and phencyclidine) and the other two are used for a positive and a negative control. A 20-μl sample is mixed with the antibody-coated red cell and anti-drug antibody cocktail and introduced into the central application well. The fluid flow along the channel linking the central application well and the test chambers is controlled by an adsorbent paper strip at the end of each chamber. The flow of fluid stops when the paper strip is saturated and this stops the reaction, hence eliminating the need for accurate timing of the assay. Appearance of an agglutination reaction indicates a negative test result.

5. TEST COMBINATIONS

Table 18.5 lists the various analytes that have been combined into dual or multianalyte assays. A limited number of multianalyte immunoassays have become established in routine clinical laboratories, and currently the main examples are HIV antibody testing in a Western blot assay format, drugs of abuse testing, and allergen testing.

6. CONCLUSIONS

Several practical hurdles limit the routine use of simultaneous multianalyte immunoassays. Cross-reactions, leading to false-positive or false-negative results on multiantibody-coated solid phases, and difficulties in optimizing the assays to cover

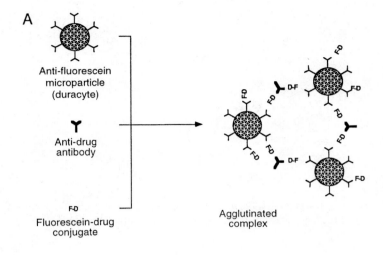

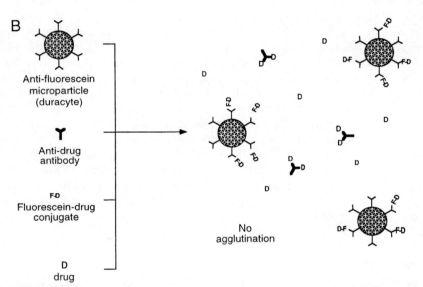

FIGURE 18.7 Agglutination reactions used in the Advisor test device (Abbott Laboratories). (A) Negative reaction, (B) positive reaction. (Reprinted from Ref. (35), courtesy of the American Association for Clinical Chemistry, Inc.)

the divergent concentration ranges for the individual analytes constitute two of the most important problems in the develpoment of routine simultaneous immunoassays. A further issue is quality control of multiple assays performed simultaneously. The chance of one assay failing in a multiassay panel would be high, and if one assay in the array fails quality control, is the analytical performance of all of the assays suspect? Subsequent repeat assays would seriously undermine any savings in personnel time and reagent costs that the simultaneous multianalyte format provides (2).

TABLE 18.5 **Simultaneous Immunoassay Test Combinations**

Assays	Reference
Dual assays	
Adenovirus type 40, adenovirus type 41	(47)
Alpha-fetoprotein, ferritin	(48)
Alpha-fetoprotein, hCG free β-subunit	(12)
Alpha 1-microglobulin, IgA-conjugated α 1-microglobulin	(21)
Albumin antibody, interleukin antibody	(49)
Beta-hCG, hCG	(50)
Carbonic anhydrase III, myoglobin	(51)
CMV antibody, herpes simplex antibody	(31)
Estrone glucuronide, pregnanediol glucuronide	(52)
Follitropin, lutropin	(8, 9, 53)
Free thyroxine, thyrotropin	(54)
Growth hormone, insulin	(7)
HIV-1 antibody, HTLV-I antibody	(5, 6)
HIV-1, HIV-2 antibody	—[a,b]
IgG, IgM	(55)
OKT3 anti-isotype and anti-idiotype antibodies	(56)
Phenobarbital, carbamazepine	(15)
Phenobarbital, phenytoin	(16)
Potato virus M, potato virus X	(10)
Prostatic acid phosphatase (PSA), PSA-α-chymotrypsin complex	(13)
Thyroxine, triiodothyronine	(57)
Treponemal antigen (TmpA), treponemal axial filament	(43)
Multianalyte assays	
Allergen-specific IgE antibodies	(32, 58)
Candida albicans antibodies	(28)
17-α-Hydroxyprogesterone, TSH, immunoreactive trypsin, CK-MM	(39)
Drugs of abuse (phencyclidine, benzodiazepines, cocaine, amphetamines, tetrahydrocannabinol, opiates, barbiturates)	(44, 45)[e]
Drugs of abuse (cocaine, methamphetamine, opiates, cannabinoid)	—[c]
Drugs of abuse (amphetamines, cocaine metabolite, cannabinoids, opiates, phencyclidine)	(35)
Follitropin, hCG, lutropin, prolactin	(33)
HIV-1 antibodies	(29)
HIV-1 antibodies, HIV-2 antibody	(28)
HIV-1, HIV-2, HTLV-I antibodies	
HIV-1/2, HTLV-I antibody	—[b]
Measles, mumps, rubella virus antibodies	(59)
Myosin light chains, troponin, CK-MB, myoglobin	—[d]

[a] Genetic Systems Corp.
[b] Sienna Biotech Inc.
[c] Drug Screening Systems.
[d] Spectral Diagnostics Inc.
[e] Panel now includes tricyclic antidepressants.

References

1. Kricka LJ. Simultaneous multianalyte immunoassays. In-Service Train Contin Educ 1992; 10:7–20.
2. Kricka LJ. Multianalyte testing. Clin Chem 1992; 38:327–8.
3. Thornton JG, Cartmill RS, Williams J, Holding S, Lilford RJ. Clinical experience with the triple test for Down's syndrome screening. J Perinat Med 1991; 19:151–4.
4. Sheldon TA, Simpson J. Appraisal of a new scheme for prenatal screening for Down's syndrome. Br Med J 1991; 302:1133–6.

5. Yamamoto K, Higashimoto K, Minagawa H, Okada M, Kasahara Y. Simultaneous detection of antibodies to HTLV-I and HIV-1 by chemiluminescent enzyme immunoassay. Clin Chem 1991; 37:1031.

6. Montagna RA, Papsidero L, Poiesz BJ. Evaluation of a solid-phase immunoassay for the simultaneous detection of antibodies to human immunodeficiency virus type 1 and human T-cell lymphotropic virus type I. J Clin Microbiol 1991; 29:897–900.

7. Morgan CR. Immunoassay of human insulin and growth hormone simultaneously using ^{131}I and ^{125}I tracers. Proc Soc Exp Biol Med 1966; 123:230–3.

8. Wians FH, Dev J, Powell MM, Heald JI. Evaluation of simultaneous measurement of lutropin and follitropin with the SimulTROPIN radioimmunoassay kit. Clin Chem 1986; 32:887–90.

9. Hemmila I, Holttinen S, Petterson K, Lovgren T. Double-label time-resolved immunofluorometry of lutropin and follitropin in serum. Clin Chem 1987; 33:2281–3.

10. Saarma M, Jarvekulg L, Hemmila I, Siitari H, Sinijarv R. Simultaneous quantification of two plant viruses by double-label time-resolved immunofluorometric assay. J Virol Methods 1989; 23:47–54.

11. Hemmila I, Markela E. Samarium (III) labelling reagent for dual label fluorescence immunoassay. Clin Chem 1990; 36:1094.

12. Pettersson K, Alfthan H, Stenman U-H, et al. Simultaneous assay of alpha-fetoprotein and free beta subunit of human chorionic gonadotropin by dual-label time-resolved immunofluorometric assay. Clin Chem 1993; 39:2084–9.

13. Leinonen J, Lovgren T, Vornanen T, Stenman U-H. Double-label time-resolved immunofluorometric assay of prostate-specific antigen and its complex with alpha-1 antitrypsin. Clin Chem 1993; 39:2089–103.

14. Hemmila I. Time-resolved fluorometric determination of terbium in aqueous solution. Anal Chem 1985; 57:1676–81.

15. Salamain M, Vessieres A, Brossier P, Jaouen G. Use of Fourier transform infrared spectroscopy for the simultaneous quantitative detection of metal carbonyl tracers suitable for multilabel immunoassays. Anal Biochem 1993; 208:117–20.

16. Dean KJ, Thompson SG, Burd JF, Buckler RT. Simultaneous determination of phenytoin and phenobarbital in serum or plasma by substrate-labeled fluorescent immunoassay. Clin Chem 1983; 29:1051–6.

17. Blake C, Al Bassam MN, Gould BJ, et al. Simultaneous enzyme immunoassay of two thyroid hormones. Clin Chem 1982; 28:1469–73.

18. Bates DL, Bailey WR. Dual enzyme assay. International Patent Appl. 1989; WO89/06802.

19. Macri JN, Spencer K, Anderson R. Dual analyte immunoassay—a new approach to neural tube defect and Down's syndrome screening. Ann Clin Biochem 1992; 29:390–6.

20. Spencer K, Macri JN, Anderson RW, et al. Dual analyte immunoassay in neural tube defect and Down's syndrome screening; results of a multicentre trial. Ann Clin Biochem 1993; 30:394–401.

21. DeMars DD, Katzmann JA, Kimlinger TK. Simultaneous measurement of total and IgA-conjugated alpha 1-microglobulin by a combined immunoenzyme/immunoradiometric assay technique. Clin Chem 1989; 35:766–72.

22. Streefkerk JG, Kors N, Boden D. Principle of a reaction for simultaneous detection of various antibodies using coloured antigen-coupled agarose beads. Protides Biol Fluids 1976; 24:811–4.

23. Kakabakos SE, Christopoulos TK, Diamandis EP. Multianalyte immunoassay-based spatially distinct fluorescent areas quantified by laser-excited solid phase time-resolved fluorometry. Clin Chem 1992; 38:338–42.

24. Ekins R, Chu F, Biggart E. Fluorescence spectroscopy and its application to a new generation of high sensitivity, multi-microspot, multianalyte immunoassay. Clin Chim Acta 1990; 194:91–114.

25. Ekins R, Chu FW. Multianalyte microspot immunoassay—microanalytical "compact disk" of the future. Clin Chem 1991; 37:1955–67.

26. Ekins RP. Multi-analyte immunoassay. J Pharm Biomed Anal 1989; 7:155–68.

27. Pappas MG. Dot enzyme-linked immunosorbent assays. In: Collins WP, Ed. Complementary Immunoassays. Chichester: Wiley, 1988:113–34.

28. Donohue J, Bailey M, Gray R, et al. Enzyme immunoassay system for panel testing. Clin Chem 1989; 35:1874–7.

29. Scillian JJ, McHugh TM, Busch MP, et al. Early detection of antibodies against rDNA-produced HIV proteins with a flow cytometric assay. Blood 1989; 73:2041–8.

30. McHugh TM, Wang YJ, Chong HO, Blackwood LL, Stites DP. Development of a microsphere-based fluorescent immunoassay and its comparison to an enzyme immunoassay for the detection of antibodies to three antigen preparations from Candida albicans. J Immunol Methods 1989; 116:213–9.

31. McHugh TM, Minner RC, Logan LH, Stites DP. Simultaneous detection of antibodies to cytomegalovirus and herpes simplex virus by using flow cytometry and a microsphere-based fluorescence immunoassay. J Clin Microbiol 1988; 26:1957–61.
32. Brown CR, Higgins KW, Frazer K, et al. Simultaneous determination of total IgE and allergen-specific IgE in serum by the MAST chemiluminescent assay system. Clin Chem 1985; 31:1500–5.
33. Renner SW. Immunoblotting and dot immunobinding. Emerging techniques in protein immunochemistry. Arch Pathol Lab Med 1988; 112:780–6.
34. Lee N, Zhang SQ, Testa D. A rapid multicolor Western blot. J Immunol Methods 1988; 106:27–30.
35. Parsons RG, Kowal R, LeBlond D, et al. Multianalyte assay system developed for drugs of abuse. Clin Chem 1993; 39:1899–903.
36. Lovgren T, Pettersson K. Time-resolved fluoroimmunoassay, advantages and limitations. In: Van Dyke K, Van Dyke R, Eds. Luminescence immunoassay and molecular applications. Boca Raton: CRC Press, 1990:233–53.
37. Gosling JP. A decade of development in immunoassay methodology. Clin Chem 1990; 36:1408–27.
38. Edwards BA, Sparks A, Voyta JC, Bronstein I. Unusual luminescent properties of odd- and even-substituted naphthyl-derivatized dioxetanes. J Biolumin Chemilumin 1990; 5:1–4.
39. Xu Y-Y, Pettersson K, Blomberg K, Hemmila I, Mikola H, Lovgren T. Simultaneous quadruple-label fluorometric immunoassay of thyroid-stimulating hormone, 17-alpha-hydroxyprogesterone, immunoreactive trypsin, and creatine kinase MM isoenzyme in dried blood spots. Clin Chem 1992; 38:2038–43.
40. Xu Y-Y, Hemmila IA. Co-fluorescence enhancement system based on pivaloyltrifluoroacetone and yttrium for the simultaneous detection of europium, terbium, samarium and dysprosium. Anal Chim Acta 1992; 256:9–16.
41. Wood V, Lam YA, McElroy WD. Complementary DNA coding click beetle luciferases can elicit bioluminescence of different colors. Science 1989; 244:700–2.
42. Fulwyler MJ, McHugh TM. Flow microsphere immunoassay for the quantitative and simultaneous detection of soluble analytes. Methods Cell Biol 1990; 33:613–29.
43. Ijsselmuiden OE, Beelaert G, Schouls LM, Tank B, Stolz E, van der Groen G. Line immunoassay and enzyme-linked line immunofiltration assay for simultaneous detection of antibody to two treponemal antigens. Eur J Clin Microbiol Infect Dis 1989; 8:716–21.
44. Buechler KF, Moi S, Noar B, et al. Simultaneous detection of seven drugs of abuse by the Triage panel for drugs of abuse. Clin Chem 1992; 38:1678–84.
45. Wu AHB, Wong SS, Johnson KG, et al. Evaluation of the Triage system for emergency drugs-of-abuse testing in urine. J Anal Toxicol 1993; 17:241–5.
46. Ekins R, Chu F. Multianalyte testing. Clin Chem 1993; 39:369–70.
47. Wood DJ, Bijlsma K, de Jong JC, Tonkin C. Evaluation of a commercial monoclonal antibody-based enzyme immunoassay for detection of adenovirus 40 and 41 in stool specimens. J Clin Microbiol 1989; 27:155–8.
48. Hoshino N, Miyai K. New screening system for simultaneous determination of two marker proteins by homogeneous enzyme immunoassay. J Clin Pathol 1992; 45:213–6.
49. Kominami G, Kawamoto H, Murai Y, Kono M. Simultaneous immunoenzymometric assay for antibodies against human interleukin-2 and human serum albumin in rat serum. J Immunoassay 1990; 11:373–85.
50. Choi MJ, Choe IS, Kang HK, Lee JS, Chug TW. Simple enzyme immunoassay for the simultaneous measurement of whole choriogonadotropin molecules and free beta-subunits in sera of women with abnormal pregnancies or tumors of the reproductive system. Clin Chem 1991; 37:673–7.
51. Vuori J, Rasi S, Takala T, Vaananen K. Dual-label time-resolved fluoroimmunoassay for simultaneous detection of myoglobin and carbonic anhydrase III in serum. Clin Chem 1991; 37:2087–92.
52. Lenton EA, King H, Johnson J, Amos S. An assessment of the dual-analyte enzyme immunoassay for ovulation timing. Hum Reprod 1989; 4:378–80.
53. Beinlich CJJ, Piper A, O'Neal JC, White OD. Evaluation of dual-label simultaneous assays for lutropin and follitropin in serum. Clin Chem 1985; 31:2014–8.
54. Desai RK, Deppe WM, Norman RJ, Govender T, Joubert SM. The simulTRAC FT4/TSH assay evaluated as a first-line thyroid-function test. Clin Chem 1988; 34:1488–91.
55. Auditore-Hargreaves K, Houghton RL, Monji N, Priest JH, Hoffman AS, Nowinski RC. Phase-separation immunoassays. Clin Chem 1987; 33:1509–16.
56. Schroeder TJ, First MR, Pouletty C, Hariharan S, Pouletty P. Rapid detection of anti-OKT3 antibodies with the Transtat assay. Transplantation 1993; 55:297–9.

57. Haynes SP and Goldie DJ. Simultaneous radioimmunoassay of thyroid hormones in unextracted serum. Ann Clin Biochem 1977; 14:12–15.
58. Lindberg RE, Anawis MA, Bailey M, *et al*. Development of the Abbott Matrix Aero assay for the measurement of specific IgE. J Immunoassay 1991; 12:465–85.
59. Condorelli F, Ziegler T. Dot immunobinding assay for simultaneous detection of specific immuno-globulin G antibodies to measles virus, mumps virus, and rubella virus. J Clin Microbiol 1993; 31:717–9.

19 | NONCOMPETITIVE IMMUNOASSAY FOR SMALL MOLECULES

FORTÜNE KOHEN
Department of Biological Regulation
The Weizmann Institute of Science
Rehovot, 76100, Israel

JOSEF DE BOEVER
Vrouwenkliniek-Poli 3
Universitair Ziekenhuis
B-9000 Gent, Belgium

GEOFF BARNARD
Regional Endocrine Unit
Department of Chemical Pathology
Southampton General Hospital
Southampton SO 16 GYD, United Kingdom

1. INTRODUCTION

All immunoassay procedures can be divided into two basic types: competitive and noncompetitive. Historically, Yalow and Berson (1), the pioneers of radioimmunoassay, developed a competitive immunoassay for the measurement of insulin in 1960. Concurrently, Ekins (2) introduced the terms "limited reagent method" and "saturation analysis" to indicate that in competitive binding reactions the concentration of the binding protein or specific antibody was insufficient to bind all the analyte. More recently, he has discussed the major disadvantages of competitive immunoassays, which include: (i) limited sensitivity and working range, (ii) slow-reaction kinetics, (iii) increased imprecision, and (iv) the development of a negative endpoint (3).

In 1968, Miles and Hales (4) introduced a noncompetitive, two-site sandwich assay for measuring compounds with more than one antigenic determinant (epitope). These excess reagent assays have been termed immunometric assays and have largely replaced the earlier competitive method for the measurement of protein hormones in biological fluids. The advantages of immunometric assays are greater sensitivity, precision, and working range of analyte (5). The major disadvantage of the two-site assay is that it is not suitable for the measurement of small molecules.

Ekins (6) has suggested that the fundamental difference between competitive and noncompetitive methods is based solely on the detection of antibody occupancy. Accordingly, we have devised a way to detect antibody occupancy (i.e., a noncompetitive method) for the measurement of small molecules using two anti-idiotypic antibodies that recognize different epitopes (idiotypes) within the hypervariable region of the primary (anti-analyte) antibody. We describe here a novel noncompetitive immunoassay procedure, which we term idiometric assay, suitable for measuring small molecules.

2. ANTI-IDIOTYPIC ANTIBODIES AS NOVEL PROBES IN IMMUNODIAGNOSTICS

The term idiotype usually designates antigenic determinants unique to a small set of antibody molecules (Ab_1). The original antibody, when used as an immunogen, can induce the production of anti-idiotypic antibodies (anti-Id) against itself. The generated anti-Id antibodies have been classified according to the location of the idiotype recognized (7). Those anti-Id antibodies recognizing epitopes at the constant region of the primary Ab_1 have been designated *allotypic* anti-Id. The anti-Id recognizing the paratope region of Ab_1 are generally classified as $Ab2\beta$ (*betatype*), and they possess the capacity of competing with the analyte for an epitope at the binding site (paratope) (see Fig. 19.1). On the other hand, those anti-Id that recognize an epitope within the framework of the variable region of the primary antibody (Ab_1), but are not sensitive to the presence or absence of the analyte at the binding site, are classified as $Ab2\alpha$ (*alphatype*) (see Fig. 19.1). In particular, the subset of α-types selected for the development of the idiometric assay will not bind to the β-type/primary antibody complex because of steric hindrance resulting from epitope proximity.

2.1. Generation of Anti-idiotypic Antibodies against Anti-hormonal Antibodies

In order to generate anti-idiotypic antibodies to anti-hormonal antibodies we devised several schemes. For instance, if the primary antibody (Ab_1) was a mouse–mouse hybridoma, then rats were used for the immunization with Ab_1. Conversely, if the primary Ab_1 was a rat–mouse hybridoma, then mice were used for immunization with Ab_1. In addition, in order to increase the immunogenicity of Ab_1, the

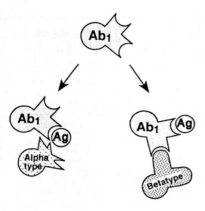

• Alphatype
• Binding to Ab_1
  is analyte **insensitive**

• Betatype
• Binding to Ab_1
  is analyte **sensitive**

FIGURE 19.1 Scheme showing the various types of anti-idiotypic antibodies generated by using the primary antibody (idiotype, Ab1) as an immunogen.

primary antibody was coupled to KLH. As another alternative, the $F(ab')_2$ dimer of Ab_1 was prepared by pepsin digestion and used as an immunogen.

Table 19.1 shows the characterization of the various hybridomas used in the generation of anti-idiotypic antibodies against anti-hormonal antibodies. These hybridomas were grown as ascites in pristane primed mice (8). The purified immunoglobulin was isolated, according to their subtype, by affinity chromatography on Sepharose–Protein A (9). The purified immunoglobulin fraction of each antibody was labeled with europium chelate (10, 11) and used as the labeled antibody in the screening of the anti-idiotypic antibodies as well as in the idiometric assay. For immunization purposes, the purified immunoglobulins served as immunogens, which were used intact, coupled to KLH (12) or as $F(ab')_2$ dimers.

Three different strains of female mice (C57 black, CD_2, and Balbc) were immunized with the immunogens derived from rat–mouse hybridomas in Freund's adjuvant as described elsewhere (10). On the other hand, Wistar-derived female rats

TABLE 19.1 Characterization of Hybridomas Secreting Anti-hormonal Antibodies

Immunogen	Hybridoma	Clone no.	Myeloma variant	Immunoglobulin subclass
Estradiol-6–BSA	Mouse/mouse	15	653	IgG_{2b}
Estradiol-6–BSA	Rat/mouse	$2F_9$	NSO	IgG_{2a}
Progesterone-11–BSA	Mouse/mouse	$1E_{11}$	NSO	IgG_1
Progesterone-3–BSA	Rat/mouse	$1A_8$	NSO	—
Progesterone-7–BSA	Rat/mouse	$2H_4$	NSO	IgG_1
Estrone-3G–BSA	Rat/mouse	$3F_{11}$	NSO	IgG_1
Pregnanediol-3αG–BSA	Mouse/mouse	44	653	IgG_{2b}

Note. Abbreviations: G, glucuronide.

were used for immunization with immunogens derived from mouse–mouse hybridomas. After 3 months of immunization, the mouse or the rat showing the highest titer of antibodies that recognized europium-labeled anti-ligand IgG was killed, and its immune cells were fused with mouse myeloma cells (NSO), using the hybridoma technique of Köhler and Milstein (13). The culture supernatants of the growing hybridomas were screened for antibody activity after 10 to 15 days, following the fusion experiment.

2.2. Screening Assays

Hybridomas secreting novel allotypic, betatypic, and alphatypic anti-idiotypic antibodies were characterized, according to the following screening strategies.

2.2.1. Screening Assay 1: Immunoglobulin Detection

In this procedure, culture supernatants of growing hybridomas were added to rabbit anti-mouse IgG-coated microtiter plates (10). After a short incubation, the plates were washed and blocked with mouse serum. Europium-labeled anti-analyte antibody was then added to each well. Immobilized IgG that bound the europium-labeled antibody was classified as a mixture of anti-idiotypes and allotypes (see Fig. 19.2).

2.2.2. Screening Assay 2: Anti-allotypic Antibody Detection

In this screening procedure, the hybridomas that gave positive results in screening assay 1 (i.e., anti-allotypes and anti-idiotypes) were captured on rabbit anti-mouse plates. After blocking with nonspecific mouse IgG, europium-labeled irrelevant anti-analyte, having the same isotype as the anti-analyte used for immunization, was added to each well. Immobilized IgGs that failed to bind the europium-labeled irrelevant anti-ligand antibody were classified as betatypes and alphatypes (see Fig. 19.3).

2.2.3. Screening Assay 3: Identification of Betatypic Analyte-Sensitive Anti-idiotypic Antibodies

In this screening procedure, the hybridomas that gave a positive result in screening 2 were added to rabbit anti-mouse coated wells. After blocking with nonspecific

Screening assay 1:
Immunoglobulin detection

To ANTI-MOUSE IgG plate:

- Add supernatants from culture
- Capture IgG
- Incubate, wash, and block with nonspecific mouse IgG
- Add Eu-labeled anti-analyte
- Incubate and wash

RESULT:

- Positives: *Anti-anti-analyte IgG*
- Negatives: Nonspecific IgG

FIGURE 19.2   Screening Assay 1.

Screening assay 2:
Anti-allotypic antibody detection

To ANTI-MOUSE IgG plate:

- Add supernatants giving a positive result in screening assay 1
- Capture IgG
- Block with nonspecific mouse IgG
- Add Eu-labeled irrelevant anti-ligand antibody belonging to the same heavy chain class as anti-analyte
- Incubate and wash

RESULT:

- Positives: *Anti-allotypic antibodies*
- Negatives: Betatypes and alphatypes

FIGURE 19.3   Screening Assay 2.

mouse IgG, europium-labeled anti-analyte ($\sim 10^7$ counts/ml) that previously had been incubated in the presence and absence of excess analyte (e.g., 50 ng/well) was added to the wells. Immobilized IgGs that failed to bind the europium-labeled anti-analyte in the presence of the analyte were classified as betatypic antibodies (see Fig. 19.4).

2.2.4. Screening Assay 4: Identification of Alphatypic Analyte-insensitive Anti-idiotypic Antibodies

The principle of this screening method is based on two-site epitope analysis that was performed for mapping the antigenic epitopes of human growth hormone (14). This screening procedure involved the binding of IgGs from the hybridomas that gave positive results in screening assay 3 (i.e., alphatypes, gammatypes, deltatypes) to rabbit anti-mouse coated plates. After blocking with nonspecific mouse IgG, europium-labeled anti-analyte that previously had been incubated in the presence and absence of culture supernatants from hybridomas secreting the strong betatypic antibodies identified in screening assay 3 was added to the microtiter plate. Immobi-

Screening assay 3:
Analyte sensitivity

To ANTI-MOUSE IgG plate:

- Add supernatants giving a positive result in screening assay 2
- Capture IgG
- Incubate, wash, and block with nonspecific mouse IgG
- Preincubate Eu-labeled anti-analyte with analyte
- Add complex
- Incubate and wash

RESULT:

- Positives: Anti-alphatypes, anti-gammatypes, anti-deltatypes, etc.
- Negatives: *Betatypes*

FIGURE 19.4   Screening Assay 3.

lized IgGs that failed to bind europium-labeled anti-analyte in the presence of betatype were identified as alphatypic antibodies (see Fig. 19.5).

2.2.5. Screening Assay 5: Epitope Analysis

In this procedure we investigated the interrelationship of the anti-idiotypic antibody binding sites on the surface of the primary antibody (Ab_1), using the two-site immunofluorometric assay (IFMA) principle. For this purpose, the anti-idiotypic antibodies identified as betatypes and alphatypes in screening assays 3 and 4 were propagated as ascites, purified on Sepharose–Protein A according to their subclass (9), and labeled with europium. Afterward, all possible combinations of these anti-idiotypic antibodies were used to construct a matrix of anti-idiotypic antibody combinations. An example is shown in Table 19.2. In this epitope study experiment, five anti-idiotypic antibodies against anti-estradiol, classified as betatypes ($1D_5$, $14H_{10}$) and as alphatypes ($14A_{10}$, $1D_7$, and $16E_9$) were utilized to construct a chessboard two-site IFMA of a 5 captured antibody × 5 europium-labeled matrix of anti-idiotypic antibody combinations. In this method, only a labeled anti-idiotypic antibody recognizing a different epitope on Ab_1 from the one recognized by the immobilized anti-idiotypic antibody, will give a positive signal, thus reflecting epitope disparity. If the labeled and the capture antibody recognize identical, overlapping, or sterically not compatible binding sites, the signal will be low or negligible.

When the data in Table 19.2 are examined, distinct patterns of binding can be distinguished, and the signals obtained varied significantly between the different combinations of antibodies. Thus, a very low signal was obtained with all combinations, of two identical antibodies (i.e., as capture and as labeled antibody). In addition, the epitope recognized by the betatypic antibody $1D_5$ overlaps with the epitope recognized with the betatypic antibody $14H_{10}$. In addition, the epitopes recognized by these betatypic antibodies ($14H_{10}$ and $1D_5$) are also recognized by the alphatypic antibody $1D_7$, resulting in a negligible signal. The data shown in Table 19.2 indicate that out of the three alphatypic antibodies $14A_{10}$, $16E_9$, and $1D_7$, only one clone—$1D_7$—because of epitope proximity, is sterically hindered from binding to the primary Ab_1 in the presence of betatype, and is thus suitable for the development of the idiometric assay. Accordingly, the use of three matched antibodies (primary antibody, alphatype, and betatype) has permitted the develop-

Screening assay 4:
Betatype sensitivity

To ANTI-MOUSE IgG plate:

- Add supernatants giving a positive result in screen 3
- Capture IgG
- Incubate, wash, and block with nonspecific mouse IgG
- Preincubate Eu-labeled anti-analyte with Betatypes identified in screen 3
- Add complex
- Incubate and wash

RESULT:

- Positives: Anti-gammatypes, anti-deltatypes, etc.
- Negatives: *Alphatypes*

FIGURE 19.5   Screening Assay 4.

TABLE 19.2 Epitope Analysis of Five Anti-idiotypic Antibodies against Anti-estradiol

Code of immobilized antibody	Code of the labeled anti-idiotypic antibody				
	$1D_5$	$1D_7$	$14A_{10}$	$14H_{10}$	$16E_9$
$1D_5$					
$+2F_9$	3,009	3,387	44,128	4,191	12,775
NSB	430	542	449	351	472
$1D_7$					
$+2F_9$	544	744	114,889	689	21,238
NSB	326	505	360	458	374
$14A_{10}$					
$+2F_9$	58,149	39,241	802	56,935	8,433
NSB	343	397	561	361	296
$14H_{10}$					
$+2F_9$	543	516	54,791	480	8,893
NSB	373	394	1,967	351	347
$16E_9$					
$+2F_9$	75,306	73,318	98,223	67,700	920
NSB	315	432	637	370	271

Note. Two-site time-resolved immunofluorometric assays (IFMAs) were used for the epitope analysis. Microtiter wells were coated with each monoclonal anti-idiotypic antibody (12 wells were used for every combination of immobilized and europium-labeled anti-idiotypic antibody). For each set of 12 wells, varying concentrations of idiotypic antibody No. $2F_9$ (200 μl, from 2.5 to 50 ng/well) were distributed into wells in duplicate (designated $+2F_9$), while the other two wells received only buffer (200 μl; designated NSB, nonspecific binding). The strips were incubated for 2 hr at room temperature, and washed. Subsequently, europium-labeled anti-idiotypic antibody (200 μl) was added to each set of 12 wells. After 2 hr incubation, the strips were washed, and the fluorescence was measured in an Arcus time-resolved fluorometer. The fluorescent signal obtained with only one concentration of $2F_9$ (10 ng) is given in the table. Note that the betatype antibodies, $1D_5$, $12B_{12}$, and $14H_{10}$, show identical patterns with the alphatype antibody, $1D_7$.

ment of a noncompetitive immunoassay method for determining antibody occupancy not based on the conventional two-site assay and appropriate for small molecules.

2.3. Development of Idiometric Assays

The availability of matched betatypic and alphatypic anti-idiotypic antibodies as well as primary antibody enabled the conception of a novel approach for the detection of antibody occupancy which we have termed idiometric assay (10). This novel method is suitable for the measurement of small molecules using noncompetitive technology. In this technique we investigated two different configurations: (a) labeled alphatype or (b) labeled primary antibody. In the labeled alphatype configuration (Fig. 19.6) the analyte is captured by the primary antibody which is adsorbed to a solid-phase matrix, creating occupied and unoccupied sites. The betatype anti-idiotypic antibody is then added to the unoccupied sites. In the third step of the reaction, the labeled alphatype is added to detect the sites occupied by the analyte only.

1. Capture of the analyte

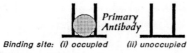

Binding site: *(i) occupied*   *(ii) unoccupied*

2. Betatype blocks unoccupied sites

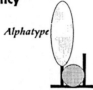

3. Alphatype detects antibody occupancy

Two assay configurations:
   1. Immobilised primary antibody and labelled alphatype
   2. Immobilised alphatype and labelled primary antibody

FIGURE 19.6   Principles of the idiometric assay.

In the labeled primary antibody format, a complex is formed between the labeled primary antibody, samples or standards, and the betatypic anti-idiotypic antibody. The complex is then added to alphatype-adsorbed microtiter plates. In this format the alphatype can be directly adsorbed to a solid-phase matrix or can be biotinylated and afterward incubated in avidin, or anti-biotin-coated plates, or with avidin-coated magnetic beads. The label on the primary antibody can be europium, or it can be an enzyme-labeled second antibody which reacts only with the allotypic epitopes of the primary antibody. In the following sections we shall give several examples for the development of idiometric assays for small molecules.

3. IDIOMETRIC ASSAYS FOR ESTRADIOL

3.1. Generation of Anti-idiotypic Antibodies against Anti-estradiol

In order to generate anti-idiotypic antibodies against anti-estradiol, Wistar-derived female rats were immunized with anti-estradiol IgG 15 (mouse–mouse hybridoma) whereas female CD_2 mice were immunized with monoclonal anti-estradiol IgG $2F_9$ (rat–mouse hybridoma). The spleen cells of the immunized rat or mouse were fused with mouse myeloma cells, and the culture supernatants of growing hybridomas were screened for antibody activity using the screening procedures described in Section 2.2. When the mouse–mouse hybridoma, clone 15, was used as an immunogen, only one clone ($1C_1$, alphatype) was obtained from the fusion experiment (see Table 19.3). On the other hand, when the rat–mouse hybridoma (clone $2F_9$) was used as an immunogen, the fusion experiment yielded 37 hybridomas that secreted antibodies against anti-estradiol (10). Of these, 8 demonstrated strong betatypic activity and 3 weak betatypic activity. From the 26 remaining hybridomas secreting anti-allotypic or alphatypic anti-idiotypic antibodies, four demonstrated alphatypic activity. One of the strong alphatypes (clone $1D_7$) and two of the strong betatypes (clone $1D_5$ and clone $14H_{10}$) were selected for the development of the idiometric assay (see Tables 19.2 and 19.3). Using these anti-idiotypic antibodies, we developed two different configurations, namely (i) labeled alphatype (10, 15–18) and (ii) labeled primary antibody for the measurement of serum estradiol in a noncompetitive manner.

3.2. Measurement of Serum Estradiol: Idiometric Assay Using Europium-Labeled Alphatype

In this procedure, affinity-purified anti-estradiol IgG was diluted in carbonate coating buffer (5 μg/ml) and 200 μl was added to the wells of polystyrene microtiter strips. After an overnight incubation at 4°C, the coating buffer was decanted, and the strips were washed twice with wash solution (10). The strips were then covered with a sealing tape and stored at 4°C until use.

Standards for estradiol (0–12,800 pmol/liter) were prepared by diluting a pooled serum (obtained from normal pregnant women) with hormone-free charcoal stripped serum. Twenty microliters of standard or sample was added in duplicate to the antibody-coated microtiter wells containing 100 μl of assay buffer. The binding reaction was performed at room temperature for 1 hr. Subsequently, the strips were washed and aspirated three times. Purified betatype (clone $14H_{10}$) was diluted 500-fold in assay buffer (10), 100 μl was added in duplicate to the microtiter wells, and binding reaction was performed at room temperature for 30 min with shaking. One hundred microliters of assay buffer containing a suitable dilution

TABLE 19.3 Characterization of Anti-idiotypic Antibodies to Anti-estradiol

Type of Anti-Id	Clone no.	Relative proximity of specific epitope to binding site
Immunogen: anti-estradiol-6–BSA (No. $2F_9$, rat–mouse hybridoma)		
Betatype	$1D_5^a$	At
	$12B_{12}$	At
	$14H_{10}^a$	At
Alphatype	$1D_7^a$	Close
	$15G_7$	Close
	$14A_{10}$	Near
	$16E_9$	Far
Allotype	$19B_{12}$	—
	$12A_3$	—
	$1B_4$	—
Immunogen: anti-estradiol-6–BSA (No. 15, mouse–mouse hybridoma)		
Alphatype	$1C_1$	—

[a] Selected for idiometric assay development, matching pair.

of europium-labeled alphatype (clone $1D_7$) was added, and the binding reaction continued for a further 2 hr. The strips were washed six times and 200 μl of enhancement solution was added to each well. The strips were agitated for 10 min and fluorescence was measured with the Arcus time-resolved fluorometer. The unknown values were derived from the calibration curves (signal vs concentration of estradiol, pmol/liter).

Calibration curves obtained at various dilutions of capture anti-estradiol antibody (clone $2F_9$) are shown in Fig. 19.7. The concentrations of serum estradiol were measured in 54 samples from patients attending an infertility clinic and compared with those by an extraction RIA with tritiated estradiol and dextran-coated charcoal separation. The linear regression equation was $y = 1.113x - 8.47$ (where y corresponds to the idiometric assay and x to RIA) with a correlation of $r = 0.97$.

3.3. Measurement of Serum Estradiol: Idiometric Assay Using Europium-Labeled Primary Antibody

A schematic diagram of the idiometric assay using the labeled primary antibody is shown in Fig. 19.8. In this procedure, the alphatype anti-idiotypic antibody (clone $1D_7$, see Table 19.3) was labeled with biotin (9), whereas the primary antibody was labeled with europium (10). As a capture antibody affinity-purified anti-biotin IgG (19) was diluted to 5 μg/ml in phosphate-buffered saline (PBS) and 200 μl was added to each well of polystyrene microtiter strips. After an overnight incubation

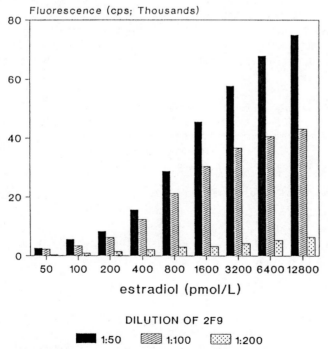

FIGURE 19.7   Effect of various dilutions of the capture antibody ($2F_9$) on the calibration curves for estradiol.

Step 1: Prepare assay tubes containing blockers, europium labeled primary antibody (clone 2F₉) and serum samples or standards

↓ Incubate 20 min

Step 2: Add betatype (clone 1D₅)

↓ Incubate 20 min

Step 3: Add 200 μl/well of this reaction mixture to anti-biotin coated microstrips which have been incubated for 1 hr with the biotinylated alphatype (clone # 1D₇) and subsequently washed

↓ a. Incubate 30 min
↓ b. Aspirate and wash 6 times

Step 4: Add 200 μl of enhancement solution/well.

↓ a. Shake the strips gently for 20 min.
↓ b. After 5 min measure fluorescence for 1 sec. in a time-resolved fluorometer.

FIGURE 19.8 A schematic diagram of the measurement of serum estradiol using the idiometric assay, europium-labeled primary antibody, and biotinylated alphatype.

at 4°C, the antibody solution was decanted from each well. The strips were blocked for 1 hr at room temperature with 0.3% ovalbumin in saline, washed twice with wash solution (10), and then covered with a sealing tape and stored at 4°C until use. Assay buffer-containing blockers was prepared by adding the displacing agents danazol and 5α-dihydrotestosterone at a concentration of 20 ng/ml and cortisol at 200 ng/ml to assay buffer (10). Estradiol standards (0–7000 pmol/liter) were prepared by using male sheep serum diluted 1:1 with assay buffer containing displacing agents. Serum samples were diluted 1:1 with assay buffer containing displacing agents and incubated at 37°C for 30 min. Standards in sheep serum or samples containing blockers (125 μl) were added to test tubes containing 375 μl of europium-labeled primary estradiol antibody (clone 2F₉, 1:5000 dilution) per tube. The reaction mixtures were incubated for 20 min and subsequently 30 μl of the betatype anti-idiotypic antibody (clone 1D₅, 1:50 dilution) was added to each test tube and the incubation was carried out for an additional 20 min. Two-hundred microliters of the reaction mixture was transferred to each well of an anti-biotin-coated microtiter strip which had been incubated for 1 hr with the biotinylated alphatype anti-idiotypic antibody (clone D₇, 100 ng/well) and subsequently washed twice. The binding reaction was performed for 30 min with shaking. The strips were then processed for time-resolved fluorescence as described in Section 3.2.

Compared to the labeled alphatype method, the labeled primary antibody method uses shorter incubation (60 to 90 min vs 4 hr). On the other hand, sensitivity (35 pmol/liter) of the two configurations is the same. The levels of serum estradiol were measured using the conditions described in Fig. 19.8 in 77 samples obtained from an infertility clinic, and compared with the values obtained by a direct RIA assay from Diagnostic Products Corporation (DPC). The linear regression equation was $y = 0.729x + 51.1$ (where y corresponds to the idiometric assay and x to RIA) with a correlation of $r = 0.96$.

4. IDIOMETRIC ASSAYS FOR PROGESTERONE

4.1. Generation of Anti-idiotypic Antibodies against Anti-progesterone

In order to generate anti-idiotypic antibodies against anti-progesterone, three different antibodies raised to three different progesterone conjugates were used as immunogens. When anti-progesterone-3–KLH conjugate was used as an immunogen, only allotypic anti-idiotypic antibodies were detected from the fusion experiment. On the other hand, when anti-progesterone-11–BSA (clone $1E_{11}$, mouse–mouse hybridoma (see Table 19.4)) was used to immunize Wistar-derived female rats, only alphatypic and allotypic anti-idiotypic antibodies were isolated from the fusion experiment (see Table 19.4). However, immunization of CD_2 mice with anti-progesterone-7–KLH conjugate and subsequent fusion of the immune cells with mouse myeloma cells yielded 40 hybridomas that secreted various types of anti-idiotypic antibodies against anti-progesterone. Of these, 3 demonstrated strong betatypic activity (see Table 19.4). From the remaining 37 hybridomas, 3 demonstrated alphatypic activity and the rest allotypic activity (see Table 19.4 and Fig. 19.9). One of the strong betatypes (clone $15F_{11}$) and the strong alphatype (clone $2E_{11}$) (see Table 19.4) were selected for the development of the idiometric assay for the noncompetitive measurement of serum progesterone.

TABLE 19.4 Characterization of Antibodies to Anti-progesterone

Type of Anti-Id	Clone no.	Relative proximity of specific epitope to binding site
Immunogen: anti-progesterone-11–BSA (clone No. $1E_{11}$)		
Alphatype	$3G_8$	Near
	$27A_6$	Far
Allotype	$18B_4$	—
	$18H_5$	—
	$27A_2$	—
Immunogen: anti-progesterone-7–BSA.KLH conjugate (clone No. $2H_4$)		
Betatype	$4E_2$	At
	$20C_3$	At
	$15F^a_{11}$	At
Alphatype	$2E^a_{11}$	Near
	$4F_4$	Close
	$14F_5$	Far
Allotype	$17H_{11}$	—
	$1A_{10}$	—
	$11G_{10}$	—

[a] Selected for idiometric assay development, matching pair.

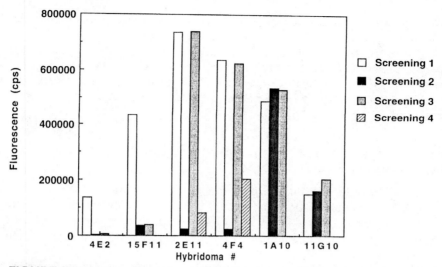

FIGURE 19.9 Screening results of antibody-secreting hybridomas derived from the fusion of mouse myeloma cells (NSO) with spleen cells of a mouse immunized with anti-progesterone-7–KLH conjugate. The antibody secreting hybridomas were screened according to the screening assays described in Section 2.2. (□) Screening Assay 1: Immunoglobulin detection. Total counts obtained when the hybridomas were screened for binding europium-labeled anti-progesterone-7–BSA (clone 2H$_4$). (■) Screening Assay 2: Anti-allotypic antibody detection. Counts obtained when the positive hybridomas from Screening Assay 1 were screened with an irrelevant europium-labeled antibody of the same isotype as anti-progesterone clone 2H$_4$. Note that hybridomas 1A$_{10}$ and 11G$_{10}$ gave positive results, indicating that these are allotypic anti-idiotypic antibodies. (▨) Screening Assay 3: Analyte sensitivity. The hybridomas that gave a negative result in Screening Assay 2 were screened in the presence or absence of excess progesterone (100 ng/well). Note that hybridomas 4E$_2$ and 15F$_{11}$ gave negative results, indicating that these are betatypic anti-idiotypic antibodies while hybridomas 2E$_{11}$ and 4F$_4$ gave positive results, indicating that these hybridomas are alphatypic anti-idiotypic antibodies. (▨) Screening Assay 4: Betatype sensitivity. The alphatypes (clones 2E$_{11}$ and 4F$_4$) identified in Screening Assay 3 were screened for epitope proximity to the paratope by testing their ability to bind to the primary antibody in the presence of the strong betatype 15F$_{11}$. Note that hybridoma 2E$_{11}$ gave a negligible signal in the presence of the betatype, while the signal obtained with hybridoma 4F$_4$ was significant. These results indicate that the epitopes of 2E$_{11}$ and 15F$_{11}$ are close to each other.

4.2. Measurement of Serum Progesterone: Idiometric Assay Using Europium-Labeled Primary Antibody

For the measurement of serum progesterone, using the labeled primary antibody method, we used the same conditions as those used for the estradiol assay (see Section 3.3). In this procedure, microtiter strips were adsorbed with anti-biotin IgG, blocked, and incubated for 1 hr with biotinylated alphatype (clone 2E$_{11}$, 100 ng/well). Serum samples were prepared by diluting them 1:1 with assay buffer containing displacing agents (see Section 3.3) and subsequently incubating them at 37°C for 30 min. Samples were sequentially reacted with europium-labeled primary antibody (clone 2H$_4$, 1:5000 dilution), followed with the betatype anti-idiotypic antibody (clone 15F$_{11}$, 1:500 dilution). The reaction mixtures were incubated for 40 min and then transferred to anti-biotin-coated strips which had been incubated with biotinylated alphatype. After a short incubation (30 min), the strips were processed for time-resolved fluorescence. Idiometric calibration curves obtained at various dilutions of betatype $15F_{11}$ are shown in Fig. 19.10.

The concentrations of serum progesterone were measured in 60 samples from patients attending an infertility clinic and compared to a direct radioimmunoassay from Diagnostic Products Corporation. The linear regression equation was $y = 0.773x + 0.229$ (where y corresponds to the idiometric assay and x to RIA) with a correlation of $r = 0.96$.

4.3. Measurement of Serum Progesterone: Idiometric Assay Using Europium-Labeled Alphatype

In this procedure affinity-purified anti-progesterone IgG (clone $2H_4$) was diluted in PBS (5 μg/ml) and 200 μl was added to the wells of polystyrene microtiter strips. After an overnight incubation at 4°C, the strips were blocked for 1 hr at room temperature with 0.3% ovalbumin in saline, washed, covered with a sealing tape, and stored at 4°C until use.

We used this configuration for measuring serum progesterone levels in ewes in order to detect ovulation. For this purpose, 25 μl of sample or standard were added in duplicate to the antibody-coated microtiter wells containing 100 μl of the betatype (clone $15F_{11}$, 1:500 dilution). The europium-labeled alphatype was diluted 10,000-fold in assay buffer, 100 μl was added in duplicate to the microtiter wells, and the binding reaction was performed at room temperature for 1 hr. The strips were then processed for time-resolved fluorescence. Representative calibration curves are shown in Fig. 19.11.

The concentration of progesterone was measured in serial plasma samples obtained from normal and hormone-treated ewes. The results were compared with those obtained by an extraction RIA with tritiated progesterone and dextran-coated

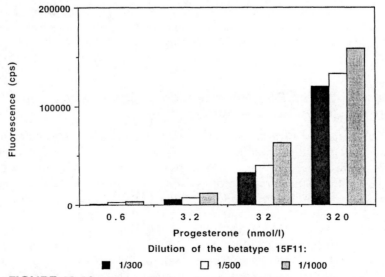

FIGURE 19.10   Idiometric assay for progesterone using labeled primary antibody: Effect of various dilutions of the betatype ($15F_{11}$) on the calibration curves.

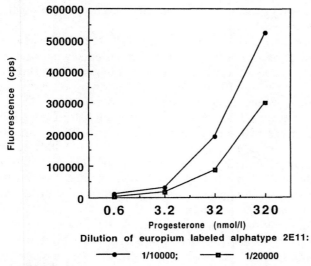

FIGURE 19.11 Idiometric assay for progesterone using labeled alphatype (2E$_{11}$): Effect of various dilutions of the labeled alphatype on the calibration curves.

charcoal separation. A good correlation was obtained between the two methods ($r = 0.95$).

5. CONCLUSIONS

In this chapter we have described the development of noncompetitive immunoassay procedures termed idiometric assays for small molecules as exemplified for estradiol and progesterone. The development of the idiometric assay has been achieved by the identification, production, and utilization of two types of anti-idiotypic antibodies induced by using the primary antibody as an immunogen. These anti-idiotypic antibodies identified as betatypes and alphatypes were selected by using a variety of screening procedures (see Figs. 19.2–19.5), and had the following characteristics:

5.1. Betatypes

These anti-idiotypic antibodies recognized an epitope at the unoccupied binding site (paratope). In addition, they were analyte sensitive and competed with the analyte for binding sites of the primary antibody. Indeed, the betatypes were used as labeled antigen in immunoassay procedures (11).

5.2. Alphatypes

These anti-idiotypic antibodies were selected on the basis that their epitopes were in close proximity to the paratope, and were unaffected by the presence or absence of the analyte. In particular, the alphatype identified for the idiometric assay could not bind to the primary antibody in the presence of the betatype due to steric hindrance (see Table 19.2).

The use of three matched antibodies (primary antibody, betatype, and alphatype) has enabled the development of a noncompetitive immunoassay method for small molecules (see Fig. 19.6). The method is an excess reagent assay, as shown by the calibration curves in Figs. 19.7, 19.10, and 19.11. The addition of excess betatype does not displace the analyte and ensures a low background.

The idiometric assays for estradiol and progesterone demonstrate good sensitivity and precision when compared with conventional direct competitive immunoassays. Since the idiometric assay is an excess reagent method, it is highly suitable for dipstick technology. In addition, the endpoint is highly flexible. The markers, the primary antibody, or the alphatype can be labeled with enzymes, radioisotopes, or fluorescent or chemiluminescent tags. Currently, we are producing reagents for the development of idiometric assays for the measurement of urinary estrone-3-glucuronide and pregnanediol-3α-glucuronide. We are also investigating the suitability of this approach for measuring large molecules (e.g., growth hormone). Interestingly, the anti-idiotypes raised against anti-estradiol IgG have been shown to bind to the estrogen receptor (20). This finding suggests that there may be structural homology between the binding site environment of antibody and the receptor.

Acknowledgments

We thank Mrs. B. Gayer, S. Lichter, J. Osher, Drs. S. Wade, D. Ayalon, and R. Limor for permission to quote collaborative work; Wallac Oz., Türkü, Finland, for the provision of equipment and reagents: Professor W.P. Collins and Dr. G. Carter for the provision of samples; and Mrs. M. Kopelowitz for excellent secretarial assistance. This work has been supported in part by the Institute of Reproductive Health, Georgetown University Medical School, Washington, DC, and the Special Programme of Research in Human Reproduction, the World Health Organization.

NOTE ADDED IN PROOF. Recently, Piran *et al.* and Self *et al.* devised new methods to measure small analytes with noncompetitive techniques (Piran, U., Riordan, W. J., Lirshin, L. A. New noncompetitive immunoassays for small analytes. Clin Chem 1995; 41:986–90; Self *et al.,* Clin Chem 1994; 40:2035–2041)

References

1. Yalow RS, Berson SA. Immunoassay for endogenous plasma insulin in man. J Clin Invest 1960 39:1157–75.
2. Ekins RP. The estimation of thyroxine in human plasma by an electrophoretic technique. Clin Chim Acta 1960; 5:453–9.
3. Ekins RP. More sensitive immunoassays. Nature 1980; 284:14–5.
4. Miles LEM, Hales CN. Labelled antibodies and immunological assay systems. Nature 1968 219:186–9.
5. Jackson TM, Ekins RP. Theoretical limitations on immunoassay sensitivity. J Immunol Methods 1986; 87:13–20.
6. Ekins RP. Current concepts and future developments. In: Collins WP, Ed. Alternative Immunoassays Chichester: Wiley, 1985:219–37.
7. Jerne NK, Rolan J, Cazenave PA. Recurrent idiotypes and internal images. EMBO J 1982; 1:243–7
8. Kohen F, Lichter S. Monoclonal antibodies to steroid hormones. In: Forti G, Lipsett MB, Eds Monoclonal Antibodies: Basic Principles, Experimental and Clinical Applications in Endocrinology New York: Raven Press, 1986:87–95.
9. Strasburger CJ, Kohen F. Biotinylated probes in immunoassay. In: Wilchek M, Bayer E, Eds. Methods in Enzymology, Vol. 184, Avidin-Biotin Technology. San Diego: Academic Press, 1990:481–96
10. Barnard G, Kohen F. Idiometric assay: A noncompetitive immunoassay for small molecules typified by the measurement of estradiol in serum. Clin Chem 1990; 36:1945–50.

11. Altamirano-Bustamante A, Barnard G, Kohen F. Direct time-resolved fluorescence immunoassay for serum oestradiol based on the idiotypic anti-idiotypic approach. J Immunol Methods 1991; 138:95–101.
12. Schick MR, Kennedy RC. Production and characterization of anti-idiotypic antibody reagents. In: Langone JJ, Ed. Methods in Enzymology, Vol. 178, Antibodies, Antigens and Molecular Mimicry. San Diego: Academic Press, 1989:36–48.
13. Köhler G, Milstein C. Continuous cultures of fused cells secreting antibody of pre-defined specificity. Nature 1975; 256:495–7.
14. Strasburger CJ, Kostyo J, Vogel T, Barnard GJ, Kohen F. The antigenic epitopes of human growth hormone as mapped by monoclonal antibodies. Endocrinology 1989; 124:1548–57.
15. Barnard G, Karsilayan H, Kohen F. Idiometric assay: The third way: A non-competitive immunoassay for the measurement of small molecules. Am J Obstet Gynecol 1992; 165:1997–2000.
16. Karsilayan H, Kohen F. Barnard G. The development of sensitive time-resolved fluorescence immunoassays for the measurement of oestradiol in serum. Com Lab Med 1992; 2:39–47.
17. Barnard G, Mor G, Amir-Zaltsman Y, Kohen F. Idiometric assay, anti-idiotypes and molecular mimicry. Com Lab Med 1992; 3:57–62.
18. Barnard G, Karsilayan H, Kohen F. Immunoassay: Current concepts and key problems. In: Advances in Hospital Technology. 1992; 1:20–26.
19. Bagçi H, Kohen F, Kusçuoglu U, Bayer EA, Wilchek M. Monoclonal anti-biotin antibodies stimulate avidin in the recognition of biotin. FEBS Lett 1993; 322:47–50.
20. Mor G, Amir Zaltsman Y, Barnard G, Kohen F. Characterization of an antiidiotypic antibody mimicking the actions of estradiol and its interaction with estrogen receptors. Endocrinology 1992; 130:3633–40.

20 | FREE HORMONE MEASUREMENTS

GYORGY CSAKO
Clinical Chemistry Service
Clinical Pathology Department
W. G. Magnuson Clinical Center
National Institutes of Health
Bethesda, Maryland

Immunoassay

1. INTRODUCTION

1.1. Definition of Free Hormones

The term "free hormone" is used at least in three different contexts in body fluids (Table 20.1). First, this term is used to describe unconjugated hormones, that is, hormones not coupled covalently to glucuronic or sulfuric acid. Examples include "free" steroids (e.g., free cortisol, androstanediol, and testosterone in urine and free estriol in serum) and free catecholamines (e.g., free epinephrine, norepinephrine, and dopamine in urine). Second, the term free hormone may refer to the nonprotein bound fraction of thyroid, steroid, and secosteroid[1] hormones. It is this context in which the term free hormone will be used in this chapter. Third, the term free hormone also is used to describe the non-(anti-insulin)antibody-bound fraction of plasma insulin. This distinction is of obvious importance in diabetics receiving heterologous insulin preparations such as pork or beef insulin, but it will not be further discussed here.

Based on the above definitions, unconjugated and non-protein-bound hormones appear to be clearly distinguished, but it is important to point out that these categories of hormones may readily overlap in biological specimens. On one hand, conju-

---

[1] In secosteroid compounds, one ring of the steroid structure is opened by breaking a bond within it (Latin *sec*[are], to cut). Secosteroids are exemplified by two families of vitamin D, namely, cholecalciferols or vitamin D_3 and ergocalciferols or vitamin D_2, in which ring B of the steroid skeleton is broken.

TABLE 20.1   Two Principal Types of Free Hormone Assays[a,b]

I. Unconjugated ("free") hormone assays	II. Non-protein-bound or unbound free hormone assays
Aldosterone (urine)[c]	Aldosterone (saliva)[c]
Cortisol (Compound F) (urine)[c]	Cortisol (Compound F)
Dehydroepiandrosterone (DHEA)[c]	Cortisol (Compound F) (saliva)[c]
11-Deoxycorticosterone (DOC)	Dihydrotestosterone-5α (DHT)[c]
Dopamine (urine)	1,25-Dihydroxyvitamin D
Epinephrine (urine)	Estradiol-17β (E$_2$)
Estradiol-17α	Estradiol-17β (E$_2$) (saliva)[c]
Estriol (E$_3$)	Estriol (E$_3$) (saliva)
Estrone (E$_1$)	Estrone (E$_1$) (saliva)
18-Hydroxycortisol (urine)	17-Hydroxyprogesterone
Norepinephrine (urine)	25-Hydroxyvitamin D
Testosterone[c]	Progesterone[c]
Progesterone (urine)[c]	Progesterone (saliva)
	Testosterone[c]
	Testosterone (saliva)[c]
	Thyroxin
	Triiodothyronine

[a] List does not include free insulin, a non-anti-insulin antibody-bound peptide hormone that represents the third type of "free" hormones.
[b] All free hormones refer to serum (plasma) unless indicated otherwise.
[c] The laboratory performing the test is listed in Ref. (1).

gated hormones, like their unconjugated counterparts, obviously can also be both free and protein bound. For instance, steroid sulfates such as dehydroepiandrosterone sulfate (DHEA-S) bind with high affinity to albumin. On the other hand, in physiologically protein-poor specimens (e.g., saliva, urine), the hormones are present almost in their entirety in the free hormone pool, and hence the concentration of total and free (non-protein-bound) hormones in these specimens may be virtually identical (2–4).

1.2. Current Issues Regarding Free Hormones

There are intriguing similarities among thyroid, steroid, and secosteroid hormones[1] in that they all are transported by specific binding proteins in the plasma[2,3] and have a similar mechanism of action (see Section 2.3). Because of recent technical

[2] Melatonin (N-acetyl-5-methoxytryptamine), a derivative of serotonin, may also be added to this list. Melatonin is postulated to be a hormone of the pineal gland opposing the action of melanocyte-stimulating hormone (MSH) in amphibia, but its physiologic role and mechanism of action are not well defined in man. About 60% of this lipid-soluble indoleamine circulates bound to albumin, while the remaining 40% is free (dialyzable). However, no specific, high-affinity binding globulin has been found for melatonin in humans.

[3] Many drugs (e.g., phenytoin, propranolol, imipramine, valproic acid) circulate bound to proteins, often in excess of 90%, in the blood. Acidic drugs are bound primarily to albumin, whereas basic drugs primarily to globulins, particularly α-1-acid glycoprotein (AAG, orosomucoid). Similar to thyroid, steroid, and secosteroid hormones, an equilibrium exists between free and protein-bound drugs. Likewise, it is widely accepted that only the free (nonprotein bound) drug in the plasma is active pharmacologically. Thus, the issues regarding the measurements of free drug concentrations are rather similar to those of free hormone measurements.

advancements, the determination of the free (i.e., non-protein-bound) form of these hormones in serum and other body fluids is increasingly common in both basic research and clinical practice. However, the ready availability of mostly free thyroxin (FT4) and, to a lesser extent, free triiodothyronine (FT3) and free testosterone (FTe) hormone determinations during the last decade generated a great debate on both the physiological role of free hormones and the validity of the methods used to measure them (5–15). Controversial issues regarding free hormones thus include both (a) theoretical (research) implications (basic endocrinology), and (b) practical (diagnostic) consequences (clinical endocrinology).

Since the clinical use of free hormone measurements assumes the validity of the free hormone hypothesis, the experimental and clinical evidence for and against this hypothesis will be discussed in this chapter. In addition, the alternative concept according to which the large protein-bound moiety of plasma hormones also is available for transport into tissues will be reviewed. Then, the issue of free hormone methodology will be addressed. A great variety of techniques are now available for routine use, but the verification of true free hormone assays remains difficult. Unjustifiably, the validity of the free hormone hypothesis often is assumed in the evaluation of these assays. Also, there is a continuing controversy regarding technical questions. The most popular methods (the so-called "one-step" assays) use hormone analogs. However, based on theoretical considerations and experimental evidence, the validity of these methods has been seriously questioned in the late 1980s.

2. OVERVIEW OF THYROID, STEROID, AND SECOSTEROID HORMONES

2.1. Chemistry

The chemical structures of representative thyroid, steroid, and secosteroid hormones are shown in Fig. 20.1. Because of their hydrophobic structure, unconjugated forms of these hormones are either poorly soluble or insoluble in water and require organic solvents such as alcohols, chloroform, ethylacetate, and dioxane for solubilization. Differential solubility of conjugated and unconjugated (free) steroids is routinely used for extraction of the free fraction by organic solvents, for instance, from urine specimens.

2.2. Physiology

The plasma half-life of thyroid, steroid, and secosteroid hormones ranges from a few minutes (most steroid hormones) through hours (cortisol, 1,25-dihydroxyvitamin D) and days (T3, vitamin D) to weeks (T4, 25-hydroxyvitamin D). These hormones regulate a wide variety of essential biological functions. The thyroid hormones primarily affect tissue metabolism. The glucocorticoids (e.g., cortisol) influence growth and development; further, they regulate tissue carbohydrate, lipid and protein metabolism, central nervous system activity, circulatory and renal function, immune response, and bone metabolism. The mineralocorticoids (e.g., aldosterone) maintain the intravascular volume by conserving sodium and eliminating

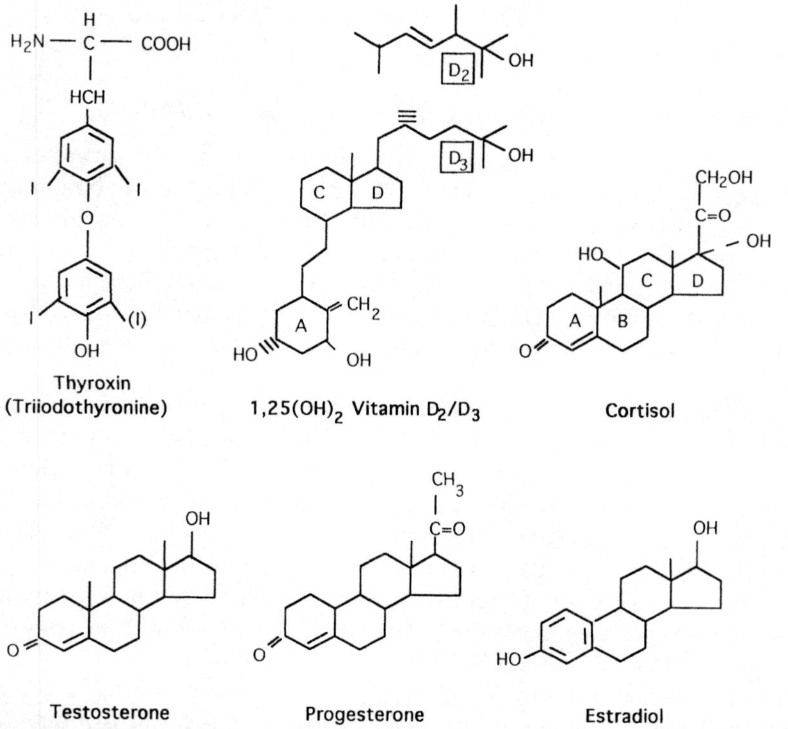

FIGURE 20.1 The chemical structure of selected thyroid, steroid, and secosteroid hormones for which free hormone assays have been developed and clinically evaluated.

potassium and hydrogen ions. The biological effect of glucocorticoids and mineralocorticoids, however, often overlaps and a sharp distinction between these steroids is inappropriate. The gonadal (sex) steroids (e.g., estradiol, progesterone, testosterone) have profound effects on genital and extragenital tissues and are essential for normal sexual development and reproduction. The biologically active 1,25-dihydroxy forms of vitamin D are true hormones that are intimately involved in calcium and phosphate metabolism.

2.3. General Mechanism of Hormonal Action

In the target cells, the thyroid and steroid hormones and vitamin D all exert their biological effect through nuclear receptor protein binding (16). First, they form an activated hormone–nuclear receptor protein complex that, after binding with specific DNA sequences, alters the expression of hormone-responsive genes. It is significant that not all tissues express all nuclear receptor proteins. If a receptor for a particular hormone is lacking from a given tissue, that hormone will be unable to act on that tissue. Different hormones such as steroids appararently share biological activities because of their ability to bind to the same receptor. The relative affinity of these hormones for each receptor determines their relative biological activity.

3. TRANSPORT OF THYROID, STEROID, AND SECOSTEROID HORMONES IN THE BLOOD

3.1. Thermodynamic Equilibrium and the Law of Mass Action

In the bloodstream, the thyroid, steroid and secosteroid hormones are extensively bound to a set of plasma proteins (Tables 20.2 and 20.3). A thermodynamic equilibrium, which depends on the production and clearance rates of hormones and on the binding properties of transport proteins, exists between the protein-bound and free (dialyzable/ultrafilterable) concentrations. The hormone binding to transport proteins is mediated by hydrophobic forces and hydrogen bonds. The resultant noncovalently bound stoichiometric complexes increasingly dissociate with rising temperature.

Individual hormone molecules constantly oscillate between the free and protein-bound pools. For instance, the dissociation half-lives of thyroxin-binding globulin (TBG), prealbumin or transthyretin (TTR), and albumin for T4 are about 39, 7.4, and <1 sec, respectively. For these, Ekins (15) estimated that individual T4 molecules in normal human serum remain free for periods of about 1.25 msec or less before rebinding for intervals of about 6.25 sec. Further, he concluded that if all FT4 molecules were suddenly removed from the blood (as may happen during capillary transit), the free thyroxin (FT4) concentration would be restored to its original level within 3 to 4 msec (15).

At the state of equilibrium, the distribution of hormone between the free and protein-bound pools is governed by the Law of Mass Action. Robbins and Rall (17) were the first to mathematically describe free hormone concentration (namely, free thyroid hormone concentration) in terms of this law. According to the Law of Mass Action, the free hormone concentration in the presence of binding proteins is defined by summation of all the factors tending to generate free hormone divided by a summation of all the factors opposing this process. In case of T4 and its three major plasma binding proteins (see Section 3.2), the free thyroxin (FT4) concentration at equilibrium is defined by

$$[FT4] = \frac{[TBG\text{-}T4] + [TTR\text{-}T4] + [Alb\text{-}T4]}{K_{TBG\text{-}T4}\,[fTBG] + K_{TTR\text{-}T4}\,[fTTR] + K_{Alb\text{-}T4}\,[fAlb]} \tag{1}$$

where the brackets signify (molar) concentration, FT4 is free (non-protein-bound) T4, TBG–T4 is TBG binding T4 (i.e., bound TBG), TTR–T4 is transthyretin (prealbumin) binding T4 (i.e., bound TTR), Alb–T4 is albumin binding T4 (i.e., bound albumin), $K_{TBG\text{-}T4}$ is the affinity constant of TBG for T4, $K_{TTR\text{-}T4}$ is the affinity constant of TTR for T4, $K_{Alb\text{-}T4}$ is the affinity constant of albumin for T4, fTBG is TBG not binding T4 (i.e., free TBG = unoccupied binding sites on TBG), fTTR is TTR not binding T4 (i.e., free TTR $\approx$ unoccupied binding sites on TTR), and fAlb is albumin not binding T4 (i.e., free albumin $\approx$ unoccupied binding sites on albumin).

Assuming that (a) in the state of equilibrium, the concentration of T4 bound to the three major plasma transport proteins approximates the total T4 concentration (i.e., both the FT4 concentration and the T4 binding to other proteins are negligible), and (b) the concentration of unoccupied binding sites on both TTR and albumin can be replaced by the plasma concentration of these proteins, Eq. (1) can be

TABLE 20.2 Principal Thyroid, Steroid, and Secosteroid Hormone-Binding Proteins in Human Plasma[a]

Hormone-binding protein	Molecular weight[b]	Number of hormone-binding sites per molecule[c]	% Binding sites normally occupied	Serum (plasma) concentration (SI units)		Half-life ($t_{1/2}$) in plasma (days)
				μmol/liter	mg/liter	
Albumin	68,000 (64,000–69,000)	6	?	515–735	35,000–50,000	15–19
Transthyretin (TTR) or thyroxin-binding prealbumin (TBPA)	55,000 (50,000–62,000)	2 (1)[d]	?	1.818–7.273	100–400	0.5–2
Thyroxin-binding globulin (TBG)	54,000 (54,000–60,000)	1	30–50	0.278–0.630	15–34	5
Transcortin or corticosteroid-binding globulin (CBG)	52,000 (50,000–58,200)	1	~50	M: 0.362–0.485 F: 0.286–0.440	18.8–25.2 14.9–22.9	?5
Sex hormone-binding globulin (SHBG) or testosterone/estradiol-binding globulin (TeBG)	104,000 (dimer) (98,000–118,000)	2	~50	M: 0.0056–0.0453 F: 0.0113–0.0737	0.59–4.72 1.18–7.67	5
Vitamin D-binding protein (DBP) or group-specific component (Gc globulin)	51,000 (51,000–58,000)	1	2–5	7.843	400	2.5

[a] Abbreviations: M, male; F, (nonpregnant) female.
[b] Molecular weight used for calculating molar concentration in serum is given first, followed by the range reported in the literature in parentheses.
[c] Total hormone-binding sites in plasma = number of hormone-binding sites per molecule × molar concentration of binding protein.
[d] Because of "negative cooperativity," usually only one of the available two binding sites is occupied.

TABLE 20.3 Free (Non-Protein-Bound) and Protein-Bound Thyroid, Steroid, and Secosteroid Hormones[a]

Hormone	% Free	Serum (plasma) concentration of free hormone	% Bound to plasma transport proteins					
			TTR	Albumin	TBG	CBG	SHBG[b]	DBP[c]
Thyroid hormones								
Thyroxin (T4)[d]	0.03	10.3–29.7 pmol/liter	10–20	8–20	70–80			
Triiodothyronine (T3)[d]	0.3	4.0–7.4 pmol/liter	5–25	5–35	40–90			
Reverse T3 (rT3)			√	√	√			
Glucocorticoids								
Cortisol (Hydrocortisone)[d,e]	3–10	17–44 nmol/liter (8am) 6–25 nmol/liter (16pm) 4–28 nmol/liter (7am)[f] 2–6 nmol/liter (22pm)[f]		5–15		75–90		
11-Deoxycorticosterone (DOC)	4			36		60		
Corticosterone	3–5			19–23		71–78		
Mineralocorticoids								
18-Hydroxycorticosterone								
Aldosterone[d]	28–37	<0.22 nmol/liter (saliva)		42–47		17–30		
Sex (gonadal) steroids								
Progesterone[e]	2–10	M: <1.6 nmol/liter F: <1.6 nmol/liter M: <0.02 nmol/liter (saliva) F: 0.02–0.38 nmol/liter (saliva)		80		17		
17-Hydroxyprogesterone				√				√

Compound		Concentration			
Dehydroepiandrosterone			√		√
Δ^4 Androstenedione	√	0.35–0.87 nmol/liter (saliva)	√		None
Δ^5 Androstenediol					
Testosterone[e]	M: 1.0–3.2[g] / F: 0.5–1.9 / PF: 0.2	M: 174–972 pmol/liter / F: 6–22 pmol/liter / PF: 8 pmol/liter	M: 40–67 / F: 18–45 / PF: 3	2–3.5 / 2–3.5	M: 33–58 / F: 55–81 / PF: 97
Dihydrotestosterone	0.5–0.9	M: 17.2–52.0 pmol/liter / F: 1.0–7.6 pmol/liter	39		60
Estrone (E$_1$)	M: 3.4		√		None
Estradiol (E$_2$)	F: 2.2–2.6	M: <1.8–2.0 pmol/liter / F: 1.8–13.2 pmol/liter	M: 79 / F: 59	M: 0.08 / F: 0.02	M: 21 / F: 38–41
Estriol (E$_3$)	11–14				
Secosteroids					
1,25-Dihydroxy-vitamin D	0.4	36–144 pmol/liter	10–15		
25-Hydroxy-vitamin D	0.03	25–125 nmol/liter	10–15		

---

[a] Abbreviations/Symbols: M, male; F, (nonpregnant) female; PF, pregnant female; √, percent binding is not available. For other abbreviations see Table 20.2.

[b] The relative binding affinity of SHBG for various steroid hormones: dihydrotestosterone > testosterone > androstenediol > estradiol > estrone.

[c] The relative binding affinity of DBP for various vitamin D structures ($D_3 > D_2$ by a factor of about 2): 25(OH)-D = 24,25(OH)$_2$-D = 25,26(OH)$_2$-D > 1,25(OH)$_2$-D ≫ vitamin D.

[d] A fraction also is bound to human red blood cells.

[e] A fraction also is bound to α_1-acid glycoprotein (AAG, orosomucoid).

[f] Saliva.

[g] In males, the free testosterone fraction peaks around 2% at the age of 20–25 years, then declines with age to about 1.3% by the age of 70–85 years.

greatly simplified. However, even this simplified equation requires knowledge of the free TBG concentration:

$$[FT4] = \frac{[\text{total T4}]}{K_{\text{TBG-T4}}[\text{fTBG}] + K_{\text{TTR-T4}}[\text{total TTR}] + K_{\text{Alb-T4}}[\text{total Alb}]} \quad (2)$$

Since the introduction of the first mathematical model for the distribution of T4, several theoretical descriptions have been published for both thyroid and steroid hormones. The newer models, though all derived from the Law of Mass Action, take into account a more complex view of hormone binding by plasma proteins (e.g., multiple interactive sites on the same binding protein like TTR for thyroid hormones, secondary binding sites on albumin, multiple competing ligands for the same binding site) (13, 18–25). Because of the great complexity of these newer models, the calculations often require computer modeling (e.g., using a program like LIGAND and TRANSPORT) (21, 25).

3.2. Biochemistry of Plasma Hormone-Binding (Transport) Proteins

The main hormone-binding (transport) proteins in plasma include albumin, TTR, and specific globulins such as thyroxin (or, more correctly, iodothyronine)-binding globulin (TBG), corticosteroid-binding globulin or transcortin (CBG), sex hormone (testosterone/estradiol)-binding globulin (SHBG), and vitamin D-binding protein (DBP) (Table 20.2) (26–33). Although all hormone-binding globulins were initially discovered extracellularly, many (e.g., CBG, SHBG, DBP) are now known to exist in a cell membrane-bound form as well. Minor hormone transport proteins in the plasma include but are not limited to α_1-acid glycoprotein (AAG or orosomucoid) for the binding of certain steroids, principally progesterone, and various lipoproteins and apolipoproteins. High-density lipoprotein (HDL) and apolipoprotein A-I bind thyroid hormones (27), whereas chylomicron remnants and low-density lipoprotein (LDL) bind dietary vitamin D (29). As to the extent of binding, lipoproteins, for instance, bind only 3 to 6% of total thyroid hormones (27). All major and most minor plasma hormone-binding proteins are synthesized primarily by the liver. However, TTR is also actively synthesized by the choroid plexus epithelial cells in the brain, and chylomicrons normally are formed in the intestinal epithelium.

Besides plasma proteins, human red blood cells also are involved in the binding (and metabolism) of hormones such as thyroxin, cortisol and testosterone. *In vivo* cortisol binding to human red blood cells, for example, approximates the sum of the unbound (free) and albumin-bound fractions. The hormone binding to red blood cells not only is important for theoretical considerations but also has direct diagnostic applications. This was the basis for the design of the first T3 uptake test (see Section 8.11). Hormone binding and metabolism by red blood cells also explain why, after blood collection, rapid separation of plasma from cells is required if accurate total steroid hormone measurements is expected. Red blood cells not only bind but also degrade cortisol to cortisone and estradiol to estrone.

Most thyroid, steroid and secosteroid transport proteins in the plasma have been characterized chemically and structurally. Using molecular biology techniques, the origin, chromosomal localization, sequence, organization, and regulation of several transport protein genes also have been elucidated (28–32). Apart from albumin and TTR, all major hormone-binding globulins are glycoproteins, containing 10–45%

carbohydrate by weight (28–33). Although various transport proteins may be composed of one (e.g., albumin, TBG, CBG), two (e.g., SHBG), or four (e.g., TTR) polypeptide chains, they are all folded into complex three-dimensional structures, often stabilized by intrachain disulfide bonds, to form the hormone-binding site(s).

3.3. Hormone-Binding Capacity, Affinity, and Specificity of Transport Proteins

The plasma transport proteins differ widely in their plasma concentration, affinity, and specificity for various hormones (Tables 20.2, 20.3 and 20.4) (26–33). Interestingly, there is no truly specific binding protein for progesterone. Also noteworthy is that because of the lack of a 17β-hydroxy group, androstenedione and estrone do not bind to SHBG (Table 20.3). Under physiologic conditions, albumin is a low-affinity but high-capacity carrier protein, whereas TTR and the specific globulins are high-affinity but relatively low-capacity carriers (Tables 20.2 and 20.3). While normally only 2 to 5% of the binding sites are occupied by hormone on DBP and only 30 to 50% of the binding sites are occupied by hormone on TBG, CBG, and SHBG (Table 20.2), 80 to 85% of total 1,25-dihydroxyvitamin D, 77% of total T4, 70 to 80% of total cortisol, and 33 to 97% of total testosterone are located on their respective high-affinity carrier globulins (Table 20.3). The T4- and/or T3-binding capacity of various thyroid hormone-binding proteins is measured for recognizing abnormalities in their binding affinity (e.g., Familial Dysalbuminemic Hyperthyroxinemia, FDH), plasma concentration, and type (e.g., anti-T4/T3-autoantibodies). In this assay, the fractional radioactivity is determined in electrophoretically separated binding proteins which, prior to analysis, have been saturated with radiolabeled T4 or T3.

On one hand, hormone transport proteins may possess exquisitely high specificity. For instance, TBG is stereospecific for T4 and binds only L-T4, whereas albumin binds both L-T4 and D-T4. On the other hand, though all transport proteins display characteristic hormone-binding profiles, the specificity of even the more specialized

TABLE 20.4 **Equilibrium Association Constants (K_a) of Various Thyroid, Steroid, and Secosteroid Hormones in Normal Human Serum at 37°C**

				K_a (liter/mol)			
	TTR[a]	Albumin	TBG	CBG	SHBG	DBP
Thyroxin (T4)	5×10^7	$0.5–1 \times 10^6$	2×10^{10}			
Triiodothyronine (T3)	2×10^7	1×10^6	2×10^8			
Reverse T3 (rT3)	?	2×10^6	2×10^9			
Cortisol		3×10^3		$3–8 \times 10^7$		
Corticosterone		1×10^4		8×10^7		
Aldosterone		$0.2–5 \times 10^4$		$0.2–4 \times 10^7$		
Progesterone		6×10^4		2×10^7		
Dihydrotestosterone		$3–4 \times 10^4$			3×10^9	
Testosterone		$3–4 \times 10^4$		0.5×10^7	1×10^9	
Estradiol		$3–6 \times 10^4$			$1–5 \times 10^8$	
1,25-Dihydroxyvitamin D3						4×10^7

[a] For abbreviations see Table 20.2.

binding globulins is never limited to a single hormone molecule (27–33). They all carry, with different affinities, structurally related hormones and their derivatives (e.g., TBG binds all T4, T3, and rT3 and SHBG binds a number of gonadal steroid hormones and their derivatives) (Tables 20.3 and 20.4).

The hormone-binding proteins also are multifunctional in the sense that they all transport substance(s) other than hormones. For illustration, the following is only a short sample of known interactions. In addition to transporting hormones, albumin, TBG, CBG, SHBG, and DBP all bind and carry free fatty acids. Albumin also is involved in the binding and transport of a wide variety of other endogenous (e.g., bilirubin) and exogenous substances (e.g., drugs). Besides carrying vitamin D and free fatty acids (FFA), DBP interacts with high affinity with G-actin, and also binds gram-negative endotoxin and a synthetic polyanionic antigen. TTR not only transports thyroid hormones, but also is capable of binding one molecule of retinol-binding protein (RBP), which, in turn, complexes with vitamin A. Besides binding progesterone, AAG is a known carrier of drugs like propranolol and lidocaine.

Obviously, if the same or nearby sites are involved in binding, either structurally related hormones and hormone derivatives or interfering nonhormonal substances will compete with a particular hormone for those binding site(s) on transport proteins, and may affect the equilibrium between this hormone and its binders in the blood. In the presence of unusually high concentrations of competing compounds, elevated free hormone concentrations may ensue. This phenomenon has been exploited for the measurement of total hormone concentrations *in vitro*. Addition of high enough concentrations of salicylates or 8-anilino-1-naphthalene-sulfonic acid (ANS) to plasma results in virtually complete displacement of thyroid and steroid hormones from high-affinity binding sites on TBG and CBG, respectively, making them accessible to direct analysis (e.g., reaction with assay antibodies). The low-affinity albumin-binding sites usually do not interfere with the measurement of total hormones. Barbital buffers (barbital ions) are used to prevent the binding of thyroid hormones to TTR during assay.

3.4. Effects of Hormone Binding by Transport Proteins

Because of their high hormone-binding capacity under physiological conditions, changes in the affinity and plasma concentration of transport proteins profoundly affect the respective total plasma hormone concentrations. These effects are particularly well documented for thyroid hormones and some steroids such as cortisol, estrogens and testosterone.

Although diseases may decrease the hormone-binding affinity of transport proteins, this change usually is genetically determined (26, 28–33). A number of variant transport proteins with decreased or increased binding affinity to the respective hormones (e.g., FDH) and the genetic "aberrations" underlying these anomalies have been described (Table 20.5) (26, 28–33). It is important, however, to emphasize that not all molecular variants possess altered hormone-binding affinity. Familial increases and decreases in the plasma concentration of transport proteins have also been reported (Table 20.5) (26, 28–33). However, variations in the concentration of transport proteins most commonly occur due to other endogenous causes, such as hormonal changes associated with growth and pregnancy or other acquired conditions such as disease and ingestion of drugs. Reduced plasma albumin and TTR concentrations are among the most common laboratory abnormalities during

TABLE 20.5 Inherited Abnormalities in the Affinity and/or Plasma Concentration of Major Thyroid, Steroid, and Secosteroid-Hormone-Binding Proteins[a]

Hormone-binding protein	Abnormality	Mode of genetic transmission
Albumin	Increase affinity for thyroid hormones: Familial Dysalbuminemic Hyperthyroxinemia (FDH) (relatively common)	Autosomal dominant
	Increased affinity for T4 only (Type I)[b]	
	T4 and rT3 (Type II)	
	T4, T3, and rT3 (Type III)	
	? T3 only (?Type IV)	
	Decreased concentration:	?
	Complete deficiency: analbuminemia (rare)	
TTR	Increased affinity for T4 (and rT3) (relatively common)	Autosomal (dominant)
	Decreased affinity for T4 (rare)	?
	Increased plasma concentration (rare)	?
	Decreased plasma concentration (rare)	?
TBG	Decreased affinity (common)	X-linked
	e.g., TBG-A (~40% of Australian Aborigines)	
	Increased plasma concentration (relatively common)	X-linked
	Decreased plasma concentration:	X-linked
	Partial deficiency—several variants (common) e.g., TBG-A (~40% of Australian Aborigines), TBG-S, TBG-San Diego	
	Complete deficiency: TBG-CD with variants (rare)	
CBG	Increased plasma concentration (rare)	?
	Decreased plasma concentration:	Autosomal codominant
	Partial deficiency (relatively common—heterozygotes only). ? Complete deficiency (single unconfirmed case)	
SHBG	Decreased plasma concentration:	?
	? Complete deficiency (single unconfirmed case)	
DBP[c]	?	?

[a] For abbreviations see Table 20.2.
[b] May be combined with increased affinity of TTR for T4.
[c] Three common genetic variants that are responsible for 6 common phenotypes and 124 other variants have been reported. The relationship of these variants to hormone binding is, however, not known.

serious acute and chronic illnesses, including malnutrition. Common causes of altered concentrations of major hormone transport globulins are listed in Table 20.6.

Besides affecting total hormone concentrations in the plasma, protein binding of hormones may produce a variety of biological effects (9, 11, 13, 15, 27–34). Although some effects are controversial, it was proposed that this binding:

(a) may enhance the solubility of hormones in biological fluids and facilitate the diffusion of hydrophobic compounds through the capillary endothelium;

(b) may facilitate uniform cellular distribution of hormones;

(c) may limit urinary loss by imparting macromolecular properties to the small hormone molecules;

(d) may protect hormones from hepatic degradation and, hence, may increase their plasma half-lives ($t_{1/2}$);

(e) provides a large reservoir of circulating hormone, which compensates for sudden changes in hormone utilization and synthesis and maintains the free hormone concentration;

TABLE 20.6   Common Acquired Causes of Altered Plasma Concentration of Major Thyroid, Steroid, and Secosteroid-Binding Globulins[a]

Increase	Decrease
	TBG
Estrogens (pregnancy, oral contraceptives, other drugs, cirrhosis of the liver, etc.)	Androgens (testosterone, oxymetholone)
	Thyroid hormones (hyperthyroidism, drugs)
Carbamazepine	Glucocorticoids
Phenothiazines (perphenazine)	Anabolic steroids (stanozolol)
5-Fluorouracil	L-Asparaginase
Clofibrate	Danazol
Methadone	Protein malnutrition (chronic illness)
Heroin	Nephrotic syndrome (protein loss)
Acute intermittent porphyria	Propranolol
	Phenytoin
	Colestipol
	CBG
Estrogens (pregnancy, oral contraceptives, other drugs, cirrhosis of the liver)	Anabolic steroids (stanozolol)
	Danazol
Tamoxifen	Nephrotic syndrome (protein loss)
Thyroid hormones (hyperthyroidism, drugs)	Hypothyroidism
Diabetes mellitus	Obesity
Phenytoin	Glucocorticoids (Cushing's, drugs)
	Septic shock
	High-carbohydrate diet
	Pernicious anemia
	Multiple myeloma
	Liver disease
	SHBG
Estrogens (pregnancy, oral contraceptives, other drugs, luteal phase of menstrual cycle, cirrhosis of the liver, etc.)	Anabolic steroids (stanozolol)
	Smoking
	Testosterone therapy in men
Thyroid hormones (hyperthyroidism, drugs)	Danazol
Phenytoin (Dilantin)	Glucocorticoids
Prolonged stress	Hyperprolactinemia
High-carbohydrate diet	Growth hormone
Diazoxide	Androgenization syndromes in women
Carbamazepine	(hirsutism, acne)
Tamoxifen	Cyproterone (anti-androgen)
	Obesity
	DBP
Estrogens (pregnancy, oral contraceptives, other drugs)	Malnutrition
	Liver disease
	Nephrotic syndrome
	Anabolic steroids (stanozolol)

[a] For abbreviations see Table 20.2.

(f) may modulate bioavailability by directly participating in hormone delivery to target cells and tissues [i] by "site-specific" enzymatic alteration of CBG and TBG, to weaken the hormonal bond, [ii] by interacting with cell surface receptors for lipoproteins as carriers of thyroid hormones, or [iii] by releasing the loosely bound hormone from albumin within selected target tissues via the general mechanism of "enhanced dissociation" (see Section 4.3);

(g) may promote selective delivery of thyroid hormones during early pregnancy (increased TBG allowing increased maternal T4 extraction by placenta);

(h) may serve, in case of SHBG, as an estrogen amplifier (estrogen increases SHBG concentration which, in turn, results in a relatively greater decrease in the free fraction of testosterone than that of estradiol);

(i) may lead, in case of AAG, to inactivation of progesterone; and

(j) may regulate, in case of TTR, distribution of thyroid hormones in the central nervous system.

3.5. Possible Non-Hormone-Binding Functions of Transport Proteins

While the complete lack of plasma albumin due to genetic deficiency (analbuminemia) apparently is of minor importance for life in humans, no verified cases of complete deficiency are known to exist for CBG, SHBG, or DBP or concomitantly for both TBG and TTR (11, 29, 31, 32).[4] This suggests a lethal mutation for these genes *in utero* and a critical role for the respective high-affinity hormone-binding proteins in embryogenesis and/or survival. Theoretically, this critical role may be related to selective hormone delivery to target tissues or to non-hormone-binding functions. The possibility that roles other than hormone transport may exist for these transport proteins in humans is rather intriguing but requires further studies.

3.6. Measurements of Transport Proteins

The plasma (serum) concentration of albumin is commonly measured by either dye-uptake [e.g., bromcresol green (BCG) or bromcresol purple (BCP)] methods or by immunochemical techniques such as immunonephelometry and immunoturbidimetry. TTR and AAG are now readily measured in serum by immunonephelometry, radial immunodiffusion, or electroimmunoassay. As to the assay of TBG, CBG, and SHBG, some techniques are indirect (also called "functional") assays that measure the capacity of these globulins to bind the respective hormone(s) such as TBG for T4, CBG for cortisol, and SHBG for testosterone, dihydrotestosterone (DHT), or estradiol ("estrogen binding globulin index"). Other techniques directly measure the protein concentration of TBG, CBG, and SHBG by immunoassays such as competitive radioimmunoassay (RIA), competitive chemiluminescent enzyme immunoassay (CEIA), particle-enhanced immunoturbidimetric assay (76), and, recently, isotopic and nonisotopic versions of two- or three-site ("sandwich") immunometric methods such as immunoradiometric assay (IRMA), immunoenzymometric assay (IEMA), and immunoluminometric assay (ILMA). At the present, no commercially available assay is known to exist for assessing the hormone-binding capacity or protein concentration of DBP.

Determination of the plasma concentration of hormone binding proteins aids in assessing alterations in plasma total hormone concentrations; further, this information is used for indirect estimation of free hormone concentrations either as an index [e.g., T4/TBG ratio, free androgen index (Te/SHBG ratio), and FT4 or FT3

---

[4] Several of these transport proteins are known, however, to normally be lacking from the plasma of certain animals.

index] or as a calculated value based on mass action law equations (see Sections 8–10).

4. THE THEORY OF FREE HORMONES AND ALTERNATIVE CONCEPTS

4.1. General Issues

The question of what constitutes the physiologically active hormone fraction in the blood obviously is the key issue in both basic and clinical endocrinology. Corresponding to the observation that thyroid, steroid, and secosteroid hormones in plasma exist in both free and protein-bound form, two different theories have been developed and are now being debated in the literature. While most "thyroidologists" accept the validity of the free hormone hypothesis, many "steroidologists" postulate that protein-bound hormones and, in particular, hormones loosely bound to albumin also enter target tissues. The following is a brief review of the two concepts of hormone delivery to target tissues.

4.2. Free Hormone Hypothesis

In 1952, Recant and Riggs (35) noted first that the non-protein-bound (free) rather than total thyroid hormone concentration may be responsible for biological activity. They observed that, despite low total thyroid hormone concentrations in the serum, their nephrotic patients were generally euthyroid. In 1957, Robbins and Rall (36) indeed showed that the disposal rate of T4 is proportional to the calculated FT4 concentration in humans. Subsequently, numerous clinical studies revealed that in most situations the calculated values for serum FT4 concentration correlate better with clinical thyroid status than do serum total T4 levels. Recent *in vivo* kinetic studies in humans confirmed a correlation between the disposal rate of T4 and the measured plasma FT4 concentration. Experimental data obtained in animals also suggested that tissue uptake of T4 and T3 occurs via the pool of free hormone. During the last decade, several investigators, including Mendel, Ekins, and their co-workers (10–15, 19, 37), provided additional evidence based on experimental data, clinical observations, and mathematical calculations for the validity of the free hormone hypothesis. Besides thyroid hormones, the concept also has been extended to steroid and secosteroid hormones (2, 10–13, 25, 29, 37–39). According to some studies, the serum FTe concentration and its indirect estimate (free androgen index = total testosterone/SHBG ratio) better represent the clinical status of androgenicity in hirsute women than does non-SHBG-bound (essentially free plus albumin-bound) testosterone (37). It is also known that the serum free (non-protein-bound) cortisol (FC) concentration and the cortisol activity remain normal during pregnancy or in women taking oral contraceptives when high CBG and, consequently, high total serum cortisol levels occur. This is in accord with earlier observations that, despite wide variations in the plasma concentration of thyroid hormone-binding proteins, the FT4 concentration (when properly measured) usually remains normal in euthyroid subjects.

In essence, the free hormone hypothesis states that when a hormone exists in the blood both in free and protein-bound form, *only the free (non-protein-bound) hormone* is transported into target tissues and exerts *physiological activity.* A corollary of this hypothesis is that the large reservoir of protein-bound hormone in the blood is passively transported by plasma proteins and is physiologically inactive.

This hypothesis assumes that, relative to the rate of hormone uptake by the tissue, the dissociation of transport protein–hormone complexes is always sufficiently rapid to maintain the free hormone concentration at its *in vitro* equilibrium value along the entire length of a capillary within the tissue vasculature (Fig. 20.2). Further, it is also implied that the free hormone concentrations are maintained irrespective of transport protein concentrations and capillary blood flow rate. From a clinical diagnostic point of view, if the free hormone hypothesis is valid, then the plasma free hormone concentration, as measured under thermodynamic equilibrium conditions *in vitro,* reliably estimates hormone availability to target tissues, and hence the patient's clinical thyroid status. This concept forms the basis of laboratory measurements of free hormones.

4.3. Protein-Bound Hormone Hypothesis

In 1964, Tait and Burstein (40) suggested that steroid hormones that are loosely bound to albumin also are available for transport to target tissues. Since then, this view has been corroborated by a number of investigators including Siiteri *et al.* (6) and Pardridge and co-workers (5, 9, 10, 12). Key points of the experimental evidence

A. Robbins - Rall model

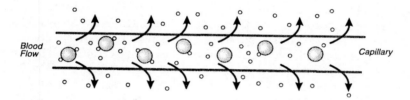

B. Tait - Burstein model

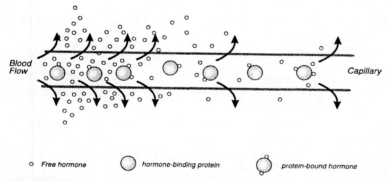

○ Free hormone   ◯ hormone-binding protein   ◯ protein-bound hormone

FIGURE 20.2   Hormone deposition along the length of a capillary in the target organ according to two different theories. (Modified with permission from R. Ekins, Measurement of free hormones in blood, Endocrine Reviews, 11, 5–46, 1990, © The Endocrine Society.)

for this hypothesis include (a) selective extraction of thyroid and steroid hormones by various tissues, (b) 10 to 90% net extraction of various thyroid and steroid hormones by the liver which greatly exceeds the fraction that is unbound *in vitro,* and (c) often 1 to 2 log orders greater nuclear receptor occupancy by various hormones than what would be predicted from the plasma concentration of unbound hormones *in vitro.* Clinically, some studies suggested that the non-SHBG bound (essentially free plus albumin-bound) testosterone concentration rather than the FTe concentration is a better marker for hyperandrogenism (41) and for the level of sexual activity (42). Expanding the original concept of albumin-bound hormones, TTR-, TBG-, and lipoprotein-bound thyroid hormones, CBG-bound corticosteroids, and SHBG-bound estradiol all have been also proposed to participate in selective hormone delivery to target tissues (13, 15, 27, 31–34).

The protein-bound hormone hypothesis summarily states that "the large pool of *protein-bound hormone* in the blood is *operationally available* for transport across microcirculatory barriers without the binding protein per se significantly exiting the plasma compartment. This process is believed to involve a mechanism of *"enhanced dissociation* of hormone . . . from the plasma protein caused by transient conformational changes about the ligand binding site within the microcirculation" (9). Assuming organ-specific dissociation of the protein–hormone complex, this concept also suggests *selective delivery* of hormones to tissues.

The protein-bound hormone hypothesis implies that the hormone is nonuniformly deposited along the capillary and that the bloodflow rate affects hormone availability to tissues (Fig. 20.2). Nevertheless, according to Pardridge (9), the central issue of this concept is that the capillary exchangeable hormone concentration, which usually is in equilibrium with the cellular hormone concentration, cannot be accurately estimated from the free hormone concentration as measured *in vitro.* This is because "enhanced dissociation," which increases the effectively transportable free hormone concentration to the level of the capillary exchangeable hormone concentration, is believed to take place only in the microcirculation (Fig. 20.3) (9). The biochemical mechanism of "enhanced dissociation" at the surface of microcirculation was proposed to involve receptors, charge selectivity, and/or local inhibitors (9).

4.4. Debate on Free and Protein-Bound Hormones

Recently, an intense debate developed between followers of the two opposing hypotheses for hormone delivery to tissues. The debated questions involve both basic and clinical endocrinology and can be summarized as follows:

(a) Which experimental techniques are valid for measuring dissociation rates of hormones from protein–hormone complexes and tissue influx rate constants for free hormones?

(b) Which mathematical models (equations) are the "best" (and likely valid) for explaining hormone delivery to tissues?

(c) Is dissociation of hormone from the protein–hormone complex always faster than tissue uptake of the hormone?

(d) What are the rate-limiting constraints in the net tissue uptake of hormones? Is it the capillary bloodflow rate (usually about 1–3 msec), dissociation of hormone from binding protein(s), influx of hormone to tissues (microvascular membrane

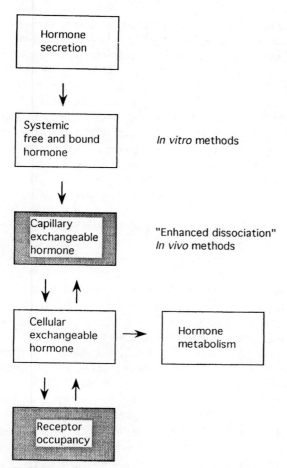

FIGURE 20.3   The driving force of thyroid/steroid/secosteroid hormone receptor occupancy according to the protein-bound hormone hypothesis. (Modified from Ref. 9, with permission.)

permeability), intracellular elimination (i.e., metabolism) of hormone, or a combination of these and other factors?

(e) What is the evidence for the existence of "enhanced dissociation"?

(f) How may hormone delivery take place with protein-bound hormone complexes?

(g) Clinically, does the free or protein-bound fraction better represent the endocrine status of the patient?

While intuitively easy to accept the validity of the free hormone hypothesis, and although substantial supportive evidence exists from both experimental and clinical work, it is important to recognize that *not* all experimental and clinical data agree with this hypothesis. For instance, examining the case of thyroid hormones, Ekins (15) pointed out that (a) the free hormone concentration immediately adjacent to the capillary wall is lower than that observed *in vitro,* and (b) because of rebinding of hormone by transport proteins, the maximal efflux rate from the capillary will be less than the intracapillary hormone dissociation rate, though the magnitude of either effect may vary between tissues. As a consequence, in contradiction to their passive role in hormone transport as proposed by the free hormone hypothesis, elevated concentrations of binding proteins with concomitant elevations in total thyroid hormone concentrations would increase the rate of hormone loss from the capillary. Indeed, in late pregnancy, high TBG concentrations and high total thyroid hormone concentrations are associated with low normal or subnormal serum concentrations of FT4 in the serum (43), a finding that is inconsistent with the traditional free hormone hypothesis. Based on a review of the literature and his own data, Ekins (15) most recently concluded that the free hormone hypothesis has not yet proven to be valid beyond doubt and, at best, represents an approximation. It is also interesting to mention that Tait and Burstein (40), the originators of the protein-bound hormone hypothesis, did not find their proposal in conflict with the free hormone hypothesis.

In an attempt to resolve some of the apparent discrepancies between the free and protein-bound hormone hypotheses, Mendel (11) recently made a distinction between the *free hormone hypothesis* and the *free hormone transport hypothesis.* According to Mendel (11), while the former hypothesis means that the free rather than the protein-bound plasma concentration affects the hormone's biological activity, the latter hypothesis means that hormones enter tissues exclusively via the pool of free hormone fraction after spontaneous dissociation of hormone–protein complexes within the vasculature. With this distinction, Mendel (11) suggested that either of the two hypotheses may be correct without requiring validity of the other. Based on experimental evidence and theoretical considerations, he concluded that (a) the free hormone hypothesis could hold even if one or more circulating protein-bound hormone pools are involved in tissue uptake of the hormone, and (b) the free hormone hypothesis is not likely valid for all hormones with respect to all tissues. While it is likely valid for thyroid hormones, cortisol, and the hydroxylated derivatives of vitamin D in all tissues, it may only be valid for many other steroid hormones (e.g., estradiol, testosterone, aldosterone) in some tissues but not in others (particularly the liver), and it is not valid at all for some steroid hormones such as progesterone (11).

While the evidence for "enhanced dissociation" as suggested by Pardridge (5) may not be entirely convincing, it appears certain that, at least in some organs and/or under some conditions, protein-bound hormones do contribute to tissue uptake of the hormone. Thus, instead of competing, the two hypotheses most likely complement each other and, depending on the type of tissue and hormone and on the plasma conditions, either or both mechanisms operate in hormone delivery to target tissues. For clinical endocrinology, the most important conclusion at the present is that, though free hormone measurements may facilitate the assessment of endocrine status under a number of conditions, the validity of the free hormone hypothesis underlying the clinical use of these measurements cannot always be assumed as a fact. The corollary of this statement is that, most likely, the measurement of certain protein-bound hormone fractions (like the so-called loosely bound hormone = free + albumin-bound hormone) rather than the free fraction may prove to be diagnostically relevant under some conditions. Obviously, further clinical (and experimental) studies are needed to bring the free hormone debate to a final conclusion.

5. HISTORY OF FREE HORMONE ASSAYS

The recognition that free hormones may represent the biologically active fraction of hormones prompted interest in developing assays for the measurement of free hormones. Since thyroid abnormalities constitute the most common endocrine disorders, it is not surprising that the free hormone hypothesis originated from the study of thyroid patients and that most of the earlier and current developmental work of laboratory technology for free hormone measurements targets the diagnosis of thyroid diseases. Accordingly, the following sections primarily refer to the measurements of free thyroid hormones, and, in particular, FT4, though most concepts are directly applicable to the measurements of other free hormones (and, in fact, free drugs) as well. The evolution of assays for FT4 was recently reviewed (44). Tables 20.7 and 20.8 summarize commercially marketed free hormone kits (essentially for FT4, FT3, and FTe), along with the design and analytical properties of the methods involved. For clarification of terminology, it is necessary to point out that all immunoassays extract free hormone from the specimen; therefore, they all are "immunoextraction" assays. Consequently, the use of this term cannot be restricted to two-step free hormone immunoassays.

From the beginning, the measurement of free hormones has been faced with two major technical challenges. The first is the difficulty to reliably measure minute quantities of a hormone (e.g., picomolar range of thyroid hormones). The second is that free hormones are measured in the presence of protein-bound hormones that are always in great excess and quickly dissociate if the initial thermodynamic equilibrium is perturbed.

6. CLASSIFICATION OF FREE HORMONE ASSAYS

Ekins (13, 15, 19) repeatedly reviewed this topic and the following brief summary is largely based on his suggestions. Based on their analytical design and calibration, free hormone assays can be subdivided at least in three ways.

I. Depending on the number of independent measurements required for the generation of a test result, the method can be:

(a) *Direct.* These methods [e.g., two-step and one-step (analog) immunoassays] involve a single measurement, and knowledge of the total hormone concentration is not needed.

(b) *Indirect.* These methods require two independent measurements, one is the total hormone concentration (e.g., total T4), the other is the fraction of hormone occurring in free form in the plasma (e.g., an equilibrium dialysis fraction) or a measurement related to it (e.g., the total hormone-binding protein capacity, such as the TBG concentration, or the unbound hormone-binding protein capacity, such as the T3 uptake)

II. Depending on the type of calibration involved, the method can be:

(a) *Absolute.* These methods are calibrated by gravimetrically determined amounts of (pure) hormone dissolved in buffer. Thus, assuming a solid physicochemical basis and optimum assay design, the results obtained by these methods are directly related to true free hormone concentrations.

TABLE 20.7 Commercial Radioisotopic Assays That Are Currently Available and/or Have Been Reported in the Literature for the Measurement of Free Thyroxin (FT4), Free Triiodothyronine (FT3), and Free Testosterone (FTe) in Serum[a,b]

Type of assay Kit	Analyte	Antibody to T4/T3[c]	Cross reactivity with (D)-T4/T3[c,d](%)	Tracer molecule	Final serum dilution[e]	Primary incubation temp.[f] (°C)	Assay system
Direct ("nontracer") equilibrium dialysis							
Direct dialysis	FT4	(Rabbit)[g]	(0.04)[g]	(^{125}I-T4)[g]	1×/13×	37	Dialysis chamber/direct RIA on dialysate
Column adsorption chromatography							
Liso-phase	FT4	(Sheep)[g]	(^{125}I-T4)[g]				Sephadex LH-20 column/direct RIA on eluate
Liso-phase	FT3	(Sheep)[g]	(^{125}I-T3)[g]				Sephadex LH-20 column/direct RIA on eluate
Microencapsulated antibody method							
LiquiSol	FT4	"Polyclonal"		^{125}I-T4	21×	37	Microcapsule dialysis (liquid-phase reaction)/centrifugation
Two-step Immunoassay							
GammaCoat	FT4	Rabbit	100–104	^{125}I-T4	21×	37	Antibody-coated tube
CoTube	FT4	Rabbit	100	^{125}I-T4	21×	37	Antibody-coated tube
RIAgnost	FT4	"Polyclonal"		^{125}I-T4$_a$	11×	RT	Antibody-coated tube
RIAgnost	FT3						Antibody-coated tube
Spectria	FT4	Rabbit		^{125}I-T4	11×	RT	Antibody-coated tube
Spiria	FT4	Rabbit	96	^{125}I-T4	2×/12×	RT	Antibody-coated latex microbeads/centrifugation (version 1)
Spiria	FT4	Rabbit	96	^{125}I-T4	2×/42×	RT	Anti-T4 antibody immunoadsorbed to a second antibody on 6.4-mm polystyrene macrobead
Phase II	FT4	Sheep	200	^{125}I-T4	6×	37	Antibody-coated solid-phase "receptacle" (SPR)/semi-automated on KinetiCount 48

Analog (one-step) immunoassay

Name	Analyte	Antibody	Value	Label	Cross-reactivity	Temp (°C)	Solid phase
Amerlex M	FT4	Sheep	82	^{125}I-T4$_a$	11×	37	Antibody-coated paramagnetic polymer particles
Amerlex M	FT3						
Coat-A-Count	FT4	n/p	n/p	^{125}I-T4$_a$	21×	37	Antibody-coated tube
Coat-A-Count	FT3	n/p	n/p	^{125}I-T3$_a$	11×	37	Antibody-coated tube
Coat-A-Count	FTe	Rabbit	n/a	^{125}I-Te$_a$	21×	37	Antibody-coated tube
Coat-Ria	FT4						
GammaCoat	FT4	Rabbit + MMC	97	^{125}I-T4$_a$	21×	37	Antibody-coated tube
GammaCoat	FT3	Rabbit	n/p	^{125}I-T3$_a$	6×	37	Antibody-coated tube
Magic	FT4	Rabbit	n/p	^{125}I-T4$_a$	15×	37	Antibody-coated paramagnetic particles
Magic	FT3	Sheep	n/p	^{125}I-T3$_a$	7×	37	Antibody-coated paramagnetic particles
Quantimmune	FT4	MMC	100	^{125}I-T4$_a$	11×	37	Antibody-coated tube
Quantimmune	FT3	n/p	?	^{125}I-T3$_a$	6×	37	Antibody-coated tube
RIA-coat	FT4						
RIA-coat	FT3						
Seria	FT4						
Seria	FT3						
SimulTRAC	FT4	Rabbit	n/p	^{57}Co-T4$_a$	3.5×	37	Antibody-coated tube
Solid-phase C.S.	FT4	Rabbit	108.5	^{125}I-T4$_a$	21×	37	Antibody-coated tube
Solid-phase C.S.	FT3	Rabbit	n/p	^{125}I-T$_a$	11×	37	Antibody-coated tube
Labeled antibody (one-step) Immunoassay							
Amerlex-MAB	FT4	(MMC)	>100[h]	^{125}I-Anti-T4	21×	37	Hapten-coupled T3$_a$ on paramagnetic particles
Amerlex-MAB	FT3	(MMC)		^{125}I-Anti-T3			Hapten-coupled T2$_a$ on paramagnetic particles
"Kinetic" RIA							
Immo Phase	FT4	Rabbit	92–108	^{125}I-T4	37×	RT	Antibody-coated porous glass particles/centrifugation
SPAC ET	FT4	MMC		^{125}I-T4	21×	37	Antibody-coated tube

(continues)

TABLE 20.7 (*Continued*)

		Analytical sensitivity[i] (pmol/liter)	Availability in the U.S.A. (1995)	Manufacturer
Direct-"nontracer") equilibrium dialysis				
Direct dialysis	FT4	1.93	Yes	Nichols Institute Diagnostics, San Juan Capistrano, CA
Column adsorption chromatography				
Liso-phase	FT4		No	Lepetit, Milano, Italy/Sclavo, Siena, Italy/Cis-International, France
Liso-phase	FT3		No	Lepetit
Microencapsulated antibody method				
LiquiSol	FT4		No[j]	Damon Diagnostics, Needham Heights, MA
Two-step Immunoassay				
GammaCoat	FT4	1.5–3.0	Yes	INCSTAR Corp., Stillwater, MN (formerly: Clinical Assays, Cambridge, MA)
CoTube	FT4	1.16	Yes	Bio-Rad Labs., Clinical Div., Hercules, CA
RIAgnost	FT4		No	Behringwerke, Marburg, Germany
RIAgnost	FT3		No	Behringwerke
Spectria	FT4		No	Famos Diagnostics, Turku, Finland
Spiria	FT4	0.6–2.5	No[l]	International Immunoassay Labs., Santa Clara, CA
Spiria	FT4			International Immunoassay Labs.
Phase II	FT4	2.6	No[j]	Medical & Scientific Designs, Inc., Rockland, MA and Vitek Systems, Hazelwood, MO
Analog (one-step) Immunoassay				
Amerlex M	FT4	0.5	No	Amersham Corp., Arlington Heights, IL/Amersham Intl. Ltd., Amersham, Bucks, U.K. (later: Johnson & Johnson Clin. Diagn., Rochester, NY)
Amerlex M	FT3		No	Amersham
Coat-A-Count	FT4	<0.13	Yes	Diagnostic Products Corp., Los Angeles, CA)
Coat-A-Count	FT3	0.3	Yes	Diagnostic Products Corp.
Coat-A-Count	FTe	0.52	Yes	Diagnostic Products Corp.
Coat-Ria	FT4			bioMerieux, Marcy l'Etoile, France
GammaCoat	FT4	0.05	Yes	INCSTAR Corp., Stillwater, MN (formerly: Clinical Assays, Cambridge, MA)
GammaCoat	FT3	0.02	Yes	INCSTAR
Magic	FT4	1.16	Yes	Ciba-Corning Diagnostics Corp., Medfield, MA
Magic	FT3	0.25	Yes	Ciba-Corning Diagnostics Corp., Medfield, MA

446

Ria-coat	FT4			Byk-Gulden Italia s.p.a., Cormano, Italy
Ria-coat	FT3			Byk-Gulden Italia
Seria	FT4		No	Serono Diagnostics Ltd., Woking, Surrey, U.K.
Seria	FT3		No	Serono Diagnostics Ltd.
SimulTRAC	FT4	0.13	Yes	Becton Dickinson Immunodiagnostics, Orangeburg, NY
Solid-phase C.S.	FT4	0.58	Yes	Becton Dickinson Immunodiagnostics
Solid-phase C.S.	FT3	<0.23	Yes	Becton Dickinson Immunodiagnostics
Labeled antibody (one-step) Immunoassay				
Amerlex-MAB	FT4	3.9	No	Amersham Corp., Arlington Heights, IL/Amersham Intl. Ltd., Amersham, Bucks, U.K. (later: Johnson & Johnson Clin. Diagn., Rochester, NY)
Amerlex-MAB	FT3		No	Amersham
"Kinetic" RIA				
Immo Phase	FT4	3.9–5.0	No[f]	Corning Medical, Medfield, MA
SPAC ET	FT4	3.9	No[f]	Byk Gulden Italia, Cormano, Italy/Byk Sangtec Diagn. (formerly: Mallincrodt), Frankfurt, Germany

[a] All assays are run at least in duplicate for unknowns (direct dialysis and column adsorption chromatography methods set up in singlet but direct RIA on the resulting dialysate/eluate is run in duplicate or triplicate).

[b] Abbreviations: MMC, mouse monoclonal (antibody); n/a, not applicable; n/p, not provided (by manufacturer); RT, room temperature; solid-phase C.S., solid-phase component system; $T3_a$, thyroxin analog; $T4_a$, triiodothyronine analog; Te_a, testosterone analog.

[c] As appropriate for the assay.

[d] Cross-reactivity (antibody specificity) usually is defined as the ratio of the amount of T3, T4, or Te required to displace 50% of the T3, T4, or Te label from the respective antibody to the amount of cross-reacting substance to give like displacement (i.e., the amount of T3, T4, or Te divided by the amount of cross-reactant at 50% tracer binding multiplied by 100 to give % cross-reactivity).

[e] Serum dilution at the time a portion of the real free hormone is physically separated or "immunoextracted" in the presence of hormone-binding proteins for assay. In case of addition of solid particle suspension, the real serum dilution is less than the one shown in the table.

[f] Incubation temperature at the time the free hormone is physically separated or "immunoextracted" in the presence of hormone-binding proteins for assay.

[g] Used in the absence of hormone-binding proteins (in direct RIA only).

[h] Cross-reactivity with (L)-T3 is 1.2%.

[i] Analytical sensitivity is defined as the lowest measurable concentration of FT3, FT4, or FTe that can be distinguished from zero. It is usually calculated from the 95% confidence limits for 20 or more replicates at the zero point of the standard curve. As available, information was collected from the package insert and/or from the literature.

[j] Product discontinued.

TABLE 20.8 Commercial Nonisotopic Assays That Are Currently Available and/or Have Been Reported in the Literature for the Measurement of Free Thyroxin (FT4) and Free Triiodothyronine (FT3) in Serum[a,b]

Type of assay Kit	Analyte	Antibody to T4/T3[c]	Cross reactivity with (D)-T4/T3[c,d](%)	Tracer molecule	Final serum dilution[e]	Primary incub. temp.[f] (°C)	Assay system
Two-step immunoassay							
Access (new)	FT4	MMC	63.0	T4$_a$-ALP	10x	37	Paramagnetic particles coated with secondary antibody: goat anti-mouse IgG Substrate: Lumi-Phos 530 Chemiluminescence
Delfia	FT4	MMC	30.1	T4-Eu	9x	RT	Microtiter strip wells coated with second antibody: rabbit anti-mouse IgG Enhancement solution Time-resolved fluorometry (TRFA)
Delfia	FT3	MMC	n/p	T3-Eu	5x	RT	Microtiter strip wells coated with second antibody: rabbit anti-mouse IgG Enhancement solution Time-resolved fluorometry (TRFA)
IMx/Axsym	FT4	Sheep	100	T3$_a$-ALP	n/p	34	Antibody-coated particles Substrate: 4-methylumbelliferyl phosphate Microparticle Enzyme Immunoassay (MEIA)
IMx/Axsym	FT3	Goat	n/p	T3$_a$-ALP	n/p	34	Antibody-coated particles Substrate: 4-methylumbelliferyl phosphate Microparticle Enzyme Immunoassay (MEIA)
Stratus	FT4	Rabbit	62.8	T4-ALP	12x	38	Glass fiber paper-bound second antibody: goat antibody to rabbit immunoglobulins Substrate: 4-methylumbelliferyl phosphate Automated on Stratus and Stratus II (plastic tabs) Fluorometry

Analog (one-step) immunoassay

ACS	FT4	Rabbit	129.0	23x	37	T4a-AE	Antibody-coated paramagnetic particles Automated on ACS:180 system Chemiluminescence
AIA-PACK	FT4	Rabbit	29.5	15x	37	T4a-ALP	Antibody-coated paramagnetic beads AIA-1200 or AIA-600 systems Substrate: 4-methylumbelliferyl phosphate Fluorescence
Amerlite	FT4				?37	T4a-HRP	? Microtiter wells coated with secondary antibody: donkey antibody to ??? Substrate: Luminol Enhanced luminescence (firefly luciferin)
Amerlite	FT3				?37	T3a-HRP	? Microtiter wells coated with secondary antibody: donkey antibody to ??? Substrate: Luminol Enhanced luminescence (firefly luciferin)
Celltech	FT4	?Polyclonal				T4a-biotin Strepavidin-HRP	Antibody-coated microtiter wells
Enzymun test (old)	FT4	Sheep	100	51x	25	T4a-HRP	Antibody-coated tube Substrate: ABTS ELISA on ES300 or 600/spectrophotometry
Enzymun test (new)	FT4	Sheep	100	51x	25	T4a-HRP Anti-T4-biotin	Streptavidin-coated tube Substrate: ABTS ELISA on ES300 or 600/spectrophotometry
Immulite	FT4	MMC	n/p	16x	37	T4a-ligand Anti-ligand-ALP	Antibody-coated polystyrene bead Substrate: Luminogen PPD Chemiluminescence
Magic Lite	FT4	Rabbit	>40	25x	RT	T4a-AE	Antibody-coated paramagnetic particles Chemiluminescence
Vidas	FT4	Rabbit	100	7x	37	T4a-ALP	Antibody-coated solid phase "receptacle" (SPR) Substrate: 4-methylumbelliferyl phosphate Enzyme-linked fluorescence assay (ELFA)
Labeled antibody (one-step) immunoassay							
Enzelsa	FT4	(MMC)				Anti-T4-HRP	Hapten-coupled T4a on paramagnetic particles Substrate: ?
Enzymun test	FT3	(Rabbit)	100	11x	25	Anti-T3-HRP T3a-biotin (polyhapten)	Streptavidin-coated tube Substrate: ABTS[f] ELISA on ES300 or 600/spectrophotometry

(continues)

TABLE 20.8 (Continued)

		Analytical sensitivity[g] (pmol/liter)	Availability in the U.S.A. (1995)	Manufacturer
Two-step immunoassay				
Delfia	FT4	1.0–2.0	Yes	Wallac Inc., Gaithersburg, MD
Delfia	FT3	5.1	Yes	Wallac Inc.
IMx	FT4	1.3	Yes	Abbott Labs, Diagnostic Div., Abbott Park, IL
IMx	FT3	3.5	Yes	Abbott Labs
Stratus	FT4	3.9	Yes	Baxter Healthcare Corp., Dade Div., Miami, FL
Analog (one-step) immunoassay				
Access	FT4	1.3	Yes	Sanofi Diagnostics Pasteur Inc., Chaska, MN
ACS	FT4	1.3	Yes	Ciba Corning Diagnostic Corp., Medfield, MA
AIA-PACK	FT4	1.3	Yes	Tosoh Medics, Inc., Foster City, CA
Amerlite	FT4	0.5	No	Amersham International/Kodak/Johnson & Johnson
Amerlite	FT3	0.42	No	Amersham International/Kodak
Celltech	FT4	2.04	No	Celltech Diagnostics, Cambridge, U.K.
				Novo Nordisk Diagnostics Ltd., U.K.
Enzymun-test (old)	FT4	2.6	No	Boehringer Mannheim Corp., Diagnostic Systems Div., Indianapolis, IN
Enzymun-test (new)	FT4	1.3	Yes	Boehringer Mannheim
Immulite	FT4	0.26	Yes	DPC Cirrus, Div. of Diagnostic Products Corp., Randolph, NJ
Magic Lite	FT4	0.7–2.57	Yes	Ciba-Corning Diagnostic Corp., Medfield, MA
Vidas	FT4	1.0	Yes	bioMerieux-Vitek Inc., Rockland, MA
Labeled antibody (one-step) immunoassay				
Enzelsa	FT4		No	Compagnie ORIS Industrie, Gif/Yvette, France
Enzymune	FT3	0.77	Yes	Boehringer Mannheim Corp., Diagnostic Systems Div., Indianapolis, IN

[a] All assays are automated or semiautomated and virtually all are run in singlets for unknowns (Delfia in duplicates) but in duplicates or triplicates for standard curve.

[b] Abbreviations: ABTS, 2,2'azino-bis-(3-ethyl-benzthiazoline-6-sulfonic acid) diammonium salt; AE, acridinium ester; ALP, alkaline phosphatase; Eu, europium; HRP, horseradish peroxidase; MMC, mouse monoclonal (antibody); n/p, not provided (by manufacturer); RT, room temperature; T3a, thyroxin analog; T4a, triiodothyronine analog.

[c] As appropriate for the assay.

[d] Cross-reactivity (antibody specificity) usually is defined as the ratio of the amount of T3 or T4 required to displace 50% of the T3 or T4 label from the respective antibody to the amount of cross-reacting substance to give like displacement (i.e., the amount of T3 or T4 divided by the amount of cross-reactant at 50% tracer binding multiplied by 100 to give % cross-reactivity).

[e] Serum dilution at the time a portion of the free hormone is physically separated or "immunoextracted" in the presence of hormone-binding proteins for assay. In case of addition of solid-particle suspension, the real serum dilution is less than the one shown in the table.

[f] Incubation temperature at the time the free hormone is physically separated or "immunoextracted in the presence of hormone-binding proteins for assay.

[g] Analytical sensitivity is defined as the lowest measurable concentration of FT3 or FT4 that can be distinguished from zero. It is usually calculated from the 95% confidence limits for 20 or more replicates at the zero point of the standard curve. As available, information was collected from the package insert and/or from the literature.

(b) *Comparative*. These methods are calibrated or, if required, can be calibrated by serum standards, the calibration of which is traceable to absolute methods. Therefore, the results obtained by comparative methods ultimately depend on the performance of absolute methods that were used for calibration of the serum standards.

III. Depending on the time point at which the measurement is taken, the method can be:

(a) *Dynamic (kinetic or rate)*. These methods measure the rate of change toward equilibrium [e.g., symmetric dialysis, kinetic (rate) RIA].

(b) *Equilibrium*. These methods take the measurement after equilibrium has been reached in the assay system (e.g., equilibrium dialysis).

Unfortunately, the terms describing various types of free hormone assays often are used inconsistently. The Committee on Nomenclature of the American Thyroid Association (ATA) (45) recently attempted to classify the various methods for thyroid function, and further suggested replacing T3U with the term thyroid hormone binding ratio (THBR). Based on the Committee's recommendation, the FT4 and FT3 methods are divided essentially into two groups (the third group refers to thyroid hormone binding):

(a) Methods which would be expected to give accurate results and measure *true free thyroid hormone concentrations*, and

(b) Methods which yield only *indirect estimates of the free thyroid hormone concentrations*.

While the Committee's critical review of available thyroid function tests certainly helped to illustrate the value and limitations of these tests and to optimize their use for patient care, as Ekins (13) noted, the Committee's recommendations themselves may generate some controversy. On one hand, the theoretical definition of a genuine free (thyroid) hormone assay may be too narrow. Any free hormone method with a verifiable physicochemical basis has the potential to accurately measure the free hormone concentration. Thus, properly designed analog methods may belong to this category. On the other hand, none of the currently available free hormone assays is capable of measuring the free hormone concentration in undiluted serum in all circumstances. In the lack of consensus, the frequency by which "correct" free hormone results are generated may not be used to make distinction between "genuine" free hormone assays that measure free hormone concentrations and those that only provide their estimates as "free hormone indices" (13).

7. PRINCIPLES OF FREE HORMONE ASSAYS

7.1. Dialysis

Dialysis methods represent the earliest attempts at free hormone measurement (46, 47). They are physicochemically well founded but are slow to perform (usually 16 to 24 hr), technically demanding, cumbersome, and labor intensive. While both direct and indirect equilibrium dialysis methods are available commercially for testing in the United States, only a single direct dialysis method for FT4 is now being marketed as a kit.

Symmetric dialysis is an indirect and dynamic (or kinetic) method. For assay, the test sample (serum) containing minute amounts of radiolabeled hormone is placed in one chamber, whereas the same serum (but with no tracer added) is placed in the second chamber. The initial rate by which the free radiolabeled hormone (preequilibrated in the test sample) is dialyzed at 37°C through a semiper-meable membrane separating the two chambers is directly proportional to the free hormone concentration in the test sample (46). Obviously, with extension of the incubation time, the tracer eventually will uniformly distribute on both sides. In the original technique, reported by Christensen (47) for FT4 in 1959, the use of undiluted serum resulted in a very low transfer rate and radioactivity (approximately 1% of initial total). Therefore, radiochemical impurities of the labeled hormone preparation strongly interfered and had to be removed in a second step from the dialysate. The use of diluted serum in a newer version of this method for free thyroid and steroid hormones considerably increased both the rate of diffusion and the amount of labeled T4 in the "dialysate" (~30% of initial total) (48, 49).

Dialysis of the radiolabeled test sample against buffer in the second dialysis chamber (i.e., indirect equilibrium dialysis) was described as a modification (50). With further modification, *flow dialysis* represents a novel indirect dynamic tech-nique for assessing free hormone concentrations (51). In this technique, the test sample (serum) enriched with a minute amount of radiolabeled hormone is dialyzed through a semipermeable membrane against continuously flowing buffer. The frac-tion of labeled hormone appearing in the outflow buffer is proportional to the free hormone concentration in the sample.

For *indirect* ("tracer") *equilibrium dialysis* (Fig. 20.4), the test serum is spiked with a minute quantity of radiolabeled hormone which rapidly distributes between the free and protein-bound hormone to match the distribution of endogenous hormone. Then, the fraction of labeled hormone that dialyzes through a semiper-meable membrane into the second compartment containing serum-free buffer is counted at equilibrium. In case of FT4, radiochemical impurities present in the tracer are separated either by $MgCl_2$ precipitation of T4 ("$MgCl_2$ method") (52) or by a second dialysis step against a buffer containing anion exchange resin ("resin dialysis method") (53). The serum sample is routinely prediluted to increase the rate of diffusion. A high dialysate to dialysand ratio is used to increase the fraction of labeled (and unlabeled) hormone in the dialysate and to reduce the interference due to radiochemical impurities of the labeled hormone.

In *direct equilibrium dialysis* (Fig. 20.4), the unaltered test serum (i.e., containing no labeled hormone) is dialyzed against buffer in the second compartment of the dialysis cell. After reaching equilibrium, the free hormone concentration in the dialysate (i.e., buffer in the second compartment) is measured by a sensitive immu-noassay, traditionally RIA (54–56). Direct equilibrium dialysis methods use minimal or no initial test sample dilution and a relatively low dialysate to dialysand ratio. It is noteworthy that FT4 results obtained by direct dialysis methods tend to be lower than those obtained by indirect equlibrium dialysis methods, suggesting that the latter may overestimate the true FT4 concentration due to radiochemical impuri-ties of labeled T4 (13, 15). Properly designed direct equilbrium dialysis may be considered a "candidate reference method" for free hormone measurements.

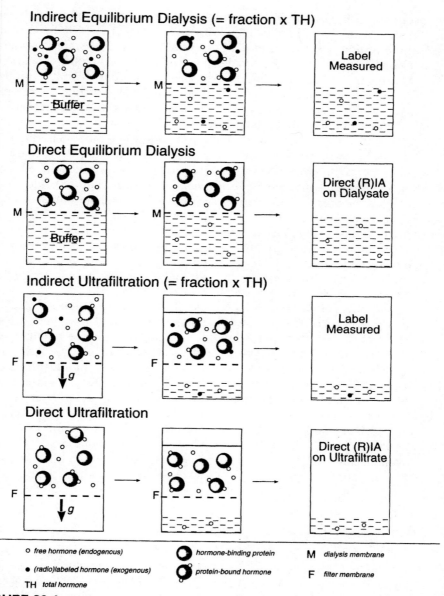

FIGURE 20.4 Basic types of equilibrium dialysis and ultrafiltration for the measurement of free hormones.

7.2. Ultrafiltration

Similar to dialysis, a fluid sample containing free hormone is separated from the serum to be tested by means of a semipermeable membrane (Fig. 20.4). However, the separation in ultrafiltration is achieved by applying centrifugal force to the test sample, which may or may not be diluted. A rigid semipermeable membrane, kept in fixed position in the centrifuge tube assembly, separates the upper compartment containing the test sample from the lower compartment collecting the ultrafiltrate. Thus, unlike dialysis, the two fluid samples usually are not in direct contact during ultrafiltration. Compared to dialysis, ultrafiltration assays are considerably faster to perform and can be completed in a few hours. However, they are also technically demanding and cumbersome for routine applications. Variable protein leakage through the semipermeable membrane under high centrifugal force represents a major problem for obtaining reliable measurements with this method.

Ultrafiltration also can be direct and indirect. In *direct ultrafiltration* (57), no radiolabeled hormone is added to the test sample and the free hormone concentration in the ultrafiltrate is measured by a sensitive immunoassay, traditionally RIA (Fig. 20.4). With proper design, this approach may also serve as a reference method for free hormone measurements. In *indirect ultrafiltration* (58), minute amounts of radiolabeled hormone are equilibrated with the test sample, and then an ultrafiltrate is generated (Fig. 20.4). The free hormone fraction (calculated from the ratio of specific radioactivity present in the ultrafiltrate and total radioactivity initially present in the test sample) multiplied by the total hormone concentration yields the free hormone concentration. While ultrafiltration techniques have been developed and used for both free thyroid and steroid hormones, no commercially marketed kits are available at the present.

Centrifugal ultrafiltration–dialysis is a novel version of indirect ultrafiltration and was originally described for the estimation of free steroid hormones such as estradiol, testosterone, and progesterone (59). The technique involves simultaneous addition of ^{3}H-steroid and ^{14}C-glucose to undiluted serum or plasma. After allowing for equilibrium, the sample is centrifuged in a sac of (semipermeable) dialysis membrane at 37°C, and the ratio of ^{3}H-steroid and ^{14}C-glucose in the ultrafiltrate is compared with the corresponding ratio in the retentate (i.e., serum retained by the membrane). Since glucose is not protein-bound, it serves as an internal standard for filtration and obviates the need to monitor the volume of ultrafiltrate. Because the ultrafiltrate remains in contact with the dialysis membrane during centrifugation, low-molecular-weight components are able to pass through the dialysis membrane in either direction (hence is the term "isodialysis") and the technique is claimed to closely mimic *in vivo* conditions.

7.3. Gel Filtration/Dialysis

Gel filtration is based on penetration of low-molecular-weight free hormones into Sephadex particles and concomitant exclusion of large protein molecules. In a way, this technique is similar in concept to dialysis: the gel particles (beads) act as tiny microdialyser units. Several techniques have been developed using this concept, but they are all cumbersome for large-scale routine applications.

Indirect gel filtration methods have been used for the determination of free thyroid hormones (60). First, minute quantities of radiolabeled hormone are equilibrated with the test sample, then the radiolabeled serum is partially fractionated on Sephadex G25 (coarse) minicolumns. After serum proteins are eluted from the column, both the protein-containing effluent and the column that still contains the low-molecular-weight (free) hormone are counted and the free hormone fraction is calculated from the ratio of activity on column and activity in effluent. Simultaneous use of ^{131}I-T4 and ^{125}I-T3 allowed simultaneous determination of FT4 and FT3 with this method (60). *Direct gel filtration* (with no tracer added to the test sample) requires sequential elution of the protein and then the free hormone fraction from the column, followed by a sensitive RIA for measuring hormone concentration in the latter eluate. Because of the lack of true thermodynamic equilibrium conditions and possible stripping of hormones from binding proteins, the direct and indirect gel filtration techniques have been largely abandoned.

Steady-state gel filtration is an indirect technique that has been used mostly for the measurements of free steroids such as cortisol, testosterone, estradiol, and progesterone (61). For assay, the test sample that has been preequilibrated with minute amounts of radiolabeled hormone (e.g., ^{3}H-steroid) is applied to a Sephadex G50 (fine) mini-glass column. Molecular sieving of the free (non-protein-bound) hormone causes the leading edge of the test sample to become progressively stripped of hormone as it advances down the column. As additional sample flows down, the net dissociation diminishes and a new equilibrium develops. Assuming a large enough serum sample, the dissociated hormone concentration in the gel eventually becomes equal to the free hormone concentration in the serum sample. Further net dissociation is thus prevented and a steady-state is reached. Elution of the column at this point gives a plateau containing the plasma proteins and hormones at their original concentration, followed by a second plateau which corresponds to the free (non-protein-bound) fraction retarded by the gel. The test is cumbersome and labor-intensive but can be completed within a few hours. The free hormone concentration is the product of the free hormone fraction and total hormone concentration.

Gel bead dialysis (Fig. 20.5) is a modification of steady-state gel filtration. This indirect method is technically simpler and more amenable to batching than steady-state gel filtration. For assay, preswollen Sephadex G25 (coarse) beads act as micro-dialysers. The test sample, minute amounts of radiolabeled hormone (e.g., ^{3}H-steroid or ^{125}I-T4), and preswollen gel beads are incubated together for a few hours. During incubation, an equilibrium is reached between free (both labeled and unlabeled) and protein-bound hormone fractions and the concentration of hormone in the bead dialysate will be equal to the free hormone concentration in the incubation medium surrounding the beads. For quantitation of the free hormone fraction, the gel beads are separated by centrifugation from the incubation mixture by means of a rigid filter. The radioactivity within the separated gel (corresponding to the free hormone fraction) is then counted. This technique was successfully used for FT4 and FTe measurements (62).

7.4. Column Adsorption Chromatography

The physicochemical basis of column adsorption chromatography (Fig. 20.5) is similar to direct dialysis and ultrafiltration. Used as a direct assay for free thyroid hormones, this method is based on chromatographic adsorption (instead of penetration, as in gel filtration) of free thyroid hormones onto lipophilic Sephadex LH-20 particles contained in polystyrene columns (63). After loading the test sample onto the column, an approximately 1-hr incubation follows at 37°C, during which the free hormone adsorbed onto the resin reaches equilibrium with the free hormone in the sample. The adsorbed free hormone fraction, which is proportional to free hormone in the sample, is then separated by sequential elutions from the column. The protein fractions are eluted by washing with buffer, whereas the adsorbed hormone is eluted with methanol and determined by a sensitive RIA. Although

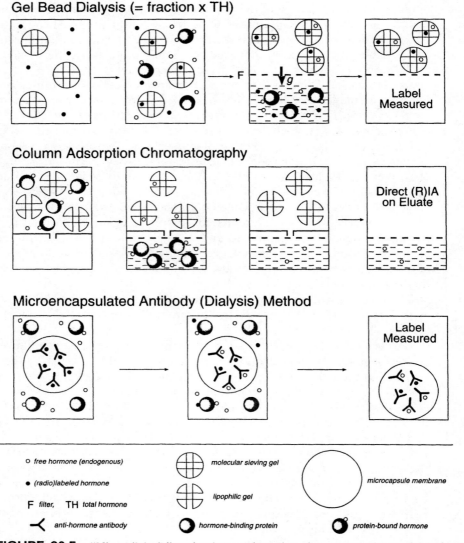

FIGURE 20.5 "Micro-dialysis" and column adsorption chromatography methods for the measurement of free hormones.

somewhat cumbersome to perform, this chromatographic separation technique is relatively quick to complete and has a solid physicochemical basis. A kit based on this principle is marketed commercially outside the United States.

7.5. Microencapsulated Antibody Assay

This direct immunoassay is an antibody displacement RIA (Fig. 20.5). It has been developed and marketed for FT4, FT3, FC, and FTe (64). In the kit, the complexes of anti-hormone antibodies and radiolabeled hormone contained within a liquid droplet are enclosed by a semipermeable membrane. The membrane pore size has been designed to physically trap inside the relatively large antibody molecules and their complexes, while allowing free diffusion of low-molecular-weight substances (<4000), such as free hormones in either direction. The microcapsules thus act as miniature dialysis systems. For assay, an aliquot of the preloaded microcapsule suspension is incubated in the test sample. Thus, all reactants (anti-hormone antibody, hormone ligand, and radiolabeled hormone ligand) are in liquid phase at all times. Further, physical retention of anti-hormone antibody molecules within the microcapsules allows dialysis and immunoassay to occur concomitantly. After a few hours of incubation, the microcapsules are separated from the incubation mixture either by centrifugation (as in the original commercially marketed version) (64) or by means of magnetic racks (as in a newer, modified version based on the incorporation of magnetizable dextran along with the antibody and labeled hormone into the microcapsules) (65). In this newer version for FT4, magnetizable cellulose also is added to the reaction mixture at the end of incubation to facilitate pelleting (65). In either version, after separation the radioactivity is counted in the sediment and the free hormone (e.g., FT4) concentration is determined from a calibration curve. Changes in TBG concentration have been shown to considerably affect the FT4 results obtained by this technique (66). Although the concept of this method is physicochemically attractive and the test is relatively easy to perform, the assay has never become a commercial success.

7.6. Kinetic (Rate) Immunoassay

This indirect immunoassay was developed for the measurement of FT4 (Fig. 20.6). It involves the use of small amount of anti-T4 antibody that has about the same affinity to T4 as TBG and is immobilized to small glass particles. For assay, the test sample is simultaneously incubated with radiolabeled T4 and antibody-coated particles in a tube. The endogenous free and exogenous labeled T4 compete for binding sites on the immobilized anti-T4 antibody. The rate of association of labeled T4 to antibody is assumed to be proportional to the FT4 concentration, and hence the radioactivity contained within the glass particles, after a specified time interval, is a measure of the FT4 concentration (67). The assay is used in conjunction with total T4 measurements in a color-coded second reaction tube. The FT4 concentration is the product of the calibrated T4 fraction, as measured by the radioactivity present in the glass particles (that are sedimented by centrifugation), and the total T4 concentration. The assay is rather robust, relatively insensitive to tracer impurities, highly reproducible, and easy to perform, but the original version of this assay (Immophase) was known to be sensitive to changes in plasma TBG concentrations (68). An improved kinetic RIA with less antibody and reduced TBG-dependence is still available in a kit format outside the United States (69).

7.7. Two-Step Immunoassay

Two-step immunoassays, also kinetic in concept, are variably called sequential, saturation, back-titration, and "immuno-extraction" assays (Fig. 20.6). They were independently developed by Ekins and Clinical Assays researchers (U.S.) for the measurement of free thyroid hormones (13, 15, 19). In the first step of the reaction, solid-phase-bound anti-hormone antibody "extracts" free hormone from the test sample, and then the plasma hormone-binding proteins are removed. In the second

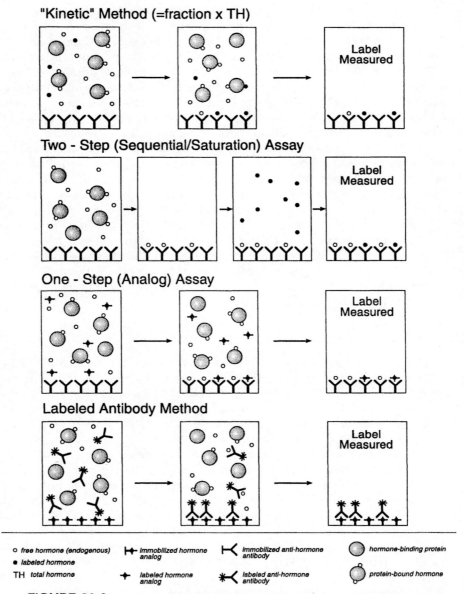

FIGURE 20.6   Common immunoassay types for the measurement of free hormones.

step (i.e., sequentially), unoccupied binding sites on the immobilized anti-hormone antibody are saturated by adding labeled hormone to the test tube ("back-titration"). While typically the labeled hormone is completely identical to the hormone to be measured, at the present there are at least two exceptions. In one commercial two-step RIA for FT4 (Table 20.7), the labeled hormone is claimed to be a T4-derivative (the same as the one used for generation of the anti-T4 antibody) and is *used to give a heightened reactivity* with the assay antibody during back-titration (70). In a commercial nonisotopic two-step immnunoassay for FT4 (Table

20.8), the labeled hormone is a T3-alkaline phosphatase conjugate that is *used to lessen the reactivity* (as compared to T4) with the assay antibody (which cross-reacts with both T4 and T3), so that only the previously unoccupied sites are filled (71). Apparently, assay formulation sometimes allows opposing solutions. It is more generally agreed that optimal design of this assay requires "small" amounts of a relatively high-affinity antibody. Small means less than 5% extraction of hormone from the sample, whereas the relatively high affinity means an affinity greater than that of TBG for the hormone. Ekins (15) proposed an antibody affinity of about 10^{11} liters/mol. When optimized, the method has been verified to perform well in most clinical situations and, because plasma-binding proteins are removed *before* the labeled hormone is added, it is little affected by variations in transport protein concentrations (45, 68, 72) and by serum dilution (8, 13, 45). On the other hand, the sequential steps are inconvenient. Because of a relatively flat dose–response curve, the precision of this method is sometimes relatively low (interassay CVs may be in the 10–15% range). Besides isotopic formulations, the assay is now commercially available in nonisotopic automated formats (Table 20.8).

7.8. One-Step (Analog) Immunoassay

In this direct competitive immunoassay type (Figure 6), a minute amount of a labeled hormone analog is incubated concurrently with the test sample and solid-phase-bound anti-hormone antibodies (hence the term, one-step assay) (8, 67, 73). If the analog shows no (or greatly reduced) binding affinity to endogenous hormone-binding proteins and the antibody does not significantly disturb the equilibrium state, the amount of labeled analog bound to the antibody is inversely proportional to the free hormone concentration. Based on theoretical considerations, optimally the assay requires an antibody with relatively high affinity to the hormone (i.e., the K_a of antibody slightly greater than K_a of TBG), but the antibody affinity for the hormone analog can be relatively low (13, 15). When this is the case, higher than usual concentrations of both antibody and analog may be used in the assay (15). Despite these theoretical considerations, several commercial one-step assays involve the use of anti-hormone antibodies with affinities slightly lower than that of the respective specific binding globulin [e.g., GammaCoat 1-step RIA for FT4 (K_a of antibody = 6.2×10^8 liter/mol), Coat-A-Count 1-step FT3 and FTe (K_a of antibody "slightly lower than that of TBG and SHBG, respectively")].

The analog assay design obviates the need for sequential incubation steps in isotopic but not in nonisotopic formulations, and hence it is simple to perform and automate. However, the presence of hormone transport proteins and substances that compete for hormone binding sites on transport proteins in the incubation mixture makes the method highly vulnerable to changes in serum constituents (13, 15, 68, 72, 74) and requires the use of hormone analogs that are truly unbound to transport proteins. Nevertheless, because of their simplicity, practicability, and favorable economy, the analog methods are now widely used, most often in a nonisotopic and automated or semiautomated format (Tables 20.7 and 20.8). Besides FT4 and FT3, an application has been also reported for FTe (Table 20.7).

7.9. Labeled Antibody Assay

This is also a direct competitive free hormone assay (Fig. 20.6), performed in one step (75, 76). The test sample and labeled anti-hormone antibody are simultaneously incubated in the presence of solid-phase-bound hormone analog. Thus, (endogenous) free hormone molecules compete with immobilized hormone analog molecules for binding sites on a limited amount of liquid-phase-labeled antibody. In case the analog is not reactive with endogenous hormone-binding proteins, the labeled antibody bound to the solid phase is inversely proportional to the free hormone concentration. Conceptually, this method resembles the classic one-step analog assays. Consequently, both the problems and the advantages of this assay type are generally similar to those of one-step (analog) immunoassays. However, as Ekins (15) pointed out, it is important to recognize that attachment of the analog to solid support creates a "macroanalog." This "macroanalog" may sufficiently differ in its physicochemical properties from the unattached analog. Thus, the performance of the labeled antibody assay may be different from that of a "classic" analog assay that involves use of the same analog in a labeled form in liquid phase. Both isotopic and nonisotopic applications of the labeled antibody assay now exist in commercially marketed kits (Tables 20.7 and 20.8). Current applications include FT4 and FT3. The labeled antibody method also is known as solid-phase antigen-linked technique (SPALT).

8. TOTAL HORMONE/TOTAL HORMONE-BINDING GLOBULIN RATIO

8.1. T4/Thyroxin-Binding Globulin Ratio

The T4/TBG ratio is an indirect method for estimating FT4 concentration (77). This ratio is derived from theoretical considerations of the Law of Mass Action. As discussed earlier, the interaction between thyroid hormones and their binding proteins conforms to a reversible binding equilibrium. Thus, the reversible interaction between T4 and its principal plasma binding protein, TBG, can be described as

$$FT4 + fTBG \overset{K_a}{\leftrightarrow} TBG\text{–}T4 \tag{3}$$

where FT4 is free (non-protein-bound) T4, fTBG is free (unbound) TBG (i.e., the unoccupied binding sites of TBG for T4), and TBG–T4 is TBG-bound T4 (i.e., the binding sites of TBG occupied by T4).

At the state of equilibrium, the interaction between T4 and TBG can be expressed by a mass action law relationship,

$$K_a = \frac{[TBG\text{–}T4]}{[FT4]\,[fTBG]}, \tag{4}$$

where K_a is the equilibrium constant for the reaction and brackets signify (molar) concentration. After rearranging this equation,

$$[FT4] = \frac{[TBG\text{–}T4]}{K_a\,[fTBG]}. \tag{5}$$

Since FT4 is negligibly small, TBG–T4 closely approximates total T4, and fTBG is total TBG − total T4. Equation (5) can be thus rewritten as

$$[FT4] = \frac{[total\ T4]}{K_a\,([total\ TBG] - [total\ T4])}. \tag{6}$$

On rearranging (dividing by total T4),

$$[FT4] = \frac{1}{K_a\left[([\text{total TBG}]/[\text{total T4}]) - 1\right]}. \tag{7}$$

Since in usual circumstances K_a is constant and the numeral 1 in the denominator can be neglected, it follows that

$$[FT4] \text{ estimate} \approx \frac{[\text{total T4}]}{[TBG]} = \textbf{T4/TBG ratio.} \tag{8}$$

When the affinity of TBG is normal and its plasma concentration only moderately altered, the T4/TBG ratio may well approximate the FT4 concentration. However, changes in the affinity of TBG and/or extreme changes in its plasma concentration will diminish the diagnostic value of this ratio (78, 79). In these situations, the T4/TBG ratio is not a substitute for the measurement of FT4.

8.2. T3/Thyroxin-Binding Globulin Ratio

The T3/TBG ratio is used analogously to the T4/TBG ratio to correct for alterations in total T3 that are related to changes in TBG concentration. However, like measured FT3 and the FT3 index (FT3I), this ratio rarely offers advantage over FT4 and its use remains limited (80).

8.3. Te/Sex Hormone-Binding Globulin Ratio or Free Androgen Index (FAI)

The Te/SHBG (or TeBG) ratio or free androgen (or testosterone) index (FAI) was originally introduced in the early 1980s for assessing the testosterone status of females with hirsutism (81). Like the T4/TBG and T3/TBG ratios, the use of the Te/SHBG ratio is based on the Law of Mass Action in a simple binding model that assumes only one binding protein (SHBG or TeBG) and one ligand (Te); that is, other binding proteins such as albumin and other (competing) steroids are ignored. The use of FAI recently has been extended by some investigators to males as well (14, 42). An analysis of the derivation of the FAI from the mass action law revealed, however, that the FAI is valid only when the binding capacity of SHBG greatly exceeds the testosterone concentration (82). Since the two are almost identical in adult males, the FAI can be used only in women and not in adult males (82).

9. TESTS BASED ON THE MEASUREMENT OF "THYROID HORMONE BINDING"

9.1. T3 Uptake Test (T3U)

The T3 uptake test (T3U) (Fig. 20.7), sometimes erroneously referred to as the "T3 test," assesses the overall binding of labeled T3 by thyroid hormone-binding proteins (77, 83). In euthyroid subjects, T3U primarily reflects the TBG concentration (and/or affinity) and saturation.

The test is performed by partitioning fixed amounts of radiolabeled T3 between binding sites on thyroid hormone transport proteins in serum and a secondary binder material such as erythrocyte membranes (84), anion exchange resin (hence the name "T3 resin uptake test"), talc, microaggregated albumin, Sephadex gel,

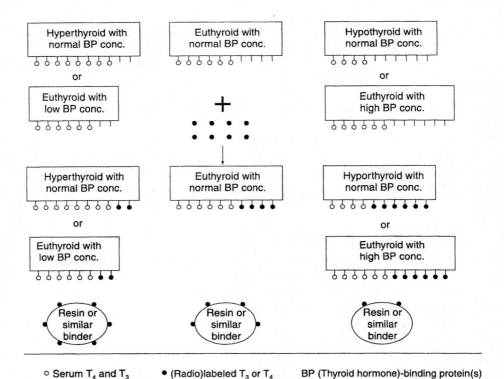

○ Serum T₄ and T₃   ● (Radio)labeled T₃ or T₄   BP (Thyroid hormone)-binding protein(s)

FIGURE 20.7   The principle and performance of the isotopic T3 (or T4) uptake test. Both the patient's thyroid status and thyroid hormone-binding capacity (i.e., the plasma concentration and affinity of thyroid hormone-binding proteins) affect the rate of labeled T3 (or T4) uptake by resin or similar binders.

charcoal, or immobilized high-affinity anti-T3 antibody. After a brief incubation, the reactants are separated and the amount of labeled hormone bound to the secondary binder (the so-called "uptake") is quantitatively determined. The uptake is inversely related to the binding of labeled T3 to transport proteins in the patient's serum. Although radiolabeled T3 is used most commonly in the test, labeled T4 may also be satisfactory ("T4 uptake test, T4U"). However, labeled T3 often is preferred because of its greater stability and relatively low affinity for TBG (and TTR) compared to T4. The relatively low affinity of T3 for TBG (and, to a lesser extent, TTR) assures that no substantial amounts of bound T4 will be replaced from these binding sites.

9.2. T Uptake Test

Recently, a variety of nonisotopic T3U and T4U assays have become available, mostly on automated instruments. These new methods all use antibodies as secondary binders and are generically named "T uptake" assays; either T3 or T4 is used as the labeled analog. Based on the label, some of them (e.g., CEDIA) are homogeneous in design; that is, they do not require separation of the reactants (85).

9.3. Thyroid Hormone-Binding Ratio (THBR)

Traditionally, the T3U (or T4U) was expressed in terms of percentage of the added (total) label activity taken up by the secondary binder. However, this approach recently has been shown to be theoretically unsound and has been replaced by calculating the result as label bound to the secondary binder divided by the residual serum protein-bound activity (45). This ratio follows more closely the Law of Mass Action and is more linearly related to the FT4 fraction over a wide range of results. The result obtained for each unknown sample also is normalized for a euthyroid reference serum or serum pool (of known per cent uptake) to minimize analytical variations. The ratio obtained by dividing the result for the patient serum by that for a reference serum is termed thyroid hormone binding ratio [THBR(T3) or (T4), depending on the labeled hormone involved]. Although centered on a ratio of 1.0, reference values for THBR may differ with laboratory and method.

9.4. FT4 and FT3 Indices (FT4I and FT3I)

Because THBR is affected by the concentration, affinity, and saturation of thyroid hormone-binding proteins, THBR alone is not a reliable indicator of thyroid function. The product of THBR (earlier T3U) and T4 concentration yields an index (the so-called "free T4 index" or FTI) (45, 83).

Because the THBR (earlier T3U) and TBG concentrations are closely and inversely related, Eq. (8) can be rewritten as

$$[FT4]\ \text{estimate} \approx [T4] \times \frac{1}{[TBG]} = [T4] \times THBR$$

$$\equiv \textbf{FT4 index}\ (\text{or } \textbf{FTI}). \qquad (9)$$

As long as the plasma concentrations of T4 and TBG change only moderately, the FT4I will be reliable for estimating the FT4 concentration, but, like the T4/TBG ratio, it fails when the T4 concentration is extremely high or low or when the affinity of TBG is altered (79).

The FT3 index [the product of THBR(T3) (earlier T3U) and total T3] is used analogously to FT4I for assessing FT3 concentrations (80).

10. CALCULATED FREE HORMONE CONCENTRATIONS

If the total hormone concentrations, binding constants, and binding site concentrations (i.e., binding protein concentrations and the number of binding sites per binding protein molecule) are known, the free hormone concentrations as well as the distribution of hormone among various binding proteins can be calculated by means of standard Law of Mass Action equations. First, Robbins and Rall (17) applied this approach to the calculation of FT4 concentration and the distribution of T4 among various T4-binding proteins. Subsequently, as detailed earlier, a number of models have been developed using computer-based solutions of mass action law equations for the calculation of both free thyroid hormones (FT4 and FT3) (13, 18–21). Similar models also are available for calculating the concentration of at least 19 free steroid hormones including testosterone and 17β-estradiol (22–25).

Under "standard" physiological conditions, the newer and improved models effectively deal with complex hormone-binding protein systems containing multiple classes of binding sites and multiple competing ligands to the same binding site. However, there are numerous conditions where the binding affinity of transport proteins is altered (see Table 20.5 and Section 14.4) and/or endogenous substances (e.g., free fatty acids) and drugs which compete with hormone binding are present in high concentrations (e.g., in patients with nonthyroidal illness; see Sections 14.3 and 15.3). These conditions can interfere with, and possibly invalidate, the free hormone calculations and may limit the application of existing models (86, 87).

11. NON-SEX HORMONE-BINDING GLOBULIN-BOUND TESTOSTERONE (NSB-Te)

The assay for NSB-Te measures the so-called loosely bound testosterone fraction (NSB-Te = albumin-bound Te + FTe), also called the "bioavailable testosterone concentration." Although this assay does not truly measure free hormone (12, 14, 37, 41, 42), its inclusion is justifiable by its close relationship to (and as a possible alternative of) FTe.

The measurement of NSB-Te is based on selective ammonium sulfate precipitation of SHBG-bound Te (41). Briefly, the test sample (unknown serum) is incubated with tracer (^{3}H-Te) at 37°C, then rapidly cooled to 0°C, and ice-cold ammonium sulfate is added to give 50% saturation. After cold centrifugation, an aliquot of the supernatant is counted. A reference tube, representing 100% non-SHBG-bound Te, is made by treating unknown serum with excess unlabeled Te at the beginning and the end of the assay. The absolute non-SHBG-bound Te is calculated as the product of percent non-SHBG-bound and total Te. While EDTA plasma may give artefactually high (up to 130%) results, heparinized plasma is suitable for the assay.

12. ASSAY PARAMETERS OF FREE HORMONE ASSAYS

12.1. Buffer (pH, Ions)

A critical assumption during the assay of free hormones is that their equilibrium with plasma binding proteins is not altered by the assay conditions. Since virtually all free hormone assays involve dilution of the test sample with buffer, it is important to ensure that the reaction buffer does not affect the preexisting equilibrium. Data obtained for FT4 in indirect equilibrium dialysis (50) illustrate the nature of problems that need to be addressed for optimizing assay buffers for free hormone measurements.

While changes in pH from 7 to 9 do not appear to influence T4 binding to human serum albumin, pH-dependent alterations of T4 binding were observed for TBG and TTR in the pH range 7.4 to 9.0 (91). The binding was very sensitive to changes in pH and was minimal around pH 8.0–8.2. The magnitue of pH effect was inversely related to the concentration of the buffer used (50).

The composition of buffer also greatly influences the equilibrium between T4 and its binding proteins. Both chloride and phosphate ions inhibit the binding of T4 to serum proteins and thus raise the FT4 concentration (50).

12.2. Incubation Temperature

It is important to recall that free hormones exist in thermodynamic equilibrium with their binding proteins *in vivo*. Thus, in order to maintain the relevance of *in vitro* free hormone measurements to *in vivo* conditions, assays should be carried out at 37°C. The importance of incubation temperature is well illustrated, for instance, by the finding that due to a decrease in the association constant of T4 for binding, the FT4 concentration doubles when the temperature rises from room temperature to 37°C (88). The affinity of TBG for T4 is much more temperature-dependent than the affinity of albumin and TTR. Therefore, the net temperature effect on the FT4 concentration in a sample will depend on the relative contribution of TBG to total T4 binding (88, 89). Because of the strong temperature dependence of binding equilibrium, the reference values for FT4 should be defined at 37°C. Room temperature incubation of FT4 assays often leads to misleading values, especially in samples with very low TBG concentration (88, 89). Tables 20.7 and 20.8 show that, ignoring the critical importance of incubation temperature, several free thyroid hormone assays are marketed, apparently for convenience, with room temperature incubations. Inadequate optimization of hormone binding assays for incubation temperature was also reported (83). Analyzing eight T3U assays, like FT4 assays, the effect of incubation temperature was most marked in high uptake (i.e., low TBG) specimens (83). Similar findings are expected for the effect of incubation temperature on the measurements of other free hormones as well.

12.3. Incubation Time

The incubation time is another critical parameter of free hormone assays. Obviously, equilibrium should be reached before measurements are taken in equilibrium assays, but rate assays also require optimization of the incubation time for best performance. Numerous examples of assays that have not been properly timed exist in the literature. The importance of proper incubation times was well illustrated in a study of eight commercial T3U kits (83).

12.4. Sample Dilution

Under physiological conditions, the plasma concentration of free hormones is maintained by parallel changes in total hormone and total binding protein concentrations. However, when the plasma is diluted even with an inert diluent such as water, the original equilibrium between the hormone and its binding protein(s) is perturbed. The dilution-related fall in free hormone concentration causes dissociation of the protein-bound hormone, in order to maintain the initial free hormone concentration according to the Law of Mass Action. In such a situation, the affinity and binding capacity of binding proteins will determine the extent of the resultant alteration (7, 13, 15). The lower the buffer capacity of binding proteins (and the higher the initial free hormone fraction), the more pronounced the dilution effect. Figure 20.8 shows that even a minimal dilution will decrease the FC concentration, while dilutions as high as 50- to 100-fold will barely affect the FT4 concentration.

As seen in Tables 20.7 and 20.8, all currently available commercial assays involve sample dilution. Even those free hormone assays which initially use undiluted serum, may lead to specimen dilution (e.g., direct equilibrium dialysis for FT4). Further, there is a confusion in the literature regarding not only the occurrence but also the degree of specimen dilution. Dilution often is identified only with initial or predilution of the specimen with the reaction buffer. Addition of reagents to the reaction mixture and dilution with the volume of dialysate (and fluid shift-related volume

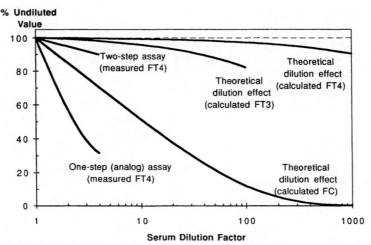

FIGURE 20.8 The effect of serum dilution on actual and/or measured free hormone concentrations. Data assume a normal human serum that contains 20 pmol/liter of FT4, 5 pmol/liter of FT3, and 340 nmol/liter of free cortisol, respectively. Experimental results were obtained by a commercial analog (one-step) RIA known to be interfered with binding of the analog to transport proteins and a commercial two-step (saturation) RIA, suggestive of 3–4% sequestration of T4 by the anti-T4 antibody. (Modified from Ekins, R. (8), with permission © American Association of Clinical Chemistry; and (13), with permission © The Endocrine Society)

increment of the dialysand) are not always recognized as contributors to the effective (or final/total) dilution of the specimen. Theoretically, sample dilution can only be avoided by preparing an ultrafiltrate for direct assay or by (immuno)absorbing with solid-phase-bound hormone-binding reagents.

Although still contested by some investigators, many experts believe that the so-called serum dilution test is capable of detecting true or "genuine" free hormone assays (7, 13, 15). In true free hormone assays, the theoretically calculated and actually measured free hormone concentrations in a set of serially diluted serum specimens should closely approximate each other. Assays that show increasing underestimation of calculated free hormone concentrations with increasing serum dilutions are considered inappropriate for use. It is important to recognize that serum dilution also causes alteration in the competitive effect of endogenous substances and drugs. These conditions for dilution effect need to be analyzed separately from those involving sera with no appreciable concentration of binding inhibitors (15).

Because of the nature of the binding protein–hormone equilibrium, samples cannot be diluted for assessing free hormone concentrations that are above the measuring range of the assay. Surprisingly, this limitation was recently ignored even in the package insert of a commercial FT4 assay.

12.5. Hormone Sequestration

All free hormone assays (even dialysis and ultrafiltration methods) isolate a fraction of free hormone and thus cause hormone sequestration (13, 15, 19, 67). Most commonly, binders such as antibody, resin, and red blood cells are involved in hormone extraction. Sequestration of this hormone fraction, like serum dilution, causes a fall in the free hormone concentration that, in turn, leads to dissociation of protein-bound hormone ("stripping") to reestablish the equilibrium. Sequestration of relatively large amounts of hormone may seriously affect the performance of a free hormone assay. The effect of hormone sequestration is best studied for FT4 immunoassays. It was suggested that an assay antibody ideally should extract less than 1% of the total T4 present in the serum specimen (13, 15, 19, 67). This extraction would insignificantly affect the hormone-binding protein equilibrium and thus the FT4 concentration. In reality, most immunoassays for FT4 now extract T4 in the range of 1 to 10%. In a recent study of patients with different serum TBG concentrations, the critical percentage of T4 stripping (the point where the percent FT4 began to decrease) was found to be related to the rate of saturation of TBG with T4. The "stripping" from TBG ranged from 2.8 to 16.7%. The higher the saturation of TBG with T4, the greater the effect of stripping on the FT4 concentration (90). Concomitant study of four different assays for FT4 disclosed TBG stripping well within critical limits (90). In the end, minimization of hormone extraction is the goal for all free hormone assays.

12.6. Hormone Analogs

The analog free hormone assays represent a novel but highly controversial approach to free hormone testing (8, 12, 13, 15, 73). The concept behind these assays is simple and physicochemically well-founded. The most commonly used analogs are those of thyroid hormones and represent conjugates of either the amino or the carboxylic (or both) groups of the alanine sidechain (Fig. 20.9). The basic assumption of analog assays is that the analog will be capable of reacting with the anti-hormone antibody but, differing sufficiently in molecular structure from the parent hormone, it will not bind to plasma proteins. Thus, the use of an analog obviates the need for sequential incubations, as required for two-step free hormone immunoassays. The concept of analog immunoassays can be extended to all free hormones (and even free drugs). In fact, solid-phase-bound hormone analogs are the basis for the design of labeled antibody free hormone assays as well (75, 76).

While the physicochemical basis of analog assays is undoubtedly firm, the analytical and diagnostic performance of the first commercial free hormone assays developed according to this concept in the early 1980s has been seriously questioned (8,

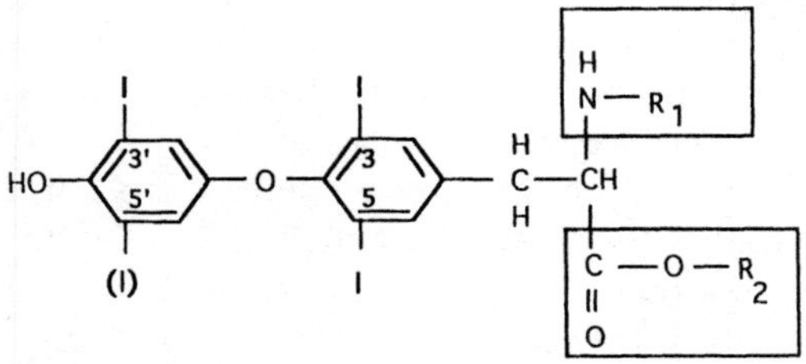

FIGURE 20.9   Substitution sites (R1 and R2) for the generation of thyroid hormone analogs. Both amino (-N-R) and carboxylic (-O-R) substitutions are known to reduce TBG-binding. T4, 3,5,3',5'-tetraiodothyronine; T3, 3,5,3'-triiodothyronine.

12–15, 73, 90). The long debate on the validity of these assays included questions about:

(a) the validity of the analog assay concept;

(b) the suitability of the analog used in the assay, including the consequences of its binding to plasma proteins;

(c) the validity of assay formulation with respect to the amount and affinity of antibody;

(d) the validity of the serum dilution test for analog assays; and

(e) the validity of general assumptions made in analog assays as analyzed by mathematical models for the complex interactions between hormone, hormone analog, binding proteins, and anti-hormone antibody.

The central issue of this debate was that, for true free hormone assays, the analogs should be virtually completely unbound to plasma proteins. If this condition is not met and the analog is merely "not significantly bound to plasma proteins," as proponents of this methodology claim, the free hormone measurements are expected to depend considerably on the serum concentration of various binding proteins, endogenous binding inhibitors (e.g., free fatty acids, FFA), and/or competing drugs. Indeed, a number of investigators observed factitiously high or low free hormone results with early analog methods (8, 13, 15, 45, 68, 72).

While first strongly rejected by proponents of the isotopic analog methods as a critical issue, binding of the T4-analog to the low-affinity but high-capacity binding sites on serum albumin turned out to be the key problem. Changes in serum albumin concentrations are among the most common biochemical abnormalities in the serum of patients with nonthyroidal illness (NTI) and the results obtained by these assays strongly and directly correlated with the serum albumin concentration. At physiologic pH, albumin binding of T4 involves a relatively nonspecific electrostatic interaction between the amino residues on albumin and the iodine–phenolic hydroxide–iodine group of T4. Thus, a T4 analog modified only on the alanine sidechain can retain its ability to bind to albumin. Ekins (13, 15) estimated that, for a minimally acceptable analog FT4 assay, less than 10% of total analog should bind to plasma proteins in the absence of antibody.

After finally acknowledging the albumin-dependence of isotopic analog assays, the manufacturers added undisclosed types of "chemical blockers" (probably substances such as salicylates and ortho-substituted phenols) and/or extra amounts of albumin as a known "sequestering agent" to the reagents. However, inclusion of these substances in the "modified" isotopic analog assays in the late 1980s did not remedy the problem and, by increasing the complexity of interactions between various components of the assay, it appeared to make the performance of some methods even worse. As pointed out earlier, labeled antibody (analog) methods carry the same concerns as classic one-step (analog) assays.

In the late 1980s, a variety of new hormone analogs have been developed for use in nonisotopic one-step immunoassays for FT4 and FT3 (Table 20.8). Either these new, fully or partially automated assays do not express the earlier noted problems, or the extent of these problems is negligibly small (91). Full validation of these new analog assays, however, has not yet been accomplished and additional critical studies are in order.

13. SPECIMENS FOR FREE HORMONE ASSAYS

13.1. Blood (Serum, Plasma)

Since there is no convincing evidence that free hormone levels in serum are different from those in plasma, for convenience, serum most often is the specimen of choice for free hormone measurements. A single report that serum obtained from silicon vacutainer tube may give falsely high results for FT4 in the GammaCoat 2-step assay has not been confirmed conclusively (67). Although plasma specimens are frequently also suitable for testing, the presence of heparin, EDTA, oxalate, or fluoride may interfere with some assays, particularly with nonisotopic immunoassays. For instance, the AIA-PACK FT4 assay is interfered with EDTA or citrate in the plasma, the Coat-A-Count one-step RIA may give falsely high FT4 and FTe results in EDTA plasma, and the Delfia two-step FT4 and FT3 methods are interfered with citrate in the plasma. Postclotting in separated serum specimens due to coagulation abnormalities or contamination with anticoagulants may be a rare source of problems because of *in situ* formation of fibrin within the analytical system of some assays.

13.2. Saliva

The measurement of free (i.e., non-protein-bound) hormones in the most commonly used specimens, serum or plasma, is complicated by the presence of a relatively large protein-bound fraction, often requiring prior separation of the two fractions. Saliva, being a natural ultrafiltrate of plasma, provides a convenient medium for the measurement of a number of hormones such as free cortisol, testosterone, estradiol, estrone, progesterone, and aldosterone (2–4, 49, 92). The total concentration of many steroid hormones in the saliva is in good agreement with the free (non-protein-bound) hormone concentration in the plasma and is independent of the salivary flow rate. The assays required for the measurement of (total) hormones in saliva are technically less demanding and often less expensive than their counterparts for serum testing. Nevertheless, the clinical usefulness of salivary hormone measurements has not yet been fully established (3, 92).

Saliva specimens can be easily and repeatedly collected by noninvasive, stress-free techniques. Patients can produce saliva in volumes sufficient for testing in less than 10 min. In fact, approximately 0.5-ml specimens can be serially obtained at intervals as short as 10 to 15 min. The specimens are clarified by centrifugation prior to testing. However, because of the relatively high ratio of protein-bound to free hormones in the blood, contamination of salivary specimens with blood during collection is of major concern. Steroid-metabolizing enzymes of the salivary glands may also interfere with the hormone measurements.

A novel device for facilitating the collection of high-quality saliva specimens contains an osmotically active substance (e.g., carbohydrate) enclosed in a pouch of semipermeable membrane (MW cut-off 12,000) to form a disc (93). By moving the device around in the mouth for about 8 min, the patient stimulates salivary flow and generates about 1.2 to 2 ml of ultrafiltrate. Since the membrane eliminates the possibility of contamination with blood (admixture of transport proteins is avoided), the ultrafiltrate is clear and can be used for analysis without centrifugation

(93). The device also allows specimen collection at home, with subsequent mailing to a testing laboratory.

13.3. Urine

In normal circumstances, urine specimens contain very low concentrations of hormone-binding proteins, and several "free" (i.e., unconjugated) steroids such as cortisol, testosterone, and aldosterone are essentially nonprotein-bound in the urine. Because the glomerular filtration and tubular reabsorption of steroid hormones are passive, the urinary free steroid excretion is directly related to the free (non-protein-bound) steroid concentration in the plasma. Consequently, measurement of some urinary free steroid hormones may obviate the need for measuring the respective free hormone in plasma (94).

Timed (such as 24-hr) urine specimens usually are collected with acid preservatives. These specimens have the advantage of condensing the changes of a period (e.g., an entire day), and hence include short-lasting events that may be missed in serum or plasma assay. On the other hand, timed urine specimens are inconvenient to collect (particularly in an ambulatory setting) and miss the peaks and troughs of the collection period. Further, urinary free steroid hormones often occur in the presence of high concentrations of related metabolites that can interfere with the analytical assay (e.g., due to antigenic cross-reactivity). Detailed analysis of techniques for urinary free hormones is beyond the scope of this chapter.

14. INTERFERENCES WITH FREE HORMONE MEASUREMENTS

14.1. Radioactive Specimens

Previously administered radionuclides such as ^{131}I, ^{32}P, ^{51}Cr, ^{99m}Tc, ^{111}In, and ^{67}Ga, for diagnostic or therapeutic purposes, will be variably present in specimens collected for free hormone measurements. By increasing the background, these radionuclides all have the potential to interfere with isotopic free hormone assays. Specimens containing radionuclides with very short half-lives may be reassayed after allowing for spontaneous decay. For instance, in case of ^{99m}Tc ($t_{1/2}$ = 6 hr) 10 half-lives (= 60 hr or ~3 days) reduce the radioactivity to <0.4% of the initial level. Alternatively, the specimen collection should be delayed to avoid or reduce radioactive contamination of the specimen. Since *in vivo* half-lifes of radionuclides are shorter than *in vitro* half-lives, delayed specimen collection always is preferred (whenever possible) over extended specimen storage.

14.2. Lipemia, Turbidity, Hyperbilirubinemia, Hemolysis

As with any other method based on the measurement of light absorption or emission, gross alterations in the appearance of the specimen, such as lipemia, turbidity, excess bilirubin, and hemolysis, all may interfere with nonisotopic free hormone assays. Lipemia and hemolysis may be the source of error in isotopic free hormone assays as well.

14.3. Endogenous Hormone-Binding Inhibitors (Free Fatty Acids, FFA) and Drugs

It has been long observed that endogeneous substances that compete for hormone binding sites may be present in the sera of certain patients (13, 15, 72, 95–97). These substances are now known to be largely identical to unsaturated (nonesterified) free fatty acids (FFA) such as oleic (18:1), linoleic (18:2), and linolenic (18:3) acids. FFA compete with both thyroid and steroid hormones for binding sites on albumin and specific binding globulins such as TBG, CBG, and SHBG. The effect of FFA is not limited to, but certainly the most extensively studied for, the measurement of FT4. Significant correlations were found between the concentrations of FFA and FT4 in practically every method, but the direction of correlation depended on the assay formulation (68, 72, 95, 98–100). Because albumin is the major FFA binder in the serum, it is not surprising that the correlations became even stronger when the FFA/albumin molar ratio was used instead of FFA alone (68, 95, 98, 100). Analog FT4 assays showed a strong negative, whereas two-step FT4 immunoassays and equilibrium dialysis showed a less prominent positive correlation between measured FT4 and FFA or FFA/albumin molar ratio. Serum FFA concentrations are most commonly elevated due to fasting (as often is the case in severe illness), diabetes, *in vivo* heparin administration, and physical exercise.

Besides endogenous hormone binding inhibitors, a number of drugs are known to interfere with free hormone, primarily FT4 (and FT3) measurements (67, 96, 97). However, most drugs appear to exert their effect *in vivo*. Drugs which are known to affect (usually *in vivo*) the measurements of FT4 and/or FT3 concentrations are listed in Table 20.9. Drugs which compete with T4 for binding sites on hormone transport proteins include phenytoin, phenylbutazone, salicylates, and furosemide. With regard to steroid hormones, danazol inhibits testosterone binding to SHBG and may cause an up to 90% increase in the concentration of FTe. In contrast, anticonvulsants such as phenytoin and carbamazepine, ketoconazole, oral contraceptives, nafarelin, and cyproterone decrease the FTe concentration. A detailed list of drug interferences is available (101).

14.4. Altered Plasma Concentration and/or Affinity of Hormone-Binding Proteins

Changes in the concentration and/or affinity of hormone binding proteins will affect the total hormone levels and may also affect the distribution of labeled hormones during free hormone measurements (68, 74, 77–79, 102–104). Many early one-step (analog) FT4 (FT3) assays [further, the T4/TBG ratio and FT4 (FT3) index] regularly showed positive correlations with increasing concentrations and/or affinity of the three major hormone-binding proteins, albumin, TTR, and TBG (Tables 20.5 and 20.6). Indirect dialysis and isotopic two-step FT4 (FT3) methods, on the other hand, generally showed little or no interference due to variations in transport proteins. The new nonisotopic one-step (analog) FT4 methods appear to be little or not affected by varying binding protein concentrations (91). However, the effect of altered affinity of binding proteins on the measured FT4 concentration has not yet been fully investigated for these new methods.

TABLE 20.9   Drugs Affecting Serum FT4 and/or FT3 Concentrations *in Vivo*

Drug	Effect	Mechanism of action
Glucocorticoids	↓ FT4 (FT3)	Inhibition of TSH secretion[a]
		Inhibition of extrathyroidal T4 → T3 conversion (large doses)
		Reduction of TBG concentration
		Increase of TTR concentration
Propranolol (large doses)	↑ FT4 ↓ FT3	Inhibition of extrathyroidal T4 → T3 conversion
Sulfonylurea drugs (e.g., propylthiouracil, methimazole)	↓ FT4 (FT3)	Inhibition of the biosynthesis and release of T4
Phenylbutazone	↑ FT4	Inhibition of the biosynthesis and release of T4
		Inhibition of thyroid hormone binding to proteins
Iodide	↓ FT4	Inhibition of the biosynthesis and release of T4
Iodinated radiographic contrast agents (e.g., iopanoic acid, sodium ipodate, sodium tyropanoate)	↑ FT4 ↓ FT3	Inhibition of extrathyroidal T4 → T3 conversion
Salicylates (>2 g/day), fenclofenic acid, furosemide	↑ FT4, ↑ FT$_3$	Inhibition of thyroid hormone binding to proteins
Amiodarone (~37% iodine content)	↑ FT4 ↓ FT3	Inhibition of extrathyroidal T4 → T3 conversion
Lithium carbonate	↓ FT4	Inhibition of the biosynthesis and release of T4
Phenytoin (diphenyl-hydantoin), carbamazepine	↓ FT4, ↓ FT$_3$	Acceleration of the clearance of T4 (and T3)
		Inhibition of thyroid hormone binding to proteins
Dopamine	↓ FT4	Inhibition of TSH secretion
Amphetamines, sulpiride benzamide, metoclopramide	↑ FT4	Increase of TSH secretion
Heparin	↑ FT4/ ↓ FT4[b]	Stimulation of plasma lipoprotein lipase to convert TG to FFA which, in turn, inhibit thyroid hormone binding to proteins

[a] TSH, thyroid-stimulating hormone (thyrotropin); TG, triglycerides; FFA, free (nonesterified) fatty acids. For other abbreviations see Tables 20.2 and 20.3.
[b] Direction of effect depends on assay principle.

14.5. Dextro Enantiomers of Thyroid Hormones

Since the anti-T4 and anti-T3 antibodies often are not stereospecific in immunoassays for free (and/or total) thyroid hormones (Tables 20.7 and 20.8), the presence of D-T4 and/or D-T3 in the patient serum may result in overestimation of the biologically fully active free L-T4 and L-T3 concentration and a spuriously high T3U or T4U. Since only the levo isomers of thyroid hormones occur naturally, this situtation may only arise by taking synthetic dextro thyroid hormones. Synthetic D-T4 (dextrothyroxin sodium) is the active ingredient of the lipid-lowering (hypocholesterolemic) drug Choloxin (Flint Labs.) in the United States.

14.6. Human Autoantibodies to Hormones and/or Hormone Analogs

The presence of anti-thyroid hormone antibodies in the sera of patients with thyroidal and nonthyroidal disoders is now a well-recognized condition (105). Some patients have autoantibody only against T4, others only against T3, and still others against both T4 and T3 (105). Depending on the relative affinities of autoantibody and assay antibody to thyroid hormones and the formulation of the immunoassay, these autoantibodies in the patient serum may cause falsely low or falsely high FT4 and/or FT3 (and total T4 and/or total T3) results, or no interference at all (105, 106). Since the patient's serum is removed before the labeled hormone added, two-step immunoassays are not interfered with these autoantibodies. Interestingly, the affinity of some human anti-T4 and/or anti-T3 autoantibodies may be even higher toward a T4 or T3 analog than toward the parent T4 or T3 molecule. In fact, most recently, human autoantibodies which only reacted with the hormone analog [possibly, the hormone (hapten)–enzyme bridge] in a T uptake test and analog FT$_4$ and FT$_3$ assays have also been reported. These phenomena, along with the one-step design (simultaneous presence of all serum components and labeled hormone analog), makes the analog-based (either classic one-step or labeled antibody) assays particularly vulnerable to interference with human anti-thyroid hormone autoantibodies. However, even in these assays, low-affinity autoantibodies may not cause interference. Prior precipitation of interfering human autoantibodies with polyethylene glycol or preabsorption of the patient serum with other physical means (e.g., affinity columns for human immunoglobulins) may eliminate or reduce these interferences. Although autoantibodies to steroid and secosteroid hormones theoretically are also possible, no such cases have yet been reported.

14.7. Human Heterophile and Immunization-Induced Antibodies

Heterophile and immunization-induced antibodies against the free (and/or total) hormone assay antibodies are known to cause falsely low or falsely high FT4 results (107, 108). The occurrence, direction (falsely high or low), and degree of interference all depend on the formulation, including the type of antibody, of a given free hormone assay. The etiology of heterophile antibodies, by definition, is unknown. In turn, unintended immunization related to therapeutic administration of specific animal antisera and immunoglobulins (e.g., passive immunization with horse anti-tetanus antibodies), consumption of foodstuff (e.g., bovine milk and meat), and prolonged exposure to animals (e.g., house pets) and animal products (e.g., meat for butchers) used to be the most common cause of the generation of specific human antibodies against bovine, sheep, goat, rabbit, and other animal immunoglobulins. Currently, most interferences are expected to occur due to human anti-mouse (immunoglobulin) antibodies (HAMAs) that are formed secondarily to the administration of diagnostic or therapeutic mouse monoclonal antibodies labeled with isotopes such as ^{99m}Tc or tagged with chemotherapeutic agents.

Prior precipitation of interfering human antibodies with polyethylene glycol, pretreatment of the patient serum with other physical means (e.g., affinity columns for human immunoglobulins), pretreatment of the patient serum with normal serum or purified immunoglobulin of the animal species involved in the assay, or, theoretically, routine inclusion of "blocking" amounts of homologous animal sera/immunoglobulins in assay reagents may eliminate or reduce the interference. For instance, normal mouse serum or immunoglobulins are needed as "blocking" agents if HAMAs are expected to be present in the patient serum. While the published data almost exclusively involve interferences caused by human anti-animal antibodies in free (and total) thyroid hormone assays, similar interferences obviously may occur in any free (and total) hormone immunoassay.

15. SELECTED ISSUES REGARDING INTERPRETATION OF FREE HORMONE RESULTS

15.1. Physiological Variations

Similar to total hormone and total hormone-binding protein concentrations, plasma free hormone concentrations may vary with age and sex (109, 110). After a long debate, it is now also accepted that the FT4 and FT3 concentrations are physiologically low-normal in late pregnancy (15, 43). Likewise, reduced FT4 concentrations were found in lactating women (111). Lower serum level of free androstenedione, testosterone, and estradiol were observed in the follicular phase of conceptional than nonconceptional cycles after ovarian stimulation with gonadotropin-releasing hormone agonist (25), indicating that appropriately cycling levels of free androgens and estradiol are important parameters of successful conception. The well-known diurnal variation in total plasma cortisol concentration is paralleled by a change in FC concentration; the levels peak around 8 to 9 AM and fall by approximately 50% 12 hr later. FTe also is highest in the morning. With a mechanism likely related to the release of FFA, prolonged physical exercise has been observed to increase the apparent FT4 concentration (100).

15.2. Effect of Timing of Therapeutic Hormone Administration

Free hormone concentrations often are measured in patients at the time when they are undergoing treatment with the same hormone. This situation is particularly common in thyroid patients, who usually receive synthetic L-T4 preparations for replacement or suppression therapy. A single oral dose of L-T4 (120 to 150 μg) transiently, but significantly, increases the serum FT4 and FT3 concentrations (112, 113). The peak responses occur approximately 3 to 4 hr postdose. Similar findings also are likely in patients receiving steroid and secosteroid hormones. Thus, free hormone measurements in patients who receive therapeutic hormone preparations should be interpreted relative to the time the last dose was given.

15.3. Nonthyroidal Illness (NTI)

The evaluation of thyroid status in patients with NTI is difficult because many thyroid function test results are decreased (72, 77, 96, 97, 114, 115). Initially, only the total T3 is low ("low T3 syndrome"), but late during the course of the disease both total T3 and total T4 are reduced ("sick euthyroid syndrome") (115). Some patients (mostly those with liver disease) initially may even have elevated total T4 levels. TSH initially is normal, but later, with progression of the severity of disease, may be slightly elevated or decreased. A long-debated question is the true thyroid status and the true concentration of free thyroid hormones in these patients. These patients often, if not always, have some reduction in their serum TTR and albumin; further, they often have elevated serum FFA levels and their serum commonly contains a variety of drugs, some of which with the potential of competing for T4 and/or T3 binding sites. Consequently, the free thyroid hormone results widely differ with the type of assay employed (8, 54, 57, 67, 68, 72, 96–100). Early isotopic one-step (analog) assays, T4/TBG ratio, and FT4 (FT3) index generally gave abnormally low results, whereas isotopic two-step and dialysis FT4 assays produced either normal or slightly elevated FT4 (FT3) results. Because of the great number of confounding factors, it is difficult to assess at the present what is the contribution of assay artifacts vs the true thyroid status of these patients to the free thyroid hormone results. Some investigators believe that patients with NTI clinically are truly slightly hypothyroid (114) and would benefit from therapy with thyroid hormones. The results of pilot studies with thyroid hormone replacement therapy in these patients are, however, conflicting. It is possible that these patients have both decreased TSH and thyrometabolic condition as a mechanism to spare their energy. The current recommendation is to postpone the laboratory evaluation of NTI patients with suspected thyroid disease to a time when fewer factors may affect their laboratory testing.

16. ANALYTICAL GOALS FOR FREE HORMONE MEASUREMENTS

While 100% accuracy is the obvious theoretical goal, the definition of universally acceptable analytical bias for routine work is now difficult for free hormone measurements. This is because of wide variations in free hormone methodology, lack of consensus regarding their validity, and consequent lack of reliable and practical reference methods. Therefore, the analytical goals presently are restricted to imprecision and the definition of detection limits (116). Since nonisotopic free hormone assays generally measure test samples in singlets, an obvious analytical goal is to either maintain or improve the imprecision of isotopic methods in which measurements usually are based on at least duplicate testing (91). The design of free hormone immunoassays for improved analytical performance is now assisted by mathematical modeling of the binding reactions (117, 118). These models also predict the limits of theoretically achievable analytical performance (e.g., precision, detection limits) (117, 118). Based on this approach, it was found that competitive one-step immunoassays provide a more favorable precision profile, a better detection limit, and a higher specificity of analyte recognition than two-step immunoassays which, in turn, require three to four times less reagents and provide a higher measuring signal (117). This latter property is favorable for the detection of analytes that occur in very low concentration (117).

Based on intraindividual variations, the imprecision goals have been already defined for FT4 (CV = 4.7%) and FT3 (CV = 3.9%). For other free hormones, for which biological variation data are not yet available, imprecision goals may be derived either from reference intervals or from the "state of the art," as judged from a stated proportion (e.g., 25%) of laboratories participating in an external survey.

The detection limits ideally should be defined by the range within which a desired CV is achievable and/or by the limits of linearity. Alternatively, a working range with 95% confidence limits of the extreme values should be calculated by using relevant imprecision data (116).

17. QUALITY CONTROL OF FREE HORMONE ASSAYS

While the general concept of internal and external quality control (proficiency testing) is not different for free hormone assays than for any other quantitative diagnostic laboratory test, there are also some peculiarities (119). One issue is that, for optimum performance, not only the integrity of the hormone of interest but also that of all respective binding proteins should be preserved in the control materials for free hormone assays. If this latter condition cannot be assured, considerable matrix effects may ensue (e.g., due to lyophilization). Second, the general lack of true reference (and definitive) methods hampers the establishment of accurate target values for free hormones. Obviously, this limitation does not affect the suitability of control preparations to monitor intra and interassay and interlaboratory precision. At the present, free hormone proficiency testing surveys of CAP are limited to FT4, FT3, and T3U (THBR).

18. CONCLUSIONS AND PERSPECTIVES OF FREE HORMONE MEASUREMENTS

Undoubtedly, immunoassays have played a key role in the development of practical and economic methods for free hormone measurements. Apart from rare attempts to use other analytical systems, all free hormone assays ultimately involve the use of antibodies. It appears certain that progress in laboratory methodology for free hormone measurements will remain intimately linked to progress in antibody and immunoassay technology, in general. Clearly, more widespread use of monoclonal, possibly genetically engineered antibodies, advanced nonisotopic technology, and complete automation will highlight the design of free hormone assays in the future. The standardization and validation of assays for free hormone measurements continue to be critical issues. The development of reference and definitive methods is a necessary first step in achieving this goal.

The clinical value of free hormone measurements ultimately depends on the validity of the free hormone hypothesis. On the other hand, accurate, precise, technically simple, and economically feasible methods are needed for the examination of this hypothesis in clinical situations. Currently available information appears to be sufficiently convincing for clinical application of free thyroid hormone measurements, but most assays involved in these measurements still require validation. Hopefully, additional clinical studies based on verifiable free hormone assays and further experimental work on hormone transport and delivery to tissues will soon establish the diagnostic usefulness and indications of other free hormone measurements as well.

Acknowledgment

The author thanks Dr. Lynn R. Witherspoon of the Ochsner Medical Foundation (New Orleans, LA) for providing valuable information.

References

1. Hicks JM, Young DS, Eds. DORA '92-93: Directory of rare analyses. Washington, DC: AACC Press, 1992.
2. McVie R, Levine LS, New MI. The biological significance of the aldosterone concentration in saliva. Pediat Res 1979; 13:755–9.
3. Kirschbaum C, Hellhammer DH (organizers). 2nd European symposium on hormone and drug assessment in saliva. [Abstracts] J Clin Chem Clin Biochem 1990; 28:649–66.

4. Swinkels LMJW, van Hoof HJC, Ross HA, Smals AGH, Benraad TJ. Concentration of salivary testosterone and plasma total, non-sex-hormone-binding globulin-bound, and free testosterone in normal and hirsute women during administration of dexamethasone/synthetic corticotropin. Clin Chem 1991; 37:180–5.

5. Pardridge WM. Transport of protein-bound hormones into tissues *in vivo*. Endocrine Rev 1981; 103–23.

6. Siiteri PK, Murai JT, Hammond GL, Nisker JA, Raymoure WJ, Kuhn RW. The serum transport of steroid hormones. Recent Progr Horm Res 1982; 38:457–510.

7. Gieseler D, Ritter M. On the validity of free hormone measurements. Anal Biochem 1983; 132:174–182.

8. Ekins R, Midgley JEM, Moon CR, Wilkins TA. Validity of analog free thyroxin immunoassays, Validity of analog free thyroxin immunoassays, Part II. Reviews and Responses. Clin Chem 1987; 33:2137–52.

9. Pardridge WM. Plasma protein-mediated transport of steroid and thyroid hormones. [Review] Am J Physiol 1987; 252(Endocrinol Metab 15):E157–64.

10. Mendel CM, Cavalieri RR, Weisiger RA, Pardridge WM. On plasma protein-mediated transport of steroid and thyroid hormones. Am J Physiol 1988; (Endocrinol Metab 2):E221–7.

11. Mendel CM. The free hormone hypothesis: a physiologically based mathematical model. Endocrine Rev 1989; 10:232–74.

12. Ekins R, Pardridge WM. Hirsutism: free and bound testosterone. Ann Clin Biochem 1990; 27:91–4.

13. Ekins R. Measurement of free hormones in blood. Endocrine Rev 1990; 11:5–46.

14. Herzog AG, Levesque LA, Isojarvi JI. Testosterone, free testosterone, non-sex hormone-binding globulin testosterone, and free androgen index: which testosterone measurement is most relevant to reproductive and sexual dysfunction in men with epilepsy? Arch Neurol 1992; 49:133–5.

15. Ekins R. Analytical measurements of free thyroxine. Clinics Lab Med 1993; 13:599–630.

16. Beato M. Gene regulation by steroid hormones. Cell 1989; 56:335–44.

17. Robbins J, Rall JE. Proteins associated with the thyroid hormones. Physiol Rev 1960; 40:415–89.

18. Prince HP, Ramsden DB. A new theoretical description of the binding of thyroid hormones by serum proteins. Clin Endocrinol 1977; 7:307–24.

19. Ekins RP. Methods for the mesurement of free thyroid hormones. In: Ekins R, Faglia G, Pennisi F, Pinchera A, Eds. Free thyroid hormones. Amsterdam: Excerpta Med, 1979:72–92.

20. Robbins J, Johnson ML. Theoretical considerations in the transport of the thyroid hormones in blood. In: Ekins R, Faglia G, Pennisi F, Pinchera A, Eds. Free thyroid hormones. Amsterdam: Excerpta Med, 1979:1–16.

21. Munson PJ, Rodbard D. Ligand: a versatile computerized approach for characterization of ligand binding systems. Anal Biochem 1980; 107:220–39.

22. Dunn JF, Nisula BC, Rodbard D. Transport of steroid hormones: binding of 21 endogenous steroids to both testosterone-binding globulin and corticosteroid-binding globulin in human plasma. J Clin Endocrinol Metab 1981; 53:58–68.

23. Sodergard R, Backstrom T, Shanrhag V, Carstensen H. Calculation of free and bound fraction of testosterone and estradiol-17β to human plasma proteins at body temperature. J Steroid Biochem 1982; 16:801–10.

24. Belgorsky A, Escobar ME, Rivarola MA. Validity of the calculation of non-sex hormone-binding globulin-bound estradiol from total testosterone, total estradiol and sex hormone-binding globulin concentrations in human serum. J Steroid Biochem 1987; 28:429–32.

25. Andersen CY, Ziebe S. Serum levels of free androstenedione, testosterone and oestradiol are lower in the follicular phase of conceptional than of non-conceptional cycles after ovarian stimulation with a gonadotrophin-releasing hormone agonist protocol. Human Reprod 1992; 7:1365–70.

26. Pearce CJ, Byfield PGH. Free hormone assays and thyroid function. Ann Clin Biochem 1986; 23:230–7.

27. Benvenga S, Gregg RE, Robbins J. Binding of thyroid hormones to human plasma lipoproteins. J Clin Endocrinol Metab 1988; 67:6–16.

28. Retetoff S. Inherited thyroxine-binding globulin abnormalities in man. Endocrine Rev 1989; 10:275–92.

29. Cooke NE, Haddad JG. Vitamin D binding protein (Gc globulin). Endocrine Rev 1989; 10:294–307.

30. Bartalena L. Recent achievements in studies on thyroid hormone-binding proteins. Endocrine Rev 1990; 11:47–64.

31. Hammond GL. Molecular properties of corticosteroid binding globulin and the sex-steroid binding proteins. Endocrine Rev 1990; 11:65–79.

32. Rosner W. The functions of corticosteroid-binding globulin and sex hormone-binding globulin: recent advances. Endocrine Rev 1990; 11:80–91.

33. Bartalena L, Robbins J. Variations in thyroid hormone transport proteins and their clinical implications. Thyroid 1992; 2:237–45.

34. Ramaker J, Wood WG. Transthyretin—an explanation of "anomalous" serum thyroid hormone values in severe illness? J Clin Chem Clin Biochem 1990; 28:155–61.

35. Recant L, Riggs DS. Thyroid function in nephrosis. J Clin Invest 1952; 31:789–97.

36. Robbins J, Rall JE. The interaction of thyroid hormones and protein in biological fluids. Recent Prog Horm Res 1957; 13:161–208.

37. Blight LY, Judd SJ, White GH. Relative diagnostic value of serum non-SHBG-bound testosterone, free androgen index and free testosterone in the assessment of mild to moderate hirsutism. Ann Clin Biochem 1989; 26:311–6.

38. Vermeulen A, Stoica T, Verdonck L. The apparent free testosterone concentration, an index of androgenicity. J Clin Endocrinol 1971; 33:759–67.

39. Bikle DD, Gee E, Halloran BP, Kowalski MA, Ryzen E, Haddad JG. Assessment of the free fraction of 25-hydroxyvitamin D in serum and its regulation by albumin and the vitamin D-binding protein. J Clin Endocrinol Metab 1986; 63:954–9.

40. Tait JF, Burstein S. *In vivo* studies of steroid dynamics in man. In: Pincus G, Thimann KV, Astwood EB, Eds. The Hormones. Physiology, Chemistry, and Applications, Vol. 5. New York: Academic Press, 1964:441–557.

41. Cumming DC, Wall SR. Non-sex hormone-binding globulin-bound testosterone as a marker for hyperandrogenism. J Clin Endocrinol Metab 1985; 61:873–6.

42. Isojarvi JI, Pakarinen AJ, Ylipalosaari PJ, Myllyla VV. Serum hormones in male epileptic patients receiving anticonvulsant medication. Arch Neurol 1990; 47:670–6.

43. Ball R, Freedman DB, Holmes JC, Midgley JEM, Sheehan CP. Low-normal concentrations of free thyroxin in serum in late pregnancy: physiological fact, not technical artefact. Clin Chem 1989; 35:1891–6.

44. Spencer CA. Thyroid profiling for the 1990s: free T4 estimate or sensitive TSH measurement. J Clin Immunoassay 1989; 12:82–9.

45. Larsen PR, Alexander NM, Chopra IJ, Hay ID, Hershman JM, Kaplan MM, et al. (Committee on Nomenclature of the American Thyroid Association). Revised nomenclature for tests of thyroid hormones and thyroid-related proteins in serum. J Clin Endocrinol Metab 1987; 64:1089–94. [Reprinted in: Clin Chem 1987; 33:2114–9].

46. Daughaday WH. The binding of corticosteroids by plasma proteins. III. The binding of corticosteroid and related hormones by human plasma and plasma fractions as measured by equilibrium dialysis. J Clin Invest 1959; 37:511–8.

47. Christensen LK. A method for the determination of free, non-protein bound thyroxine in serum. Scand J Clin Invest 1959; 11:326–31.

48. Ross HA. A dialysis rate method for measurement of free iodothyronine and steroid hormones in blood. Experientia 1978; 34:538–9.

49. Swinkels LMJW, Meulenberg PMM, Ross HA, Benraad TJ. Salivary and plasma free testosterone and androstenedione levels in women using oral contraceptives containing desogestrel or levonogestrel. Ann Clin Biochem 1988; 25:354–61.

50. Spaulding SW, Gregerman RI. Free thyroxine in serum by equilibrium dialysis: effects of dilution, specific ions and inhibiitors of binding. J Clin Endocrinol Metab 1972; 34:974–82.

51. Moll GW, Rosenfield RL, Helke JH. Estradiol-testosterone binding interactions and free plasma estradiol under physiological conditions. J Clin Endocrinol Metab 1981; 52:868–74.

52. Sterling K, Brenner MA. Free thyroxine in human serum: simplified measurement with the aid of magnesium precipitation. J Clin Invest 1966; 45:153–63.

53. Ingbar SH, Braverman LE, Dawber NA, Lee YG. A new method for measuring the free thyroid hormone in human serum and an analysis of the factors that influence its concentration. J Clin Invest 1965; 44:1679–89.

54. Helenius T, Liewendahl K. Improved dialysis method for free thyroxin in serum compared with five commercial radioimmunoassays in nonthyroidal illness and subjects with abnormal concentrations of thyroxin-binding globulin. Clin Chem 1983; 29:816–22.

55. Clerico A, Strigini F, Del Chicca MG, Paoletti AM, Melis GB, Fioretti P. Apparent free cortisol concentration in normal men, non-pregnant, pregnant and postmenopausal women. J Nucl Med Allied Sci 1982; 26:181–5.

56. Nelson JC, Tomei RT. Direct determination of free thyroxin in undiluted serum by equilibrium dialysis/radioimmunoassay. Clin Chem 1988; 34:1737–44.
57. Tikanoja SH, Liewendahl BK. New ultrafiltration method for free thyroxin compared with equilibrium dialysis in patients with thyroid dysfunction and nonthyroidal illness. Clin Chem 1990; 36:800–4.
58. Vlahos I, MacMahon W, Sgoutas D, Bowers W, Thompson J, Trawick W. An improved ultrafiltration method for determining free testosterone in serum. Clin Chem 1982; 28:2286–91.
59. Hammond GL, Nissker JA, Jones LA, Siiteri PK. Estimation of the percentage of free steroid in undiluted serum by centrifugal ultracentrifugation-dialysis. J Biol Chem 1980; 255:5023–6.
60. Finucane JF, Griffiths RS. A rapid and simple method for simultaneous measurement of serum free thyroxine and triiodothyronine fractions. J Clin Pathol 1976; 29:949–54.
61. Wheeler MJ, Nanjee MN. A steady state gel filration method on microcolumns for the measurement of percentage free testosterone in serum. Ann Clin Biochem 1985; 22:185–9.
62. Lavoie R, Bergeron J, de Laclos BF, Forest J-C. Determination of free testosterone fraction of human serum by gel bead dialysis. Clin Biochem 1989; 22:451–6.
63. Romelli PB, Pennisi F, Vancheri L. Measurement of free thyroid hormones in serum by column adsorption chromatography and radioimmunoassay. J Endocrinol Invest 1979; 2:25–40.
64. Buehler RJ. Applications of microencapsulated antibody in free hormone radioimmunoassays. In: Albertini A, Ekins RP, Eds. Free hormones in blood. Amsterdam: Elsevier Biomed Press, 1982:121–7.
65. Wallace AM, Aitken S, Duffy FA, Fraser WD, Beastall GH. Measuring free thyroxin by using magnetic antibody-containing microcapsules. Clin Chem 1990; 36:614–9.
66. Hashimoto T, Ishibashi K, Nagahara M, Matsubara F. Unforeseen effect of thyroxine binding globulin when using the microencapsulated antibody method to determine free thyroxine (FT4): misleading results due to circulating unsaturated thyroxine binding globulin. J Clin Chem Clin Biochem 1990; 28:175–9.
67. Witherspoon LR, Shuler SE. Estimation of free thyroxine concentration: clinical methods and pitfalls. J Clin Immunoassay 1984; 7:192–205.
68. Csako G, Zweig MH, Glickman J, Ruddel M, Kestner J. Direct and indirect techniques for free thyroxin compared in patients with nonthyroidal illness. III. Analysis of interference variables by stepwise regression. Clin Chem 1990; 36:645–50.
69. Plebani M, Perobelli L, Burlina A. New method ("SPAC ET") for free thyroxin in serum evaluated. Clin Chem 1986; 32:680–3.
70. Izembart M, Sala M, Baldet L, Schlumberger M, Deltour G. Multi-center study of a new technique for measuring free thyroxin in serum. Clin Chem 1989; 35:2137–9.
71. Piketty M-L, Bounaud M-P, Bounaud J-Y, Lebtahi R, Valat C, Askienazy S, Begon F, Besnard J-C. Multicentre evaluation of a two-step automated enzyme immunoassay of free thyroxine. Eur J Clin Chem Clin Biochem 1992; 30:485–92.
72. Bayer MF. Effective laboratory evaluation of thyroid status. Med Clin North Am 1991; 75:1–26.
73. Midgley JEM, Ekins R. Continuation of misrepresentations of analogue free hormone assays. Ann Clin Biochem 1990; 388–92.
74. Stockigt JR, Barlow, JW, White EL, Csicsmann JN. Influence of altered plasma binding of free and total thyroid hormone levels. In: Albertinin A, Ekins RP, Eds. Free Hormones in Blood. Amsterdam: Elsevier Biomedical Press, 1982:223–30.
75. Christofides ND, Sheehan CP, Midgley JEM. One-step, labeled-antibody assay for measuring free thyroxin. I. Assay development and validation. Clin Chem 1992; 38:11–18.
76. Sheehan CP, Christofides ND. One-step, labeled-antibody assay for measuring free thyroxin. II. Performance in a multicenter trial. Clin Chem 1992; 38:19–25.
77. Wilke TJ. Estimation of free thyroid hormone concentrations in the clinical laboratory. Clin Chem 1986; 32:585–92.
78. Attwood EC, Atkin GE. The T4:TBG ratio: a re-evaluation with particular reference to low and high serum TBG levels. Ann Clin Biochem 1982; 19:101–3.
79. Nelson JC, Tomei RT. Dependence of the thyroxin-binding globulin (TBG) ratio and the free thyroxin index on TBG concentrations. Clin Chem 1989; 35:541–4.
80. Konno N, Nakazato T, Hagiwara K, Taguchi H. A comparison of measurements of serum free T3 concentration by equilibrium dialysis, free T3 index, and T3:TBG ratio in thyroidal and nonthyroidal illnesses. Acta Endocrinol 1983; 103:501–8.
81. Marthur RS, Moody LO, Landgrebe S, Williamson HO. Plasma androgens and sex hormone-binding globulin in the evaluation of hirsute females. Fertil Steril 1981; 35:29–35.

82. Kapoor P, Luttrell BM, Williams D. The free androgen index is not valid for adult males. J Steroid Biochem Mol Biol 1993; 45:325–6.

83. Witherspoon LR, Shuler SE, Garcia MM. The triiodothyronine uptake test: an assessment of methods. Clin Chem 1981; 27:1272–6.

84. Hamolsky MW, Stein M, Freedberg AS. The thyroid hormone-plasma protein complex in man. II. A new in vitro method for study of "uptake" of labeled hormonal components by human erythrocytes. J Clin Endocrinol Metab 1957; 17:33–44.

85. Horn K, Castineiras MJ, Ortola J, Kock R, Perriard FC, Bittner S, et al. The determination of thyroxine and thyroxine uptake with new homogeneous enzyme immunoassays using Boehringer Mannheim/Hitachi analysis systems. Eur J Clin Chem Clin Biochem 1991; 29:697–703.

86. Fresco G, Curti G, Biggi A, Fontana B. Comparison of calculated and measured free thyroid hormones in serum in health and in abnormal states. Clin Chem 1982; 28:1325–9.

87. Keane PM, Walker WHC, Thornton G, Rodbard D. Studies of thyroxine binding to plasma proteins in health and disease. Clin Biochem 1986; 19:52–7.

88. van der Sluijs Veer G, Vermes I, Bonte HA, Hoorn RKJ. Temperature effects on free-thyroxine measurements: analytical and clinical consequences. Clin Chem 1992; 38:1327–31.

89. Ross HA, Benraad TJ. Is free thyroxine accurately measurable at room temperature? Clin Chem 1992; 38:880–6.

90. Nagakawa T, Matsumura K, Taakeda K, Shinoda N, Matsuda A, Matsushita T, Tagami T. Effect of stripping thyroxin from thyroxin-binding globulin on the measurement of free thyroxin in serum by equilibrium dialysis and by radioimmunoassay. Clin Chem 1990; 36:313–8.

91. Zweig MH, Csako G. New automated nonisotopic immunoassays for free thyroxin: effect of albumin and thyroxin-binding globulin concentrations. Ann Clin Biochem 1992; 29:551–5.

92. Vining R, McGinley R. The measurement of hormones in saliva: possibilties and pitfalls. J Steroid Biochem 1987; 27:81–94.

93. Schramm W, Smith RH. An ultrafiltrate of saliva collected in situ as a biological sample for biologic evaluation. Clin Chem 1991; 37:114–5.

94. Klopper A. The choice between assays on blood or on urine. In: Loraine JA, Bell ET Eds. Hormone assays and their clinical application. Edinburgh: Churchill Livingstone, 1976:73–86.

95. Mendel C, Frost PH, Cavalieri RR. Effect of free fatty acids on the concentration of free thyroxine in human serum: the role of albumin. J Clin Endocrinol Metab 1986; 63:1394–9.

96. Kaplan MN, Hamburger JI. Nonthyroidal causes of abnormal thyroid function test data. J Immunoassay 1989; 12:90–9.

97. Cavalieri RR. The effects of nonthyroid disease and drugs on thyroid function tests. Med Clin North Am 1991; 75:27–39.

98. Csako G, Zweig MH, Glickman J, Ruddel M, Kestner J. Direct and indirect techniques for free thyroxin compared in patients with nonthyroidal illness. I. Effect of free fatty acids. Clin Chem 1989; 35:102–9.

99. Sapin R, Shlienger JL, Grunenberger F, Gasser F, Chambron J. In vitro and in vivo effects of increased concentrations of free fatty acids on free thyroxin measurements as determined by five assays. Clin Chem 1990; 36:611–3.

100. Liewendahl K, Helenius T, Naveri H, Tikkanen H. Fatty acid-induced increase in serum dialyzable free thyroxine after physical exercise: implication for nonthyroidal illness. J Clin Endocrinol Metab 1992; 74:1361–5.

101. Young DS. Effects of drugs on clinical laboratory tests, 3rd ed., and 1991 supplement to 3rd ed. Washington, DC: AACC Press, 1990/1991.

102. Borst GC, Eil C, Burman KD. Euthyroid hyperthyroxinemia. Ann Intern Med 1983; 98:366–78.

103. Bikle DD, Gee E, Halloran B, Haddad JG. Free 1,25-dihydroxyvitamin D levels in serum from normal subjects, pregnant subjects and subjects with liver disease. J Clin Invest 1984; 74:1966–71.

104. Sapin R, Gasser F. Free thyroxin in familial dysalbuminemic hyperthyroxinemia, as measured by five assays. Clin Chem 1988; 34:598–9.

105. Sakata S, Nakamura S, Miura K. Autoantibodies against thyroid hormones or iodothyronine. Implications in diagnosis, thyroid function, treatment, and pathogenesis. Ann Intern Med 1985; 103:579–89.

106. John R, Henley R, Shankland D. Concentrations of free thyroxin and free triiodothyronine in serum of patients with thyroxin- and triiodothyronine-binding autoantibodies. Clin Chem 1990; 36:470–3.

107. John R, Henley R. Antibody interference in free thyroxine assays. Ann Clin Biochem 1992, 29:472–3.

108. Lai LC, Day JA, Peaston RT. Spuriously high free thyroxine with the Amerlite MAB FT4 assay. J Clin Pathol 1994; 47:181–2.

109. Roti E, Gardini E, Minelli R, Bianconi L, Flisi M. Thyroid function evaluation by different commercially available free thyroid hormone measurement kits in term pregnant women and their newborns. J Endocrinol Invest 1991; 14:1–9.

110. Nelson JC, Clark SJ, Borut DL, Tornei T, Carlton EI. Age-related changes in serum free thryoxine during childhood and adolescence. J Pediatr 1993; 123:899–905.

111. Iwatani Y, Amino N, Tanizawa O, Mori H, Kawashima M, Yabu Y, Miyai K. Decrease of free thyroxin in serum of lactating women. Clin Chem 1987; 33:1217–9.

112. Carpi A, Toni MG, De Gaudio C. Effect of a single oral dose of L-thyroxine (150 μg) on serum thyroid hormone and TSH concentrations in clinically euthyroid goitrous patients. Thyroidol Clin Exp 1992; 4:69–73.

113. Ain KB, Pucino F, Shiver TM, Banks SM. Thyroid hormone levels affected by time of blood sampling in thyroxine-treated patients. Thyroid 1993; 3:81–5.

114. Midgley JE, Sheehan CP, Christofides ND, Fry JE, Browning D, Mardell R. Concentrations of free thyroxin and albumin in serum in severe nonthyroidal illness: assay artefacts and physiological influences. Clin Chem 1990; 36:765–71.

115. Docter R, Krenning EP, de Jong M, Hannemann G. The sick euthyroid syndrome: changes in thyroid hormone serum parameters and hormone metabolism. Clin Endocrinol 1993; 39:499–518.

116. Browning MCK. Analytical goals for quantities used to assess thyrometabolic status. Ann Clin Biochem 1989; 26:1–12.

117. Kellacker H, Besch W, Woltanski K-P, Diaz-Alonso JM, Kohnert K-D, Ziegler M. Mathematical modelling of competitive labelled-ligand assay systems. Theoretical re-evaluation of optimum assay conditions and precision data for some experimentally established radioimmunoassay systems. Eur J Clin Chem Clin Biochem 1991; 29:555–63.

118. Blomberg KR, Engblom SO. Mathematical theory of complex ligand-binding systems applied to free triiodothyronine immunoassays. Anal Chem 1991; 63:2581–6.

119. Burrin JM. Quality assurance of hormone analyses. Ann Clin Biochem 1988; 25:340–5.

21 AUTOMATION OF IMMUNOASSAYS

DANIEL W. CHAN
Departments of Pathology and Oncology
Johns Hopkins University School of Medicine
and Division of Clinical Chemistry
Johns Hopkins Hospital
Baltimore, Maryland 21287

1. INTRODUCTION

1.1. Meeting the Challenges of Today's Clinical Laboratory

In the 1990s, the clinical laboratory is faced with many challenges (Table 21.1). These include the chronic shortage of qualified technologists, reengineering, space limitation in the hospital, and decreased available resources for the laboratory. External forces also produce challenges such as health care reform, managed care competition, cost compression, and increased regulation of the testing laboratory. Despite these challenges, the users expect the laboratory to provide better services.

In order to meet these challenges, the clinical laboratory needs to become more efficient by incorporating creative solutions and adapting to changes. One solution is automation and system integration. Since most clinical laboratory procedures are labor-intensive, automation will reduce the dependency of the labor requirement. Furthermore, smaller clinical laboratories could justify performing a larger menu of tests "in-house" rather than sending them to outside laboratories. With the

Immunoassay

483

**TABLE 21.1 Challenges of Today's
Clinical Laboratory**

1. Reengineering
2. Limited laboratory space
3. Limited available resources
4. Health care reform
5. Cost compression
6. Increased laboratory regulations

availability of automated devices, certain laboratory tests may be relocated to "near patient," i.e., point-of-care, whether at the bedside or at an outpatient location.

1.2. History of Immunoassay Automation

During the last 20 years, major advances have been achieved in automating routine, general clinical chemistry procedures. Discrete and random access analyzers provided a wide spectrum of chemistry tests around the clock to meet the demands of rapid testing. Recently, more attention has been focused on automating the sample-handling and processing steps, especially with the concern of infectious specimens from patients with hepatitis or acquired immunodeficiency syndrome (AIDS).

Automation of specialized procedures, for example, immunoassay, has lagged behind, especially for heterogeneous immunoassay, i.e., an assay requiring a physical separation of the bound and unbound antigens. The homogeneous immunoassay, i.e., an assay requiring no physical separation of bound and unbound antigens, can be adapted to general chemistry analyzers, however, the heterogeneous immunoassay requires a dedicated analyzer.

The first attempt was to automate radioimmunoassay (RIA). Several systems were introduced in the late 1970s. These systems included the Centria (Union Carbide), Concept 4 (Micromedic), ARIA II (Becton–Dickinson), and Gammaflow (Squibb). These systems, with limited throughput and testing menu, were not as reliable and cost-effective as the users wanted. Automation of immunoassay would not be successful until nonisotopic systems became available.

This chapter is based on two recent publications by Chan, entitled "*Immunoassay Automation: A Practical Guide*" (1) and "*Immunoassay Automation: An Updated Guide to Systems*" (2). The focus is on the concept, principle, issues, and performance of automated immunoassay systems. The detailed descriptions of specific automated systems are cited in the references. For the latest model of a particular system, literature should be requested from the manufacturer of the system. In the ever-changing world of automated immunoassay systems, this approach may have longer lasting value.

2. AUTOMATION OF IMMUNOASSAY

2.1. The Concept of Automation

The total laboratory testing process starts with the ordering of laboratory tests. A complete test menu should include instructions for a particular blood collection device and barcode label for positive identification. The sample should be centrifuged in a closed system and transferred onto the automated system for direct sampling. The actual testing procedure may include a separation step of the bound from unbound antigen if it is a heterogeneous immunoassay. No physical separation step is needed if it is a homogeneous immunoassay. The detection system could be multiapproach, e.g., spectrophotometry and fluorimetry. Finally, electronic data processing and quality control should facilitate verification and reporting of results. Computer terminals located at the user's site will shorten the turnaround time of testing and reporting.

The traditional idea of automation is to adapt reagent to an automated instrument for a central clinical laboratory. Such instrumentation mechanized all the necessary steps in an immunoassay procedure, e.g., pipetting, incubation, washing, and detecting the signal. The automated system performs a large variety of test mixes at the same time with fairly high throughput.

In a broader sense, the concept of automation could include disposable devices designed for quick, mostly qualitative tests, e.g., ICON (Hybritech, Inc.) and test pack (Abbott Labs) for pregnancy testing. These devices use membrane technology with immobilized monoclonal antibodies. A qualitative result is indicated within a few minutes by the presence of color development. Quantitative results are read on a photometer. These devices are self-contained "automation in a box" without instrumentation. Most of these devices are intended for use in the "point of care testing."

In reality, all types of automation may be applicable in a clinical laboratory, whether large or small. A large clinical laboratory may perform all tests on the day shift. During the evening shift, its testing may resemble a medium-size clinical laboratory, while on the night shift, it is more like a small clinical laboratory.

2.2. The Components of Automation

An automated system consists of instrument, reagent, and computer. These three components are interdependent. The format of the reagent will determine the design of the instrument. The limits of the instrument design may require modification of the reagent and the immunoassay procedure. The computer program could optimize the reaction conditions, the sequence of reagent addition, and the order of sample testing. It will expedite data processing and management as well as result reporting. A system will not be successful unless all three components are functioning well as a unit. Therefore, we should consider the issues of automation as an integrated system.

2.3. Issues of Automation

Immunoassay is an analytical procedure involving antigen and antibody binding reaction. After the binding takes place, separation of bound antigen and antibody complex from unbound antigen is needed before the unknown antigen can be quantified. The following are some of the important issues to be considered.

2.3.1. Competitive or Immunometric Assay

Traditional RIA is based on the principle of competitive binding. The radioactive-labeled antigen competes with the unlabeled antigen for a limited amount of binding sites on the antibody. "Sensitivity," as defined by the minimum detectable amount, is affected by the affinity constant of the antibody, the nonspecific binding, the specific activity of the labeled antigen, and the experimental error in the measurement of bound and unbound antigen. In the development of an immunoassay, the competitive approach conserves the use of antibody in the assay since the antibody concentration is limited.

Immunometric assay could be optimized for better sensitivity than the competitive immunoassay. Maximal sensitivity can be achieved with a large concentration of labeled antibody with high specific activity, low nonspecific binding by the labeled antibody, high affinity constant of the labeled antibody, and small experimental errors in measuring the bound labeled antibody.

The decision on whether to use a competitive or immunometric assay will depend on the size of the analyte. The choice for small analytes is the competitive immunoassay, while for large analytes it is the immunometric assay. Immunometric assay provides both the sensitivity and the specificity needed for peptide hormones, e.g., parathyroid hormone (PTH) and adrenocorticotropin (ACTH). The specificity of measuring the intact molecule of PTH could exclude the PTH c-terminal fragments which accumulate in renal disease.

2.3.2. Sample Management

The sample management system is becoming increasingly important as the concern of infectious specimens rises. A random access device is preferable since test requests vary with each individual patient. Furthermore, random access will allow the laboratory to perform testing continuously and eliminate the batching and scheduling of tests.

A sample management system could include sample processing and introduction to the instrument. Positive identification, e.g., barcode label, should be applied at the blood-collection step. The primary blood-drawing tube could be centrifuged and transferred to the testing step. The concept of centrifugation along the axis of the tube allows direct sampling through the top of the tube. Another approach is the use of an automated cap-removal device. Either approach will allow the sample management system to be fully automated.

The sample introduction system should be designed to minimize carryover. Carryover is not a major problem for general chemistries since the physiological ranges of most analytes are rather limited. However, carryover could be a significant problem for hormones and tumor markers. It is not uncommon to have a 10^5-fold difference in the values of tumor markers. An ideal target for carryover is less than 1 part per million. To minimize carryover, the design (shape, size, and materials) of the sampler is important. Adding a washing step in between each sampling may help reduce carryover.

2.3.3. Signal Detection

The type of signal detection system is determined by the signal or the label of the reagent. The choice should be based on technical performance and economic considerations. A system should be able to achieve the sensitivity of most clinically important analytes with acceptable precision, and should be easy to build, relatively inexpensive, common, and easy to troubleshoot. Three types of detection systems that fit these criteria have been used in most automated systems.

Spectrophotometry is probably the most popular type of detection. Enzyme immunoassay (EIA) could be homogeneous or heterogeneous. In the heterogeneous assay, the two most frequently used enzymes are alkaline phosphatase and peroxidase.

Fluorimetry is used widely for both homogeneous and heterogeneous immunoassay. Some systems use enzymes to convert a substrate to a fluorescent product, while others use both spectrophotometry and fluorimetry in the same system. In theory, fluorimetry is capable of detecting as little as 10^{-14} mol of a compound, while spectrophotometry can only detect 10^{-8} mol. In practice, the sensitivity is much reduced due to the background noise from the endogenous fluorophores, e.g., bilirubin, protein, and lipids. Time-resolved fluorescence technique such as the DELFIA system developed by Wallac may reduce this problem somewhat.

Luminometry is gaining popularity rather quickly. Luminescence immunoassay (LIA) has the potential of achieving the highest sensitivity. Most LIAs are heterogenous assays. Taking advantage of the inherent sensitivity, manufacturers have developed an ultrasensitive TSH assay which is capable of measuring TSH down to 0.005 mIU/liter.

2.3.4. Data Management

The data management system is the command center. Table 21.2 lists the desirable characteristics of a data management system.

In order to manage the automation effectively, the data management system should control as many steps as possible in the total testing process. The system should be designed to be user-friendly, and should allow a technologist to perform the crucial daily functions efficiently.

A real-time, on-line quality control (QC) system allows the technologist to make a quick decision on the acceptability of the laboratory result. In this verification step, an "exception" list of results could be generated for further investigation. Results not on the exception list will be allowed to pass through to the reporting step. The rules for the exception list should be user-defined.

Sample identification should be done by a barcode device with a unique identifying label generated as early as possible in the history of the sample. This label will provide positive identification throughout the testing process. It should contain all the testing information and provide a link to the patient identification. An automated system should be able to communicate with the host computer with a bidirectional interface. A buffer to store laboratory data will be important in the event that the host computer is "down."

TABLE 21.2   Desirable Characteristics of a Data Management System

1. Management of all steps in the total testing process
2. User-friendly
3. On-line quality control
4. Sample identification—barcode label
5. Patient identification—report
6. Data reduction—selection of models
7. Troubleshooting of instrument malfunction
8. Lab management functions—workload recording, turnaround time, and QA productivity

Diagnostics of instrument malfunction are important for troubleshooting purposes. Troubleshooting can be performed by the operator or with remote diagnostics through modem or satellite connection to the manufacturer. Modern instruments should contain built-in sensors for the proper operation of the system. One example is a "detector of short-sample" by the pipettor. Continuous monitoring and self-adjusting may be necessary for truly "walk-away" automation.

Other management functions will be useful for a laboratory to evaluate the testing data, workload recording, turnaround time, productivity, quality assurance, and efficiency of the operation. However, these management functions are less critical and should not interfere with the daily operating routines.

2.3.5. Disadvantages of Automated Systems

Automation has its disadvantages. The most obvious disadvantage is the need for capital equipment acquisition. Most fully automated systems use dedicated reagents. The closed system "locks in" the laboratory to use all the reagents from the same manufacturer, even though they may not have the same quality. The choice of tests is also limited by that particular system. The commitment for an automated system is usually 3–5 years. While the quality of reagents may change, the instrument may also become obsolete.

The throughput of most automated systems using heterogenous assays are between 30 and 120 tests/hr. The limited throughput, as well as the reliability issue, forces many laboratories to acquire more than one system. The total dependency of an automated system means that the entire immunoassay system may be shut down. All instruments require maintenance and service. Finally, one should not overlook the human factor. Most instruments are advertised as "walk-away." However, as technologists walk away from the instrument, they are concerned about the outcome of the testing—what if the instrument malfunctions and none of the results are acceptable?

3. AUTOMATED IMMUNOASSAY SYSTEMS

3.1. Homogeneous Immunoassay Systems

Homogeneous immunoassay requires no physical separation of bound and unbound antigen. The major advantage is the ability to adapt the reagent to the existing clinical chemistry analyzer, (for example, the enzyme-multiplied immunoassay technique (EMIT) by Syva). The automated homogeneous immunoassay systems use small sample size and low reagent volume, and provide fast turnaround time. The calibration curve is stable from several days to weeks. This allows the laboratory to perform tests at all hours without having to recalibrate the system. The efficiency is enhanced by saving technical time, quality control, and reagent expenses.

Most homogenous immunoassays take advantage of the size difference between unbound antigen (small) and antigen-bound antibody complex (large). The differences in the size may limit the spectral changes. This will in turn limit the dynamic range of the assay and, to a certain extent, the sensitivity. Since there is no separation of the patient sample from the final signal detection, the sensitivity may be further compromised. Interferences from the patient's sample may cause high background signal or compete with the binding site. Some tests require sample pretreatment to eliminate interferences. For example, digoxin assay requires an acid precipitation (TDx) before analysis. In general, small analytes such as drugs, thyroid, and steroid hormones which are present in relatively high concentrations will work well using homogeneous immunoassay systems.

3.1.1. Open System

An open system consists of a general purpose instrument designed to perform chemistry tests. Immunoassay reagent could be adapted to the instrument if it could use the same sample delivery and the detection device, and require no physical separation of unbound from bound antigen (homogeneous). For example, the BMC/ Hitachi 747 and 911 analyzers are designed to perform routine chemistry tests (for glucose, cholesterol, alkaline phosphatase, etc.). The EMIT reagent could be adapted to this instrument because it uses the same pipetting device and the spectrophotometric detection step.

Because immunoassay may require more reagent or reaction steps than the simpler chemistry test, not all general chemistry instruments could be used for homogeneous immunoassay. For example, the "cloned enzyme-donor immunoassay" (CEDIA) reagent for Vitamin B_{12} and folate uses reagent components which require four reagent-addition steps. The Hitachi 704 analyzer is not designed to handle so many steps, whereas the Hitachi 911 analyzer is. The open systems do have the advantage of the user's choice of reagent and potential competitive edge of more than one reagent. With the introduction of Clinical Laboratory Improvement Amendment (CLIA) of 1988 and the FDA approval process, open systems will have to specify the reagent and the instrument combination in the FDA approval process. Examples of these systems are shown in Table 21.3A.

3.1.2. Closed System

A closed system is one that uses specific reagents designed for a particular instrument. Generally, the same company produces both the instrument and the reagent, although there are a few exceptions. For example, the popular TDX ana-

TABLE 21.3

Instrument	Reagent
A. Open homogeneous immunoassay systems	
Hitachi 747, 911	CEDIA, EMIT
Olympus AU5000	EMIT
Miles Chem 1	EMIT
Roche Cobas/Mira	EMIT
Beckman Array	Nephelometric
B. Closed homogeneous immunoassay systems	
Abbott TDX, ADX	FPIA[a]
Dupont ACA	PETINIA[b]
Roche Cobas	FPIA[c]

[a] Ref. (3).
[b] Ref. (4).
[c] Ref. (5).

lyzer made by Abbott Diagnostics (3) uses fluorescent polarization immunoassay (FPIA) reagents made by Abbott. Because there are so many TDX analyzers for the testing of therapeutic drugs, FPIA reagents made by other companies have become available. The DuPont ACA analyzer (4) uses the particle-enhanced turbidimetric inhibition immunoassay (PETINIA). The advantage of a closed system is that the overall quality of performance can be better controlled by the company. The disadvantage is usually higher price of the reagent. Examples of these systems are shown in Table 21.3B (5).

3.1.3. Combined Homogeneous Immunoassay System

A combined homogeneous immunoassay system (Table 21.4) uses both "open" and "closed" reagents and has the ability to measure both small and large molecules. Most of these systems are available for research use only. They incorporate a unique approach so that both large and small molecules can be measured in a homogeneous format. In addition to immunoassay, electrochemiluminescence (ECL) technology (6) has been applied to the detection of nucleic acids using the Origen analyzer. The coupled particle light scattering (Copalis) system (7) could be used to detect markers on the cell surface in addition to the coupled particles for immunoassay. It uses a flow cytometry approach. The optical fiber evanescent wave fluoroimmunosensor (OIB) immunoassay developed by Boehringer Mannheim (8) uses conventional competitive or immunometric assay with fluorescent conjugates. The fluorescence produced by the evanescent wave generated by the molded polystyrene optical fiber is detected by an immunosensor. This allows short reaction time of less than 5 min while achieving sensitivity comparable to that of conventional immunoassay.

3.2. Heterogeneous Immunoassay Systems

A heterogenous immunoassay is more versatile. It can measure both small and large analytes. With a physical separation step, it eliminates most interfering substances present in the patient's sample before quantification. The separation step together with the potential of using larger sample size improves sensitivity. The immunometric assay tends to have a broader dynamic range of the standard curve. The peptide hormones and tumor markers are ideally measured by immunometric assay, for example, human chorionic gonadotropin (hCG). The heterogeneous immunoassays are more labor-intensive and time-consuming, and require a dedicated immunoassay analyzer.

TABLE 21.4   "Combined"
Homogeneous Immunoassay Systems

Instrument	Reagent	Detection
Sienna Biotech	Copalis	Flow cytometry[a]
BMC-OIB	FIA	OIB[b]
IGEN-Origen	LIA	ECL[c]

[a] Ref. (7).
[b] Ref. (8).
[c] Ref. (6).

TABLE 21.5   Semiautomated Immunoassay Systems

Company	Instrument	Reagent[a]	Separation[b]	Test[c]	Reference
Kodak	Amerlite	LIA	CW	H, T	9
Hybritech	Photon QA	EIA	CB	T	10
Abbott	Commander	EIA	CB	ID	11

[a] EIA, enzyme immunoassay; LIA, luminescent immunoassay.
[b] CB, coated bead; CW, coated well.
[c] H, hormone; T, tumor marker; ID, infectious disease.

3.2.1. Semiautomated Immunoassay Systems

An automated instrument could be built on multiple blocks. These building blocks may be either linked by computer program or mechanically attached. In most semiautomated systems, these blocks function separately, for example, the pipetting of reagent, the incubation of the reaction mixture, the bound/free separation by washing the solid phase, the signal detection, and the data management steps. These systems are operating in batch concept, i.e., testing of all samples for the same analyte. Most fully automated heterogeneous immunoassay systems are relatively slow, with throughput between 30 and 120 tests/hr. Therefore, a high-volume testing laboratory may benefit from using a semiautomated system which takes care of the most labor-intensive steps, leaving the less time-consuming steps for the technologist. Examples are shown in Table 21.5 (9, 10).

3.2.2. Fully Automated Immunoassay Systems

Fully automated immunoassay systems link all the separate components of the semiautomated systems and allow the testing to be completed from sample addition to result reporting. Depending upon the ability of the system to select sample for analysis on demand, the fully automated system can be further subdivided into batch, selective, and continuous access systems. The batch immunoassay systems (11, 12) have been (so far) the primary working systems in the clinical laboratory (Table 21.6A). These systems are small in size and relatively slow in throughput, and are being replaced by the random access systems. The selective systems are similar to the batch systems; however, they have the ability to perform more than one test for a given specimen (13–16). Selective systems are useful for laboratories with a relatively large test volume (Table 21.6B). Because of their inability to test continuously, the selective systems are also being replaced with the truly continuous, random access systems (17–29). These systems vary in their throughput from 30 to 150 tests per hour (Table 21.6C).

4. PERFORMANCE OF IMMUNOASSAY SYSTEMS

4.1. Defining Goals and Objectives

The first step in the evaluation of an automated immunoassay system is to define the goals and objectives of automation (Table 21.7).

Automation is the way to consolidate workstations and thereby reduce the labor requirements and both the number and the skill level of the technologist. Most

TABLE 21.6

Company	Instrument	Reagent[a]	Separation[b]	Test[c]	Ref.
	A. Batch-automated immunoassay systems				
Abbott	IM$_x$	FIA	PF	A	11
Baxter	Stratus II	FIA	CF	H, D, T	12
	B. Selective-automated immunoassay systems				
BMC	ES-300 AL	EIA	CT	A	13
Bio-Rad	Radius	EIA	CW	H	14
BioMerieux	VIDAS	FIA	CW	A	15
Syva	Vista	FIA	MP	A	16
	C. Continuous-access immunoassay systems				
Abbott	AxSym	FIA & FPIA	PF	A	17
Becton–Dickinson	Affinity	EIA	CT	H	18
Behring	Opus Magnum	FIA	CF/MF	A	19
Biotrol	System 7000	EIA	MP	A	20
Ciba-Corning	ACS-180 Plus	LIA	MP	A	21
Diagnostic Products Corporation (DPC)	Immulite	LIA	CB	H	22
DuPont	ACA Plus	EIA	MP	A	23
Miles	Immuno 1	EIA	MP/TB	A	24
Roche	Cobas Core	EIA	CB	A	25
Sanofi	Access	LIA	MP	A	26
Serono	SR-1	EIA	MP	H	27
Tosoh	AIA-1200DX	FIA	MP	A	28
Wallac	AutoDELFIA	tFIA	CW	A	29

[a] EIA, enzyme immunoassay; FIA, fluorescent immunoassay; LIA, luminescent immunoassay; FPIA, fluorescent polarization immunoassay; tFIA, time-resolved FIA.

[b] PF, particle filter; CF, coated filter paper; CT, coated tube; CW, coated well; MP, magnetic particle; MF, multiple-layer film; CB, coated bead; TB, turbidimetric.

[c] A, all; H, hormone; D, drug; T, tumor.

automated systems can achieve calibration stability in 2–4 weeks. This allows more frequent testing without the increased cost of daily calibration. The random access feature of automation should eliminate the "batch" concept. There will be no scheduling of tests. This will enhance the turnaround time.

Automation generally improves the technical performance (precision and sensitivity) of the assay. Most assays could be performed in a single tube rather than in duplicate. This reduces not only the total assay time but also the cost of reagent.

TABLE 21.7 Goals and Objectives of Automation

1. Improve laboratory efficiency
2. Reduce total cost, including personnel
3. Reduce space by consolidating workstations
4. Increase test frequency by continuous testing
5. Improve turnaround time
6. Improve assay performance

The total cost of the testing should be reduced, as the savings in labor and reagents could offset the cost of the instrument. The overall goal of automation is to improve the efficiency of testing.

4.2. Technical Performance

Technical performance is the first step in the evaluation of an automated immunoassay system. The system should be tested in the order of precision, sensitivity, accuracy, patient comparison with another method, and lot-to-lot variation.

4.2.1. Precision

Precision, or more appropriately imprecision, is probably the most important technical aspect of the system. Automation should improve precision to the point that single testing is acceptable. Both within-run and between-run precision should be evaluated. Between-run precision is a more realistic performance indicator since patient samples are analyzed from day to day. The acceptable level of precision is about 5–10% CV in the useful concentration ranges. For random access systems, the precision should be determined in the random access versus batch mode to determine whether there are any differences.

Since precision is the most important aspect of the technical performance, identifying and controlling the source of imprecision is quite important. Table 21.8 lists the sources of imprecision. The reagent components of a system could affect the extent of imprecision, e.g., the affinity constant and the concentration of the antibodies used in the reagent. For immunometric assays, the antibody conjugate will determine the amount of signal generated. The stability and the consistency of the substrate will affect the enzyme reaction and the final color production. The accurate assignment of the calibrator value and the stability of the calibrator are important. Other components that affect the precision are diluent, wash solution, quench solution, and quality control samples. The matrices, pH, ionic strength, and lyophilization process also influence the overall precision.

The binding of antigen and antibody is influenced by the incubation time, temperature, pH, the separation step, and the washing of unbound antigen (competitive assay) or the antibody (immunometric assay). If the separation step involves a membrane device, the nonspecific binding to this membrane may be an area of concern. Adequate washing of the membrane is important.

The enzyme–substrate reaction is affected by conditions similar to the antigen–antibody reaction. However, the effect of temperature and time may be more crucial than the antigen–antibody reaction. Furthermore, the stability of both the enzyme

---

TABLE 21.8   Sources of Imprecision

1. Reagent: antibodies, calibrator, diluent, wash solution, substrate, quality control
2. Antigen–antibody reaction: timing, temperature, separation, washing
3. Enzyme–substrate reaction: timing, temperature, quenching
4. Pipetting: calibration, setting, reproducibility, carryover
5. Interference: nonspecific, heterophilic antibodies, high-dose hook effect
6. Detection: radioactive counter, spectrophotometer, fluorometer, or luminometer
7. Data reduction: curve-fitting algorithm

and the substrate is less than that of the antibody. The color development is also subject to spectral interferences.

Imprecision could be introduced at the detection step. The selection of inappropriate curve-fitting models for data reduction could affect the imprecision. For example, the use of the logit–log model to linearize the standard curve could post imprecision at both ends of the curve. Pipetting is one step in the automation that affects the precision directly.

Interferences could cause imprecision. Nonspecific interferences such as hemolysis, lipemia, and icterus, as well as specific interferences such as heterophilic antibodies, will affect both accuracy and precision. Samples with extremely high concentrations of analyte will affect precision in two ways. First, the high concentration of this sample could carry over into the next sample. Second, it may cause a high dose hook effect. The apparently low value will be rather imprecise.

4.2.2. Sensitivity

Sensitivity is usually defined as the detection limit of an assay. Several approaches to the determination of sensitivity do not yield the same result.

The minimum detectable dose (MDD) is calculated from the mean ± 2 SD of 20 replicates of the zero calibrator response, performed within a run. It is usually calculated from the response (signal) and read-off the calibration curve to obtain the MDD. This approach usually gives the best (lowest) MDD possible and is the accepted industry standard. The MDD calculated in this manner is unrealistic and usually irreproducible from day-to-day. The value of MDD between days is usually higher than the within-run MDD.

Another approach is to use patient samples with zero analyte concentration in determining sensitivity since calibrator does not always resemble patient material. A patient's serum is diluted with the assay diluent to below the detection limit of the assay. The sensitivity is determined at the dilution for which the percentage of recovery found is no longer close to 100% of the expected value. Recently, the term "biological detection limit" was introduced in the area of prostate-specific antigen testing (30).

4.2.3. Accuracy

Analytical accuracy is the ability of a system to determine the true value of the analyte. Methods include recovery, linearity, parallelism, interference, carryover, and calibration stability.

Recovery is an indirect assessment of accuracy. It tests the system's ability to measure a known amount of analyte. The experiment is done by adding a known amount of analyte (A) to a sample with concentration B, and measuring the total concentration (C). The percentage of recovery can be calculated by $100\% \times (C - B)/A$.

The dilution experiment is an assessment of the relative recovery of the system. Diluent is usually the assay buffer or the zero calibrator. In addition, saline or another patient sample could also be used to assess the matrix effect. The linearity is an indication that the responses are proportional and the final concentrations calculated from the curve are linearly related. Good parallelism indicates that the assay fulfills one of the fundamental principles of immunoassay, i.e., the unknown antigen gives the same response as the standard antigen.

4.2.4. Interference

Calculation of analyte concentrations beyond the range of the calibration curve may indicate assay problems such as the high dose hook effect in an immunometric assay or the presence of interferences. At extremely high analyte concentrations, the antibody-binding sites may be saturated with antigens, making the antibodies unavailable to form a sandwich, i.e., antibody–antigen complexes. The end result is the severe underestimation of the analyte concentration. This is a particular problem with analytes which could be present in wide concentration ranges (e.g., choriogonadotropin and many tumor markers).

Heterophilic antibodies have been reported to cause false-positive results in immunometric assays (31 and Chapter 7). Since most monoclonal antibodies are developed from a hybridoma using the mouse system, the presence of anti-mouse antibodies in a patient's serum will lead to false-positive results. To minimize this problem, mouse serum has been added to the reaction medium to absorb mouse antibodies. Some assays use other scavenger antibodies or use Fab fragments rather than the whole immunoglobulins in the immunoassay. Genetically engineered chimeric antibody with a combined mouse and human immunoglobulin molecule has also been used. In addition to the problem of endogenous antibodies, immunotherapy of cancer patients with mouse toxin-labeled antibodies generates human anti-mouse antibodies (HAMA) which cause interference (32). High titers of rheumatoid factors could also cause false-positive results in immunometric assays (for details see Chapter 7).

Other nonspecific interferences such as lipemia, hemolysis, and icterus may affect separation and detection using spectrophotometric, luminometric, or fluorometric measurement. Substances may be present in the serum that cross-react with the antigen–specific antibody. In the digoxin assay, digoxin-like immunoreactive substances (DLIS) have been identified to cause false-positive results in neonates, pregnant women, and patients with renal or liver diseases (33).

4.2.5. Carryover

Carryover is a potential problem for the automated immunoassay system. For most analytes of immunoassay, the physiological ranges are quite broad. Carryover is particularly troublesome for some tumor markers and choriogonadotropin analysis. One would require a carryover rate of less than one part per million.

4.2.6. Calibration Stability

The stability of calibration curve can be determined by the daily QC results over a period of weeks or months. Trend analysis and other statistical analyses may be helpful. Some assays require running one calibrator with each run. The signal generated by this calibrator is compared to the stored curve. The ratio is calculated. The variation of this factor may be a useful indicator of the extent of shift in the calibration curve. If the QC values show a declining trend, calibration may be in order; however, the bias introduced during the recalibration may be a significant component of the overall imprecision of the system.

4.2.7. Method Comparison

Despite the potential shortcomings of method comparison, it is still useful if one realizes the limitations for such comparison. If the reference method is a definitive method, the result of the method comparison could be used to establish the analytical accuracy of the new method. When the clinically defined patient samples are used in the method comparison, the clinical accuracy of the new method can be established. The comparison to the reference method can be used to identify outliers if the reference method has good precision. When the current method is the reference method, one can decide whether the reference ranges need to be changed. With a good correlation coefficient but slope not equal to unity, one can adjust the reference ranges by the slope factor. If the correlation coefficient is poor, i.e., significantly less than 1.0, it will be difficult to assess the reference ranges.

4.2.8. Lot-to-Lot Variation

Whenever possible, the technical performance of multiple lots of reagents should be evaluated. A recommended protocol is shown in Table 21.9.

To check-in a new lot of reagent, one should record the lot number of all components. In the event of inconsistent performance, the component information will facilitate troubleshooting of the causes. The most frequent lot change is the tracer in the RIA and the conjugate in the EIA. This may produce rather dramatic changes in the absolute absorbance or the amount of radioactivity. When the calibrator lot changes, shifts in QC and patient results may be observed. The tolerance limit of the manufacturers vary from 5 to 10% or 1 to 2 SD of the difference between lots.

The signal of the calibrator is a good indicator of lot-to-lot variation of the conjugate. The slope of the calibration curve changes significantly according to the signal. This may affect the sensitivity, linearity, and precision of the assay. For qualitative assays, the positive or negative result will depend greatly on the differences in the absorbance of the zero and the positive cut-off calibrator. Minimum acceptable absorbance value should be set for such assays, e.g., the EMIT assay for drugs of abuse, to avoid false-positive results.

The parameters generated from the data reduction of the calibration curve could be evaluated. These parameters include the slope, intercept, coefficient of correlation, and the standard error estimate. Such parameters could be recorded for quality control and troubleshooting purposes. If there is any indication of nonlinearity, e.g., a patient specimen with high analyte value is shown to have a much lower value with the new lot of reagent, a linearity study should be performed. If both the primary and secondary wavelengths are used, one should compare patient results obtained by both wavelengths.

4.3. Clinical Performance

The goal of a clinical evaluation is to assess the ability of a system to provide accurate test results in a timely fashion for clinical need. The need could be disease-screening, diagnosis, or management.

TABLE 21.9 Protocol for Checking Lot-to-Lot Variation

1. Record lot numbers of all components.
2. Evaluate the absolute and the differences in signal of the calibrator.
3. Evaluate the characteristics of the calibration curve.
4. Evaluate the QC shifts.
5. Compare patient results between the old and new lots.
6. Check linearity, if necessary.

4.3.1. Predictive Value of a Diagnostic Test

The determination of reference values is rather time consuming and requires a large healthy population ($n = 120$ or more). Statistical analysis using the mean ± 2 SD for a population with Gaussian (normal) distribution is the most frequently used method. For non-Gaussian distribution, the percentile method is probably the simplest approach. For tests with relatively specific applications, e.g., CK-MB in the diagnosis of acute myocardial infarction (AMI) or tumor markers in the diagnosis and management of cancer, a decision level is more appropriate than the upper limit of the normal population. The decision level can be determined using a predictive value model.

The predictive value model includes sensitivity, specificity, and efficiency of a test. By varying the decision level, sensitivity and specificity will change in opposite directions. A higher decision level will reduce the sensitivity while increasing the specificity. An optimal decision level can be selected based on the highest possible efficiency.

A useful approach to evaluate multiple tests for the same analyte is the receiver operating characteristic (ROC) curve. The ROC curve can be constructed by plotting sensitivity versus $1-$ specificity or true positive rate versus false positive rate. The advantage of a ROC curve is the display of the performance over the entire range of decision levels. One can pinpoint the decision level at which the optimal sensitivity and specificity can be achieved. By superimposing the ROC curves of more than one test method, one can select the best methodology. A better test is one that displays higher true positive rate and lower false-positive rate. Examples are shown in Fig. 21.1. Prostate-specific antigen (PSA) is better than prostatic acid

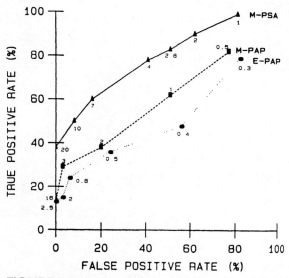

FIGURE 21.1 Receiver-operating characteristic (ROC) curves for PSA, M-PAP, and E-PAP. PSA, prostate-specific antigen; PAP, prostatic acid phosphatase assayed by an immunological mass assay (M) or an enzymatic (E) assay. The data for all 128 patients with prostatic disease are plotted, with several quantitative decision levels (as indicated in the figure) for each assay. Units are μg/liter for M-PAP and PSA, and U/liter for E-PAP. Reprinted, with permission, Ref. (34).

phosphatase (PAP) in the diagnosis of prostatic cancer (34). The preparation of a ROC curve has been discussed in detail by Zweig and Robertson (35).

4.3.2. Distribution of Patient Values

The predictive value model is difficult for use with analytes which are not diagnostic for a single disease. Most, if not all, tumor markers are elevated in more than one disease condition. Carcinoembryonic antigen (CEA) has been shown to be elevated in colorectal, lung, breast, and pancreatic carcinoma as well as in benign conditions. The reference values for CEA in healthy population are higher for smokers than nonsmokers. Using the predictive value model, it is necessary to select a population which includes disease and nondisease groups. The clinical question asked should be used to define the disease group. The outcome of the sensitivity and specificity will depend greatly on the inclusion of the number and groups of patients. In this situation, the actual distribution of patient values may be more informative. The distribution of tumor marker values is usually shown as the percentage of patients with elevated values using various cut-off values in as many groups of healthy, benign, and cancerous patients. These groups are selected based on past experience with other similar markers. An example is CA 549 for breast cancer (36) (Table 21.10).

4.3.3. Disease Management

Disease management is mainly for analytes like tumor markers which are used in the monitoring of treatment and progression of cancer. To determine the success

TABLE 21.10 Distribution of CA 549 Values[a]

Diagnosis	No. patients	No. (and %) of patients with CA 549 values (kilo-units/liter)					
		0–8	>8	>11	>15	>20	>25
Normal women	100	85(85)	15(15)	5 (5)	0 (0)	0 (0)	0 (0)
Nonmalignant							
Benign liver	42	19(45)	23(55)	11(26)	3 (7)	0 (0)	0 (0)
Benign breast	69	63(91)	6 (9)	1 (1)	1 (1)	0 (0)	0 (0)
Pregnancy	30	26(87)	4(13)	0 (0)	0 (0)	0 (0)	0 (0)
Nonbreast metastatic cancer							
Endometrial	8	7(88)	1(12)	1(12)	1(12)	1(12)	0 (0)
Colon	41	25(61)	16(39)	7(17)	3 (7)	1 (2)	1 (2)
Lung	40	22(55)	18(45)	13(33)	11(28)	6(15)	6(15)
Prostate	30	13(43)	17(57)	12(40)	5(17)	5(17)	3(10)
Ovarian	60	22(37)	38(63)	30(50)	21(35)	15(25)	10(17)
Breast cancer							
Adjuvant	88	61(69)	27(31)	10(11)	6 (9)	4 (5)	0 (0)
Metastatic							
Complete remission	16	11(69)	5(31)	3(19)	1 (6)	1 (6)	1 (6)
Partial remission	52	12(23)	40(77)	33(63)	27(52)	22(42)	16(31)
No response (progressive)							
Local	12	5(42)	7(58)	5(42)	3(25)	2(17)	2(17)
Metastasis	94	7 (7)	87(93)	83(88)	79(84)	73(78)	69(73)

[a] Reprinted, with permission, from Ref. (36).

of surgery, one would expect that an elevated marker prior to surgery should fall after a successful operation. The extent of the decrease in the marker value will depend on the pretreatment tumor involvement. After a successful initial treatment, one would expect that the marker value will be steady, possibly within the reference values of healthy individuals. When the marker value starts to trend upward, it may indicate the recurrence of cancer. To monitor the effectiveness of cancer therapy, one would expect that the marker value should increase with progression of cancer. With the regression of cancer, the marker value should decrease. For stable patients, the marker value should not change.

4.4. Operational Performance

An important benefit of automation is enhancing the efficiency of the laboratory operation. Two major issues are the improvement of the system operation and the impact of automation on the laboratory operation.

4.4.1. System Operation

The important features of a data management system were discussed previously. An automated system should require minimum servicing, both scheduled and unscheduled. Reliability of an automated system is critical since automation usually means consolidation of procedures into a system. Therefore, malfunction of the system could shut down the entire immunoassay laboratory.

It is difficult to compare throughput of various systems. Most available systems listed the maximal throughput, which is between 30 and 180 tests/hr. One should also evaluate the throughput in terms of patient samples/hr and samples/working day. If the system is a batch analyzer, one should evaluate how many batches can be performed in a shift. It is more realistic to evaluate the throughput based on your own workload and the physician's ordering pattern. The throughput based on patient samples will depend on the calibration and quality control frequencies as well as the batch size. The less frequent the calibration and quality control of a system, the closer the real throughput of patient samples to the theoretical throughput.

4.4.2. Impact of Automation

The impact of automation on laboratory operation is mainly on the mechanization of the testing procedure and the consolidation of workstations. The random access feature of the automation will facilitate the workflow and improve the turnaround time.

To evaluate an automated system, one should examine the steps of testing which are mechanized. A totally automated system including all the steps of the total testing process is possible by combining computer technology for order entry and result-reporting with a robotic device for sample application and analysis. Automation will change the function of a technologist from technician to data manager and quality control officer. Through workstation consolidation, it will reduce the labor requirement, as well as the skill level and number of workers.

The ability to perform multiple assays is the advantage of an automated system. Therefore, the major benefit of automation is in the consolidation of workstations. The reduction in bench space and personnel should be evaluated. The disadvantage of consolidation is the total dependency on the system. In the event of malfunction, the entire immunoassay testing will be shut down. One should consider back-up systems to ensure continued testing. The extent of such consolidation will depend on the degree of random accessibility. A selective system capable of analyzing multiple tests in a batch format will achieve intermediate consolidation, e.g., the ES-300 analyzer by BMD. A truly random access system with a broad menu and high throughput should allow maximum consolidation into one workstation for immunoassay testing, e.g., the AIA-1200 analyzer by Tosoh Medics. This type of system should eliminate scheduling of analytical runs. Tests will be performed as the sample arrives in the laboratory. The turnaround time should be improved.

4.5. Economic and Human Issues

With the changing health care delivery system, the laboratory is under considerable pressure to reduce costs. Four aspects of the cost improvement will be examined in the economic performance of an automated immunoassay system.

4.5.1. Productivity

Productivity is defined as the output of product per full-time equivalent (FTE) of laboratory personnel. The product could be measured by the number of tests or work units. The higher the work unit per FTE, the higher the productivity. The work unit per FTE is a better indicator than the number of tests per FTE, since tests vary in their complexity. In the process of arriving at the final productivity, one should examine other testing support activities. These include calibration, quality control, duplicate testing, dilution of high samples, and repeat testing due to malfunction of the system. A system which requires frequent calibration, quality control, and repeat testing will result in lower productivity of patient results. An automated system should have a calibration curve that is stable for at least 2 weeks. The calibration stability may vary with different analytes.

4.5.2. Labor Requirement

The labor component represents the greatest potential in the cost improvement. Both the skill level and the number of FTE needed to operate the system will be affected by automation. With a given level of product output, the smaller the labor denominator, the higher the productivity. Automation demands different skills and training, but not necessarily less skill. The number of technologists should be reduced due to the consolidation of workstations. Any reduction in the labor requirement is not beneficial unless this saving can be turned into additional productivity. If the savings in technologist time is fragmented and difficult to convert to a significant block of time, the anticipated increase in productivity will be hard to realize.

4.5.3. The System Cost

The cost of acquiring and operating a system includes instrument, reagent, disposables, maintenance, service contract, and quality control.

Laboratorians often negotiate the price for the instrument and reagent, while other operating costs are not appreciated. Examples include the service contract, maintenance, disposables, and quality control. The annual service contract is often priced at about 10% of the instrument cost. Unscheduled downtime could be costly for both the laboratory and the hospital.

Disposable items could be costly on a daily basis if a system uses disposable cuvettes, pipettes, tips, etc. Quality control is essential but does not generate revenue. The cost of QC is determined by the frequency of QC and the QC material. The cost of reagent should be analyzed not only per test, but also per patient. A number of factors affect reagent usage and hence reagent cost. Examples are single versus duplicate testing, frequency of calibration, QC, retesting of samples with values outside the assay dynamic range, and malfunction of the system. The other factor is waste; it is usually between 5 and 20%.

In most closed systems, the instrument cost is less important to the manufacturer since the reagents and disposables must also be purchased from them. In general, purchase of the system is probably the most economical approach since the manufacturer will most likely give you a better reagent price. In other situations, it may be more advantageous to rent or lease. For example, during this time of rapidly changing technology, it may be wiser to rent so that your system will not be obsolete before the end of its useful life.

4.5.4. The Total Cost

One should consider the total cost to include quality assurance and impact on the health-care provider. The impact of turnaround time and the level of laboratory service on the hospital is difficult to measure. One indicator is the length of stay of patients in the hospital. Any avenue to reduce the length of stay will save the hospital money. An automated system could provide more frequent testing and better turnaround time. This may lead to faster diagnosis and workup of the patient. It will expedite the discharge of the patient and shorten the length of stay of the patient.

4.5.5. Human Issues

Finally, one should not forget about human issues in automation. The first issue is safety. A system should be designed to ensure safety of the operator. Safety issues relate to injury due to mechanical moving parts, infections from biological hazards (e.g., AIDS, hepatitis virus), and potential fire hazards. Computer programs for the operation of the system should be "user-friendly." Psychological factors should be considered for a walk-away instrument. For example, error messages should be indicated as soon as a problem occurs. An audible alarm should be used to alert the operator of such an occurrence.

5. FUTURE TRENDS

The design of the future automated immunoassay system will be dependent upon the need of the testing location, the quality expectation, and the technological advances.

Where will the testing of patients be done in the future? In central clinical laboratories, decentralized locations, physician's office, or the patient's home? It is possible that a trained technologist could perform laboratory tests in the patient's home using a portable testing device. Alternatively, a sample can be collected by the patient and transported to a testing center. Reports could be transmitted by fax or electronic mail.

Outpatient testing could be performed at a testing center in a convenient location away from the patient's home. It depends on the desired turnaround time, the complexity of the test, and the cost. I believe that the turnaround time issue will be less critical in the future as more automation will include preanalytical variables such as order entry, sample collection, transportation, processing, and result reporting. At the present time, such preanalytical variables often cause significant delays in the testing process.

For in-patients, a hospital laboratory needs a system with a large menu and continuous access to different samples and tests. A commercial laboratory needs an automated system with higher throughput since most of the testing is routine in nature. The continuous access feature is less critical. I believe that more centralization of laboratory testing will occur to improve efficiency. Therefore, the need of such high throughput instruments will increase.

System integration will be the next level of automation. Since an individual system may not fulfill all the needs of a particular laboratory, multiple systems of the same or different type could be linked together with a common sample processor. The data generated by the different instruments could be reported by a common data management system. Furthermore, a totally integrated immunoassay system would be able to perform all the steps in the total testing process.

Technological advances in immunoassay automation will result in miniaturized systems with better sensitivity and faster testing time, for example, the BMC system using optical fiber evanescent wave fluoro-immunosensor. Multiple analytes could also be performed simultaneously using different labels, for example, the time-resolved fluorescence system (DELFIA). The other approach is the use of different particle sizes, for example, the Copalis system. The laser detector of the flow cytometer could produce signals at different positions based on the size of the particle.

Finally, automated immunoassay systems should be designed to meet the clinical need and expectation of the user. It should include as many steps as possible in the total testing process. A system composed of individual modules may be the best approach. In one extreme, such modules may be a disposable unit to perform a single test. On the other hand, the module may be able to perform a group of tests suitable for a unique clinical setting, e.g., emergency room, critical care unit, and outpatient clinic for a specific medical discipline. Clinical settings would be the determining factor of the test menu on a particular system, rather than the traditional laboratory disciplines, i.e., chemistry, microbiology, and hematology. Such modular systems would be most suitable for the changing needs of the clinical laboratory in the 1990s and beyond.

References

1. Chan DW, Ed. Immunoassay Automation: A Practical Guide. San Diego: Academic Press, 1992:1–367.
2. Chan DW, Ed. Immunoassay Automation: An Updated Guide to Systems. San Diego: Academic Press, 1996:1–309.
3. Wong SH. TDx systems. In: Chan DW, Ed. Immunoassay Automation: A Practical Guide. San Diego: Academic Press, 1992:317–41.
4. Litchfield W, Craig AR, Frey WA, Leflar CC, Looney CE, Luddy M. Novel shell/core particle for automated turbidimetric immunoassays. Clin Chem 1984; 30:1489–93.

5. Goldsmith BM. Cobas-Fara II analyzer. In: Chan DW, Ed. Immunoassay Automation: A Practical Guide. San Diego: Academic Press, 1992:129–35.
6. Blackburn GF, Shah HP, Kenten JH, Leland J, Kamin RA, Link J, et al. Electrochemiluminescence detection for development of immunoassays and DNA probe assays for clinical diagnostics. Clin Chem 1991; 37:1534–9.
7. Bodner AJ, Britz J. Copalis system. In: Chan DW, Ed. Immunoassay Automation: An Updated Guide to Systems. San Diego: Academic Press, 1996:253–276.
8. Mahoney W, Lin JN, Brier RA, Luderer A. Real-time immunodiagnostics employing optical immunobiosensor. In: Chan DW, Ed. Immunoassay Automation: An Updated Guide to Systems. San Diego: Academic Press, 1996:231–252.
9. Faix JD. Amerlite immunoassay system. In: Chan DW, Ed. Immunoassay Automation: A Practical Guide. San Diego: Academic Press, 1992:117–27.
10. Frye RF. The Photon-ERA immunoassay analyzer. In: Chan DW, Ed. Immunoassay Automation: A Practical Guide. San Diego: Academic Press, 1992:269–92.
11. Chou PP. IMx system. In: Chan DW, Ed. Immunoassay Automation: A Practical Guide. San Diego: Academic Press, 1992:203–19.
12. Kahn SE, Bermes EW. Stratus II immunoassay system. In: Chan DW, Ed. Immunoassay Automation: A Practical Guide. San Diego: Academic Press, 1992:293–316.
13. Sagona MA, Collinsworth WE, Gadsden RH. ES-300 immunoassay system. In: Chan DW, Ed. Immunoassay Automation: A Practical Guide. San Diego: Academic Press, 1992:191–202.
14. Russel J, Edwards R. Radius immunoassay system. In: Chan DW, Ed. Immunoassay Automation: An Updated Guide to Systems. San Diego: Academic Press, in press.
15. Ng R. VIDAS system. In: Chan DW, Ed. Immunoassay Automation: An Updated Guide to Systems. San Diego: Academic Press, 1996:51–62.
16. Li TM. The Vista immunoassay system. In: Chan DW, Ed. Immunoassay Automation: a Practical Guide. San Diego: Academic Press, 1992:343–49.
17. Painter P. The AxSym system. In: Chan DW, Ed. Immunoassay Automation: An Updated Guide to Systems. San Diego: Academic Press, 1996:13–28.
18. Chan DW, Kelley C. Affinity immunoassay system. In: Chan DW, Ed. Immunoassay Automation: A Practical Guide. San Diego: Academic Press, 1992:83–94.
19. Shoemaker B. The Opus Magnum system. In: Chan DW, Ed. Immunoassay Automation: An Updated Guide to Systems. San Diego: Academic Press, 1996:29–43.
20. Dellamonica C, Frier C. Routine use of a Biotrol System 7000 in a private laboratory. J Clin Immunoassay 1992; 15:242–5.
21. Klee G. The Ciba Corning ACS 180 automated immunoassay system. In: Chan DW, Ed. Immunoassay Automation: An Updated Guide to Systems. San Diego: Academic Press, 1996:63–102.
22. Witherspoon L. The DPC IMMULITE automated immunoassay system. In: Chan DW, Ed. Immunoassay Automation: An Updated Guide to Systems. San Diego: Academic Press, 1996:103–130.
23. Vaidya HC, Zuk PJ, Ballas RA. ACA plus accessory for the ACA discrete clinical analyzer. In: Chan DW, Ed. Immunoassay Automation: An Updated Guide to Systems. San Diego: Academic Press, 1996:131–144.
24. Ehresman DJ, Jacob L. Immuno 1 automated immunoassay system. In: Chan DW, Ed. Immunoassay Automation: An Updated Guide to Systems. San Diego: Academic Press, 1996:145–166.
25. Huber PR. Cobas Core immunoassay system. In: Chan DW, Ed. Immunoassay Automation: An Updated Guide to Systems. San Diego: Academic Press, 1996:167–184.
26. Guitard M. The Access immunoassay system. In: Chan DW, Ed. Immunoassay Automation: An Updated Guide to Systems. San Diego: Academic Press, 1996:185–200.
27. Demers LM. SR1 immunoassay system. In: Chan DW, Ed. Immunoassay Automation: A Practical Guide. San Diego: Academic Press, 1992:277–92.
28. Chan DW. AIA-1200 immunoassay system. In: Chan DW, Ed. Immunoassay Automation: A Practical Guide. San Diego: Academic Press, 1992:95–115.
29. Gudmundsson TV, Olafsdottir E. AutoDELFIA system. In: Chan DW, Ed. Immunoassay Automation: An Updated Guide to Systems. San Diego, Academic Press, 1996:215–230.
30. Vessela RL, Noteboom J, Lange PH. Evaluation of the Abbott IMx automated immunoassay of prostate specific antigen. Clin Chem 1992; 38:2044–54.
31. Boscato LM, Stuart MC. Heterophilic antibodies: a problem for all immunoassays. Clin Chem 1988; 34:27–33.
32. Kricka LJ, Schmerfeld-Pruss D, Senior M, Goodman DB, Kaladas P. Interference by human antimouse antibody in two-site immunoassays. Clin Chem 1990; 36:892–4.

33. Soldin SJ. Digoxin-issues and controversies. Clin Chem 1986; 32:2–12.
34. Rock RC, Chan DW, Bruzek DJ, Waldron C, Oesterling J, Walsh P. Evaluation of a monoclonal immunoradiometric assay for prostate-specific antigen. Clin Chem 1987; 33:2257–61.
35. Zweig MH, Robertson EA. Clinical validation of immunoassay: a well-designed approach to a clinical study. In: Chan DW, Ed. Immunoassay: A Practical Guide. San Diego: Academic Press, 1987:97–128.
36. Chan DW, Beveridge RA, Bruzek DJ, Damron DJ, Bray KR, Gaur PK, *et al.* Monitoring breast cancer with CA 549. Clin Chem 1988; 34:2000–4.

22 THIN-FILM IMMUNOASSAYS

SUSAN J. DANIELSON

Johnson & Johnson Clinical Diagnostics
Rochester, New York

1. INTRODUCTION

Techniques in clinical diagnostics have undergone many advances in recent years as clinical chemistry workloads have increased, due to increased numbers of both analytes and specimens. Assay methods for important analytes have been streamlined by increased automation, resulting in improved performance and increased convenience for the user. At the same time, there has been an increasing demand for assays with equivalent performance which can be carried out in small laboratories, doctors' offices, and other decentralized settings by personnel with limited formal technical training. The approach referred to as dry reagent chemistry has satisfied both of these needs. Miniature analytical elements have been developed for the quantitative analysis of serum analytes. These assays integrate several conventional analytical steps, including chemical and physical reactions as well as separation steps, into one element. Generally no reagent preparation or sample pretreatment is necessary, and only sample application is required to initiate an analysis. The sample volume is small, and the analysis is usually completed in a few minutes. This technology allows both low- and high-volume testing to be cost-effective because of the stability of the dry format and the unit-dose reagent packaging. In addition, these elements are easily stored and disposed of following use. The instrumentation required is generally uncomplicated, and the technology adapts well to small instruments.

Immunoassay

1.1. Early Dry Reagent Clinical Assays

One of the earliest dry reagent clinical assays was a test for glucose in urine (1). This test, introduced in 1957, used glucose oxidase/peroxidase chemistry and contained all the reagents necessary for the assay dried in paper pads. The element was dipped into the urine specimen to dissolve the dry reagents and initiate the reaction events, which led to color formation within a minute. The results were semiquantitative, because the color generated on the element was compared to a color chart to determine the approximate glucose concentration. Several other tests were subsequently developed for other urine analytes (2). These tests were then extended to the measurement of glucose in blood, and quantitation became feasible in these elements with the introduction of appropriate instrumentation (3). The detection methodology that was developed for these purposes has most commonly utilized reflectance and front-face fluorescence measurements. The success of these early products stimulated the development of a variety of analytical elements for a large number of blood analytes based on single-element and multilayer technology. The layered coating technology, introduced by the Eastman Kodak Company in 1978 (4, 5), in which classical clinical chemical assays were transformed into coated, multilayered thin-film elements, is an extension of technology used in the photographic industry. These assays have greatly simplified the operations performed by the customer, while the element and assay designs have become substantially more complex.

1.2. Dry Reagent Immunoassays

Immunoassay technology has also advanced over the past several years with improvements in antibody and label production, separation techniques, and convenience for the customer. One approach has involved the development of immunoassays based on single- or multilayer dry reagent devices (6, 7). Single-layer immunoassays have all the reagents contained in one phase, while multilayer immunoassays have assay reagents segregated into layers or zones that collectively constitute the analytical element. Reagents used in these assays have generally been adapted from conventional solution immunoassays. Multilayer elements can accommodate both homogeneous and heterogeneous immunoassay formats. Separation of the antibody-bound label from the free label can be accomplished by diffusion or by liquid transport in the multilayer formats. Self-contained, single-layer immunoassays can generally accommodate only homogeneous immunoassays because there is no means for separation of bound from free label. When all of the reagents are incorporated into the element, antibody-binding and signal-generating reactions proceed simultaneously. Thus there is no opportunity for altering individual steps in a reaction sequence. Increased flexibility in reaction time has been built into the Dade Stratus (8), Behring OPUS (9), and Johnson & Johnson Clinical Diagnostics (J&JCD) VITROS Immuno-Rate (10) assays, all of which incorporate a defined incubation time, prior to addition of substrate, to initiate the enzymatic reaction and to remove unbound material from the area observed by the reflectometer or photometer.

The majority of the single-element and multilayer immunoassay systems described in the literature are based on a competitive binding format for low-molecular-weight analytes. Assays for small molecules are easier to design because these materials migrate more readily through multilayer films. High-molecular-weight proteins can be excluded or retarded by the sieving effects of the matrix. This can complicate the design of elements for these analytes. In addition, the measurement of high-concentration, high-molecular-weight analytes usually requires the incorporation of high levels of expensive immunomaterials into the element in order to avoid the high dose hook effect (11). This phenomenon affects all sandwich assays, but is of particular concern for undiluted assays. In spite of these complications, a variety of dry reagent immunoassays have been developed for high-molecular-weight analytes (12, 13).

The small dimensions of the multilayer systems constrain the useable sample volume, but provide the advantage of minimizing diffusion distances required for reactants. For example, an element which is 1 mm thick, with an 80% void volume and a 1-cm^2 detection area, can accomodate a maximum sample size of 80 μl. Most of the existing systems have even smaller dimensions and thus require even smaller sample volumes. Many assays utilize only a 10-μl sample. The small dimensions of these elements also constrain the removal of large excesses of reagents such as those used in immunometric assays or single-step sandwich assays for high-concentration analytes. An advantage of these small elements is that effective diffusion distances are much shorter than in conventional microtiter plate immunoassays. For example, reactants have to migrate less than 1/100th the radius of a conventional microtiter plate well to reach an immobilized antibody in these elements. Burke estimates, using the Einstein equation for Brownian motion, that the time required for a protein with a diffusion coeffecient of 5×10^{-7} cm^2/sec to travel through a 100-μm-thick layer is only 20 sec (6). This decrease in diffusion time translates into shorter required analysis times.

The purpose of this chapter is to describe the basic features of dry reagent analytical elements and provide an overview of their operation. The development of dry reagent assays has proven to be considerably more complex than the development of solution assays. Optimization data from solution experiments are generally not applicable to dry reagent systems, because analyte concentration, diffusion, and reaction rates are generally different in thin-film analytical elements than in solution. In the design of dry reagent immunoassays variables such as matrix composition, layer thickness, wetting agents, drying time, and manufacturing process variables during layer casting must be considered in addition to the standard solution variables of antibody and label concentration and binding parameters (7). The successful development of these assays in the dry format has frequently required the invention of new approaches, methods, and materials. The different approaches that have been followed are described with a focus on novel solutions to specific problems encountered in the development of these dry reagent immunoassays.

2. BASIC FEATURES OF DRY REAGENT ASSAYS

The goal in the design of dry reagent assays is generally to achieve a self-contained analytical device. These elements can have multiple functional zones that exist as single layers or which have been combined into one layer during the construction of the assay. All of these elements have a support zone, a reflective zone, an analytical zone, and a sample application zone (14). The support zone is often provided by a transparent, thin, rigid, plastic material such as poly(ethylene terephthalate) that serves as a foundation for the element. Alternatively, the support layer can be opaque and provide the reflective function.

These assays are generally monitored by reflectance spectroscopy or front-face fluorescence, which requires the presence of a reflective surface. This surface functions by reflecting light emitted or not adsorbed by a dye in the element to a detector. The reflective function is generally constructed by introducing reflecting or scattering centers into the element. Commonly used materials include pigments such as titanium dioxide (TiO_2) or barium sulfate ($BaSO_4$), reflective materials such as metals or foils, fibrous materials including paper and fabrics, or particulate materials such as polymer beads or short fibrous rods. The primary requirement of a reflective material is that its absorbance of electromagetic radiation in the spectral region of interest be negligible.

The analytical function of the dry chemistry can be very complex and consist of multiple chemical reaction and physical function zones. Specific reaction zones, separation zones, masking zones including radiation blocking zones, and trapping zones including selectively permeable barriers can all be included. These zones may be incorporated as separate layers or may be integrated in various combinations into a single layer. Layers that constitute the analytical function have been prepared from a variety of materials including film-forming polymers, fibrous materials, or nonfibrous porous materials.

The sample application zone can be designed to trap cells, crystals, and other particulates as well as proteins and other high-molecular-weight materials in addition to rapidly spreading the applied sample. Some sample application zones have also been designed to incorporate the reflectance function as well. A variety of materials have been used for the construction of these zones, including blush polymers, polymer beads, fabrics, membranes, and paper.

2.1. Sample Delivery

In the absence of a sample application zone, a drop of blood or serum applied to a dried film of hydrophilic polymer comprising the analytical function of these elements tends to form a bead of fluid on the surface even when surfactant has been added to minimize surface tension. The result is that the fluid enters the element very slowly. In addition, chromatographic effects can lead to undesirable washing of incorporated reagents away from the sample application area. The primary purpose of a sample application zone is to counteract the surface tension of the applied sample in order to rapidly spread it laterally after application. This rapid spreading phenomenon, relative to underlayer penetration, makes this technology relatively insensitive to changes in applied sample volume.

Early attempts to apply a uniform concentration of analyte to an element's reagent area used an approach called sample confinement (15). This approach utilized a barrier placed on top of the element to confine the applied sample to a predefined region of the element's surface. Specialized spreading systems, based on wettable capillary matrices, subsequently evolved. This approach is based on two principles (6). The first is that minimization of the surface tension in a very porous layer will allow a sample to fill this zone quickly, thus providing a level reservoir from which the underlying reagent layers can draw liquid. The second is that the osmotic pressure of rehydration in the underlying layers greatly exceeds the capillary retention forces in a porous spreading layer, which results in fluid being pulled into these layers from the porous layer. This concept is shown in Fig. 22.1.

2.1.1. Blush Polymer Spreading Layer

Experiments conducted in the early 1970s by Pryzbylowicz and Millikan of the Eastman Kodak Company, aimed at improving sample spreading, led to the idea that a spreading layer could be coated as a slurry over the thin-film reagent layers and formed in place during drying. From this idea, they (16) invented the integral blush polymer spreading layer that has formed the basis of the multilayer thin-film technology of J&JCD. This spreading layer is prepared by dissolving a nonswelling, water-insoluble polymer, such as cellulose acetate, in a low-boiling, good solvent for the polymer, such as acetone. A higher-boiling "nonsolvent," such as toluene, which is a poor solvent for the polymer, is then added. This slurry is then coated onto the reagent layers and dried under controlled conditions. Following drying, an isotropically porous structure remains, which is typically about 100 to 300 μm in thickness, with 60 to 90% void volume and average pore sizes ranging from 1.5 to 3.0 μm. After incorporation of pigments such as TiO_2 or $BaSO_4$, these structures were found to have diffuse reflecting properties ideal for reflection densitometry. It was found that a variety of other materials can also be added to the formulation, including carbon black for opacity, plasticizers to prevent cracking, and surfactants to promote spreading.

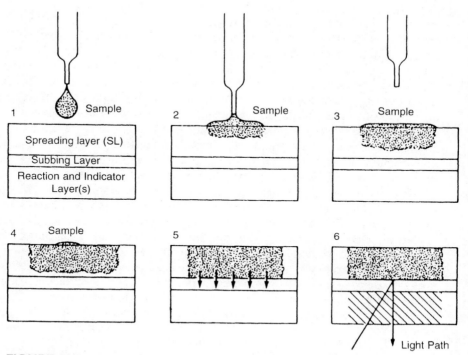

FIGURE 22.1 Sample spreading in a porous spreading layer. Reprinted from *Clin. Biochem.* 16, Shirey, TL, Development of a layered-coating technology for clinical chemistry, Copyright 1983, 147–55, with kind permission from Elsevier Science Ltd., The Boulevard, Langford Lane, Kidlington OX5 1GB, UK.

2.1.2. Particulate Spreading Layers

The direct incorporation of immunoreagents into a nonaqueous formula, such as the blush polymer described above, was found to present some problems because of their relative tendency to denature in the organic solvents used in this process. In addition, the void spaces in these blush polymers were not large enough to accommodate very high-molecular-weight analytes, antibodies, labels, and immune complexes. In an effort to produce a spreading layer with a higher degree of porosity, which could be coated under aqueous conditions, it was discovered that mixtures of plastic spheres ($d = 1$–100 μm) could be coated in the presence of certain types of adhesive to give coherent layers with the desired porosity and performance (17). Liquid transport is facilitated in these spreading layers by the capillary action of the liquid being drawn through the interconnected spaces within the particulate structure of the layer. This approach results in the generation of sample spreading layers which are similar to the blush polymer spreading layer in their ability to distribute liquid sample uniformly in a constant volume per unit area throughout the reagent layers and also in their relative insensitivity to applied sample volume.

These particulate layers are generated *in situ* by coating and drying a metered coverage of an aqueous slurry of particles and adhesive over the reagent layers. The particles are inert, stable to the heat of drying, impermeable, and nonswellable in aqueous solutions in order to ensure structural integrity and retention of the void spaces upon application of sample. Beads that are near neutral buoyancy, such as polystyrene, are preferred because of their stabilization of the coating slurry. The adhesive polymers typically have a glass transition temperature (T_g) that is at least 30°C less than the heat-stability temperature of the heat-stable particles. This enables the adhesive to be rendered flowable without adversely affecting the particles. The attachment of the adhesive to the surface of the particles is facilitated in this state. As the drying process occurs, capillary pressure forces develop between adjacent particles, tending to draw flowable adhesive to these regions. This enhances the concentration of the adhesive at the junction of the particles, resulting in the formation of a coherent particulate structure. The amount of binder must be sufficient to ensure adequate adhesive strength, but it cannot be present at levels high enough to decrease void volume and impede fluid flow. In addition, the adhesive must remain insoluble following the initial drydown in order to preserve the structural integrity of the spreading layer following rewetting by the applied sample.

Adhesives can be prepared as latexes in the presence of surfactants. This approach offers the advantage of maintaining the adhesive in a finely divided discrete form and prevents undesired coalescence and agglomeration of the adhesive and particles in the coating slurry. In addition, the use of the adhesive in latex form promotes the concentration of the adhesive at discrete surface areas during drying. The use of latexes also makes possible the use of water-insoluble adhesives in aqueous dispersions. An example of a polymer that has sufficient water insolubility to be useful as an adhesive for the preparation of these spreading layers is Poly(*n*-butyl acrylate co-2-acrylamido-2-methylpropanesulfonic acid-co-2-acetoacetoxyethyl methacrylate). Photomicrographs of cross sections of blush polymer and particulate bead spreading layers are shown in Fig 22.2.

2.1.3. Particulate Spreading Layers with Reactive Groups

Koyama *et al.* (Konishiroku, Japan) (18) have described the use of particulate polymer beads that contain cross-linkable reactive groups, such as glycidyl methacry-

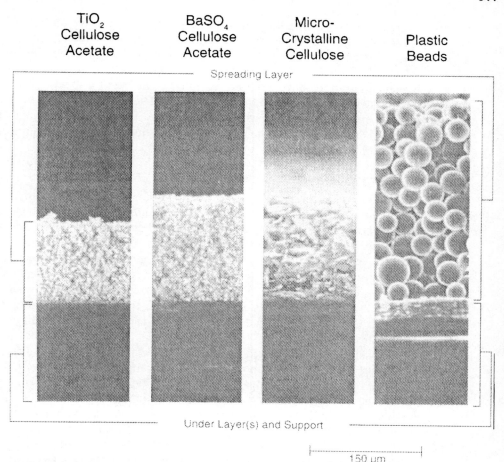

FIGURE 22.2 Photomicrographs of cross sections of blush polymer and particulate bead spreading layers.

late, in order to form isotropically porous spreading layers which do not require the separate addition of binder. The cross-linking can occur between epoxide groups on adjacent beads or between different kinds of reactive groups (e.g., epoxide groups and amino groups) on adjacent beads. In addition to epoxide groups, other reactive groups are available for the formation of chemical bonds between adjacent particles having the same reactive group, including aziridyl, formyl, hydroxymethyl, thiol, and carbamoyl groups. Several combinations of different reactive groups capable of forming chemical bonds between adjacent beads are also mentioned. These particles have diameters of 1 to 350 μm and generate spreading layers containing void volumes of 25 to 85%. The preferred polymer particles are heat stable with T_gs of 40°C or higher. The bound particulate structure has been designed to be impermeable and nonswellable in the presence of aqueous fluids. These particulate layers are generated by coating a stable dispersion of reactive particles in a solvent which does not dissolve the particles. This is followed by removing the solvent at a temperature below the T_g of the polymers and, at the same time, promoting the chemical cross-linking of adjacent particles. Surfactants can be added to aid in the stabilization of the reactive particle dispersions. Catalysts such as acids or bases are often added to the dispersions to promote chemical bond formation.

Koyama and Kikugawa have also described an alternative approach (19) in which reactive epoxide groups have been grafted onto cellulose or polypropylene fibers, resulting in the generation of cross-linkable fibers. These materials are then coated and dried in order to form porous spreading layers. Enzymes and antibodies can be covalently immobilized via the same reactive groups prior to formation of the coated particulate layer.

2.1.4. Preformed Spreading Layers

Kitajima et al. (Fuji, Japan) (20) have described the use of fabric spreading layers which are laminated to an underlying coated thin-film reagent layer. A variety of fabrics have been used, including both natural and synthetic fibers. These fabrics have been treated with surfactants, wetting agents, and hydrophilic polymers to improve the wettability of the layer such that an applied sample will be absorbed into the layer quickly. An advantage of this approach is that sensitive assay reagents can be impregnated into the spreading layer prior to lamination under mild conditions that will not cause activity loss. In addition, the possibility of undesirable extraction of reagents from already coated underlayers into the spreading layer is reduced by this approach.

Plain weave fabrics, which are formed by weaving warp and weft yarns alternately, are preferred for the preparation of these liquid sample spreading layers. Cotton (canequim, broadcloth, and poplin), other natural fibers (kapok, flax, hemp, ramie, silk), or synthetic fibers (viscose rayon, cupro-ammonium rayon, cellulose acetate, vinylon and polyethylene terephthalate) woven in a similar manner have been described. These fabrics are subsequently processed to introduce the desired degree of hydrophilicity by the incorporation of a variety of surfactants, wetting agents (e.g., glycerine or polyethylene glycol), or hydrophilic polymers (e.g., gelatin or polyvinyl alcohol) at levels ranging from about 0.1 to 10% per unit weight of fabric. These materials can be incorporated by dipping or spraying followed by drying. The proper level of reagent processing is determined experimentally for each fabric and application since levels which are too high can cause deterioration of the sample-spreading action.

These multilayer elements can be constructed as sheets by a lamination process in which the fabric spreading layer is firmly adhered to a reagent layer. This is achieved by forcing the two layers into close contact with each other by passing them between a pair of pressed rollers to form a uniform laminate. An adhesive layer, consisting of a hydrophilic polymer, may also be included to strengthen the adhesion force between the layers. The fabric layer is laminated to the reagent layer by application of pressure before the hydrophilic polymer of the adhesive layer is dried or after this layer is wetted with water or an aqueous surfactant solution.

Other functions can be introduced into the element by modification of the spreading layer fabric prior to its lamination onto the reagent layer. Kitajima et al. (21) have described an element containing a very thin water-permeable, radiation-blocking layer. This layer is composed of a metal or metal alloy that has been vacuum deposited on the spreader fabric prior to lamination. The thickness of the deposited metal film layer is only about 50 to 500 Å. This barrier layer functions to block light transmitted from the porous spreading layer and as a reflective surface for colorimetric analysis.

2.1.5. Sample Spreader

The OPUS immunoassay system (Behring Diagnostics) uses a sample application device to facilitate sample spreading in their immunoassay elements (22). This "spreader grid" is part of an injection-molded plastic holder for the thin film. It consists of multiple, pyramid-shaped projections which rise from a flat surface and are 100 μm high. When this structure is placed in contact with the top layer of the film, a structure with a high degree of capillarity results, thus achieving the same results as the spreading layers described previously.

2.2. Instrumentation

Chemical reactions in dry reagent elements are generally monitored by reflectance or fluorescence spectroscopy. The instrumentation ranges in size from hand-held devices to large freestanding instruments. Many of the hand-held instruments are microprocessor-controlled and are designed to monitor a specific chemistry. These instruments usually allow the customer to store calibration curves and time reactions, and to report clinical values. Benchtop, manual, or semiautomated instrumentation makes possible the execution of multiple assays. Fully automated instrumentation is also available where the operator only has to provide the samples and select the desired tests.

2.2.1. Diffuse Reflectance Spectroscopy

Chemical reactions in dry reagent elements are most commonly monitored by diffuse reflectance spectroscopy (14). The principle of reflectance spectroscopy is illustrated in Fig. 22.3. These elements can be illuminated by either a direct or a diffuse light source. Both sources of light will provide specular and diffuse reflection. Specular reflection is defined as the reflection from the surface of the element, where the angle of incidence equals the angle of reflectance. It is not a good indicator of the progress of reactions occurring within the element and thus is of minimal value in making these measurements. Diffuse reflection, which arises from the interaction of light with various chemical and physical factors within the reaction volume of the element, is the major component of the measurement. These interactions include the absorption, transmission, and scattering properties of the illuminated element. A layer in which a chromophore is being generated or degraded is illuminated at a suitable wavelength in order to make a measurement. The amount of diffuse light recovered in an element which contains a reflective function is used to measure the progress of the reaction.

The intensity of diffuse light reflected by the reaction layers of the element is compared to a known reference standard and is commonly expressed as percent reflectance (%R). Equation (1) defines %R.

$$\%R = (I_s/I_r)\ R_r \tag{1}$$

In this equation, I_s is the reflected light from the sample, I_r is the reflected light from the standard reflector, and R_r is the percent reflectivity of the standard. Reflectance measurements are comparable to transmittance measurements in absorption spectroscopy. These measurements do not have a linear relationship to

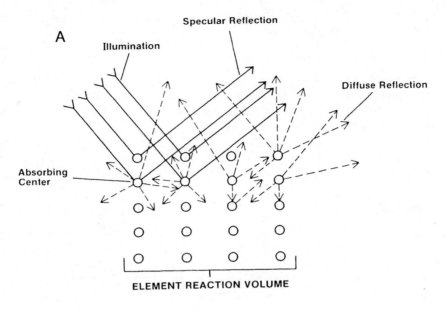

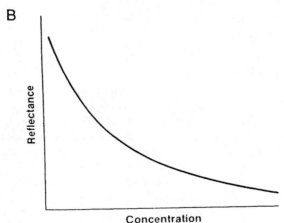

FIGURE 22.3   (A) Principle of reflectance spectroscopy. (B) Relationship of concentration to reflectance measurements. Reprinted with permission from Churchill-Livingstone, Inc., from V. Marks and K.G.M.M.Alberit (Eds), "Clinical Biochemistry Nearer the Patient" (1985).

concentration as shown in Fig. 22.3, but several algorithms have been developed to linearize the relationship between $\%R$ and analyte concentration in order to make the measurements more useful. Two of these algorithms, the Kubelka–Munk and the Williams–Clapper equations, are shown in Fig. 22.4. The algorithm which gives the best result depends on many factors, including the type of illumination, the reflectance characteristics of the element, and the instrument geometry (14).

Williams and Clapper's algorithm (23) was developed as a way of linearizing plots of dye reflection density versus dye concentration in photographic prints. Although dry chemistry elements are optically more complex, their properties are similar to the photographic systems studied by Williams and Clapper. Adaptation

A. Kubelka-Munk Equation

$$C \propto K/S = \frac{(1-R)^2}{2R}$$

C	=	concentration
K	=	absorption coefficient
S	=	scattering coefficient
R	=	% reflectance

B. Williams Clapper Equation

$$D_T = -0.194 + 0.469D_R + \frac{0.422}{1 + 1.179\, e^{3.379\, D_R}}$$

D_R	=	Log R
C	=	$\beta[D_T - D_B]$
C	=	concentration
β	=	reciprocal absorptivity
D_R	=	transmittance density
D_B	=	blank density
D_R	=	reflectance density
R	=	reflectance

FIGURE 22.4 Examples of algorithms used to linearize reflectance measurements versus concentration curves.

of their algorithm for use in a multilayer thin-film assay is described in more detail in Curme *et al.* (4).

2.2.2. Front-Face Fluorescence Spectroscopy

Front-face fluorescence spectroscopy can be used to measure fluorescence generated or destroyed during the course of a reaction in dry chemistry elements (24). In this analysis, sample irradiation and fluorescence monitoring occur on the same side of the element. The irradiating light is passed through a filter or monochromator to select the correct wavelength for illumination. A portion of the fluorescence and reflected, irradiating light is collected by the detection system with the aid of the element's reflective zone. An angle of irradiation is selected which minimizes the reflection of the excitation light. The fluorimeter detector segregates fluorescence from reflected, excitation light by a filter or a monochromator. This allows measurement of the fluorescent light only. Unlike reflectance measurements, the measured fluorescence is linear with the fluorophore concentration, in the absence of self-quenching.

2.3. Construction of Dry Reagent Elements

Dry reagent elements are constructed by trapping materials ranging from low-to high-molecular-weight molecules. The approaches generally involve the simultaneous trapping of components in layers as they are being formed or the trapping of components in preformed matrices. Film casting, which uses technology developed for use in the photographic industry, is used to trap reagents as a layer is being formed. Saturation techniques are used to trap components in a preformed matrix. Single layer elements can be prepared by multisaturation techniques. Multilayer elements are constructed by casting multiple layers of film upon a support or by stacking multiple layers of preformed matrices upon a support. Integrated elements can also be constructed by the combined use of coating and saturation techniques.

In layered coatings, physical or chemical reactions can be physically separated as shown in Fig. 22.5 (25). The products of reactions in one layer can proceed to another layer, where subsequent reactions can occur. Each layer of a multilayered coating can provide a unique environment that makes possible reactions comparable to those occurring in solution as well as reactions that would not be possible in solution. Interferents can be left behind, altered, or inactivated in upper layers. Reactions or signals can be enhanced by optimizing the chemical environment in the appropriate layer. This layered format makes possible a several-step sequence of reactions with no operator involvement or expensive automation.

The technology of photography has resulted in the development of black and white film with as few as one layer, and color instant film, which contains as many as 15 layers. Each layer serves a specific physical or chemical function in image development and stabilization. It is possible to coat multiple uniform layers (1–5 μm in thickness) simultaneously using hopper coating techniques which are

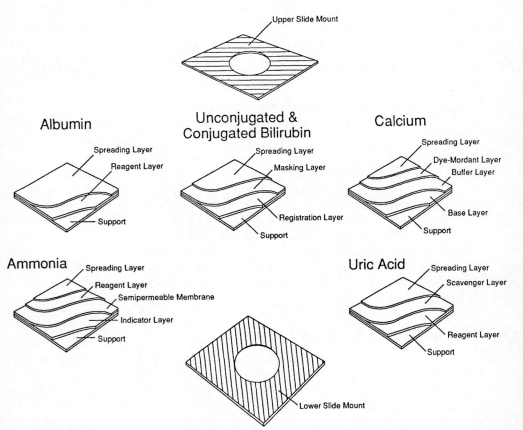

FIGURE 22.5 Examples of physical and chemical reaction layers which have been incorporated into J&JCD VITROS thin-film elements.

well known in the photographic industry. Discrete layers, in which multilayer component migration is minimized or eliminated, can be readily formed with the proper
selection of components for each layer, including solvent and dispersion medium.
Photographic technology has also provided pigments, dyes, adhesives, and mordants
which have been useful in the development of thin-film clinical elements.

2.3.1. Multilayer Film Casting

A variety of naturally occurring and synthetic polymers have been used for the
casting of multilayer coatings. The primary requirements are that the polymer form
a porous film or be adaptable to membrane formation, be functionally water-
insoluble in order to maintain layer integrity during use, and be readily rehydrated
from a dried film (6, 14). Thin films are prepared by a metered application of
viscous solution through a slot-extrusion orifice to a plastic film support moving at
a constant velocity, followed by drying at a downstream location.

Gelatin (denatured collagen) is a natural polymer that is commonly used because of its emulsifying action and other desirable chemical and physical attributes.
Other polymers that have been used include polyacrylamide, poly(vinyl alcohol),
hydroxypropylmethyl-cellulose, methylcellulose, poly(vinyl acetate), agarose, algi-
nate, and carrageenan. The tertiary and quaternary structures of thermoreversible
gels are held together principally by hydrogen bonding. Hydrophilic additives can
be included in the liquid mixture which is coated to act as a solid diluent once the
water is removed. These additives often compose the majority of the coating solution
with the gelling polymer present only at a high enough concentration to generate
a discrete layer. In addition, cross-linking agents may be added to the coating melt
to increase the integrity of the cast layers.

The film porosity is directly dependent on water content and is controlled by
such factors as the molecular weight of the polymer, the degree of cross-linking,
and the concentration of the polymer in the casting medium. The quantities of
reagents available during analysis are controlled by their concentration in coating
mixture, the thickness of the film wetted by the sample, and their solubility in the
sample. The composition and thickness of the layers can be used to adjust reaction
times to a certain degree. The primary mode of fluid transport in these layers is
diffusion. Most gel media are not suitable for facilitating interaction of large molecules such as high-molecular-weight analytes, antibodies, and immune complexes,
because they exhibit insufficient porosity at polymer levels required to maintain
structural integrity of the coated layer during use.

2.3.2. Saturation Techniques

An alternative to film casting involves trapping or immobilizing components in
a preformed matrix by saturation techniques (26, 27). In this approach, the matrix
of choice is saturated with a solution containing the desired reagents and then is
allowed to dry. The availability of reagents during analysis is controlled by the
concentration of reagents in the saturation solution, the thickness and porosity of
the matrix, the absorptivity of the solution by the matrix fibers, and the solubility
of the reagents in the applied sample (6). Preformed matrices that have been used
include paper, woven fabrics, and a variety of porous membranes. These materials
consist of mostly void volume. Fluid transport is driven by capillary forces with no
molecular weight selectivity if the matrix has been treated properly to inhibit surface

adsorption. These matrices offer an advantage over film-cast layers in that washing with larger volumes of applied fluid can remove excess reagents.

Multiple functions and incompatible reagents can be introduced into a single layer by a multistep saturation process in which solvents are selected to prevent unwanted interactions between components (28). The solvents of successive saturations are selected to prevent the dissolution of reagents deposited by previous saturations. This approach was utilized in the development of the Apoenzyme Reactivation Immunoassay System (ARIS) assays.

3. EXAMPLES OF THIN-FILM IMMUNOASSAYS

3.1. Bayer ARIS Assays

One of the first single-element immunoassay systems to be developed was the ARIS system (Bayer Corporation, Elkhart, IN (formerly Miles Laboratories, Inc.)) (29). This method is homogeneous and is based on the reactivation of apoglucose oxidase by its cofactor, flavin adenine dinucleotide (FAD), as shown in Fig. 22.6. The analyte is linked to FAD through a bridging arm and is capable of reactivating apoglucose oxidase. The enzyme reactivation is blocked when the analyte–FAD conjugate is bound to an antibody. Analyte from a patient sample competes with the conjugate for a limited number of antibody sites. The reactivated glucose oxidase produces hydrogen peroxide, which, in the presence of peroxidase, oxidizes the indicator 3,3′,5,5′-tetramethylbenzidine (TMB) to a blue-colored product. Glucose oxidase activity is directly proportional to the analyte concentration. The rate of color formation in the analytical element is monitored at 740 nm by reflectance spectroscopy using the rapid-scanning Seralyzer Reflectance Photometer. The reflectance is measured every 5 sec, and the results are converted to a K/S ratio using the Kubelka–Monk equation (Fig. 22.4). The rate of change in K/S over 20 sec is used to prepare a calibration curve and determine unknown concentrations. Tests for carbamazepine, phenobarbital, phenytoin, and theophylline (30) are currently available on the Seralyzer.

3.1.1. Element Construction and Assay Performance

The analytical elements are constructed in a two-step impregnation process on filter paper in order to prevent reaction of the FAD–analyte conjugate with the apoglucose oxidase or the antianalyte antibody prior to application of the patient sample (31). In the first step, the filter paper is passed through an aqueous solution containing antibody specific for the analyte, excess apoglucose oxidase complexed with goat antiserum to glucose oxidase, peroxidase, glucose, and buffer. The glucose oxidase antibody enhances the reactivation of glucose oxidase by the analyte–FAD conjugate at 37°C where the reaction is run. After drying, the paper is passed through a second solution containing the analyte–FAD conjugate and the substrate tetramethylbenzidine in an organic solvent such as acetone or propanol. This is followed by another drying step. The treated paper is cut into 0.5 × 1-cm sections and mounted with double-sided adhesive on polystyrene supports. The reagent strips are stored in a capped bottle with desiccants.

The test is performed by pipetting 30 μl of a manually diluted sample onto the test strip and placing the strip in the analyzer within 4 sec of sample application

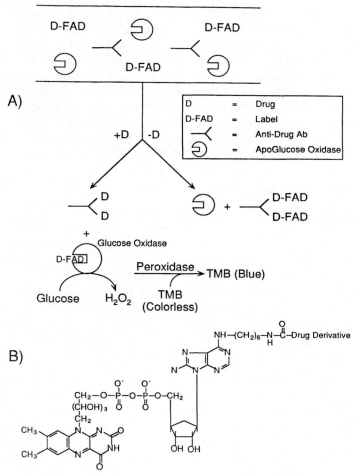

FIGURE 22.6   (A) Principle of the apoenzyme reactivation immunoassay system (ARIS). (B) Structure of an analyte–FAD conjugate.

(30). The test result is displayed on the analyzer's display panel after an 80- to 90-sec incubation. Calibration of these immunoassays is recommended every 2 weeks or whenever a new bottle of strips is opened. Ambient moisture can be a source of error by acting to initiate the holoenzyme regeneration in the absence of analyte, resulting in positive biases. It is necessary for the reagent strip to be used promptly after removal from the desiccated storage bottle. This system requires proper pipetting techniques for dilution and sample application. ARIS assays have been found to have acceptable precision with within-run CVs < 6% and between-run CVs < 8%.

3.1.2. Adaptations for Digoxin Measurement on the Seralyzer

The ARIS approach is not sensitive enough to allow the measurement of digoxin, which is present in serum at nanomolar concentrations. The approach, which was developed to quantify this analyte (32), involves a combination of liquid and dry reagents and the quantitation of color changes in a dry reagent element by reflectance using the Seralyzer analyzer. There is an initial sample extraction step with a single-test "sample processor," followed by analysis with the dry chemistry strip. In this assay, an excess of a monoconjugate of β-galactosidase with a Fab' fragment of a digoxin monoclonal antibody binds the digoxin in the sample. The conjugate that is not complexed with digoxin is subsequently removed by binding to a capture phase consisting of digitoxigenin bound to polyacrylamide beads via a spacer arm. Following the separation of the capture phase from the assay solution, the β-galactosidase activity of the assay solution is determined by reflectance spectroscopy on a reagent strip which contains the substrate dimethylacridinone galactoside.

3.2. Dade International Stratus Assays

The Stratus immunoassay system (Dade International, Miami, FL) uses a hybrid approach that combines solid-phase, immobilized antibody with radial chromatographic separation. This technique is known as radial partition immunoassay (33). This immunoassay system was first introduced by the American Dade Division, American Hospital Supply, in 1982 with tests for eight therapeutic drugs and thyroxine (8). The current system, Stratus II, was introduced in 1989 by Baxter Diagnostics, Inc. (Miami, FL), which acquired the technology. Approximately 30 tests are currently available for measurement of both large and small molecules in the areas of therapeutic drug monitoring, reproductive endocrinology, thyroid function, general endocrinology, cardiac disease, anemia, and allergy testing (34). The Stratus II is an automated batch immunoassay analyzer which has on-board dilution. It contains three onboard dispensing stations for fluid handling, including sample, conjugate, and substrate dispensers. Several different immunoassay methodologies are accommodated on this system, including competitive or sequential saturation immunoassays for the measurement of low-molecular-weight molecules and sandwich immunoassays for the measurement of high-molecular-weight molecules. In general, these assays have been found to have acceptable performance and correlate well with other commercially available immunoassays.

The reaction is conducted on a glass-fiber solid phase. These reaction tabs contain a preimmobilized antibody raised against the analyte. When the sample is applied, the analyte binds to the immobilized antibody. Once the other steps in the reaction sequence have occurred, unbound enzyme-labeled analyte is radially eluted to the periphery of the reaction tab with a wash solution that also contains substrate to initiate the enzymatic reaction. The amount of enzyme conjugate remaining in the center of the element following the wash is quantitated using a fluorigenic substrate and a front-surface fluorimeter as shown in Fig. 22.7.

3.2.1. Assay Construction

An antibody reaction tab is prepared by immobilizing an immune complex containing an antibody directed against the analyte to be measured onto a 1-in.-square piece of glass fiber (8, 33). The immune complex is created by titrating the antigen-specific antibody with an appropriate secondary antibody. An aliquot of the premixed immune complex is pipetted onto the glass fiber membrane and allowed to dry, thus noncovalently immobilizing the complex in a 10- to 15-mm reaction zone. The glass-fiber matrix was selected because of its desirable properties. It was found to be porous and inert with minimal background absorbance and

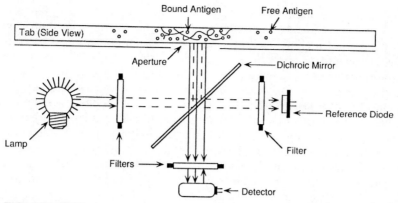

FIGURE 22.7 Front-face fluorimeter used for analysis of Dade Stratus assays. Reprinted from Ref. (8), with permission from Clinical Chemistry.

fluorescence. It also has good fluid capacity, good dimensional wet stability, and a large surface area which facilitates immobilization of antibody.

The enzymes used in these assays are either *Escherichia coli* or calf intestinal alkaline phosphatase (ALP). The substrate chosen was 4-methylumbelliferyl phosphate, which is converted to 4-methylumbelliferone in the presence of the ALP enzyme. Specific inhibitors of human alkaline phosphatase are added to the substrate solution to eliminate interference from human alkaline phosphatase.

For competitive immunoassays, the sample containing the antigen of interest is premixed with the enzyme-labeled antigen and is spotted on the center portion of the element. For sequential saturation immunoassays, the sample is prediluted if necessary and then spotted on the element. After allowing time for this binding reaction to occur, the enzyme-labeled antigen is added and binds to unoccupied antibody binding sites. For sandwich assays, sample is applied to the element, and then, following an incubation period, an enzyme-labeled second monoclonal antibody is applied. The chromatographic separation step and substrate addition step are the same for all the assay types described.

3.3. Johnson & Johnson Clinical Diagnostics VITROS Assays

The VITROS clinical chemistry thin-film layered coating technology (Johnson & Johnson Clinical Diagnostics, Rochester, NY (formerly Eastman Kodak Company)) was developed to adapt clinical chemical analyses to a dry film format (4, 5, 25). In this format reagents are incorporated into one or more layers of hydrophilic polymer and coated on top of a transparent plastic base. An isotropically porous, polymer-spreading layer is coated over the reagent layer(s). In the analysis, a 10- to 11-μl drop of serum is applied to the postage stamp-sized reaction chip. When a drop of serum is applied to the spreading layer, it spreads uniformly and rapidly through the layer until the capillary pores are filled. After this rapid spreading process has occurred, the hydrophilic polymer underlayers rapidly swell to several times their dry volume. This introduction of water into the system initiates the reactions that lead to color formation. The rate of color formation varies with the concentration of the analyte and is measured by reflection spectroscopy.

Tests for over 40 analytes are currently available in this thin-film format on J&JCD VITROS clinical chemistry analyzers including: colorimetric endpoint assays, rate assays for clinically important enzymes, and ion selective electrodes for electrolyte determination in serum or plasma. Urine and CSF assays are also available. Patient results are reported within 5 min of sample application. The VITROS 250 analyzer is designed for small laboratories, clinics, and satellite locations or as a companion to the larger VITROS 950 analyzer. It includes immunoassay and auto-dilution capability. In general, the results of numerous studies have shown excellent precision and agreement with conventional methods. These dry elements have been found to be extremely stable with calibration required only after 6 months or with a new lot of elements. Research on the effects of interferences on various clinical chemistry systems have shown the VITROS system to be least affected by hemolytic, icteric, and lipemic samples (35).

3.3.1. Early Immunoassays

Frickey *et al.* (36) described an immunoassay element that consists of a gelatin reagent layer and a polystyrene bead (d = 5–20 μm) spreading layer coated over a transparent film base. In this format, radial or horizontal separation of bound and free label occurs during sample spreading so that a separate wash step is not required. The reagent layer contains peroxidase, leuco dye, and glucose in a hardened gelatin matrix. The spreading layer contains immobilized antibody directed against the analyte. The label, a glucose oxidase–analyte conjugate, is a separate lyophilized reagent. Sample and diluent are added to the lyophilized enzyme label and, following reconstitution, a 10-μl aliquot is applied to the element. Competition between analyte and labeled analyte for a limited number of immobilized antibody-binding sites occurs during spreading of the applied sample. The rate of dye formation is measured by reflection densitometry at the center of the applied spot. The amount of enzyme label bound to antibody and thus the rate of dye formation is inversely proportional to the analyte concentration. The need to very closely control the spreading time of the applied sample in order to achieve the bound/free separation during spreading is a limitation of this system. In addition, the glucose oxidase/peroxidase-coupled detection system did not exhibit sufficient sensitivity to allow detection of analytes below a concentration of 1×10^{-8} M.

3.3.2. Incorporation of the Label into the Element

In most competitive binding assays it is necessary to keep the labeled analyte apart from the analyte-specific antibody prior to introduction of the analyte in the patient sample in order to allow the assay to be conducted in a reasonable length of time. In many assays the label is combined with the sample prior to contact with the element. This approach requires the customer to maintain supplies of additional reagents and, in some cases, to perform additional manipulations. Even if the label addition is performed by the analyzer, throughput can be slowed. Systems that utilize multiple preformed matrices can supply the label incorporated into a layer which is separate from the antibody. The multiple saturation technique described above can also be used to prevent prebinding of label and antibody.

Dappen *et al.* (37) have developed an alternative approach of applying the labeled analyte to the spreading layer of the element using a gravure-coating process followed by rapid drying. The gravure-coating cylinder transfers fluid to the surface of bead spreading layers via cells with micrometer dimensions. The label penetrates only slightly into the spreading layer, thereby minimizing its interactions with immobilized antibody, which has been coated in a layer located below the spreading layer prior to application of sample. Using this approach, it is possible to achieve dose–response curves that are identical to those obtained when the label is added to the patient prior to conducting the assay.

3.3.3. J&JCD VITROS Immuno-Rate Assays

J&JCD VITROS Immuno-Rate assays (10) are multilayer, thin-film immunoassay elements that contain all the reagents necessary for the measurement of a wide range of analytes in undiluted serum or plasma with no sample pretreatment. These assays have been designed for use on the VITROS 250 and 950 Chemistry Systems. Competitive and noncompetitive binding enzyme immunoassays are conducted in the same thin-film format. The assays are stable on the analyzer for 1 week at room temperature. Tests are complete in less than 8 min.

3.3.3.1. Competitive Binding Immunoassays

Assays have been described for phenytoin (38), phenobarbital (39), and digoxin (40) in this format. The structure of the element and the steps involved in conducting a competitive binding immunoassay are shown in Fig. 22.8. The element is composed of a transparent plastic support layer, a reagent layer, an antibody layer, and a porous reflective spreading layer consisting of 20- to 40-μm polymer beads. Analyte-specific antibody, which has been covalently immobilized on 1-μm beads, is coated in a thin polymer layer directly underneath the spreading layer, or is incorporated directly into the spreading layer. An analyte–enzyme conjugate, which has been designed to compete with the analyte for a limited number of immobilized antibody binding sites, is located in a thin layer (coated by the gravure process) on top of the spreading layer. A leuco dye is also present in the spreading layer. Buffer and other reagents necessary for enzyme detection are coated in a separate cross-linked gelatin layer located directly on top of the support.

Upon application of an 11-μl sample of undiluted serum or plasma, the analyte label in the top of the spreading layer dissolves and competes with analyte in the sample for antibody binding sites. Following a 5-min incubation at 37°C, a second fluid (12 μl)-containing enzyme substrate is slowly added approximately 4 mm from the initial sample application site. This fluid washes away unbound analyte label from the detection area and initiates the enzymatic reaction leading to color formation. The concentration of enzyme label that is bound to the antibody in the central observation area is determined by measuring the rate of dye formation at 670 nm by reflection spectroscopy during a second 2.5-min incubation at 37°C. The enzyme used in these assays is horseradish peroxidase (HRP). Blue color is generated by the oxidation of the triarylimidazole dye in the presence of hydrogen peroxide as shown in Fig. 22.8. In competitive binding immunoassays, the rate of dye formation is inversely related to the concentration of analyte in the applied sample. The concentration of analyte in the patient sample is determined by comparison of the sample rate with a standard curve of known analyte concentration versus rate. The standard curve is established using patient samples of known analyte concentration. Within-run CVs of less than 5% have been reported for these assays, and the results have been found to correlate well with a variety of commercial assays (38–40).

3.3.3.2. Noncompetitive Sandwich Immunoassays

A sandwich enzyme immunoassay has been developed for the measurement of C-Reactive Protein

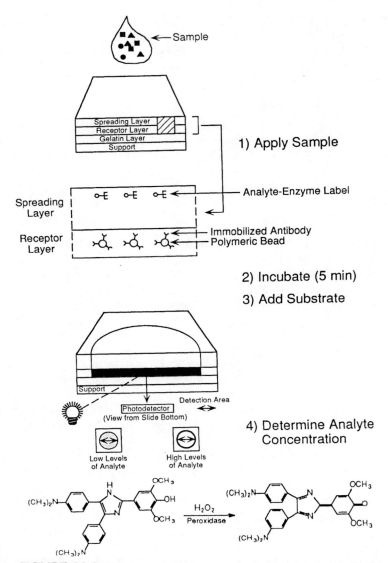

FIGURE 22.8 Principle of competitive binding J&JCD VITROS Immuno-Rate assays.

(CRP) in human serum using the same thin-film multilayer format described for competitve immunoassays (13). In this assay the polymer receptor layer contains a monoclonal anti-CRP antibody labeled with HRP and a derivative of phosphoryl-choline (PC) covalently bound to the surface of polystyrene copolymer beads. Leuco dye is also present in this layer.

The assay is conducted by applying 11 μl of undiluted patient serum to the slide. The slide is incubated in the analyzer at 37°C for 5 min to allow the sandwich to form. Twelve microliters of wash fluid containing hydrogen peroxide is then applied to the slide to remove unbound Mab–HRP conjugate from the observation area and to initiate the dye formation reaction. The amount of PC–CRP–Mab–HRP sandwich formed is determined by measuring the amount of dye formed in the observation area using reflection spectroscopy. This assay was found to correlate well with the Behring nephelometric method. Within-run imprecision was found to be <7%. The assay range was 5 to 200 mg/liter CRP with no high dose hook effect up to 500 mg/liter CRP (13).

3.3.4. New Materials

The successful development of undiluted assays for the measurement of analytes in serum over a wide range of concentrations, ranging from 10^{-4} to 10^{-9} M, has required the invention of new materials, methods to incorporate them into the thin-film format, and algorithms to measure the progress of reactions in the element. In the development of competitve binding immunoassays, it is necessary to optimize the position of the dose–response curve in order to maximize the rate of color change over the desired concentration range. This can be accomplished by achieving the correct balance between the relative affinity of the immobilized antibody for the analyte and for the analyte–enzyme label. New and improved haptens, linkers, and conjugation chemistries have been developed for the preparation of enzyme labels. Antibodies have been screened and selected based on optimized performance in these elements.

3.3.4.1. Enzyme Labels

3.3.4.1.1. New Conjugation Techniques
The traditional approach for digoxin label preparation, i.e., oxidation of the digoxin terminal monosaccharide residue to a dialdehyde followed by attachment to enzyme amines, did not generate satisfactory peroxidase labels for these undiluted thin-film assays (41) . Traditional approaches resulted in labels that contained a substantial fraction of peroxidase (>80%) which could not be bound by digoxin antibody but which contributed to unacceptably high background rates in the element. The successful preparation of digoxin labels for these assays required the preparation of a new digoxin derivative. Further improvement was observed with the introduction of additional amine attachment sites by the preparation of amine-enriched peroxidase. The new digoxin diacid derivatives were coupled to the amine-enriched peroxidase by mixed anhydride coupling chemistry. The use of these materials made possible the development of a digoxin assay in this format.

3.3.4.1.2. New Linkers
Novel extended linkers, which were designed to provide improved recognition of analytes by analyte-specific antibodies, were used to generate improved peroxidase labels for a variety of analytes including phenytoin, phenobarbital, and carbamazepine (42). It was found that labels prepared from valerate or 5-carbon linkers did not bind tightly enough to the antibodies. However, when the linker length was increased to 13 atoms, the binding of the labels to a variety of antibodies improved substantially. Optimization of the coupling chemisty and the analyte/enzyme substitution ratio also improved the performance of the labels in these assays.

3.3.4.2. Reactive Solid Supports
Another key element of these assays is the solid support that is used for the immobilization of the analyte-specific antibodies. Covalent attachment of the antibody to the solid support is preferable to adsorption because of the potential of displacement by surfactants which are added to the

coated element to promote spreading of proteins present in the patient sample. Small ($d = 1$ μm), uniformly sized, copolymeric latex particles have been found to offer a very reactive substrate for the immobilization of antibodies (43). These particles are prepared from styrene and a variety of novel carboxylic acid-containing monomers by surfactantless, emulsion polymerization. The structure of these monomers has been modified to provide hydrolytic stability and to achieve the desired hydrophobic/hydrophilic balance. Because these beads are hydrophobic, they have a high protein adsorption capacity and are nonporous in aqueous media. This ensures that all reactions will occur at the surface of the beads.

Coupling protocols for the covalent attachment of antibodies have been developed, whereby complete attachment of added antibody can be achieved with 100% covalent binding. The performance of these novel carboxylic acid polymer beads was compared to that of beads prepared using acrylic acid as the reactive monomer in thin-film immunoassays for thyroxine, phenytoin, phenobarbital, and digoxin. The new carboxylic acid beads were found to be 10-fold more immunoreactive with an equivalent amount of bound antibody (44).

In addition to the carboxy group, a variety of other novel reactive copolymers have also been incorporated into these beads, which has made possible the efficient coupling of antibodies under mild conditions, thus maximizing the retention of antibody activity. Copolymeric latex particles have been prepared from styrene and polymerizable monomers which contain pendant activatable 2-substituted ethylsulfonyl or vinylsulfonyl groups (45). These beads and coupling chemistry have been optimized such that a very high percentage of the offered antibody is bound and more than 90% is bound covalently. This approach provides the added advantage of not requiring a separate reagent for activation of the beads.

3.4. Behring Diagnostics OPUS Assays

The OPUS immunoassay system (Behring Diagnostics Systems, Westwood, MA) is a benchtop, continuous-access immunoassay analyzer that operates in random-access, stat, preset panel, and batch mode (9, 46). The OPUS utilizes single-unit test modules that contain all the reagents needed for each test. Two types of test modules are used: a multilayer film test module and a fluorogenic enzyme-linked immunosorbent assay (ELISA) test module. The multilayer test module (Fig. 22.9) uses a combination of multilayer film technology and competitive binding immunoassays with fluorescent detection for the analysis of low-molecular-weight analytes and some thyroid function assays. The fluorogenic ELISA test module (Fig. 22.10) incorporates sandwich and sequential binding formats for the measurement of higher-molecular-weight analytes or antibodies and some low-concentration small molecules. Tests are currently available for therapeutic drug monitoring, endocrinology, fertility panels, infectious disease markers, tumor markers, and cardiac markers. Test modules are stored at 2–8°C with a shelf life of at least 6 months. Reagents can be stored on board the instrument for 7 days. The calibration curve is stable for at least 2 weeks for the fluorogenic ELISA assays and for 6 weeks for the multilayer film immunoassays. The average test time is 6 to 18 min. The recently introduced OPUS Magnum allows storage on the instrument of up to 36 separate assays (360 test modules) and a throughput of up to 190 assays per hour.

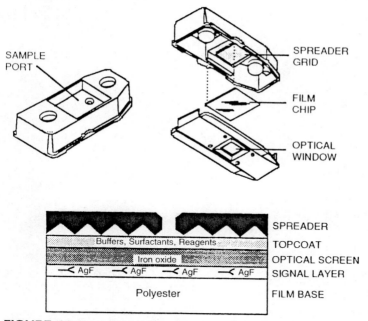

FIGURE 22.9 Behring OPUS multilayer film test module. Reprinted from D. W. Chan (Ed), "Immunoassay Automation: A Practical Guide" (1992) with permission from Academic Press, Inc.

3.4.1. Multilayer Film Assays

These assays consist of a coated, multilayer film chip encased in a plastic test module. The assay uses a 10-μl sample of undiluted serum or plasma and requires no external reagents or sample pretreatment (except for total triiodothyronine (T3) which requires a dilution step). The method is based on a ligand-displacement assay principle, and the bound/free separation is achieved by diffusion (47). Assays have been developed for several therapeutic drugs in this format, including theophylline, phenytoin, phenobarbital, carbamazepine, valproic acid, gentamicin, and tobramycin (48). Tests for thyroxine and thyroid hormone uptake have also been described (9).

3.4.1.1. Element Construction
The thin-film multilayer structure of the Opus immunoassay system is shown in Fig. 22.9. A very thin signal layer (1 μm) is coated onto a polyester film base. This layer contains a preformed complex between a monoclonal antibody and a rhodamine–hapten conjugate completely entrapped in an agarose matrix. The next layer is a screening layer (10 μm) which consists of an agarose matrix. This matrix contains the red pigment, iron oxide, which serves as a light blocker. If necessary, buffer components, detergents, and displacement agents are coated in the top agarose layer (10 μm). The top layer also acts as a filter so that proteins and other high-molecular-weight molecules cannot reach the signal layer and interfere with the immunoreaction. This layer is kept in close contact with a sample-spreading device (described in Section 2.1.4). The multilayer film is sandwiched between the spreader and a flat plastic bottom, which has an aperture for making the optical measurement.

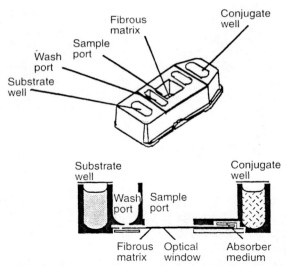

FIGURE 22.10   Behring OPUS fluorgenic ELISA test module. Reprinted from D. W. Chan (Ed), "Immunoassay Automation: A Practical Guide" (1992) with permission from Academic Press, Inc.

3.4.1.2. Assay Principles   The reaction is initiated by the application of 10 μl of serum or plasma to the spreader opening. Liquid fills the void volume of the spreader grid and then rehydrates the agarose layers. The sample antigen travels from the top layer, through the screen layer, and into the signal layer, where it displaces labeled antigen from the binding sites of the antibodies. The displaced label then diffuses freely throughout the coating. Because the volume of the signal layer accounts for only 2% of the total volume, an effective bound/free separation is achieved by diffusion away from the signal layer. The red pigment in the screening layer, which is located above the signal layer, blocks the detection of the label outside the signal layer. At equilibrium , the amount of antibody-bound labeled antigen in the signal layer is inversely proportional to the amount of analyte in the serum sample.

Antibodies have been selected for this test that have very fast dissociation rates so that assay kinetics are fast enough to allow reporting of results in a reasonable amount of time (47). The theophylline test has been reported to reach equilibrium in <4 min at 37°C with the signal remaining stable for more than 20 min. The thyroxine assay is slower, reaching 90% of equilibrium after 12 min, because of the slower dissociation rate of the more strongly binding antibody required for this assay.

3.4.1.3. New Materials   The OPUS uses highly efficient fluorophores as direct labels (47). Three potential drawbacks to the use of fluorescent labels in undiluted serum or plasma were taken into consideration in the selection process. Human serum and plasma exhibit substantial intrinsic fluorescence, especially if the sample is applied without dilution. In addition, a second source of background fluorescence is encountered from impurities and additives to the film base onto which the layers are coated. Another factor that must be considered in the construction of undiluted assays is the binding of the labels to serum proteins, especially albumin. This binding can lead to reduced accuracy of the assays. The first two sources of fluorescence were found to be minimized by the selection of certain xanthine dyes (e.g., Rhodamine B and Rhodamine 6 G), which have adsorption maxima at higher wavelengths (near 550 nm or higher). These fluorophores required further modification to improve fluorescence efficiency and to reduce their hydrophobicity, which resulted in strong binding to serum proteins. The rotation of the amino groups was eliminated by ring closure with the result being a new material with a quantum yield of 0.9 in aqueous solution and with absorption and emission maxima at 550 and 580 nm, respectively. In addition, two sulfonic acid groups and a hydrophilic spacer, between the fluorophore and the hapten, had the effect of reducing the albumin-binding constant of a theophylline derivative 40-fold relative to a theophylline–fluorescein conjugate.

3.4.2. Fluorogenic ELISA Format Assays

The fluorogenic ELISA assays are based on the capture of test-specific antigens or antibodies on an insoluble solid phase (9, 46) (Fig. 22.10). The test module consists of a 1 1/2-in. plastic unit with individual foil-covered wells containing enzyme conjugate and substrate. The reaction zone contains antibody immobilized on a fibrous glass matrix. In the operation of this assay, the specimen is pipetted onto the fibrous matrix and allowed to incubate in order to allow the binding of the analyte to the immobilized antibody. The enzyme conjugate is then pipetted onto the reaction zone, followed by an additional incubation step to form a sandwich immune complex. Substrate is then dispensed into the wash port and migrates through the reaction zone by capillary action. The enzyme conjugate converts the substrate into a fluorescent product while unbound conjugate is simultaneously washed away from the reaction zone. The resulting fluorescence is measured, and the amount is either directly or inversely related to the concentration of the analyte depending on the type of ELISA methodology used.

Quantitative tests have been developed in this format for digoxin, hCG, TSH, and FSH. Qualitative tests for cytomegalovirus and toxoplasma have also been developed. An approach has also been described that combines the immunoassay element described above and a filter device. This would make possible the analysis of whole blood samples (22).

3.5. Fuji Dri-Chem Assays

A variety of approaches for the development of thin-film immunoassays have been proposed in published descriptions from Fuji Photo Film Company, Ltd. (Minami-Ashigara, Japan). Some of these approaches use a combination of wet and dry chemistry. All have combined the use of coated thin-film layers with preformed spreading layers which have been laminated onto the film layers. Recently, workers at Fuji have published extensively on a homogeneous thin-film immunoassay.

3.5.1. Early Immunoassay Approaches

In 1981, Hiratsuka et al. (49) described an immunoassay for insulin using photochemical element for detection. Insulin is labeled with a carbocyanine dye that acts as a photographic spectral sensitizer or fogging agent. Insulin, labeled insulin, and anti-insulin antibody, previously pretreated with a second antibody, are combined and incubated prior to being spotted on the element.

The reaction product is applied to a thin-film element that contains a polyacrylamide bound/free separation layer and a silver halide layer coated on top of a transparent support. The unbound insulin passes through the separation layer and comes into contact with the silver halide layer. The optical density, which results following exposure to light and subsequent photographic development, is quantitated using a densitometer.

Hiratsuka has also disclosed an immunoassay (50) in which the competitive binding reaction between the labeled and unlabeled immunoreactant (for a limited number of microparticle immobilized antigen or antibody binding sites) takes place in solution prior to spotting on a multilayer thin film. The analytical element consists of a porous spreading layer and a water-absorbing detection layer coated on top of a transparent support. An assay for antibodies to human IgG is described in which glucose oxidase (GOD) is used as the labeling enzyme. Following a 5-min incubation of the GOD–anti-IgG conjugates with the serum sample and immoblized IgG, a 30-μl aliquot is applied to a membrane filter layer that has been laminated onto the element. The microparticles are trapped in this layer but the label migrates through this layer to a plain weave cloth layer that contains glucose. The hydrogen peroxide that is generated migrates into a gelatin layer which contains the reagents to form a quinoneimine dye through an oxidative coupling reaction. The color formed is measured at 540 nm by reflection spectroscopy.

Another competitive, multilayer immunoassay has also been described by Sudo *et al.* (51). In this scheme, the spreading layer contains analyte-specific antibody immobilized on one population of agarose beads and an enzyme substrate immobilized on a second population of the same beads. The label can react with the immobilized enzyme substrate only when it is not bound to immobilized antibody. The reagent layer, located below this layer, contains a detection reagent composition for coupling with an enzymatic reaction product produced by the reaction between the enzyme label and the immobilized enzyme substrate.

An assay for thyroxine has been described using this approach. The spreading layer contains immobilized T4 antibody and galactose oligomer imbibed into a glass fiber filter. The galactose detection layer consists of a coated layer of gelatin containing galactose oxidase, peroxidase, 1,7-dihydroxynapthalene, 4-aminoantipyrine, and surfactants. A thin color shielding layer (15 μm), consisting of gelatin and TiO_2, is located between this layer and the spreading layer. The assay is conducted by applying a sample containing T4, which has been spiked with T4-β-galactosidase label, and a displacement agent to the element. The label competes with T4 in the patient sample for antibody binding sites. The unbound label reacts with the immobilized substrate to generate galactose, which migrates to the detection layer where it reacts to generate color. Following incubation at 37°C for 8 min, the amount of color generated is measured at 500 nm by reflection spectroscopy. The amount of color formed is directly proportional to the amount of T4 in the sample.

3.5.2. Homogeneous Immunoassay

A homogeneous, multilayer thin-film immunoassay approach that can be used for the measurement of both large and small analytes has also been developed (12, 52). The label consists of analyte-specific antibody conjugated to α-amylase from *Bacillus subtilis*, and insoluble starch is included as the substrate. The insoluble starch cannot be digested efficently by the antibody–enzyme conjugate when it is complexed with high-molecular-weight antigen. The activity of the enzyme is inversely proportional to the amount of high-molecular-weight antigen that is present in the patient sample. Assays for low-molecular-weight analytes are conducted in the same format by preparing polymerized analyte (53) which competes with the low-molecular-weight antigen for antibody binding sites. The polymerized analyte behaves like high-molecular-weight antigens by preventing the digestion of the insoluble starch when bound to the antibody–amylase label (in the absence of low-molecular-weight antigen in the patient sample). In this assay, enzyme activity is directly related to antigen concentration.

The structure of the slide for these assays is shown in Fig. 22.11. The slide consists of a developing zone for immunological and enzymatic reactions, a barrier zone, and a color developing zone. The antibody–amylase label and blue starch are incorporated into a preformed porous spreading layer. Following application of a diluted sample containing antigen, the reagents are reconstituted and the antigen can complex with the label. Only the unbound label reacts with the insoluble substrate in this layer. The digested low-molecular-weight starch migrates through the barrier zone to the color developing zone. The low-molecular-weight starch is further digested in this zone to glucose by glucoamylase contained in this layer. The amount of glucose present is quantitated via glucose oxidase and peroxidase

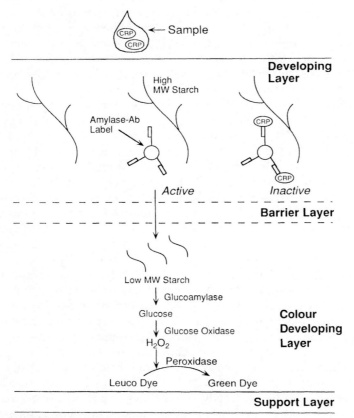

FIGURE 22.11   Fuji Dri-Chem homogeneous immunoassay for C-Reactive Protein.

in the presence of a leuco dye. The green color that results is quantitated by reflectance spectroscopy.

The serum sample is diluted 20- to 220-fold with a diluent buffer, which contains a specific inhibitor to human serum amylase, prior to application of a 10-μl aliquot to the slide. The slides are incubated at 37°C in the Fuji Dri-Chem 5500 analyzer. Absorbance readings are taken at 4 and 6 min and the difference between the two is measured. Tests for CRP, ferritin, α-fetoprotein, and theophylline have been described using this approach. The CRP assay has been compared to the Hoechst turbidometric method and the theophylline assay to the Syva EMIT assay. Both of these assays have been found to correlate well with these methods (12).

3.6. Konishiroku Assays

Workers at Konishiroku Photo Industry Company, Ltd. (Tokyo, Japan), have generated several patents and patent applications describing a variety of thin-film immunoassay elements. These elements are based on thin-film coatings together with porous particulate spreading layers. The porous, beaded layer generally consists of the reactive particles described previously. Two approaches are described below.

Yasoshima *et al.* (54) describe an immunoassay method using a multilayer element which consists of three porous layers of particulate beads coated over a transparent support. The bottom layer consists of poly(styrene-co-n-butyl methacrylate-co-glycidyl methacrylate) particles ($d = 21 \ \mu$m), which have been dried at an elevated temperature to form a crosslinked, porous layer (described in Section 2.1.2). The second layer, which is designed to be a blocking layer, consists of the same beads which have been imbibed with a fluoresence blocking dye or pigment. The same particles are also used in the top layer with analyte-specific antibody adsorbed onto them prior to coating. A test for α-fetoprotein is described utilizing a fluorescein-conjugated α-fetoprotein as the label. The assay is conducted by applying a 10-μl aliquot of a sample containing a fixed concentration of the label onto the element. Following incubation at 37°C for 20 min, the fluorescence is measured on either the top or the bottom of the element to get a measurement of either the antibody-bound or the free label. Results are given that show discrimination in levels of α-fetoprotein between 5 x 10^{-8} and 2 x 10^{-6} *M* by either measurement.

Ito *et al.* (55) have disclosed another immunoassay element that consists of a porous beaded layer coated over a gelatin layer on top of a transparent support. An assay for human IgG is described. Anti-IgG antibody and an antifluorescein antibody which has been designed to quench the fluorescence of the label are immobilized separately on the epoxide-containing beads described above. These beads are combined in the appropriate ratios with BSA-treated beads and applied to a support to prepare a dried film. A reagent layer, consisting of fluorescein-labeled human IgG, is coated in a cross-linked gelatin layer over a transparent support. The bead reaction layer, described above, is peeled from its support and applied to the top of the gelatin layer to construct the element. An assay for human IgG is described in which 10-μl aliquots, containing varying levels of IgG, are applied to the element. The fluorescence is measured from the spotted side of the element following incubation at 37°C for 20 min. At low levels of IgG, the label is bound preferentially to the IgG antibody and the measured fluorescence intensity is high. At high levels of IgG, more of the label is bound to the fluorescein antibody and the measured fluorescence intensity is lower.

4. CONCLUSION

A variety of approaches for the development of dry reagent immunoassays have been described. The majority of the assays currently available in this format are for low-molecular-weight analytes because these assays have been easier to design. In addition, many of the assays that have been developed utilize a hybrid approach combining wet and dry chemistry. Frequently, the immunological reaction is conducted in solution and the detection reaction is conducted in the dry element. This approach allows flexibility in the optimization of these reactions for a wider analyte concentration range. However, the hybrid approach requires the customer to maintain a supply of space-consuming liquid reagents and also requires additional manipulations to be performed by the customer or the analyzer. The goal of developing self-contained dry reagent immunoassays for analytes that span a wide range of concentrations and molecular weights has been difficult and has required the development of specialized new technology. It is expected that as these assays become available they will alter immunoassay testing practices, much as dry reagent clinical assays have altered clinical chemistry testing.

References

1. Free AH, Adams EC, Kercher ML, Free HM, Cook MH. Simple specific test for urine glucose. Clin Chem 1957; 3:163–8.
2. Free HM, Collins GF, Free AH. Triple-test strip for urinary glucose, protein and pH. Clin Chem 1960; 6:352–61.
3. Mazzaferri EL, Lanese RR, Skillman TG, Keller MP. Use of test strips with colour meter to measure blood-glucose. Lancet 1960; 1:331–3.
4. Curme HG, Columbus RL, Dappen GM, Eder TW, Fellows WD, Figueras J, Glover CP, Goffe CA, Hill DE, Lawton WH, Muka EJ, Pinney JE, Rand RN, Sanford KJ, Wu TW. Multilayer film elements for clinical analysis: general concepts. Clin Chem 1978; 24:1335–42.
5. Spayd RW, Bruschi B, Burdick BA, Dappen GM, Eikenberry JN, Esders TW, Figueras J, Goodhue CT, LaRossa DD, Nelson RW, Rand RN, Wu TW. Multilayer film elements for clinical analysis: applications to representative chemical determinations. Clin Chem 1978; 24:1343–50.
6. Berke CM. A primer for multilayer immunoassay. In: Ngo TT, Ed. Nonisotopic Immunoassay. New York: Plenum, 1988:303–12.
7. Boguslaski R, Carrico R. Multilayer film immunoassay. In: Price CP, Newman DJ, Eds. Principles and Practices of Immunoassays. Stockton Press, 1992:543–62.
8. Giegel JL, Brotherton MM, Cronin P, D'Aquino M, Evans S, Heller H, Knight WS, Krishnan K, Sheiman M. Radial partition immunoassay. Clin Chem 1982; 28:1894–8.
9. Lehrer M, Miller L, Natale J. The OPUS system. In: Chan DW, Ed. Immunoassay Automation: A Practical Guide. San Diego: Academic Press, 1992; 245–67.
10. Danielson SJ, Daiss JD, Hilborn DA, Mauck LA, Oenick MDB, Ponticello IS, Sutton RC, Wu A. Development of enzyme immunoassays in thin film format. 18th National Meeting Clinical Ligand Assay Society, 1992; 105–7.
11. Fernando SA, Wilson GS. Studies of the 'hook' effect in the one step sandwich immunoassay. J Immunol Methods 1992; 151:47–66.
12. Ashihara Y, Hiraoka T, Makino Y, Shinoki H, Hora N, Sudo Y, Ogawa M, Tanimoto T, Ninomiya T, Nishizono I, Kasahara Y. Immunoassay for determining low- and high-Mr antigens with a dry multilayer film. Clin Chem 1991; 37:1525–6.
13. Wu A, Harmoinen A, Chambers D, Fagnan K, Ferrara L, Kennel N, Mauck L, Novros J, Oenick M, Smolowyk A, Sprague L, Thomas G. Comparison of a thin-film immunoassay for C-reactive protein (CRP) with a turbidometric method. Clin Chem 1994; 40:1018.
14. Walter B. Construction of dry reagent chemistries: use of reagent immobilization and compartmentalization techniques. Methods Enzymol 1988; 137:394–420.
15. Natelson S. Automatic chemical analyzer. 1968; US Patent No. 3,368,872.

16. Przybylowicz EP, Millikan AG. Integral analytical element. 1976; US Patent No. 3,992,158.
17. Pierce ZR, Frank DS. Element, structure and method for the analysis of transport of liquids. 1981; US Patent No. 4,258,001.
18. Koyama M, Kikugawa S. Analytical element and method of use. 1984; US Patent No. 4,430,436.
19. Koyama M, Kikugawa S. Analytical element. 1985; US Patent No. 4,551,307.
20. Kitajima M, Arai F, Kondo A. Multilayer analysis sheet for analyzing liquid samples. 1981; US Patent No. 4,292,272.
21. Kitajima M, Arai F, Kondo A. Multilayered integral element for the chemical analysis of the blood. 1981; US Patent No. 4,255,384.
22. Grenner G. Biological diagnostic device and method of use. 1990; US Patent No. 4,906,439.
23. Williams FC, Clapper FR. Multiple internal reflections in photographic color prints. J Opt Soc Am 1953; 43:595–9.
24. Walter B. Dry reagent chemistries. Anal Chem 1983; 55:498A–514A.
25. Shirey TL. Development of a layered-coating technology for clinical chemistry. Clin Biochem 1983; 16:147–55.
26. Liotta LA. Enzyme immunoassay with two-zoned device having bound antigens. 1984; US Patent No. 4,446,232.
27. Greenquist AC. Multizone analytical element having labeled reagent concentration zone. 1989; US Patent No. 4,806,311.
28. Greenquist AC, Rupchock PA, Tyhach RJ, Walter B. Preparing homogeneous specific binding assay element to avoid premature reaction. 1984; US Patent No. 4,447,529.
29. Tyhach RJ, Rupchock PA, Pendergrass JH, Skjold C, Smith PJ, Johnson RD, Albarella JP, Profitt, JA. Adaptation of prosthetic-group-label homogeneous immunoassay to reagent-strip format. Clin Chem 1981; 27:1499–504.
30. Ng RH. Immunoassay systems for the physician's office. In: Chan DW, Ed. Immunoassay Automation: A Practical Guide. San Diego: Academic Press, 1992:351–63.
31. Rupchock P, Sommer R, Greenquist A, Tyhach R, Walter B, Zipp A. Dry reagent strips used for determination of theophylline in serum. Clin Chem 1985; 31:235–41.
32. Sommer RG, Belchak TL, Bloczynski ML, Boguslawski DL, Clay DL, Corey PF, Foltz MM, Fredrickson RA, Halmo BL, Johnson RD, Marfurt KL, Runzheimer H-V, Morris DL. A unitized enzyme-labeled immunometric digoxin assay suitable for rapid testing. Clin Chem 1990; 36:201–6.
33. Evans S, Kirchick H, Goodnow T. Radial partition immunoassay. In: Price CP, Newman DJ, Eds. Principles and Practices of Immunoassays. Stockton Press, 1992; 610–43.
34. Kahn SE, Bermes EW, Jr. Stratus II immunoassay system. In: Chan DW, Ed. Immunoassay Automation: A Practical Guide. San Diego: Academic Press, 1992; 293–316.
35. Glick MR, Ryder KW, Jackson SA. Graphical comparisons of interferences in clinical chemistry instrumentation. Clin Chem 1986; 32:470–5.
36. Frickey PH, Sanford KJ, Dappen GM, Thunberg AL, Sundberg MW, Danielson SJ. Heterogeneous immunoassay utilizing horizontal separation in an analytical element. 1987; US Patent No. 4,670,381.
37. Dappen GM, Hassett JW, Heinle JF. Analytical element coated by a gravure process. 1992; European Patent Application 517,338.
38. Oenick M, Hilborn D, Danielson S, Mauck L, Byrne D, Thomas G, Specht C, Hassett J, Angie K. Measurement of phenytoin in human serum by multilayered slide enzyme immunoassay. Clin Chem 1993; 39:1234.
39. Hilborn D, Oenick MB, Danielson S, Mauck L, Angie K, Byrne D, Hassett J, Thomas G, Specht C. Measurement of phenobarbital in serum by multilayered slide immunoassay. Clin Chem 1993; 39:1232.
40. Mauck L, Brigito A, Findling K, Graby C, James J, Pratt L. Multilayered slide immunochemical method for the measurement of digoxin in human serum. Clin Chem 1993; 39:1229.
41. Danielson SJ, Detty MR, Alexandrovich SK. Improved labels for use in digoxin multilayer enzyme immunoassays. Clin Chem 1987; 33:923.
42. Danielson SJ, Brummond BA, Oenick MDB, Ponticello IS, Hilborn DA. Labeled drug hapten analogues for immunoassays. 1994; US Patent No. 5,298,403.
43. Sutton RC, Danielson SJ, Findlay JB, Oakes FT, Oenick MDB, Ponticello IS, Warren HC III. Biologically active reagents prepared from carboxy-containing polymer, analytical element and methods of use. 1992; US Patent No. 5,147,777.
44. Danielson SJ, Ponticello N, Sutton R, Oenick M, Swartz J. Novel carboxylic acid copolymer beads and their use in thin-film immunoassays for thyroxine, phenytoin, phenobarbital and digoxin. Clin Chem 1992; 38:1096.

45. Sutton RC, Danielson SJ. Water-insoluble reagents, elements containing same and methods of use. 1993; US Patent No. 5,177,023.
46. Velazquez FR, MD. The P.B. Diagnostics' OPUS immunoassay system. J Clin Immunoassay 1991; 14:126–32.
47. Grenner G, Inbar S, Meneghini FA, Long EW, Yamartino EJ Jr. Bowen MS, Blackwood JJ, Padilla AJ, Maretsky D, Staedter M. Multilayer fluorescent immunoassay technique. Clin Chem 1989; 35:1865–8.
48. Jandreski MA, Shah JC, Garbinclus J, Bermes EW Jr. Clinical evaluation of five therapeutic drugs using dry film multilayer technology on the OPUS immunoassay system. J Clin Lab Anal 1991; 5:415–21.
49. Hiratsuka N, Mihara Y, Masuda N, Takushi M, Miyazako M. Method for immunological assay using multilayer analysis sheet. 1982; US Patent No. 4,337,065.
50. Hiratsuka N. Competitive binding immunoassay process. 1989; US Patent No. 4,868,131.
51. Sudo Y, Masuda N, Miura K. Multilayered element for quantitative analysis of immunoreactant. 1990; US Patent No. 4,975,366.
52. Ashihara Y, Nishizono I, Tanimoto T, Tsuchiya H, Yamamoto K, Kido Y, Mlyagawa E, Kasahara Y. Enzyme inhibitory homogeneous immunoassay for high molecular weight antigen (I). J Clin Lab Anal 1988; 2:138–42.
53. Sudo Y, Ashihara Y, Hiraoka T, Nishizono I, Kageyama S, Tanimoto T. Dry-type analytical element for immunoassay. 1992; US Patent No. 5,093,081.
54. Yasoshima S, Koyama M, Okaniwa K. Immunoassay method for measuring immunological antigen in fluid sample. 1986; US Patent No. 4,613,567.
55. Ito T, Kawakatsu S, Onishi A, Ishikawa M. Analytical element and method for determining a component in a test sample. 1989; US Patent No. 4,868,106.

23 | IMMUNOBLOTTING TECHNIQUES

JAIME RENART
M. MARGARITA BEHRENS
MARGARITA FERNÁNDEZ-RENART
JOSÉ L. MARTÍNEZ
Instituto de Investigaciones Biomédicas del CSIC
and Departamento de Bioquímica de la UAM
Madrid, Spain

1. INTRODUCTION

Blotting techniques are used to study a macromolecule simultaneously with respect to size and/or isoelectric point and another specific character, usually binding of a specific antibody.

The first of these techniques was developed E. M. Southern (1), who took advantage of the already known capability of DNA to bind in its denatured state to nitrocellulose. Molecular biology benefitted from this development, since characterization of DNA could now be done by gel electrophoresis and hybridization instead of electron microscopy.

In the 1970s it was believed that RNA could not bind to nitrocellulose membranes, and therefore an alternative method was devised by G. R. Stark and coworkers that employed diazo-paper to covalently bind RNA or DNA (2). The next step was to use the same principle to study proteins.

As the molecular weight of proteins is, on average, much lower than that of nucleic acids, their separation by electrophoresis must be carried out in polyacrylamide gels, which unfortunately allow very poor diffusion of macromolecules off the gel. To overcome this difficulty, two approaches were developed almost simultaneously. In the first approach, composite polyacrylamide/agarose gels were prepared with a reversible crosslink to allow diffusion by standard blotting techniques after degrading the acrylamide matrix (3). In the second approach, proteins were transferred off the gel by electrophoresis (4). Diazo-paper was used in the former approach, while nitrocellulose membranes were used in the latter. Subsequently it was shown that electrophoretic transfer can also be done to diazo-paper (5).

Protein blotting techniques are currently known as "Western" blotting (6), a name derived from the previously coined "Northern" blots (RNA bound to the support) versus "Southern" blots (DNA bound to the support). Whereas the Northern and Southern blotting techniques detect specific RNA or DNA sequences by hybridization with radioactive or nonradioactive probes, Western blotting generally detects the presence of different proteins by incubating the membrane with specific antibodies directed against them.

Today, blots are applied to membranes and not to derivatized paper. The range of detection methods is considerably larger than before, which makes the technique flexible and powerful.

2. PRINCIPLES

2.1. Gel Electrophoresis

As mentioned above, proteins are separated by gel electrophoresis before blotting. Any system can be used, which affords the capability to take advantage of every improvement of resolution.

The most commonly used electrophoretic technique is one-dimensional slab gel electrophoresis, in which a number of samples are run together so that comparisons between samples can be made easily. In a first attempt, the method of choice is the discontinuous system in the presence of sodium dodecyl sulfate (SDS), as developed by Laemmli (7). With this method, denatured proteins are separated according to their molecular weight.

For better resolution of complex mixtures of proteins, two-dimensional gel electrophoresis, developed by O'Farrel (8), is advisable. In this method, the first dimension consists of an isoelectric focusing in the presence of high concentrations of urea. Once the proteins are focused to their respective isoelectric point, the gel rod is placed atop a slab denaturing gel. An electrophoretic step is then run, producing individual spots of proteins separated according to differences in isoelectric point and size.

Even better resolution can be obtained from both one- and two-dimensional gel electrophoresis when the gel has a linear gradient of acrylamide monomer. In this case, the low-molecular-weight proteins are well resolved in sharper bands.

2.2. Blotting Supports

Nitrocellulose was the first support to be used. Currently, manufacturers offer a wide variety of support media. Nitrocellulose is still used, although with better performance than before. Nylon membranes, both neutral and charged, with larger mechanical resistance have been developed. Interaction of proteins with nitrocellulose appears to be due mainly to hydrophobic forces, and a new, very hydrophobic membrane made of polyvinylidene difluoride (PVDF) with high capacity and adsorption properties has been developed.

3. THE BASIC PROTOCOL

A simplified flowchart of a blotting experiment is shown in Fig. 23.1. Proteins are transferred from the gel to the support electrophoretically. The gel and the membrane are put together in close contact in a suitable buffer and current is applied. Two different setups are used today: the tank transfer and the semidry transfer.

3.1. Tank Transfer

Blotting is performed in a tank of buffer with the gel in a vertical position completely submerged between two electrodes. Figure 23.2 depicts the transfer device as well as the correct location of gel and membrane with respect to the electrodes. Since the current heats the buffer, some commercial apparatuses incorporate a cooling system.

3.2. Semidry Transfer

In this setup, blotting is done horizontally and buffer is needed only to wet some pieces of filter paper that are placed between the electrodes and the gel and membrane. The stack is then placed between two large electrodes. Figure 23.3 illustrates this type of transfer. Precautions need to be taken to exclude a y air bubbles between the gel and the membrane, and also to avoid touching the membrane with bare hands, as the traces of lipids that result can block the transfer.

The transfer buffers used in both setups are the same and depend on the type of membrane used, as shown in Table 23.1.

3.3. Experimental Conditions

Although some specific solutions, buffers, etc., are given in this chapter, readers should note that there are as many specific protocols as researchers in a given field. In general, the use of one or another protocol is a matter of personal taste and the requirements of a particular situation.

Time and current settings depend on the type of transfer. In the tank system, 1 hr at 100 V is sufficient, although good results are obtained at lower voltages for extended periods of time (e.g., overnight). For the semidry system, currents of $0.2-0.8$ mA/cm^2 of gel area and short times (around 1 hr) are used. Care must be taken to avoid excessive heating, mainly in the graphite electrode apparatuses, which lack any cooling system.

Before continuing with the detection of the proteins, the extent of the transfer can be assessed by reversible staining of the blot. This can be done with the dye Ponceau S (9). After staining, photographs can be taken and/or molecular-weight standards can be marked with indelible ink. Destaining is achieved by soaking the

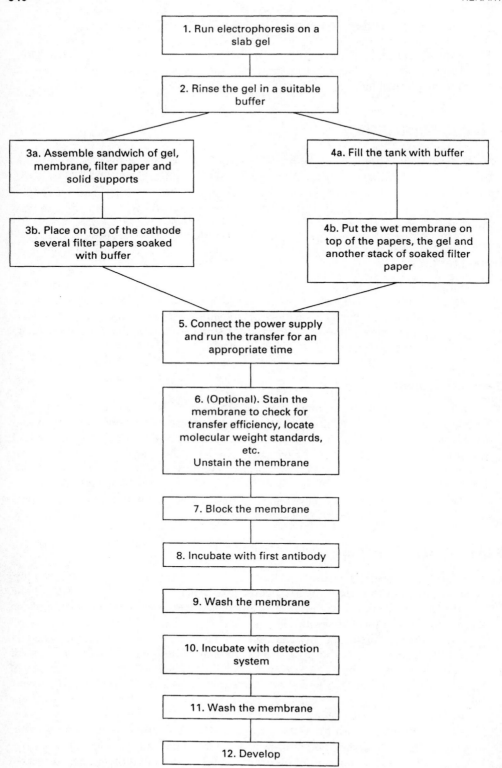

FIGURE 23.1   Simplified flowchart of a blotting experiment.

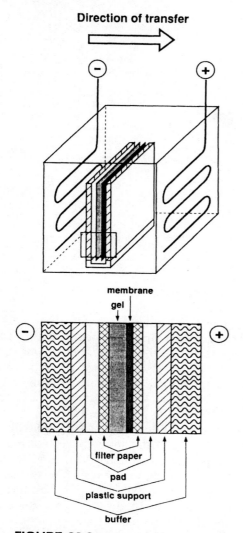

Direction of transfer

membrane
gel

filter paper
pad
plastic support
buffer

FIGURE 23.2 Diagram of a transfer tank. The upper part of the figure shows the general setup, with the location of the electrodes in the inner walls of the tank. The lower part of the figure is a magnification of the transfer assembly.

membrane in water. If needed, permanent staining of the blots can be done with india ink (10) or colloidal metals (11). These methods, however, cannot be used with nylon membranes.

Another important step in the blotting procedure is the quenching of any active group that could remain in the membrane after the transfer; otherwise, these groups could bind proteins used for detection, thereby increasing background. Different buffers are used according to the type of membrane and the type of detection method used. Some commonly used buffers are shown in Table 23.2. Although bovine serum albumin has been used as a universal protein for blocking, it may contain trace contaminants of immunoglobulins, which could eventually increase

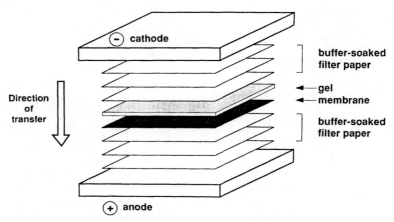

FIGURE 23.3   Diagram of a semidry transfer setup.

background. Hence, it is more convenient to use casein or nonfat dry milk, which are inexpensive and give consistently low backgrounds.

The blocking reaction and subsequent incubations are done in small volumes. The common procedure is to use plastic bags (first developed to store food in freezers), which are conveniently heat-sealed to the appropriate size of the blot. The amount of solution used is 50–100 μl/cm^2. The bags are gently rocked end over end at the appropriate temperature (1 hr at room temperature is a good choice). Another possibility is to use special glass cylinders developed for commercially available hybridization ovens.

Incubation with the specific antibody is done under the same conditions described above, with a suitable dilution of the antibody. If the antibody has not been used before, dilution has to be determined empirically, although typical ranges are 1:100 to 1:1000 for polyclonal antibodies, 1:10 to 1:100 for hybridoma supernatants, and 1:1000 or more for ascites fluid-containing monoclonal antibodies. Incubation times depend on the affinity and specificity of the antibody; usual protocols describe incubations from 1 hr at room temperature to overnight at 4°C.

TABLE 23.1   Transfer Buffers According to Membrane Used

Type of membrane	Transfer buffer
Nitrocellulose	0.025 M Tris 0.152 M glycine 20% methanol
PVDF membranes	0.025 M Tris 0.152 M glycine 10–15% methanol 0.1% SDS
Nylon membranes	0.025 M Tris 0.152 M glycine

TABLE 23.2 Blocking Buffers According to Membrane and Detection System

Membrane type	Colorimetric detection	Luminescence detection
Nitrocellulose	0.1% Tween 20 Tris-buffered saline (TTBS)	
PVDF		0.2% Casein in TBS
Neutral nylon	10% Nonfat dry milk in TBS	
Positively charged nylon		6% Casein, 1% polyvinyl-pyrrolidone in Tween 20 Tris-buffered saline (TTBS)

4. DETECTION METHODS

There are two main ways to detect immunocomplexes. The two types of detection systems are illustrated in Fig. 23.4. One strategy uses protein A or protein G from different strains of staphylococci (12, 13) (method 1 in Fig. 23.4A). Another method employs a second antibody that is directed against the primary antibody (methods 2–4 in the figure). In either case, protein A or G or the secondary antibody must be labeled, either with radioactivity or with enzymes. Another method (method 3 in the figure) employs secondary biotinylated antibodies and a bridging system based on avidin/streptavidin.

Proteins A or G are relatively unspecific reagents that react with many, but not all, classes of immunoglobulins. Table 23.3 shows the species-specificity of these two proteins, as well as their affinities for some monoclonal antibodies.

Proteins A and G have the advantage of being general reagents that can be used with several immunocomplexes. However, as shown in Table 23.3, not all immunoglobulins are recognized. This is especially inconvenient with rat immuno-globulins (a common source of monoclonal antibodies), which are recognized poorly by protein G and not at all by protein A. Secondary antibodies are more versatile in that it is possible to simultaneously detect two (and theoretically more) analytes by using two primary antibodies (e.g., from mouse and rabbit), two secondary labeled antibodies (e.g., anti-mouse and anti-rabbit), and two different detection methods.

4.1. Radioactivity

Radioiodination is a common way to label proteins A or G or secondary antibodies (methods 1 and 2 in Fig. 23.4). A suitable isotope is ^{125}I, which is easily detected by autoradiography and has a relatively long half-life (60 days); further, its low energy minimizes radiation hazards. However, iodination reactions must to be done in a well-operating hood because I_2 is volatile and is uptaken very efficiently by the thyroid.

There are three main types of iodination protocols: those based in acylating reagents, such as the Bolton–Hunter procedure (14); those based on chemical oxidation of I^- with chloramine T (15); and those based on enzymatic oxidation of I^- with lactoperoxidase (16). All methods are reliable and give highly specific activities. The enzymatic iodination has the advantage of iodinating only surface residues, due to steric hindrance between lactoperoxidase and the protein to be

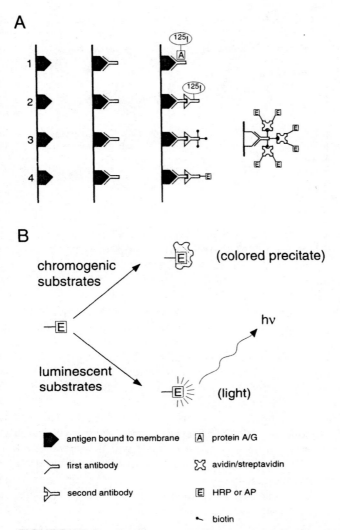

FIGURE 23.4 Diagram of the different detection methods. In (A), the steps (from left to right) of four different methodologies are shown. Method 1: Detection of the immunocomplex with iodinated protein A or G. Method 2: Detection of the immunocomplex with an iodinated second antibody. Method 3: Use of biotinylated secondary antibody. A further step is needed to allow binding of the avidin/streptavidin-conjugated enzyme to the complex. Method 4: Detection of the immunocomplex with an enzyme-linked secondary antibody. (B) The two alternative types of substrates for detecting the enzyme conjugates. If chromogenic substrates are used, a colored precipitate is developed; if luminescent substrates are used, the light produced can be detected with autoradiography.

labeled. Nevertheless, labeled proteins A and G as well as several secondary antibodies are now commercially available.

4.2. Enzyme-Based Systems

The most common methods for detecting the antigen–antibody complexes today are based on a secondary antibody with an enzyme conjugated to it, either directly

TABLE 23.3 Specificity of Proteins A and G from Staphylococci

Species	Protein A[a]	Protein G[b]	Monoclonals	Protein A[a]	Protein G[b]
Human	+ + + +	+ + + +	Human IgG1	+ + + +	+ + + +
Horse	+ +	+ + + +	Human IgG2	+ + + +	+ + + +
Cow	+ +	+ + + +	Human IgG3	−	+ + + +
Pig	+ + +	+ + +	Human IgG4	+ + + +	+ + + +
Sheep	+/−	+ +	Rat IgG1	−	+
Goat	−	+ +	Rat IgG2a	−	+ + + +
Rabbit	+ + + +	+ + +	Rat IgG2b	−	+ +
Chicken	−	+	Rat IgG2c	+	+ +
Hamster	+	+ +	Mouse IgG1	+	+ + + +
Guinea pig	+ + + +	+ +	Mouse IgG2a	+ + + +	+ + + +
Rat	+/−	+ +	Mouse IgG2b	+ + +	+ + +
Mouse	+ +	+ +	Mouse IgG3	+ +	+ + +

[a] From Richman *et al.* (43).
[b] From Åkerström *et al.* (13).

or via an avidin(streptavidin)–biotin arm. In the latter case, sensitivity is increased, since many reporter enzyme molecules can bind to each secondary antibody molecule.

The enzymes most commonly used are horseradish peroxidase (HRP) or alkaline phosphatase (AP), conjugated directly to the second antibody (method 4 in Fig. 23.4A) or conjugated with avidin (to use with a biotinylated secondary antibody; method 3 in Fig. 23.4). Conjugation of these enzymes to the antibody molecules is usually done with glutaraldehyde, periodate, or techniques described in other chapters of this book, or by biotinylation with succinimide esters of biotin. These reactions will not be discussed here; many conjugates are commercially available. Readers interested in these procedures should refer to the manual by Harlow and Lane (17). A note of caution when using the avidin–biotin system is that the reaction may also detect biotin-binding proteins in the extract, giving false-positive results independent of the first antibody.

As will be shown later, chromogenic and luminescent substrates for both enzymes (see Fig. 23.4B) produce either a colored precipitate or light as end-products.

The blot is incubated with a dilution of the second antibody (commercial products are used at dilutions of 1 : 1000 to 1 : 3000). After washing, the enzyme is visualized with chromogenic or luminescent substrates.

4.2.1. Horseradish Peroxidase

Peroxidases (EC 1.11.1.7) are a class of enzymes that oxidize a substrate using H_2O_2:

$$RH_2 + H_2O_2 \rightarrow R + 2H_2O.$$

Several substrates that produce a colored precipitate upon oxidation have been developed. The most common one is 4-chloronaphthol, although it is not very sensitive. HRP is also able to oxidize luminol, and therefore the antigen–antibody complex can be detected by luminescence. The main substrates and their reaction products are shown in Fig. 23.5 and described in Table 23.4.

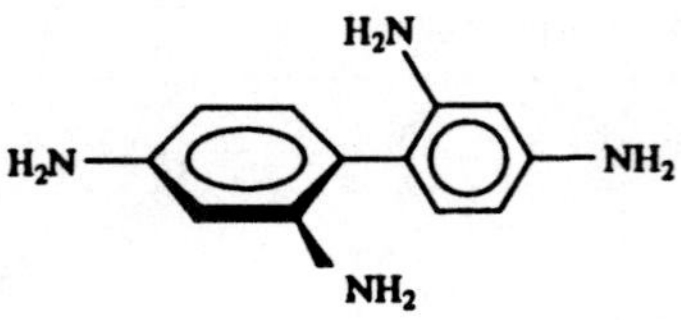

3,3'-diaminobenzidine
(DAB)

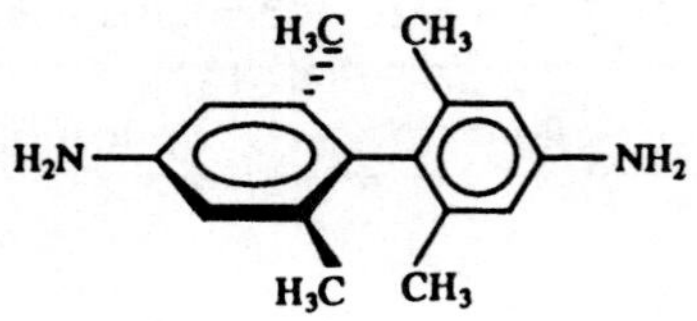

3,3',5,5'-tetramethylbenzidine
(TMB)

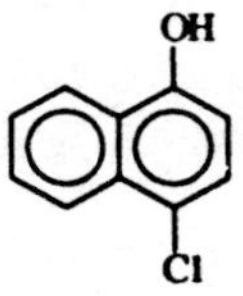

4-Chloro-naphtol
(4CN)

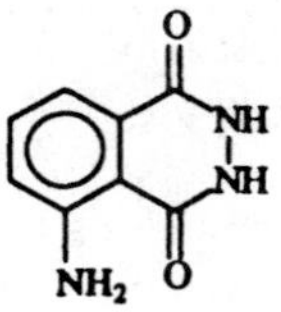

5-amino-2,3-dihydro-1,4-
phtalazine dione
(Luminol)

FIGURE 23.5 Common substrates for horseradish peroxidase. The first three, diaminobenzidine, tetramethylbenzidine, and 4-chloronaphthol, are chromogenic; luminol is luminescent.

4.2.2. Alkaline Phosphatase

Alkaline phosphatase (EC 3.1.3.1) hydrolyzes a phosphomonoester bond at alkaline pH:

$$R\text{-}O\text{-}P\text{-}OH + H_2O \rightarrow R\text{-}OH + P_i.$$

As in the case of HRP, substrates have been developed that, upon hydrolysis of the phosphate anion, either result in dark precipitates or give luminescent prod-

TABLE 23.4 Detection Reagents for Peroxidases

Detection	Reagent	Reaction	Comments
Chromogenic	4-Chloronaphthol (4CN)	Purple precipitate	Not very sensitive
	Diaminobenzidine (DAB)	Dark brown precipitate	Carcinogenic; reaction enhanced by $NiCl_2$
	Tetramethylbenzidine (TMB)	Dark purple stain	Less toxic than DAB
Luminescent	Luminol	Oxidation releases light	Very sensitive; *p*-iodo-phenol increases light output

ucts; the primary ones are shown in Fig. 23.6 and described in Table 23.5. The most common alkaline-phosphatase-based method is that of BCIP/NBT. The indoxyl derivative formed by the hydrolysis of BCIP is oxidized to indigo and the released protons reduce NBT to a formazan precipitate. For luminescent detection, dioxetane

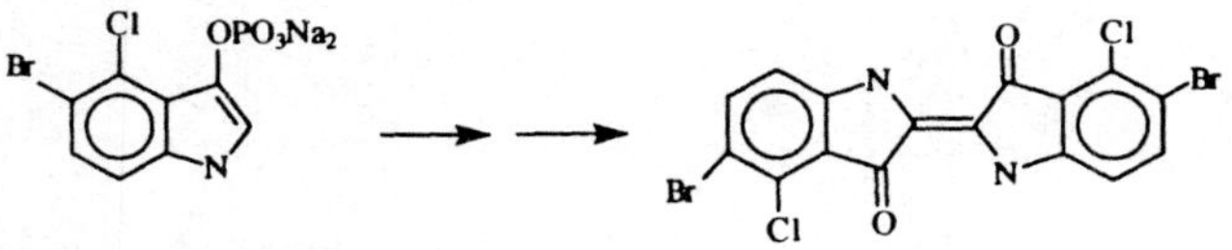

5-Bromo-4-Chloro-3-indolyl phosphate (BCIP)

(indigo derivative)

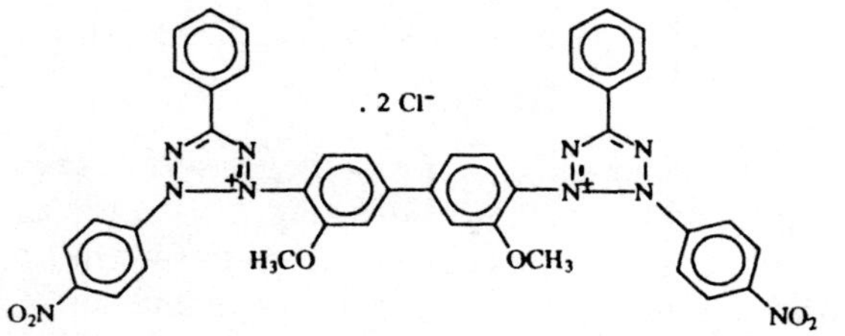

2,2'-di-p-nitrophenyl-5,5'-diphenyl(-3,3'-dimethoxy-4,4'-biphenylene) ditetrazolium chloride (Nitroblue tetrazolium, NBT)

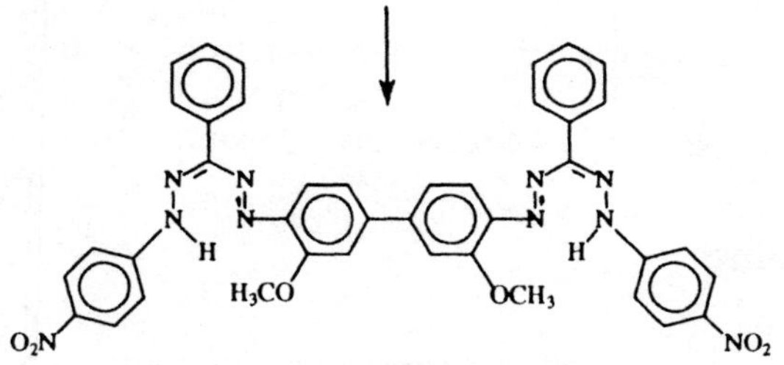

formazan derivative of NBT

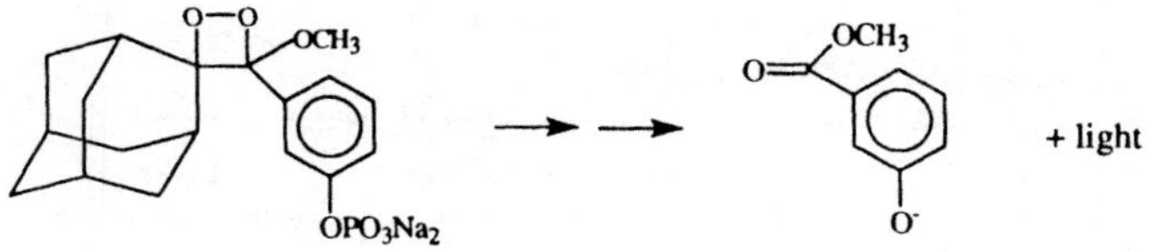

+ light

3-(2'-spiroadamantane)-4-methoxy-4-
(3"-phosphoryloxy)-phenyl-1,2-dioxetane
(AMPPD)

FIGURE 23.6 Common substrates for alkaline phosphatase. The chemical structure of BCIP and NBT is shown. Colored precipitate production is triggered by the hydrolysis of the phosphomonoester bond of BCIP. In the case of the adamantane derivative AMPPD, hydrolysis by alkaline phosphatase gives unstable products that decompose with production of light.

TABLE 23.5   Detection Reagents for Alkaline Phosphatases

Detection	Reagent	Reaction	Comments
Chromogenic	BCIP/NBT	Hydrolysis product of BCIP is oxidized (to an indigo derivative) by NBT, which is reduced to a formazan derivative, giving dark-blue–gray precipitate	Sensitive
Luminescent	AMPPD and derivatives	Hydrolysis product is unstable and decomposes with emission of light	Sensitive

derivatives have been developed that emit light upon hydrolysis of the phosphate group by the enzyme and consequent degradation of the unstable product formed.

4.3. Technical Considerations

The choice of detection method depends mainly on the sensitivity required. If the first antibody has high affinity and gives clean and strong signals, the chromogenic methods can be used to obtain good results. The next step toward more sensitivity is to use the avidin–biotin variation, which introduces an amplification step. Finally, luminescent methods are the most sensitive, although they need preliminary trials for optimization.

Another point to be considered is that, in general, proteins in the blot are denatured, so only antibodies that recognize denatured epitopes will react. Varshavski *et al.* (18) have made the observation that sensitivity is greatly enhanced by heating the wet blot. This suggests that there is some renaturation during incubation, and therefore heating unmasks epitopes that otherwise would remain unrecognized.

4.4. Reuse of Blots (Reprobing)

It is sometimes convenient to "erase" the signals obtained in a blotting experiment and reuse the blot to detect a different antigen. Different buffers have been proposed, all of them creating conditions that destabilize antigen–antibody interactions, as shown in Table 23.6.

TABLE 23.6   Buffers for Erasing Blots (Reprobing)

Reagent	Treatment	Source
0.05 M Na-phosphate buffer, pH 7.6, 2% SDS, 0.1 M 2-mercapto-ethanol	60°C, 60 min	Symington *et al.* (44)
0.05 M Na-phosphate buffer, pH 7.6, 0.154 M NaCl, 10 M urea, 0.1 M 2-mercaptoethanol	60°C, 30 min	Renart *et al.* (3)
0.01 M Tris-Cl, pH 7.6, 3 M NaSCN	37°C, 60 min	Reiser and Wardale (5)
0.04 M Glycine-Cl, pH 2.2, 30% (v/v) 2,2′-dimethylformamide	Room temperature, dipping	Geysen *et al.* (19)
0.04 M Glycine-Cl, pH 2.2, 2% (w/v) SDS	60°C, 30 min	Geysen (45)
0.1 M Glycine-Cl, pH 2.2	Room temperature, 90 min	Legocki and Verma (46)

After reincubating the blot with an appropriate buffer, it can be used again. An interesting alternative, developed by Geysen *et al.* (19), is "double staining." In this technique, the first antigen is stained with HRP and diaminobenzidine as chromogen. Since the colored product formed is insoluble, it is possible to desorb the immunocomplex without affecting the signal. The blot is stained again with another chromogen, such as 4-chloronaphthol, whose signal can be distinguished from that of diaminobenzidine. Nitrocellulose can be reprobed once, PVDF membranes many times.

5. SPECIALIZED USES AND APPLICATIONS

Although the protocols described above utilize antibodies to detect the antigen bound to the membrane, this is by no means the only procedure by which to specifically detect a protein. Actually, any reagent that can interact with a polypeptide is a potential detection system provided the specificity is adequate. In this section we discuss different ways of detecting proteins and specialized variations of the basic protocol.

5.1. Dot Blots

Dot blot refers to the deposition of a protein solution directly onto the membrane (20). If the volume to be added to the membrane is small (ca. 5 μl), the solution can be applied directly with a capillary micropipette. For larger volumes or when making quantitative measurements, dot-blot or slot-blot apparatuses are available that give uniform-size dots or slots, therefore allowing the comparison of intensity of staining.

Since in the dot-blot systems the molecular weight information is lost, this technique is especially well suited for probing a given antigen with different sera (as in the screening of monoclonal antibodies), or for quantitation of a given protein in a mixture by serial dilutions. Due to this limitation, dot blots can be used only if the specificity of the antibody is known; that is, it reacts only with the antigen of interest. All the techniques for detection discussed above can be applied to a dotted membrane.

5.2. Epitope Characterization

The classical studies of Atassi (21) and Lerner (22) show that antibodies react with small, well-defined areas of the surface of proteins (epitopes). Therefore, antibodies can be used as molecular probes to map and dissect these epitopes on proteins. The mapping of these epitopes has been facilitated by the use of blotting techniques, since blotting gives double or triple specificity: size and antigen recognition or size plus isoelectric point and antigen recognition. Proteases and chemicals can cleave proteins in a specific manner. After blotting these fragments, they can be revealed with a single monoclonal antibody, thereby determining its specificity, or with a battery of them, in which case the conformation of the protein can be studied provided the specificity of the monoclonals is known. Needless to say, in this type of study, cloning and sequencing of the antigen greatly facilitates the analysis, as shown by Scammell *et al.* for bovine prolactin (23).

5.3. Antibody Isolation

This technique, developed by Olmsted (24), takes advantage of the reversible immobilization of a given antibody when it is bound to its cognate antigen in a blot. After detecting the antigen of interest, the membrane is cut and the antibody eluted from it, using buffers that are of low pH or contain chaotropic agents. Care must be taken to neutralize or dialyze the eluant immediately after releasing the antibody, so as to protect it from the extreme conditions needed for elution.

Several extensions of the technique are worth mentioning; Talian *et al.* (25) used the technique to conjugate fluorophores under conditions in which the antigen-binding site is protected. Cox *et al.* (26) have used it to generate sera that lack antibodies to specific proteins.

All of these procedures rely on the irreversible binding of the antigen to the support. This is true if diazo-paper is used; however, it is not necessarily so in the case of membranes, even though the binding is very strong. In any case, preliminary experiments should be carried out to ascertain this point.

5.4. cDNA Library Screening

cDNA libraries can be constructed in expression vectors (27). These vectors normally have a cloning site at the end of the coding sequence of a bacterial protein gene. The gene should be under the control of a strong inducible promoter. The first of this type of vector was λgt11 (28), in which the cloning site is at the end of the β-galactosidase gene. In general, one out of six of the inserted sequences should be in phase with respect to β-galactosidase gene. Inducing the promoter prompts bacteria to synthesize the fusion protein encoded by β-galactosidase and the inserted DNA. The colonies can be lysed *in situ* and transferred to nitrocellulose membranes (29). Detection with a specific antibody allows for the easy selection of the cDNA coding for the protein.

A classical immunoassay application for this purpose is also available. Erlich *et al.* (30) bound F(ab')$_2$ fragments (from anti-β-galactosidase antibodies) to diazo-paper and made a blot from bacterial colonies expressing the enzyme. The complexes were detected with antibodies and ^{125}I-labeled protein A.

5.5. Protein Isolation for Microsequencing

Blotting of proteins onto PDVF membranes has been used for isolating and handling proteins for automatic microsequencing (31). Using this method, the recovery of a single band from an SDS–polyacrylamide gel is easy, so that sequencing of one specific protein from a complex mixture is possible. The membranes have high capacity, bind proteins strongly, and are inert to most organic solvents.

5.6. Glycoprotein Detection and Analysis

Lectins are proteins that bind complex sugar chains with relatively high affinity ($K_d \approx 10^{-5}$ M^{-1}) and with high specificity (32). They can be used, therefore, to identify and partially characterize glycoproteins on blots. A convenient detection system is to use biotinylated lectins and avidin-conjugated enzymes, as described in previous sections. Another possibility is to use digoxigenin-labeled lectins and detect them with anti-digoxigenin Fab fragments conjugated with alkaline phosphatase (33, 34).

Specificity of the reaction can be assessed by incubating blots with the lectin in the presence of small oligosaccharides which effectively compete with the glycoprotein–lectin interaction.

5.7. Enzyme Detection

Once proteins are attached to membranes in a noncovalent manner, they can be renatured by interchanging SDS with guanidinium chloride and then eliminating the latter. This procedure was developed by Celenza and Carlson (35) to assay protein kinases in the blot by incubating the membrane with $[\gamma$-^{32}P]ATP. Ferrel and Martin (36) have explored the method further. Nevertheless, two important points must be kept in mind: first, not all proteins renature under the conditions described; second, one can detect only monomeric enzymes, unless the gel electrophoresis is done under native conditions.

Although this is an elegant application of blotting techniques, one point is worth mentioning: This enzyme assay uses no substrate, so only autophosphorylation reactions are detected, and these could also occur in phosphorylated intermediaries of non-protein-kinase enzymes. Saturation of the blot with a putative substrate (casein, for instance) should only be valid if the enzyme does not autophosphorylate, a property of almost all protein kinases.

For the benefit of readers interested in *in situ* detection of enzyme activity, more interesting possibilities arise when the detection is made directly in the gel and not in the blot. In some cases, substrates can be copolymerized with the matrix, and with washing give very low backgrounds.

Another procedure has been described in which a complex mixture of proteins is blotted and incubated with a "pure" protein kinase and $[\gamma$-^{32}P]ATP. Under these conditions, substrates for this kinase are identified (37). The method allows the subsequent study of the identified substrate by the standard protocol with specific antibodies, or by digesting the protein with proteases and studying phosphorylated peptides.

5.8. South-Western Blotting

This technique, which borrows its name from Southern and Western blotting, takes advantage of the specificity of interactions between DNA and proteins. In its first version, recombinant phages expressing fusion proteins were plated and transferred to nitrocellulose membranes, as was the case for the cDNA library screening method mentioned earlier. However, instead of using antibodies to detect the proteins, short fragments of labeled DNA were used (after renaturing the proteins, as described in the last section) (38). In this way, only the phages with a fusion protein specifically recognizing the DNA fragment were detected by autoradiography.

The same type of analysis can be done with proteins separated by gel electrophoresis, after transfer to a membrane (39).

5.9. Shift-Western Assays

Gel retardation assays (often called "band shifting assays") are a powerful technique for studying DNA–protein interactions. A fragment of DNA with a protein bound to it migrates slower in a native polyacrylamide gel than the DNA fragment alone. If the DNA is labeled, one uses the difference in migration to detect interactions of the DNA with proteins (40).

Detection of the proteins by blotting the complexes was already known (41). The Shift-Western technique (42) takes advantage of the different binding specificities of different supports: nitrocellulose binds proteins but does not bind double-stranded DNA. By transferring the retardation-assay gel to stacked nitrocellulose (closest to the gel) and charged membranes, the protein responsible for the retardation binds to one membrane and the DNA to the other. The protein blot can be probed with specific antibodies and the DNA blot hybridized, obtaining a full characterization of the macromolecules involved.

6. CONCLUSIONS

Since the initial descriptions of blotting procedures in 1975 and 1979, these techniques have become invaluable to the cell and molecular biologist as well as the immunologist, because they afford the capability to detect antigens not only by the specificity of the antibodies used to detect then, but also by the information obtained by gel electrophoresis.

References

1. Southern EM. Detection of specific sequences among DNA fragments separated by gel electrophoresis. J Mol Biol 1975; 98:503–17.
2. Alwine JC, Kemp DJ, Parker BA, Reiser J, Renart J, Stark GR, Wahl GM. Detection of specific RNAs or specific fragments of DNA by fractionation in gels and transfer to diazobenzyloxymethyl paper. Methods Enzymol 1979; 68:220–42.
3. Renart J, Reiser J, Stark GR. Transfer of proteins from gels to diazobenzyloxymethyl-paper and detection with antisera: a method for studying antibody specificity and antigen structure. Proc Natl Acad Sci USA 1979; 76:3116–20.
4. Towbin H, Staehelin T, Gordon J. Electrophoretic transfer of proteins from polyacrylamide gels to nitrocellulose sheets: procedure and some applications. Proc Natl Acad Sci USA 1979; 76:4350–4.
5. Reiser J, Wardale J. Immunological detection of specific proteins in total cell extracts by fractionation in gels and transfer to diazophenylthioether paper. Eur J Biochem 1981; 114:569–75.
6. Burnette WN. "Western blotting": electrophoretic transfer of proteins from sodium dodecyl sulfate-polyacrylamide gels to unmodified nitrocellulose and radiographic detection with antibody and radioiodinated protein A. Anal Biochem 1981; 112:195–203.
7. Laemmli UK. Cleavage of structural proteins during the assembly of the head of bacteriophage T4. Nature 1970; 227:680–5.
8. O'Farrel PH. High-resolution two-dimensional gel electrophoresis of proteins. J Biol Chem 1975; 250:4007–21.
9. Salinovich O, Montelaro RC. Reversible staining and peptide mapping of proteins transferred to nitrocellulose after separation by sodium dodecyl sulfate-polyacrylamide gel electrophoresis. Anal Biochem 1986; 156:341–7.
10. Hancock K, Tsang VCM. India ink staining of proteins on nitrocellulose paper. Anal Biochem 1983; 133:157–62.
11. Moeremans M, Daneels G, De Mey J. Sensitive colloidal metal (gold or silver) staining of protein blots on nitrocellulose membranes. Anal Biochem 1985; 145:315–21.
12. Langone JJ. Protein A of *Staphylococcus aureus* and related immunoglobulin receptors produced by streptococci and pneumococci. Adv Immunol 1982; 32:157–251.
13. Åkelström B, Björk L. A physico-chemical study of protein G, a molecule with unique immunoglobulin G-binding properties. J Biol Chem 1986; 261;10240–7.

14. Bolton AE, Hunter WM. The labeling of proteins to high specific radioactivities by conjugation to a ^{125}I-containing acylating agent. Biochem J 1973; 133:529–39.
15. McConahey PJ, Dixon FJ. Radioiodination of proteins by the use of the chloramine-T method. Methods Enzymol 1980; 70:210–3.
16. Morrison M. Lactoperoxidase-catalyzed iodination as a tool for investigation of proteins. Methods Enzymol 1980; 70:214–20.
17. Harlow E, Lane D. Antibodies: a laboratory manual. Cold Spring Harbor, NY: Cold Spring Harbor Laboratory, 1988.
18. Swerdow PS, Finley D, Varshavsky A. Enhancement of immunoblot sensitivity by heating of hydrated filters. Anal Biochem 1986; 156:147–53.
19. Geysen J, De Loof A, Vandesande F. How to perform subsequent or "double" immunostaining of two different antigens on a single nitrocellulose blot within one day with an immunoperoxidase technique. Electrophoresis 1984; 5:129–32.
20. Hawkes R, Niday E, Gordon J. A dot-immunobinding assay for monoclonal and other antibodies. Anal Biochem 1982; 119:142–7.
21. Atassi MZ. Antigenic structures of proteins. Eur J. Biochem 1984; 145:1–20.
22. Lerner RA. Antibodies of predetermined specificity in biology and medicine. Adv Immunol 1984; 36:1–44.
23. Scammell JG, Luck DN, Valentine DL, Smith M. Epitope mapping of monoclonal antibodies to bovine prolactin. Am J Physiol 1992; 263:E520–5.
24. Olmsted JB. Affinity purification of antibodies from diazotized paper blots of heterogeneous protein samples. J Biol Chem 1981; 256:11955–7.
25. Talian JC, Olmsted JB, Goldman RD. A rapid procedure for preparing fluorescein-labeled specific antibodies from whole anti-serum. Its use in analyzing cytoskeletal architecture. J Cell Biol 1983; 97:1277–82.
26. Cox JV, Schenk EA, Olmsted JB. Human anticentromere antibodies: distribution, characterization of antigens, and effect on microtubule organization. Cell 1983; 35:331–9.
27. Sambrook J, Fritsch EF, Maniatis T. Molecular cloning: a laboratory manual, 2nd ed. Cold Spring Harbor, NY: Cold Spring Harbor Laboratory, 1989.
28. Young RA, Davis RW. Efficient isolation of genes by using antibody probes. Proc Natl Acad Sci USA 1983; 80:1194–8.
29. Benton WD, Davis RW. Screening λgt recombinant clones by hybridization to single plaques in situ. Science 1977; 196:180–2.
30. Erlich HA, Cohen SN, McDevitt HO. A sensitive radioimmunoassay for detecting products translated from cloned DNA fragments. Cell 1978; 13:681–9.
31. Matsudaira P. Sequence from picomole quantities of proteins electroblotted onto polyvinylidene difluoride membranes. J Biol Chem 1987; 262:10035–8.
32. Goldstein IJ, Hayes CE. Carbohydrate-binding proteins of plants and animals. Adv Carbohyd Chem Biochem 1978; 35:127–340.
33. Haselbeck A, Schikaneder E, Eltz H, Hösel W. Structural characterization of glycoprotein carbohydrate chains by using digoxigenin-labeled lectins on blots. Anal Biochem 1990; 44:25–30.
34. Becker B, Salzburg M, Melkonian M. Blot analysis of glycoconjugates using digoxigenin-labeled lectins: an optimized procedure. BioTechniques 1993; 15:232–5.
35. Celenza JL, Carlson M. A yeast gene that is essential for release from glucose repression encodes a protein kinase. Science 1986; 1175–80.
36. Ferrell JE, Martin GS. Thrombin stimulates the activities of multiple previously unidentified protein kinases in platelets. J Biol Chem 1989; 264:20723–9.
37. Valtorta F, Schiebler W, Jahn R, Ceccarelli B, Greengard P. A solid-phase assay for the phosphorylation of proteins blotted on nitrocellulose membrane filters. Anal Biochem 1986; 158:130–7.
38. Vinson CR, LaMarco KL, Johnson PF, Landschulz WH, McKnight SL. In situ detection of sequence specific DNA binding activity specified by a recombinant bacteriophage. Genes Dev 1988; 2:801–6.
39. Francis-Lang H, Price M, Polycarpou-Schwarz M, Di Lauro R. Cell-type-specific expression of the rat thyroperoxidase promoter indicates common mechanisms for thyroid-specific gene expression. Mol Cell Biol 1992; 12:576–88.
40. Garner MM, Revzin A. A gel electrophoresis method for quantifying the binding of proteins to specific DNA regions: application to components of the *Escherichia coli* lactose operon regulatory system. Nucleic Acids Res 1981; 9:3047–60.
41. Granger-Schnarr M, Lloubes R, De Murcia G, Schnarr M. Specific protein-DNA complexes: immunodetection of the protein component after gel electrophoresis and Western blotting. Anal Biochem 1988; 174:235–8.

42. Demczuk S, Harbers M, Vennström B. Identification and analysis of all components of a gel retardation assay by combination with immunoblotting. Proc Natl Acad Sci USA 1993; 90:2574–8.
43. Richman DD, Cleveland PH, Oxman MN, Johnson KM. The binding of staphylococcal protein A by the sera of different animal species. J Immunol 1982; 128:2300–5.
44. Symington J, Green M, Brackman K. Immunoautoradiographic detection of proteins after electrophoretic transfer from gels to diazo-paper: analysis of adenovirus encoded proteins. Proc Natl Acad Sci USA 1981; 78:177–81.
45. Geysen J. Desorption of antibodies for reuse of blots. In: Bjeruum OJ, Heegard NHH, Eds. Handbook of Immunoblotting of Proteins. Boca Raton, FL: CRC Press, 1988:213–20.
46. Legocki RP, Verma DPS. Multiple immunoreplica technique: screening for specific proteins with a series of different antibodies using one polyacrylamide gel. Anal Biochem 1981; 111:385–92.

24 DEVELOPMENT OF IN-HOUSE IMMUNOASSAYS

ELEFTHERIOS P. DIAMANDIS
Departments of Pathology and
Laboratory Medicine
Mount Sinai Hospital
Toronto, Ontario, Canada M5G 1XS

THEODORE K. CHRISTOPOULOS
Department of Chemistry and
Biochemistry
University of Windsor
Windsor, Ontario, Canada N9B 3P4

MOHAMMAD J. KHOSRAVI
Diagnostic Systems Laboratories
Toronto, Ontario, Canada

1. INTRODUCTION

Although many companies manufacture and distribute immunoassay kits for research applications, it is not possible to cover all the needs of individual researchers. Additionally, many research-oriented immunoassay kits are expensive and are not suitable for studies in which relatively substantial numbers of samples will be analyzed. For these reasons, many researchers frequently consider setting up in-house immunoassay methodologies.

Before embarking into such a project the researcher must be familiar with the general principles of analytical chemistry, the nature of the reagents to be used, and their limitations and possible pitfalls. The researcher should be in a position to judge the validity of all results because, when working with biological samples it is very common to encounter problems usually associated with a small percentage of samples. For example, results could be analytically invalidated in cases of hyperbilirubinemia, hyperlipidemia, and drug consumption, in autoimmune disease sera and pregnancy, in patients with cancer, etc. In some cases unreliable results could not be explained even after lengthy and costly investigations.

The set-up of a particular immunoassay method could take a very short or a very long time depending on the availability and quality of the necessary reagents, especially of the antibodies. The researcher must also define the needs and set-up goals and objectives for the problem at hand. For example, the required sensitivity (detection limit) must be clearly defined. In general, the best attainable sensitivity with the current state of the art detection methodologies is approximately 1 amol of analyte ($\sim$600,000 molecules) per assay. With 100 μl sample volume, this corresponds to an analyte concentration of 10^{-14} mol/liter. However, such detection limits can only be achieved with antibodies of very high affinity and with noncompetitive immunoassay techniques. In general, easily attainable sensitivities are in the order of 10^{-8}–10^{-11} mol/liter of analyte. For sensitivities in the range 10^{-11}–10^{-13} mol/liter, the researcher is advised to use high-affinity antibodies (affinity constants $\geq 10^{10}$ mol^{-1} liter) and detection techniques based on chemiluminescence or time-resolved fluorometry. However, with appropriate antibodies and assay optimization, ultrasensitive immunoassays could also be developed using conventional colorimetric enzyme immunoassay reagents but at the expense of limiting the measurement range of the assay.

Once a method is set-up it is imperative to study the analytical characteristics of the assay, e.g., within-run and day-to-day precision, recovery, specificity (cross-reactivity studies), dilution linearity, dynamic range and comparison with other techniques. The robustness of the assay, i.e., its ability to perform consistently over long periods of time with different operators should also be examined. The stability of reagents, standards, and samples for the analyte of interest is of paramount importance in producing meaningful results.

In general, the researcher who is interested in setting up an immunological assay is advised to be always alert in order to spot any unexpected or suspect results and design simple experiments to investigate the problems. One should not rush into analyzing samples just after achieving a decent calibration curve. In the authors' experience, representative calibration curves could be obtained during the first few days of experimentation but reliable results with real samples are usually obtained weeks or months after the initiation of the project.

2. DEVELOPMENT OF AN IMMUNOASSAY METHOD

2.1. Solid Phase

Immunoassays can be homogeneous (not requiring a separation step) or heterogeneous. Research methods are usually heterogeneous and require a solid phase which will facilitate bound/free separation of label. A detailed description of solid-phases is presented in Chapter 9. Although in immunological assays many shapes/types of solid phases are used, e.g., tubes, beads, microspheres, and magnetic particles, the easiest to use in an in-house immunoassay development are the microtiter wells. These are available either as solid 96-well plates or in the form of 8- or

12-well strips. Many manufacturers make excellent products, most composed of polystyrene of high protein-binding capacity. In many cases, the polystyrene protein-binding capacity is increased by irradiation; this is done by the manufacturer. For absorption and fluorescence spectroscopy clear wells are used. For chemilumines-cence and for time-resolved fluorescence immunoassays based on reflectance mea-surements, opaque, white, or black microtiter wells are used. Such wells are pro-duced by adding titanium-containing compounds to the polystyrene plastic.

Microtiter plates are the easiest to handle and use for in-house development because of the availability of a wide range of auxiliary equipment, e.g., multichannel pipettes, washers, and readers. One of the critical steps of the assay, the washing, can be easily and reproducibly performed with inexpensive washing/aspirating devices, either fully automated or manual.

Antibodies can be covalently bound to the solid phases but in the authors' experience this requires more time and expense without always leading to improved results. For in-house developments, the simple noncovalent adsorbtion of antibodies to microtiter wells is recommended. However, when the passive adsorption fails, covalent binding may have to be evaluated.

For antibody coating to polystyrene wells, many authors recommend carbonate buffers at pH 9–9.5. We recommend a 50 mmol/liter Tris buffer, pH 7.80, which, in our experience, gives equivalent or superior results. A step-by-step coating proce-dure is given in the example that follows. In general, one polystyrene well has a capacity of ~50 ng of antibody or less but researchers usually coat with 1 μg of antibody per well when the antibody is inexpensive. One can easily reduce this amount to 500 or 200 ng/well without any noticable change in performance. For very expensive monoclonal antibodies it is advisable to coat the solid phase with a secondary antibody, e.g., a goat anti-mouse antibody, and then add the primary antibody of interest (see example later in this chapter). In this case, it is possible to consume as little as 10–20 ng/well without any antibody waste. Some researchers collect the liquid after the noncovalent coating and reuse it after a preconcentration step, but in this case one has to verify with experimentation that the reused antibod-ies are fully active. For more discussion refer to Chapter 9.

Once the antibody is pipetted into the wells (100–200 μl per well) it is usually left for 14–24 hr at room temperature to complete the adsorption. Coating can be accelerated at higher temperatures and coating times of 1 hr at 37°C have been found to be successful. However, in order to achieve long-term reproducible results it is always advisable to use a consistent coating protocol, i.e., ~16 hr coating time at room temperature. After coating, the wells are washed twice to remove any unbound or loosely bound antibodies and are blocked with 250 μl of a 1% bovine serum albumin solution for 30 min. If the wells are not to be used immediately, they could be stored at 4°C in the blocking solution for up to 1 week. Storage of the wells with the coating antibody solution for long periods (>2 days) results in deterioration of precision. Best results are obtained with freshly coated plates (e.g., coat overnight and use the next day).

Many companies dry the antibody-coated wells after stabilization with a sucrose solution in order to provide long-term stability at room temperature. For in-house assays, this procedure is not recommended because uncontrolled drying or storage in unsealed bags without dessicant will cause plate deterioration and loss of assay performance.

For antigen coating similar principles apply. Antigen is usually coated for competitive-type assays or when antibodies against an analyte of interest are being quantified. If the antigen is not a protein, it must first be covalently conjugated to a carrier protein, e.g., bovine serum albumin (BSA) or bovine thyroglobulin before coating. When coating antigens, it is recommended to coat on a trial basis at pH between 4 and 10 because of the wide variability of coating with pH for some antigens. We recommend acetate (pH 4–6), phosphate (pH 6–7), Tris (pH 7–9), and carbonate (pH 9–10) buffers at a concentration of 50 mmol/liter and antigen concentrations of 50–500 ng/100 μl coating buffer.

Solutions containing antibodies and antigens for coating are usually prepared in glass or stainless steel cups and tubes because plastic adsorbs some coating proteins. Also, the plastic pipette tips that are used for coating are blocked with BSA and rinsed with water before use. The coating buffer must be absolutely free of any protein other than the coating protein otherwise the coating will be ineffective.

2.2. Antibodies

Antibodies are the most important reagents of an immunological assay. Their affinity and specificity will determine the overall sensitivity and specificity of the assay. Usually, antibodies with affinity constants $>10^9$ mol^{-1} liter should be used. For in-house assay development the researcher may have produced the monoclonal or polyclonal antibody, or the antibody could be donated or purchased. It should be remembered that many companies do not sell their best antibody clones but retain them for their kits. This is the reason that in-house assays sometimes cannot match the performance of commercial kits for the same analyte.

One of the best practices when trying to develop an in-house assay is to bring-in as many different antibodies as possible, both monoclonal and polyclonal, and evaluate them in combination. Many companies and antibody brokers offer free samples for evaluation. About 100 μg is usually enough for an initial screen. Antibodies may come as affinity-purified monoclonals or polyclonals, ascites fluid, immunoglobulin fractions, or unpurified antisera. Although purified preparations are preferred because they can be conjugated or coated more efficiently, this is not always necessary. Alternatively, ascites fluid or antiserum can be affinity-purified with protein A or G chromatography using simple commercial kits. Details are given in Chapter 5. For coating purposes, the more purified the antibody is, the more amount of antibody binding is achieved. If there is extraneous protein, competition for coating between the specific antibody and the irrelevant proteins will occur. If the extraneous proteins are not immunoglobulins, nonpurified antibodies (e.g., ascites) can be efficiently coated without purification using secondary antibody-precoated wells. In order to coat polyclonals, these must be purified at least to the stage of obtaining an immunoglobulin fraction. For direct conjugations to detectable moieties (e.g., enzymes, Eu^{3+}, chemiluminescent labels, biotin) the more purified the antibody fraction, the less the consumption of the labeling reagent and the less the background signal. However, for research purposes, direct labeling is not recommended because it is labor intensive and time consuming, it needs expertise, and it may lead to antibody inactivation.

Among the preferred approaches for research, the two most suitable strategies are: (a) the biotin–streptavidin system, in which the detection antibody is biotinylated and the detectable moiety, e.g., an enzyme is conjugated to streptavidin (this format is suitable for double monoclonal as well as monoclonal–polyclonal assays); and (b) the secondary antibody technique, in which the detection antibody is not labeled at all. The detectable moiety in this case is present on a secondary antibody. This format is suitable for monoclonal–polyclonal assay configurations.

In Chapter 11 biotin-labeling strategies have been presented in detail. Streptavidin-labeled reagents and secondary antibody-labeled reagents suitable for immunoassays are available from many manufacturers. In our laboratory we have used enzyme-labeled streptavidin and secondary antibodies from Jackson Immunoresearch. The same products from different manufacturers do not always have the same performance.

Modifications of the two basic techniques mentioned above can be adapted to competitive-type assays and assays for measuring specific antibodies against antigens (1–3).

Once the antibodies are available, and appropriate standards can be prepared, the best strategy to start an experimentation is first to decide on the assay format, e.g., (a) or (b) above, or both, and try all combinations between the available antibodies. For example, if two monoclonals (M_1, M_2) and two polyclonals (P_1, P_2) are available, and the polyclonals are not purified, the initial screen would include the following coating antibody-detection antibody combinations: (1) M_1–M_2; (2) M_1–P_1; (3) M_1–P_2; (4) M_2–M_1; (5) M_2–P_1; (6) M_2–P_2. A small portion, e.g., 50 μg of M_1 and M_2, is biotinylated as described in Chapter 11 or elsewhere (1), to be used as detection antibodies in combinations 4 and 1, respectively. For combinations 2, 3, 5, and 6, use of the secondary antibody technique would be the preferred strategy. For example, if the polyclonal antibody is from rabbits, one can use a goat anti-rabbit antibody conjugated to a detectable moiety, e.g., an enzyme.

This initial screen will usually reveal one or more acceptable sandwich combinations which can then be used for optimization in the next step. Part of the optimization will include sample volume, incubation times and temperature, and reagent dilutions. These aspects will be addressed below.

2.3. Labeling Systems

Currently, there are a number of nonisotopic detection techniques that are used for immunological assays. The major labeling systems include chemiluminescent labels, e.g., acridinium esters, lanthanide ions, and enzymes, mainly horseradish peroxidase (HRP) and alkaline phosphatase (ALP). These enzymes can be detected further with the use of colorimetric, chemiluminogenic, fluorogenic, or time-resolved fluorimetric techniques. The various detection/labeling systems are covered in other chapters of this book. Research reagents and instrumentation are available for all of the above technologies. However, some of these technologies require special instrumentation, e.g., microplate-based luminometers, fluorometers, time-resolved fluorometers, and spectrophotometers. In general, it is not efficient to use standard laboratory equipment to measure fluorescence, absorbance, etc., because the volumes used in immunoassay are generally small (<250 μl). Moreover, transferring many samples for analysis is time consuming. An initial investment to buy a specialized reader (e.g., an absorbance microplate reader) will be the preferred option.

In this chapter we will focus on the use of only one labeling system, but the principles mentioned apply to other technologies as well. In the proposed system, HRP will be the detectable label and the substrate will be 3, 3', 5, 5'-tetramethylbenzidine (TMB). With this system, one can usually achieve analyte sensitivities of the order 10^{-11}–10^{-12} mol/liter and two orders of magnitude of dynamic range.

2.4. Assay Configurations

The possible assay configurations in immunoassays are covered in Chapter 10. For research applications, the following configurations are preferred (Fig. 24.1). Configuration A is particularly attractive when two monoclonal antibodies are available. When only polyclonal antibodies are available, it is also possible to use them as in configuration A. This may also work when only one polyclonal is used for coating and detection. The other configurations can be used only if the coating antibody and the detection antibody are from different species. Configurations B and C can be modified to work with biotinylated polyclonal detection antibody and labeled streptavidin, especially when problems with anti-species antibodies in the sample are encountered. These problems are sometimes severe because they may link the coating antibody and the detection antibody, leading to false-positive results (2) (see also Chapter 7).

The direct coating with the monoclonal antibody (Figs. 24.1 A and 24B) is usually preferred when antibodies costing <$100 per milligram are used. For more expensive antibodies, configuration C is the method of choice because the coating polyclonal antibody is cheaper than $50 per milligram and the primary monoclonal antibody consumption is usually 10–30 times less in comparison to direct coating. When operating configuration C, it is not necessary to preform the coating antibody–

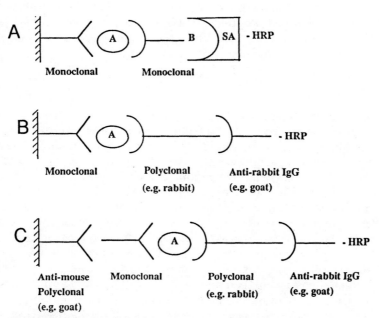

FIGURE 24.1 Preferred research assay configurations based on the heterogeneous noncompetitive immunoassay principle. A, analyte; B, biotin; SA, streptavidin; HRP, horseradish peroxidase. Monoclonal antibodies are considered to be mouse immunoglobulins. For more explanations see text.

primary antibody complex formation in advance. The primary antibody and sample can be pipetted at the same time. However, care must be taken that the primary antibody is not in excess over the coating antibody because, in this case, there will be loss of antigen bound to excess primary antibody during the washing. In general, configuration C has similar or better sensitivity than configuration B.

One should avoid coating with a secondary antibody and then using primary and detection antibodies from the same species because of background problems. In this case, some detection antibody would bind to the solid phase even after careful blocking, thus increasing background signal.

For in-house procedures we usually select a two-step assay format in which the sample is incubated with the coating antibody or primary antibody (as in configuration C) in the first step, followed by washing and addition of the detection antibody in the second step. This usually results in better sensitivity, especially with monoclonal–polyclonal assay configurations and avoids the possible problems of the high-dose hook effect described in detail in the literature (4).

2.5. Reagents/Washing/Incubation Times/Sample/Standards

The coating antibody should always be diluted in protein-free solutions, preferably in glass tubes, for the reasons already discussed. When using assay configuration C (Fig. 24.1), the primary antibody diluent may contain carrier protein and other constituents (see example below) but not mouse IgG or mouse serum because this will exhaust the binding capacity of the secondary antibody coated to the wells. Goat serum (10%) is usually added to this diluent to block human anti-goat antibodies present in some human sera (2). Mouse serum (5%) is also added when configurations A and B are used to block the presence of human anti-mouse antibodies in some patient sera (Chapter 7). The problem of anti-species antibodies is more severe when double-monoclonal configurations are used and are less of a problem in configurations B and C. In some instances, KCl, 0.5–1 mol/liter, may be used to increase the ionic strenght of diluents containing antibodies. High ionic strength reduces nonspecific binding effects of antibodies due to ionic interactions. The detection antibodies are always diluted in solutions containing a carrier protein, usually bovine serum albumin (BSA).

We have formulated a general detection antibody diluent consisting of a 50 mmol/liter Tris buffer, pH 7.80, and 60 g/liter of BSA. This diluent is also supplemented with mouse serum (5%) in configuration A, or goat serum (10%) in configurations B and C. The presence of these additives reduces nonspecific binding of the labeled or unlabeled rabbit detection antibody. If the detection antibody is from goat the addition of goat serum in this diluent is not recommended because it will increase the background signal due to nonspecific binding of goat IgG, detected in the next step with a labeled anti-goat antibody. The BSA carrier protein reduces the nonspecific binding of the antibodies used. The labeled antibody is usually diluted in a solution containing serum (5–10%) or IgG from the species where the antibody was raised. For example, in configuration A mouse serum is used in the biotinylated antibody diluent, and goat serum is used in conjugations B and C. The unlabeled IgG from the same species reduces the nonspecific binding of the labeled antibody.

The streptavidin–HRP conjugate diluent should contain 6% BSA in order to reduce nonspecific binding of the streptavidin conjugate. Care should be taken to use BSA free of biotin or biotinylated proteins, otherwise the streptavidin will be blocked and become unreactive. Similarly, the labeled antibody stock or labeled streptavidin, as well as their diluents for the assay, should be free from sodium azide as it is a strong inhibitor or HRP activity. This is more critical for a one-step assay format in which the standards should be prepared without use of sodium azide.

The wash solution is a weakly buffered solution (e.g., 5–10 mmol/liter Tris buffer, pH 7.80) containing 0.15 mol/liter NaCl and 0.05% of Tween 20, a nonionic detergent. The detergent facilitates efficient washing; however, wash solution consisting only of distilled or even tap water was found to be equally satisfactory in some cases. The frequency of washing depends on the step. It is important to keep the wells moist at all times; if they dry out, the washing may not be effective, leading to high backround. After coating, blocking, and sample incubation, one or two washes are enough. After the detection antibody incubation, three washing steps are recommended and after the labeled reagent addition, five or more washes are preferred. A soaking cycle during washing is beneficial.

The incubation times during an immunoassay vary with the nature of the solid phase, shaking, temperature, and concentration of analyte and other reagents. In general, the first step (sample incubation) requires about 1–4 hr to reach equilibrium or to achieve good sensitivity. The second step (detection antibody incubation), in the presence of approximately 50–100 ng of antibody per well, needs 1/2 to 1 hr. The third step, involving SA-ALP or SA-HRP, requires 15 min when the conjugate is present at amounts of 3–5 ng per well. More incubation increases the nonspecific binding leading to high background signals. In assay configuration C (Fig. 24.1) the labeled antibody incubation step is usually 1/2–1 hr when the antibody is present at amounts of 10–20 ng per well.

The substrate incubation time depends on the enzyme substrate but usually it is between 10 and 30 min, depending on the measuring range and sensitivity requirements. Longer incubations may sometimes improve the detectability but at the expense of limiting the measuring range. In the presence of high background signals, prolonged substrate incubation does not improve the signal to noise ratio.

For most applications all steps can be carried out at room temperature using intense mechanical shaking.

The complexity of the sample will determine if there will be many or few problems during assay development. Complex samples such as serum and urine, the composition of which may vary from person to person, usually create difficulties. One must pay a lot of attention to the sample collection and storage to ensure preservation of the analyte of interest. For initial experiments, fresh samples are preferred. The possible difficulties associated with sample composition, collection, and storage fall beyond the scope of this chapter. However, it is advisable to select patients who are normal, positive, and negative (if possible) for the analyte of interest to check the validity of the results. For example, for the evaluation of a PSA assay, one should run female sera in order to check the negativity of the assay. Positive sera from prostate cancer patients should also be measured. If positive or negative controls from patients are not available, it may be possible to find cell lines or recombinant vectors producing the protein of interest or cell lines with the gene of interest deleted.

The preparation of appropriate standars is a major factor in achieving accurate results. We usually use a standard diluent based on 50 mmol/liter Tris buffer, pH 7.80, containing 6% BSA. It is important to establish the stability of the analyte of interest in the standard and sample matrix. No meaningful results can be obtained if the sample analyte is deteriorating to a variable degree with time. For new analytes, appropriate standards may not be available. This is not an absolute limitation. Sometimes it is possible to use a high patient sample, which is given an arbitrary concentration, and then dilute it to obtain a series of standards (5). Absolute standardization may require months or years with the advent of newly discovered analytes. Alternatively, one can use recombinant proteins or cell lines producing the analyte to construct calibration curves. Again, patient results may be relative to an arbitrary standard but they can still be interpretable.

3. A PRACTICAL EXAMPLE—AN ELISA FOR p53

The p53 tumor suppressor gene product is a 53-kDa protein which is now considered a cell cycle regulator (6). This gene is mutated in many different cancer types and the mutant protein accumulates in the cell, presumably due to stabilization. Increasing evidence exists that p53 mutant protein accumulation in the tumor is an unfavorable prognostic indicator (7). Thus, the measurement of this protein in the tumor has practical value. In most studies conducted so far immunohistochemistry or DNA sequencing are used to assess the status of p53 gene and protein. A quantitative ELISA-type assay has been commercialized by one manufacturer, but the kit is relatively expensive. Thus, some investigators are discouraged from using it, especially in studies involving more than 40–50 samples.

Monoclonal and polyclonal antibodies for p53 are well-characterized and commercially available from many sources. These are currently used for immunohistochemistry. In the following text we present a stepwise approach to set up an ELISA for p53 protein.

3.1. Assay Configuration

Configuration C (Fig. 24.1) was selected based on criteria described earlier in this chapter. Initial coating with a goat anti-mouse immunoglobulin economizes valuable monoclonal anti-p53 antibody. The use of monoclonal–polyclonal sandwich assay will allow development of the assay without the need for modification of any of the reagents used.

3.2. Coating of Microtiter Wells

We use clear polystyrene eight-well strips as solid-phase. The coating buffer is a 50 mmol/liter Tris, pH 7.80, containing 0.5 g of sodium azide per liter. The coating antibody is a goat anti-mouse immunoglobulin, Fc fragment specific, obtained from Jackson ImmunoResearch West Grove, PA. Prepare a 5 μg/liter coating antibody solution, in a glass, pipet 100 μl per well, cover with parafilm to avoid evaporation, and let stand overnight at room temperature. The next day, wash the strips two or three times and block them by adding 200 μl per well of the blocking solution. This is a 50 mmol/liter Tris buffer, pH 7.80, containing 10 g bovine serum albumin and 0.5 g sodium azide per liter. The plates can be stored covered at 4°C in the blocking solution for about 1 week or they can be used 1 hr after blocking.

3.3. p53 Standards

There is no p53 standard available. For this reason, we cultured a cell line that is known to overexpress p53 and use the cell lysate to produce the standards. This cell line, COLO 320 HSR(+), is available from the American Type Culture Collection (Rockville, MD). We lysed approximately 10^7 cells in 0.3 ml lysis buffer (for details see Ref. 8) and arbitrarily assigned a value to this solution. We then made several dilutions in 6% BSA solution to obtain calibrators with arbitrary concentrations of 0, 2, 5, 20, 50, and 200 units/liter. These standards were kept frozen at $-70°C$.

3.4. p53 Antibodies

Newly developed antibodies could be obtained from researchers free of charge. The monoclonal anti-p53 antibody used here for coating was a tissue culture supernatant (~30 μg antibody/ml) available from Oncogene Sciences (Uniondale, NY). This antibody is known as PAb240 and binds mutant p53 protein. The detection antibody is a rabbit polyclonal anti-p53 antibody, called CM-1, and is available from Dimension Laboratories, Mississauga, Ontario, Canada. The horseradish peroxidase (HRP)-conjugated goat anti-rabbit antibody was from Jackson Immunoresearch.

3.5. HRP-Substrate and Stopping Solution

A variety of detection reagents have been described for HRP determination, but TMB is by far the most popular chromogenic substrate. The main reason for this popularity is the comparably excellent sensitivity of TMB, as well as its long-term stability and availability. High-quality one- or two-reagent systems from several manufacturers are available. We routinely use the two-reagent system (reagents A and B) available from KPL, Inc. (Maryland, U.S.A.). These reagents are mixed in equal proportions prior to use. Reagent A contains TMB at a concentration of 0.4 g/liter in a solution of dimethylformamide and deionized water. Reagent B contains 0.02 g/liter hydrogen peroxide in a citric acid buffer. Because TMB is a suspected carcinogen, the users are advised to handle these reagents with care and avoid any contact with skin. Also avoid exposure of these reagents to excessive heat or direct sunlight during storage and incubation. Store tightly sealed at 4°C when not in use. The stop solution is a 2 M H_2SO_4 solution. It can be stored at room temperature. Avoid contact with skin or clothes. The reaction catalyzed by HRP is shown in Fig. 24.2.

HRP catalyzes the transfer of hydrogen from a variety of hydrogen donors (e.g., TMB) to hydrogen peroxide according to the principle shown in Fig. 24.2. This apparently occurs by oxidation of the enzyme by peroxide which is, in turn, reduced to its original state through a two-step successive interaction with the hydrogen donor (8, 9). Generally, the appearance of the oxidized donor is measured after the addition of a stopping solution. In the case of TMB, the stopping sulfuric acid solution not only inhibits further color development but also converts the blue oxidation product of TMB to a yellow derivative which has a significantly higher molar absorptivity at 450 mm.

3.6. Assay Procedure

Wash the coated wells and pipette in each well 100 μl of monoclonal anti-p53 antibody and 50 μl of standards or samples (e.g., breast tumor extracts). The

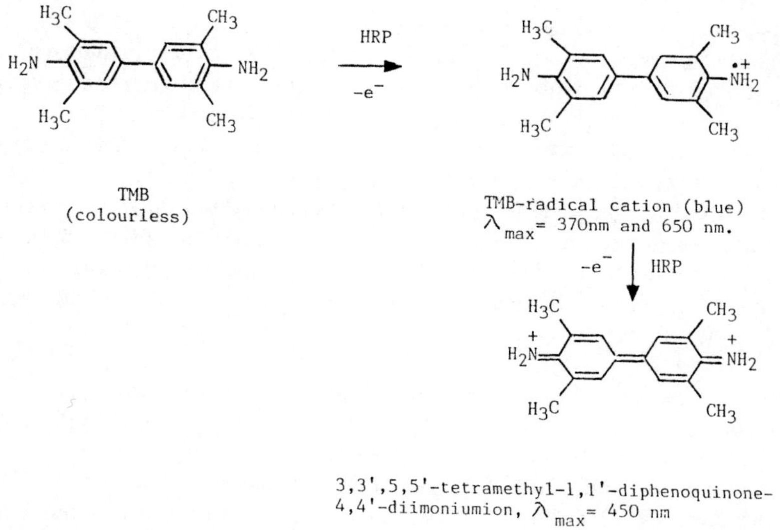

FIGURE 24.2   HRP-catalyzed indicator reaction using tetramethylbenzidine as substrate. (Reprinted, with permission, from Ref. (9).)

monoclonal anti-p53 PAb240 antibody ($\sim$30 μg/ml ascites fluid) should be diluted 50-fold in 6% BSA before addition. The wells are then incubated at 37°C for 3 hr with continuous shaking. During this step, the PAb240 binds to the solid phase through the goat anti-mouse antibody and at the same time binds p53. In this step, the PAb240 antibody must be tried at various dilutions to optimize the amount. Too much or too little antibody will affect sensitivity. Alternatively, it is possible to incubate the PAb240 alone, wash, and then add the p53 standard.

After incubation, wash the wells three times and add 100 μl/well of CM-1 polyclonal antibody at 5000-fold dilution and incubate for 1 hr at room temperature with continuous shaking. Again, one must incubate for variable lengths of time at various dilutions of CM-1 to achieve the best results, i.e., low background, appropriate signal, and measuring range. The wells are then washed six times and 100 μl/well of a 5000-fold diluted goat anti-rabbit–HRP conjugate is added. Similarly, the optimum incuabtion time and conjugate dilution must be found by comparative experimentations. After incubation for 1 hr, wash the wells six times, add 100 μl/well of the substrate solution prepared as above, and incubate for 10–30 min, depending on the need for sensitivity and range. Finally, stop the reaction by adding 100 μl/well of the stopping solution (2 M H$_2$SO$_4$) and read absorbance as outlined below.

To minimize potential assay drift due to variations in the substrate incubation time, care should be taken to add the stopping solution into the wells in the same order and rate used to add the substrate solution. This consideration assumes greater importance when analyzing a large number of samples.

3.7. Absorbance Measurements

For absorbance measurement in EIA, several techniques including kinetics and single-wavelength, two-point, and dual-wavelength measurements have been described. Most of the currently available microtiter plate readers are equipped with specialized software capable of operating in any of the above measurement modes as well as additional manipulations. However, for EIA, and especially with manual handling, absorbance measurements at two different wavelengths (dual-wavelength model) may be most appropriate. In this approach, the first measurement usually corresponds to the maximum absorbance of the chromogen after its enzymatic conversion, and the second measurement is taken at a wavelength near the baseline. The latter provides a blank reference value for each individual well which includes not only baseline absorbance, but also absorbance due to dust and other exogeneous materials that could randomly adhere to the outside of the wells and contribute to imprecision. The microplate readers conveniently subtract the second absorbance reading from the first measurement and relate the difference to the analyte concentration.

Another advantage of dual-wavelength measurement is a significant improvement in assay sensitivity and thus precision and accuracy of values falling between the first (zero) and the second standard of the assay. In the example given in Fig. 24.3 for single wavelength measurement, the absorbances of the zero standard and the second standard (2 U/liter of p53) with 10,000-fold dilution of the HRP anti-rabbit conjugate were 0.073 and 0.18, respectively. This corresponds to an apparent signal-to-noise ratio of 2.47-fold and a calculated lower detection limit of 0.27 U/liter (at 2 SD above the mean), assuming an imprecision of 10% at the 2 U/liter of p53 level. On the other hand, substrating the baseline absorbance, which is typically

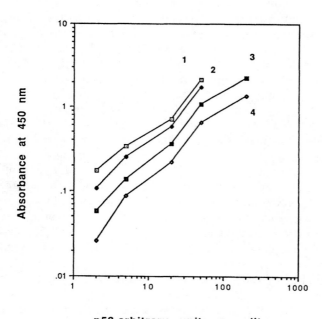

p53, arbitrary units per liter

FIGURE 24.3 Calibration curve for the ELISA p53-assay. The HRP-conjugated goat anti-rabbit IgG was used at four dilutions as follows: 1, 5000-fold; 2, 10,000-fold; 3, 20,000-fold; and 4, 40,000-fold. The zero standard gave absorbances of 0.087, 0.073, 0.060, and 0.056, respectively. These readings were substracted from all other readings. Best sensitivity is achieved at dilutions of 5000–10,000-fold. The dynamic range is extended at higher dilutions but at the expense of sensitivity. For more details see text.

around 0.045 absorbance units, from the above measurement gives corrected absorbance readings of 0.028 and 0.135 for the zero and the second standard, respectively. With this simple manipulation, the signal-to-noise ratio increases from 2.47- to 4.82-fold and, as expected, the sensitivity increases to detecting 0.10 U/liter of p53.

In our laboratory, we routinely employ the dual absorbance measurement principle. For the TMB substrate system, the maximum absorbance measurement is taken at 450 nm with the baseline reference reading set at 600–660 nm. The corrected absorbance values are then used to construct the standard curve and determine the unknown values.

If dual-wavelength analysis is not possible, then the use of single-wavelength reading at 450 nm is recommended.

3.8. Results

A calibration curve for the p53 assay is shown in Fig. 24.3. The assay can be evaluated by analyzing tumor extracts for p53 as has been presented elsewhere (10). Although it is relatively simple to perform the set-up, this assay was not commercially available for years. Even the one assay currently available commercially is not used widely because of its cost. The assay developed with off-the-shelf reagents costs significantly less and can be used to conduct extensive clinical trials as has been shown by our group (11). Its comparison to immunohistochemistry techniques has been discussed recently (12). This assay has been improved further (13).

4. CONCLUSIONS

The principles behind the set-up of immunological assays are simple. Proper selection of the assay design will allow the researcher to set up assays without the need to perform relatively cumbersome procedures such as purifications and conjugations. In the example given, all reagents used were commercially available and were used at such dilutions so that cost is minimized. Following the example of p53, it is possible to set up assays for new analytes in order to promote research projects.

References

1. Diamandis EP, Christopoulos TK. The biotin-(strept)avidin system: Principles and applications in biotechnology. Clin Chem 1991; 37:625–36.
2. Angelopoulou K, Diamandis EP. Autoantibodies against the p53 tumor suppressor gene product quantified in cancer patient serum with time-resolved immunofluorometry. Cancer J 1993; 6:315–21.
3. Khosravi MJ, Morton RC. Novel application of streptavidin-hapten derivatives as protein-tracer conjugate in competitive-type immunoassays involving biotinylated detection probes. Clin Chem 1991; 37:58–63.
4. Khosravi MJ. Shifting the 'Hook Effect' in one-step immunometric assays. Clin Chem 1990; 36:169.
5. Angelopoulou K, Diamandis EP, Sutherland DJA, Kellen JA, Bunting PS. Prevalence of serum antibodies against the p53 tumor suppressor gene protein in various cancers. Int J Cancer 1994; 58:480–7.
6. Goldberg DM, Diamandis EP. Models of neoplasia and their diagnostic implications: A historical perspective. Clin Chem 1993; 39:2360–74.
7. Harris CC, Hollstein M. Clinical implications of the p53 tumor suppressor gene. N Engl J Med 1993; 329:1318–27.

8. Tijssen P. Properties and preparation of enzymes used in enzyme immunoassays. In: Practice and Theory of Enzyme Immunoassays. Amsterdam: Elsevier, 1985:181.

9. Porstmann B, Porstmann T. Chromogenic substrates for enzyme immunoassay. In: Ngo TT, Ed. Nonisotopic Immunoassay. New York: Plenum Press, 1988:57–84.

10. Hassapoglidou S, Diamandis EP, Sutherland DJA. Quantification of p53 protein in tumor cell lines, breast tissue extracts and serum with time-resolved immunofluorometry. Oncogene 1993; 8:1501–9.

11. Levesque M, Katsaros D, Yu H, Diamandis EP, Zola P, Sismondi P, Giordina G. p53 protein overexpression is associated with poor outcome in patients with well or moderately differentiated ovarian carcinoma. Cancer 1995; 75:1327–38.

12. Diamandis EP, Levesque M. Assessment of p53 overexpression by non-immunohistochemistry methods. J Pathol 1995; 175:93–4.

13. Levesque MA, D'Costa M, Angelopoulou K, Diamandis EP. Time-resolved immunofluorometric assay of p53 protein. Clin Chem 1995; 41:1720–9.

INDEX